APPLIED PHARMACOLOGY
for the
VETERINARY TECHNICIAN

THIRD EDITION

D=Dexter (Right)
S=sinister (left)
ex: OS

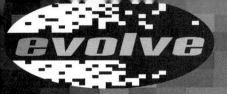

The Latest *Evolution* in Learning.

Evolve provides online access to free learning resources and activities designed specifically for the textbook you are using in your class. The resources will provide you with information that enhances the material covered in the book and much more.

Visit the Web address listed below to start your learning evolution today!

► **LOGIN:** *http://evolve.elsevier.com/Wanamaker/*

Evolve Student Learning Resources for Wanamaker: *Applied Pharmacology for the Veterinary Technician,* Third Edition offers the following features:

- **Image Collection**
  Each image from the text is accessible in a single location and presented in printable, high-resolution format.

- **Interactive Exercises**
  Challenging review questions and dosage calculations composed by the authors test students' knowledge of material in the text.

- **WebLinks**
  This exciting resource lets you link to hundreds of websites carefully chosen to supplement the content of the textbook. The WebLinks are regularly updated, with new ones aded as they develop.

- **Outlines**
  Text content is arranged in concise outlines to aid in study.

Think outside the book... *evolve.*

APPLIED PHARMACOLOGY
for the
VETERINARY TECHNICIAN

3

THIRD EDITION

Boyce P. Wanamaker, DVM, MS
Director,
Veterinary Technology Program,
Columbia State Community College,
Columbia, Tennessee

Kathy Lockett Massey, LVMT
Veterinary Technology Department,
Columbia State Community College,
Columbia, Tennessee

with 144 illustrations

SAUNDERS
An Imprint of Elsevier

SAUNDERS
An Imprint of Elsevier Inc.

11830 Westline Industrial Drive
St. Louis, Missouri 63146

APPLIED PHARMACOLOGY FOR THE VETERINARY TECHNICIAN

NOTICE

Pharmacology is an ever-changing field. Standard safety precautions must be followed, but as new research and clinical experience broaden our knowledge, changes in treatment and drug therapy may become necessary or appropriate. Readers are advised to check the most current product information provided by the manufacturer of each drug to be administered to verify the recommended dose, the method and duration of administration, and contraindications. It is the responsibility of the licensed prescriber, relying on experience and knowledge of the patient, to determine dosages and the best treatment for each individual patient. Neither the publisher nor the author assumes any liability for any injury and/or damage to persons or property arising from this publication.

Previous editions copyrighted 2000, 1996.

International Standard Book Number 0-7216-0382-3

Publishing Director: Linda L. Duncan
Senior Editor: Liz Fathman
Managing Editor: Teri Merchant
Editorial Assistant: John N. Dedeke
Publishing Services Manager: Pat Joiner
Project Manager: Gena Magouirk
Designer: Julia Dummitt

Printed in USA.

Last digit is the print number: 9 8 7 6 5 4 3 2 1

This book is dedicated to:
Tippy, Mammy, Meghan, and the other dogs of my past and future
for their unwavering loyalty, affection, and companionship.
Doris and Preston, my parents, for a lifetime of encouragement,
discipline, and love.
Karen, my wife, for her emotional support and editorial assistance.
The students with whom I have had the pleasure to share knowledge
through the years.

B.W.

Thanks to God for the loving miracle of my parents,
Harry and Bettie Lockett, who chose me to share their lives with.
To my children, Eric and Darla, you are the light of my life.
Try to give back to the world more than you take.
To Dr. Wanamaker for his patience.
To Dr. Frankie Locklar for teaching me about tolerance
and other life lessons.
To all the technicians and students I've worked with, don't ever forget
that we are not just helping animals, but people too. If an animal can
make a person laugh, our job may have a twofold purpose.
Perhaps mirth is the epitome of human health.

K.M.

Preface

Applied Pharmacology for the Veterinary Technician is designed for both the graduate technician and the student. As a teaching and reference book, its purpose is to help veterinary technicians become familiar with the many veterinary pharmacologic agents and their uses, adverse side effects, and dosage forms. We feel it is very important for the technician to understand the uses of pharmacologic agents and to have the ability to provide client education under the supervision of the attending veterinarian. A key feature of this publication is a format intended to provide easy and quick access to chapter information. Each chapter is introduced with learning objectives, a chapter outline, and key terms with simple definitions. "Technician's Notes" throughout the text provide helpful hints and important points we feel technicians should be aware of to avoid errors and increase efficiency.

New features have been added to the third edition to further aid the student and technician in the study and application of pharmacology. Chapter 1 has been amended with information on the Minor Use and Minor Species Animal Health Act of 2001. Chapter 19 is entirely new and outlines the importance of inventory control for the veterinary technician. Other key additions include a discussion of drug interactions, information on inhalation anesthetics, a user-friendly comparison of flea and heartworm products, and additional review questions in each chapter.

Our intent in writing this book has been to combine the comprehensiveness of a veterinary pharmacology textbook with the coverage of pharmacologic fundamentals needed by veterinary technicians. No longer will veterinary technician educators have to draw from two sources for this type of coverage. The scope and organization of the information in this book should make it a useful reference for the practicing technician as well.

Boyce P. Wanamaker, DVM, MS
Kathy Lockett Massey, LVMT

Acknowledgments

I offer a special thanks to my original co-author, Christy Pettes, for her superb work on editions one and two. Without her efforts there would not be an edition three.

I also acknowledge the hard work and unique talents brought to edition three by my new co-author, Kathy Massey.

I would like to recognize the assistance of Jennifer Brookover for her help in composing new questions and reviewing old ones.

Finally, I would like to express my appreciation to Paul Porterfield for his helpful suggestions.

Boyce P. Wanamaker

I would like to thank:
Boyce Wanamaker, DVM, Columbia State Community College;
Mary Kirby, LVMT, Columbia State Community College;
Bill Henson, DVM, Henson Animal Clinic, Corinth, Mississippi;
Jim Jackson, DVM, Jackson Animal Clinic, Corinth, Mississippi;
Forrest Cutlip, DVM, Milan Animal Hospital, Milan, Tennessee;
C.F. Locklar, Jr., DVM, Maury County Veterinary Hospital, Columbia, Tennessee;
Martha Locklar, CPA, Maury County Veterinary Hospital, Columbia, Tennessee;
Steve Grubbs, DVM, PhD, Princeton, New Jersey;
Robert Myers, DVM, Maury County Veterinary Hospital, Columbia, Tennessee;
Christi Cartwright, LVMT, Maury County Veterinary Hospital, Columbia, Tennessee.

Kathy Lockett Massey

Contents

1 General Pharmacology, 1

Introduction, 2
Drug Sources, 3
Pharmocotherapeutics, 3
Pharmacokinetics, 4
  Routes of Administration, 6
  Drug Absorption, 7
  Drug Distribution, 9
  Biotransformation, 10
  Drug Excretion, 11
Pharmacodynamics, 13
Drug Interactions, 14
Drug Names, 16
Drug Labels, 16
Development and Approval of New
  Drugs, 18
  Regulatory Agencies, 18
  *Steps in the Development of a New
    Drug, 19*
Federal Laws Relating to Drug Development
  and Use, 20
  *The Animal Medicinal Use Clarification
    Act, 20*
  Compounding of Veterinary Drugs, 21
  The Veterinary Feed Directive, 22
  *The Minor Use and Minor Species Animal
    Health Act, 22*
Dispensing Versus Prescribing Drugs, 22
Marketing of Drugs, 22

2 Routes and Techniques of Drug Administration, 25

Introduction, 26
Dosage Forms, 26
Drug Preservatives and Solvents, 33
Drug Administration, 33
  Oral Medications, 34
  Parenteral Medications, 36
  Inhalation Medications, 44
  Topical Medications, 45

Medication Orders, 46
Controlled Substances, 47
Client Education, 48

3 Practical Calculations in Pharmacology, 51

Introduction, 52
Mathematics Fundamentals, 52
Systems of Measurement, 53
  The Metric System, 53
  Conversion between Metric Units, 53
  The Apothecary and Household Systems, 55
Dosage Calculations, 56
Solutions, 57
Percent Concentrations, 58
  Calculations Involving Concentrations, 58
Milliequivalents, 59
Calculations Involving IV Fluid
  Administration, 59
  *Calculations for Constant Rate Infusion
    Problems, 59*

4 Drugs Used in Nervous System Disorders, 67

Introduction, 68
Anatomy and Physiology, 69
Autonomic Nervous System, 73
  *How Drugs Affect the Autonomic Nervous
    System, 76*
Classes of Autonomic Nervous System
  Agents, 76
Cholinergic Agents, 76
  Direct-Acting Cholinergics, 77
  *Indirect-Acting Cholinergics
    (Anticholinesterase) Agents, 77*
Cholinergic Blocking Agents (Anticholinergic), 77
Adrenergic (Sympathomimetic) Agents, 78
Adrenergic Blocking Agents, 79
Central Nervous System, 79
Tranquilizers, 80

Phenothiazine Derivatives, 80
Benzodiazepine Derivatives, 80
Xylazine Hydrochloride, 81
Detomidine Hydrochloride, 81
Medetomidine, 82
Barbiturates, 82
*Long-Acting Barbiturates (Oxybarbiturates,
8 to 12 Hours), 82*
*Short-Acting Barbiturates (Oxybarbiturates,
45 Minutes to 1.5 Hours), 83*
*Ultrashort-Acting Barbiturates
(Thiobarbiturates, 5 to 30 Minutes), 83*
Dissociative Agents, 84
Opioid Agonists, 84
Naturally Occurring Narcotics, 85
Synthetic Narcotics, 85
Opioid Antagonists, 86
Neuroleptanalgesics, 87
Drugs to Prevent or Control Seizures, 87
Inhalant Anesthetics, 88
Miscellaneous Central Nervous System Drugs, 91
Propofol, 91
*Glyceryl Guaiacolate or Guaifenesin
(Guailaxin, Gecolate), 91*
Chloral Hydrate/Magnesium Sulfate, 91
Central Nervous System Stimulants, 92
Doxapram, 92
Pentylenetetrazol (Metrazol), 92
Caffeine, 92
Amphetamines, 92
Neuromuscular Blocking Drugs, 92
Behavioral Pharmacotherapy, 93
Pharmacotherapeutic Agents, 93
Antianxiety Medications, 93
Benzodiazepines, 93
Azapirones, 94
Antidepressants, 94
Tricyclics, 94
Serotonin Reuptake Inhibitors, 94
Monoamine Oxidase-B Inhibitors, 94
Synthetic Progestins, 95
Euthanasia Agents, 95

**5 Drugs Used in Respiratory System
Disorders, 99**
Introduction, 100
Respiratory Anatomy and Physiology, 100

Respiratory Defense Mechanisms, 102
Principles of Respiratory Therapeutics, 102
Inhalation Therapy for Respiratory
Disease, 103
Categories of Respiratory Drugs, 103
Expectorants, 103
Guaifenesin (Glyceryl Guaiacolate), 103
Mucolytics: Acetylcysteine, 104
Antitussives: Centrally Acting Agents, 104
Butorphanol Tartrate, 104
Hydrocodone Bitartrate, 104
Codeine, 105
Dextromethorphan, 106
Temaril-P, 106
Bronchodilators, 106
Cholinergic Blockers, 107
Antihistamines, 107
Beta-2-Adrenergic Agonists, 107
Methylxanthines, 107
Decongestants, 108
Antihistamines, 108
Corticosteroids, 108
Miscellaneous Respiratory Drugs, 109
Respiratory Stimulants, 109

**6 Drugs Used in Renal and Urinary
Tract Disorders, 111**
Introduction, 112
Physiologic Principles, 113
Renal Failure, 116
Common Drugs for the Treatment of Renal
Dysfunction and Associated
Hypertension, 117
Diuretic Drugs, 117
Loop Diuretics, 117
Osmotic Diuretics, 117
Thiazide Diuretics, 117
Potassium-Sparing Diuretics, 117
Carbonic Anhydrase Inhibitors, 118
Cholinergic Agonists, 118
Anticholinergic Drugs, 118
Adrenergic Antagonists, 119
Alpha-Adrenergic Antagonists, 119
Beta-Adrenergic Antagonists, 119
Angiotensin-Converting Enzyme Inhibitors, 119
Vasodilators and Calcium Channel Blockers, 120

Antidiuretic Hormone, 120
Urinary Acidifiers, 120
Xanthine Oxidase Inhibitors, 121
Urinary Alkalizers, 121
Pharmacotherapy of Renal Failure
    Complications, 121
Pharmacotherapy of Urinary
    Incontinence, 121
Miscellaneous Renal Drugs, 123
    Urinary Tract Analgesics, 123
    Tricyclic Antidepressants, 123
    Glycosaminoglycans, 123
Technician's Role, 123

7 Drugs Used in Cardiovascular
    System Disorders, 125
Introduction, 126
Anatomy and Physiology of the Heart, 126
Compensatory Mechanisms of the
    Cardiovascular System, 129
Basic Objectives in the Treatment of
    Cardiovascular Disease, 131
Categories of Cardiovascular Drugs, 131
Positive Inotropic Drugs, 131
    Cardiac Glycosides (Digitalis), 131
    Catecholamines, 132
    Bipyridine Derivatives, 133
Antiarrhythmic Drugs, 133
    Class IA, 134
    Class IB, 135
    Class IC, 135
    Class II, 135
    Class III, 136
    Class IV, 136
    Other Class IV Antiarrhythmics, 137
Vasodilator Drugs, 137
    Hydralazine, 138
    Nitroglycerin Ointment, 138
    Prazosin, 139
    Angiotensin-Converting Enzyme
        Inhibitors, 139
Diuretics, 139
    Furosemide, 139
    Thiazides, 140
    Spironolactone, 140
Dietary Management of Heart Disease, 140

Ancillary Treatment of Heart Failure, 141
    Bronchodilators, 141
    Oxygen Therapy, 141
    Sedation, 141
    Aspirin, 141
    Thoracocentesis and Abdominocentesis, 141

8 Drugs Used in Gastrointestinal
    System Disorders, 143
Introduction, 144
Anatomy and Physiology, 144
Regulation of the Gastrointestinal
    System, 147
Vomiting, 148
Emetics, 148
    Centrally Acting Emetics, 148
    Locally Acting Emetics, 149
Antiemetics, 149
    Phenothiazine Derivatives, 150
    Procainamide Derivatives: Metoclopramide,
        150
    Antihistamines, 151
    Anticholinergics, 151
    Butyrophenones, 152
Antiulcer Medications, 152
    H_2 Receptor Antagonists, 152
    Proton Pump Inhibitors, 153
    Antacids, 154
    Gastromucosal Protectants, 154
    Prostaglandin E-1 Analogs, 155
Diarrhea, 155
Antidiarrheal Medications, 155
    Narcotic Analgesics, 155
    Anticholinergics/Antispasmodics, 156
    Protectants/Adsorbents, 156
Laxatives, 157
    Saline/Hyperosmotic Agents, 157
    Bulk-Producing Agents, 157
    Lubricants, 157
    Surfactants/Stool Softeners, 158
    Irritants, 158
Gastrointestinal Prokinetics/Stimulants, 158
    Dopaminergic Antagonists, 158
    Serotonergic Drugs, 159
    Motilin-Like Drugs, 159
    Direct Cholinergics, 159

Acetylcholinesterase Inhibitors, 159
Digestive Enzymes, 160
Miscellaneous Gastrointestinal Drugs, 160
  Antibiotics, 160
  Antiinflammatory Agents, 161
  Antifoaming Agents, 161
Oral Products, 161
  Dentifrice and Cleansing Products, 161
  Fluoride Products, 162
  Perioceutic Agents, 162
  Polishing Paste, 162
  Disclosing Solution, 162

9 Drugs Used in Hormonal, Endocrine, and Reproductive Disorders, 165
Introduction, 166
Anatomy and Physiology, 166
  Pituitary Gland, 166
  Control of the Endocrine System, 168
Hormonal Drugs Associated with Reproduction, 170
Gonadotropins and Gonadal Hormones, 170
  Gonadotropins, 170
  Estrogens, 171
  Androgens, 171
  Progestins, 172
Prostaglandins, 173
  Dinoprost Tromethamine, 174
  Fenprostalene, 174
  Fluprostenol, 174
  Cloprostenol Sodium, 175
Drugs Affecting Uterine Contractility, 175
  Oxytocin, 175
  Ergot, 176
  Prostaglandins, 176
  Corticosteroids, 176
  Miscellaneous Reproductive Drugs, 176
Pheromones, 176
Thyroid Hormones, 177
Drugs Used to Treat Hypothyroidism, 177
  Levothyroxine Sodium (T_4), 177
  Liothyronine Sodium, 178
  Thyroid-Stimulating Hormone, 178
Drugs Used to Treat Hyperthyroidism, 178
  Methimazole, 178

Carbimazole, 178
Ipodate, 179
Propylthiouracil, 179
Radioactive Iodine, 179
Propranolol, 179
Agents for the Treatment of Diabetes Mellitus, 179
  Insulin, 179
  Oral Hypoglycemic Agents, 183
Hyperglycemic Agents, 183
Hormones that Act as Growth Promoters, 184
Sex Steroids, Synthetic Steroid Analogs, and Nonsteroidal Analogs, 184
Growth Hormone: Bovine Somatotropin, Bovine Growth Hormone, 185
Anabolic Steroids, 185
  Stanozolol, 185
  Boldenone Undecylenate, 186
  Nandrolone Decanoate, 186

10 Drugs Used in Ophthalmic and Otic Disorders, 189
Ophthalmic Agents, 190
Mydriatics and Cycloplegics, 191
  Phenylephrine Hydrochloride, 191
  Atropine Sulfate, 191
  Homatropine Hydrobromide, 192
  Cyclopentolate Hydrochloride, 192
  Tropicamide, 192
  Epinephrine, 192
Miotics, 192
  Pilocarpine, 192
  Carbachol, 193
  Echothiophate Iodide, 193
Other Agents that Reduce Intraocular Pressure, 193
  Carbonic Anhydrase Inhibitors, 193
  Mannitol, 193
  Glycerol, 193
Topical Anesthetics, 194
  Proparacaine Hydrochloride, 194
  Tetracaine and Tetracaine Hydrochloride, 194
Ophthalmic Stains, 194
Collagen Shields, 195
Topical Ophthalmic Antiinfectives, 195
  Antiviral Agents, 195

Antifungal Agents, 195
Antibacterial Agents, 195
Topical Ophthalmic Antiinflammatory Agents, 196
   Nonsteroidal Agents, 196
   Topical Corticosteroid Agents, 196
Agents for the Treatment of Keratoconjunctivitis
  Sicca, 196
   Cyclosporine, 196
   Artificial Tear Products and Ocular
    Lubricants, 196
Otic Drugs, 197
Topical Otic Antiinfective Agents, 197
   Gentamicin Sulfate, 197
   Chloramphenicol, 198
   Neomycin Sulfate, 198
   Enrofloxin, 199
Antiparasitics, 199
   Pyrethrins, 199
   Rotenone, 199
   Ivermectin, 199
Drying Agents, 200
Cleaning Agents, 200
Miscellaneous Otic Agents, 200
   Tris-EDTA, 200
   Silver Sulfadiazine, 200

11 Drugs Used in Skin Disorders, 203
Introduction, 204
Anatomy and Physiology, 204
Topical Antiseborrheics, 206
   Sulfur, 206
   Salicylic Acid, 206
   Coal Tar, 208
   Benzoyl Peroxide, 208
   Selenium Sulfide, 208
Topical Medications Mixed with Water, 209
   Aluminum Acetate, 209
   Magnesium Sulfate, 209
   Bath Oils, 209
Topical Antipruritics, 209
   Nonsteroidal Antipruritics, 209
   Topical Corticosteroids, 210
Astringents, 210
Antiseptics for the Skin, 210
   Alcohols, 210
   Propylene Glycol, 210

   Chlorhexidine, 210
   Acetic Acid, 211
   Iodine, 211
   Benzalkonium Chloride, 211
Wound Healing, 211
Topical Wound Dressings, 212
   Healing Stimulators, 212
   Wound Cleansers, 212
   Protectants, 213
Other Drugs Used in Dermatologic Therapy, 213
   Systemic Corticosteroids, 213
   Topical Antibacterial Agents, 213
   Topical Antifungal Agents, 214
   Fatty Acid Supplements, 214
Counterirritants, 215
Caustics, 216
Miscellaneous Drugs, 216

12 Antiinfective Drugs, 219
Introduction, 220
Mechanism of Action, 220
Penicillins, 222
   Pharmacokinetics, 222
   Pharmacodynamics, 222
Cephalosporins, 225
   Pharmacokinetics, 226
   Pharmacodynamics, 226
Tetracyclines, 227
   Pharmacokinetics, 228
   Pharmacodynamics, 228
Aminoglycosides, 229
   Pharmacokinetics, 229
   Pharmacodynamics, 229
Fluoroquinolones, 231
   Pharmacokinetics, 231
   Pharmacodynamics, 231
Other Antiinfectives, 231
   Chloramphenicol, 231
   Florfenicol, 232
   Macrolides and Lincosamides, 232
   Vancomycin, 233
   Spectinomycin, 233
   Polymyxin B and Bacitracin, 234
   Sulfonamides, 234
   Nitrofurans, 234
Antifungal Drugs, 235

Polyene Antifungal Agents, 235
Imidazole Antifungal Agents, 235
Antimetabolic Antifungal Agents, 236
Superficial Antifungal Agents, 236
Other Antifungal Agents, 236
Antiviral Drugs, 237
Acyclovir, 237
Interferon Alfa-2A, Human
   Recombinant, 237
Disinfectants/Antiseptics, 237
Alcohols, 238
Ethylene Oxide, 238
Formaldehyde, 239
Chlorines and Iodines, 239
Phenolics: Saponated Cresol, Semisynthetic
   Phenols, 240
Quaternary Ammonium Compounds:
   Cationic Detergents, 240
Biguanide Compounds, 240
Other Disinfectants, 241

13 Antiparasitic Drugs, 243
Introduction, 244
Endoparasites, 245
Antinematodal, 253
Benzimidazoles, 253
Organophosphates, 253
Tetrahydropyrimidines, 254
Imidazothiazoles, 254
Avermectins, 254
Other Agents, 255
Anticestodal, 255
Bunamidine (Scolaban), 255
Epsiprantel (Cestex), 256
Antitrematodal, 256
Clorsulon (Curatrem), 256
Albendazole (Valbazen), 256
Praziquantel (Droncit), 256
Antiprotozoal, 256
Drugs for Treating Coccidia and Other
   Protozoans, 256
Drugs for Treating Giardia, 256
Drugs for Preventing Giardia, 257
Drugs for Treating Babesia, 257
Heartworm Disease, 257
Adulticides, 257

Melarsomine Dihydrochloride (Immiticide),
   257
Microfilaricides, 259
Preventatives, 259
Ivermectin (Heartgard, Heartgard Plus,
   Heartgard for Cats), 259
Milbemycin Oxime (Interceptor, Sentinel),
   259
Moxidectin (ProHeart), 259
Selamectin (Revolution), 260
Diethylcarbamazine Citrate (Carbam,
   Filaribits, Filaribits Plus), 260
Ectoparasites, 260
Application Systems, 260
Prediluted Sprays, 260
Emulsifiable Concentrates, 262
Shampoos, 262
Dusts, 262
Foggers, 263
Monthly Flea and Tick Products, 263
Insecticides, 264
Pyrethrins, 264
Synthetic Pyrethroids, 264
Chlorinated Hydrocarbons, 265
Carbamates, 265
Organophosphates, 265
Formamidines, 265
Synergists, 266
Repellents, 266
Insect Growth Regulators ([IGRs], Insect
   Growth Hormones), 266
Other Insecticides, 266

**14 Drugs Used to Relieve Pain and
   Inflammation, 269**
Introduction, 270
Anatomy and Physiology, 271
Nonsteroidal Antiinflammatory Agents, 272
Salicylates, 274
Pyrazolone Derivatives, 274
Flunixin Meglumine (Banamine), 275
Dimethyl Sulfoxide, 275
Acetaminophen, 276
Propionic Acid Derivatives, 276
Other Nonsteroidal Antiinflammatory Drugs, 277
Etodolac, 277

Deracoxib, 277
Tepoxalin, 277
Opioid Analgesics, 278
Opioid Agonists, 278
Opioid Agonists-Antagonists, 279
Opioid Partial Agonists, 279
Antihistamines, 279
H_1 Blockers, 280
H_2 Blockers, 280
Muscle Relaxants, 280
Methocarbamol (Robaxin-V), 280
Other Muscle Relaxants, 281
Corticosteroids, 281
Injectables, 283
Oral, 283
Topical, 284
Local, Regional, and Topical Anesthetic
Agents, 284
Injectable, 286
Topical, 286

**15   Therapeutic Nutritional, Fluid, and
Electrolyte Replacements, 289**
Introduction, 290
Anatomy, Physiology, and Chemistry, 290
Distribution of Body Water and
Electrolytes, 290
Composition of Body and Therapeutic
Fluids, 291
Osmotic Pressure and Tonicity of
Fluids, 292
Principles of Fluid Therapy, 295
Indications for Fluid Therapy, 295
Fluid Balance, 296
History, Physical Examination, and
Laboratory Findings, 296
Determining the Amount of Fluid to
Administer, 296
Routes of Fluid Administration, 298
Rate of Administration, 300
Monitoring Fluid Administration, 301
Preparing Fluid Administration
Equipment, 302
Types of Solutions Used in Fluid
Therapy, 304
Crystalloid Solutions, 304

Physiologic Saline, 304
Lactated Ringer's Solution, 304
Dextrose 5% in Water, 305
Ringer's Solution, 305
2.5% Dextrose in Half-Strength (0.45%)
Saline/Potassium Added, 305
Multisol-R/Normosol-R, 305
Normosol-M in 5% Dextrose, 305
Plasma-Lyte/Plasma-Lyte M in 5%
Dextrose, 305
Colloid Solutions, 305
Hypertonic Solutions, 306
Fluid Additives, 306
Sodium Bicarbonate, 306
Potassium Chloride, 307
Calcium Supplements, 308
50% Dextrose, 308
Vitamin Supplements, 309
Oral Electrolyte Preparations, 309
Parenteral Nutrition, 310
Parenteral Vitamin/Mineral Products, 310
Water-Soluble Vitamins, 311
Vitamin B Complex, 311
Thiamine Hydrochloride (Vitamin B_1),
311
Vitamin B_{12} (Cyanocobalamin), 311
Fat-Soluble Vitamins, 312
Vitamin A, 312
Vitamin D, 312
Vitamin E, 312
Vitamin K, 312

**16   Blood-Modifying, Antineoplastic, and
Immunosuppressant Drugs, 315**
Introduction, 316
Blood-Modifying Drugs/Agents, 316
Hematinics, 316
Iron Compounds, 317
Erythropoietin, 318
Androgens, 318
Blood Substitutes, 318
Anticoagulants, 319
Heparin, 319
Ethylenediamine Tetraacetic Acid
(EDTA), 321
Coumarin Derivatives, 321

Acid Citrate Dextrose (ACD) Solution and
Citrate Phosphate Dextrose Adenine
(CPDA-1), 322
Antiplatelet Drugs, 322
Hemostatics/Anticoagulant Antagonists, 322
Topical Agents, 322
Parenteral Agents, 322
Fibrinolytic (Thrombolytic) Drugs, 323
Antineoplastic Drugs, 323
Alkylating Agents, 325
Antimetabolites, 327
Plant Alkaloids (Mitotic Inhibitors), 327
Antibiotic Antineoplastic Agents, 327
Platinum Drugs, 328
Miscellaneous Antineoplastic Agents, 328
Asparaginase, 328
Glucocorticoids, 328
Biologic Response Modifiers, 329
Monoclonal Antibodies, 329
Interferon, 329
Other Biologic Response Modifiers, 329
Immunosuppressive Drugs, 330
Azathioprine, 331
Cyclosporine, 331
Metronidazole, 331
Cyclophosphamide, 332
Corticosteroids, 332
Other Immunosuppressive Agents, 332

17   Immunologic Drugs, 335
Principles of Vaccination, 336
Common Vaccine Types that Produce
    Active Immunity, 337
Inactivated, 337
Live, 337
Modified Live, 337
Recombinant, 338
Toxoid, 338
Common Vaccine Types that Produce
    Passive Immunity, 339
Antitoxin, 339
Antiserum, 339
Other Types of Vaccines, 339
Autogenous Vaccine, 339
Mixed Vaccine, 339
Administration of Vaccines, 339

Biologic Care and Vaccine Failure, 341
Adverse Vaccination Responses, 341
Vaccinations for Preventive Health
    Programs, 342
Canine, 342
Equine, 342
Feline, 342
Bovine, 342
Others, 344
Immunotherapeutic Drugs, 344
Immunostimulants, 346
Complex Carbohydrates, 346
Immunomodulatory Bacterins, 349

**18   Miscellaneous Therapeutic
    Agents, 355**
Alternative Medicines, 356
Chondroprotectives, 356
Polysulfated Glycosaminoglycans, 356
Nutraceuticals, 356
Glucosamine and Chondroitin Sulfate, 357
Echinacea, 357
Garlic, 358
Ginseng, 358
Fatty Acids, 358
Brewer's Yeast, 358
Probiotics, 358
Bioflavonoids, 358
Fiber, 358
Ginkgo, 358
St. John's Wort, 358
Saw Palmetto, 358
Superoxide Dismutase, 359
Coenzyme Q, 359
Aloe Vera, 359
S-Adenosylmethion (SAMe), 359
Miscellaneous Antidotes, 359
Activated Charcoal, 359
Calcium EDTA, 359
Methylene Blue, 360
Acetylcysteine, 360
Dimercaprol, 360
Pralidoxime Chloride, 361
Penicillamine, 361
Sodium Thiosulfate, 361
Ethanol, 362

Fomepizole, 362
Antivenin Polyvalent (Crotalidae)/Antivenin
    (Micrurus fulvius) Coral Snake, 362
Vitamin K-1 (Phytonadione), 362
Thiamine HCl, 363
Reversal Agents, 363
    Atipamezole HC1, 363
    Flumazenil, 363
    Naloxone HC1, 363
    Tolazoline HC1, 363
    Yohimbine HC1, 364
Lubricants, 364

19 **Inventory: The Veterinary
        Technician's Role, 367**
Introduction, 368
Inventory, 369
The Time Equation, 371
Turnover, 371
    Calculating Turnover Rate, 371
Controlling Inventory, 371
A Proactive Inventory Control System, 372
Keeping Accurate Records, 375
Inventory Records, 376
    Reorder Quantity, 379
    Rabies Vaccine, 379
Organizing Inventory, 379
    Pharmacy and ICM Office, 379
    Organizing Inventory in the Veterinary
        Hospital, 379
    Staff Memos, 379
    Special Conditions, 381
Physical Inventory, 381

Monthly Inventory Versus Rotating
    Inventory, 381
Purchasing Information, 381
    Incoming Freight, 383
    FOB Rules, 383
    Receiving Freight, 384
    Stocking Shelves, 384
    Vendors, 384
    Communicating with Sales Representatives,
        385
    DEA Forms, 385
    Special Orders, 386
    Human Pharmacy, 386
Computers and Inventory, 386
The Job of ICM, 386

Appendix A   Common Abbreviations Used
              in Veterinary Medicine, 389

Appendix B   Weights and Measures, 391

Appendix C   Resource Information, 393

Appendix D   Controlled Substances
              Information Summary, 397

Bibliography, 399

Review Question Answers, 403

APPLIED PHARMACOLOGY
for the
VETERINARY TECHNICIAN

THIRD EDITION

INTRODUCTION
DRUG SOURCES
PHARMACOTHERAPEUTICS
PHARMACOKINETICS
  Routes of Administration
    ORAL
    PARENTERAL
    INHALATION
    TOPICAL
  Drug Absorption
  Drug Distribution
  Biotransformation
  Drug Excretion
PHARMACODYNAMICS
DRUG INTERACTIONS
DRUG NAMES
DRUG LABELS
DEVELOPMENT AND APPROVAL OF
  NEW DRUGS
  Regulatory Agencies
    THE FOOD ANIMAL RESIDUE
      AVOIDANCE DATABANK
  Steps in the Development of a New
    Drug
    PRELIMINARY TRIALS
    PRECLINICAL (ANIMAL SAFETY) TRIALS
    CLINICAL TRIALS
    SUBMISSION OF A NEW ANIMAL DRUG
      APPLICATION
    FINAL REVIEW BY THE FDA
    PRODUCT MONITORING
    THE GREEN BOOK
FEDERAL LAWS RELATING TO DRUG
  DEVELOPMENT AND USE
  The Animal Medicinal Use Clarification
    Act
  Compounding of Veterinary Drugs
  The Veterinary Feed Directive
  The Minor Use and Minor Species
    Animal Health Act
DISPENSING VERSUS PRESCRIBING
  DRUGS
MARKETING OF DRUGS

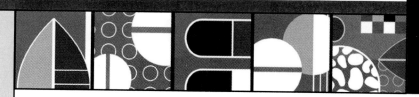

CHAPTER **1**

General Pharmacology

LEARNING OBJECTIVES

After studying this chapter, you should be able to:

1. Define terms relating to general pharmacology
2. List common sources of drugs used in veterinary medicine
3. Outline the basic principles of pharmacotherapeutics
4. Define the difference between prescription and over-the-counter drugs
5. Describe the events that occur after a drug is administered to a patient
6. List and describe the routes of administration of drugs
7. Define biotransformation, and list common chemical reactions involved in this process
8. List routes of drug excretion
9. Discuss in basic terms the mechanisms by which drugs produce their effects in the body
10. Discuss the mechanisms of clinically important drug interactions
11. Discuss the different names that a particular drug is given
12. List the items that should be on a drug label
13. List the steps and discuss the processes involved in gaining approval for a new drug
14. List the government agencies involved in the regulation of animal health products
15. Describe reasons for dispensing rather than prescribing drugs in veterinary medicine
16. Discuss the primary methods of drug marketing

1

KEY TERMS

ADVERSE DRUG REACTION An undesirable response to a drug by a patient. It may vary in severity from mild to fatal.

AGONIST A drug that brings about a specific action by binding with the appropriate receptor.

ANTAGONIST A drug that inhibits a specific action by binding with a particular receptor.

COMPOUNDING Any manipulation (e.g., diluting or combining) to produce a dosage-form drug other than that manipulation provided for in the directions for use on the labeling of the approved drug product.

DRUG A substance used to diagnose, prevent, or treat disease.

EFFICACY The extent to which a drug causes the intended effects in a patient.

EXTRALABEL USE The use of a drug that is not specifically called for on the Food and Drug Administration (FDA)-approved label.

HALF-LIFE The amount of time (usually expressed in hours) that it takes for the quantity of a drug in the body to be reduced by 50%.

MANUFACTURING The bulk production of drugs for resale outside of the veterinarian-client-patient relationship.

METABOLISM (BIOTRANSFORMATION) The biochemical process that alters a drug from an active form to a form that is inactive or that can be eliminated from the body.

PARENTERAL The route of administration of injectable drugs.

PARTITION COEFFICIENT The ratio of the solubility of substances (e.g., gas anesthetics) between two states in which they may be found (e.g., blood and gas or gas and rubber goods).

PRESCRIPTION (LEGEND) DRUG A drug that is limited to use under the supervision of a veterinarian because of potential danger, difficulty of administration, or other considerations. The legend designating a prescription drug states: "Caution: Federal law restricts this drug to use by or on the order of a licensed veterinarian."

REGIMEN A program for administering a drug that includes the route, the dose (how much), the frequency (how often), and the duration (for how long) of administration.

RESIDUE An amount of a drug still present in animal tissue or products (e.g., meat, milk, or eggs) at a particular point (slaughter or collection).

VETERINARIAN-CLIENT-PATIENT RELATIONSHIP The set of circumstances that must exist between the veterinarian, the client, and the patient before dispensing prescription drugs is appropriate.

WITHDRAWAL TIME The amount of time that it takes for a drug to be eliminated from animal tissue or products after stopping its use.

INTRODUCTION

Veterinary technicians are an essential part of the efficient health care delivery team in veterinary medicine. One of the important roles that veterinary technicians carry out is the administration of **drugs** to animals on the order of a veterinarian. Because this role may have serious consequences on the outcome of a case, it is mandatory that technicians have a thorough knowledge of the types and actions of drugs used in veterinary medicine. They should have an understanding of the reasons for using drugs, called *indications*, and the reasons for not using drugs, called *contraindications* (pharmacotherapeutics). They should also know what happens to drugs once

they enter the body (pharmacokinetics); how drugs exert their effect (pharmacodynamics); and how adverse drug reactions manifest themselves (toxicity). Because veterinarians dispense a large amount of drugs, technicians must also be well versed in the components of a valid **veterinarian-client-patient relationship,** the importance of proper labeling of dispensed products, and client education on the proper use of the products to avoid toxic effects or residue. Finally, technicians should have a basic understanding of the laws that apply to drug use in veterinary medicine and the concept of the marketing of veterinary drugs. In short, veterinary technicians need a working knowledge of the science of veterinary pharmacology.

DRUG SOURCES

The traditional sources of drugs are plant (botanical) and mineral. Plants have long been a source of drugs. The active components of plants that are useful as drugs include alkaloids, glycosides, gums, resins, and oils. The names of alkaloids usually end in *–ine*, and the names of glycosides end in *–in* (Williams and Baer, 1990). Examples of alkaloids include atropine, caffeine, and nicotine. Digoxin and digitoxin are examples of glycosides. Bacteria and molds (e.g., *Penicillium*) produce many of the antibiotics (penicillin) and anthelmintics (ivermectin) in use today. Animals once were important as a source of hormones, such as insulin, and as a source of anticoagulants, such as heparin. Today, most of the hormones are synthesized in a laboratory. Mineral sources of drugs include the electrolytes (sodium, potassium, and chloride); iron; selenium; and others. Laboratories are now one of the most important sources of existing drugs because chemists are finding methods of reproducing the drugs apart from plant and animal sources. Advances in recombinant deoxyribonucleic acid (DNA) technology have also made it possible to produce animal and human products (e.g., insulin) in bacteria in large quantities.

PHARMACOTHERAPEUTICS

Veterinarians are challenged with assessing a patient to determine a diagnosis and arrive at a plan of treatment. If the plan of treatment includes the use of drugs, the veterinarian must choose an appropriate drug and a drug regimen. The choice of a drug is determined by using one or more of the broadly defined methods called *diagnostic, empirical,* or *symptomatic.* The diagnostic method involves an assessment of a patient, including a history, physical examination, laboratory tests, and other diagnostic procedures, to arrive at a specific diagnosis. Once the diagnosis is determined, the causative microorganism or altered physiologic state is revealed to allow the choice of the appropriate drug. The empirical method calls on the use

of practical experience and common sense to make the drug choice. In other instances, drugs are chosen to treat the symptoms or signs of a disease if a specific diagnosis cannot be determined. In veterinary medicine, the comparative cost of a drug may also be an important consideration in choosing an appropriate drug. Once the drug to be used in the treatment has been determined, the next step for the veterinarian is to determine the plan for administering the drug. This plan, called a **regimen,** includes details about the following:

The route of administration
The amount to be given (dosage)
How often to give the drug (frequency)
How long to give the drug (duration)

Every drug has the potential to cause harmful effects if given to the wrong patient or according to the wrong regimen. Some medications have greater potential for causing harmful outcomes than others. According to the FDA, when a drug has potential toxic effects or must be administered in a way that requires trained personnel, that drug cannot be approved for animal use except under the supervision of a veterinarian. In such a case, the drug is classified as a **prescription drug** and must be labeled with the following statement: "Caution: Federal law restricts the use of this drug to use by or on the order of a licensed veterinarian." This statement is sometimes referred to as the *legend,* and the drug is called a *legend (prescription) drug.* Labels that state "for veterinary use only" or "sold to veterinarians only" do not designate prescription drugs. Technicians should be aware that prescription drugs have often been approved by the FDA for use in specific species or for specific diseases or conditions. Veterinarians have some discretion to use a drug in ways not indicated by the label if they take the responsibility for the outcome of this use. Using a drug in a way not specified by the label is called **extralabel use.**

Federal law and sound medical practices dictate that prescription drugs should not be dispensed indiscriminately. Before prescription drugs are issued or extralabel use is undertaken, a valid veterinarian-client-patient relationship must exist.

For this relationship to exist, certain conditions must be met. These include, but are not limited to, the following:

The veterinarian has assumed responsibility for making clinical judgments about the health of the animal(s) and the need for treatment, and the client has agreed to follow the veterinarian's instructions.

The veterinarian has sufficient knowledge of the animal(s) to issue a diagnosis. The veterinarian must have recently seen the animal and be acquainted with its husbandry.

The veterinarian must be available for follow-up evaluation of the patient.

Drugs not having enough potential to be toxic or that do not require administration in special ways do not require the supervision of a veterinarian for administration. These drugs are called *over-the-counter* drugs because they may be purchased without a prescription. Drugs having the potential for abuse or dependence by people have been classified as *controlled substances*. Careful records of the inventory and use of these drugs must be maintained, and some of these drugs must be kept in a locked storage area.

When a drug and its regimen have been determined, veterinary technicians are often directed to administer the drug through verbal or written orders. Technicians have several important responsibilities in carrying out these orders:

1. Making sure that the correct drug is being administered
2. Administering the drug by the correct route and at the correct time
3. Observing the animal's response carefully to the drug
4. Questioning any medication orders that are not clear
5. Creating and affixing labels accurately to medication containers
6. Explaining administration instructions to clients
7. Recording appropriate information in the medical record

Technicians should be aware that even when the correct drug is administered in a correct manner, an unexpected adverse reaction might occur in a patient. All **adverse reactions** should immediately be reported to the veterinarian.

PHARMACOKINETICS

Pharmacokinetics is the complex sequence of events that occurs after a drug is administered to a patient (Figure 1-1). Once a drug is given, it is available for absorption into the bloodstream and delivery to the site where it will exert its action. After a drug is absorbed, it is distributed to various fluids and tissue in the body. It is not enough for the drug simply to reach the desired area, however. It must also accumulate in that fluid or tissue at the required concentration to be effective. Because the body immediately begins to break down and excrete the drug, the amount available to the target tissue becomes less and less over time. The veterinarian must then administer the drug repeatedly and at fixed time intervals to maintain the drug at the site of action in the desired concentration. Some drugs are administered at a high dose (loading dose) until an appropriate blood level is reached. Then the dose is reduced to an amount that replaces the amount lost through elimination. Doses of other drugs are at the replacement level throughout the regimen. Underdosing leads to less-than-effective levels in tissue, and overdosing may lead to toxic levels (Figure 1-2). Drug levels can be measured in blood, urine, cerebrospinal fluid, and other appropriate body fluids to help a veterinarian determine whether it is achieving an appropriate level. The cost of this procedure, however, usually restricts its use to research settings.

The primary factors that influence blood concentration levels of a drug and a patient's response are:

1. The rate of drug absorption
2. The amount of drug absorbed
3. The distribution of the drug throughout the body
4. Drug metabolism or biotransformation
5. The rate and route of excretion

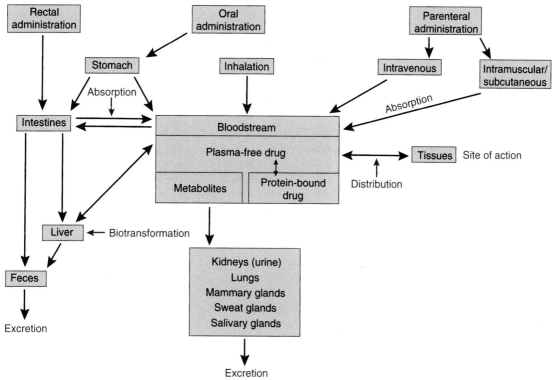

FIGURE 1-1
Outline of the possible sequence of events that a drug may follow in an animal's body.

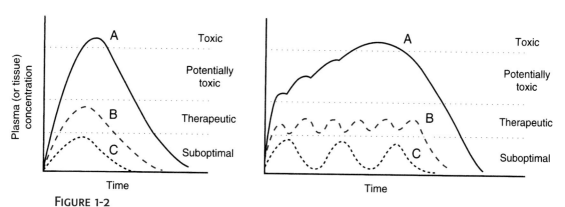

FIGURE 1-2
The effect of dose amounts on the effectiveness of a drug. (From Jenkins WL: In Ettinger SJ, editor: Textbook of veterinary internal medicine, diseases of the dog and cat, Philadelphia, 1983, WB Saunders.)

These factors are explored after the discussion of the drug administration routes.

Routes of Administration

A drug is of no use unless it can be delivered to a patient in a form and at a site that is appropriate. The way in which a drug is administered to an animal patient is influenced by several factors:

The pharmaceutic form of the drug available
The physical or chemical properties (irritation) of the drug
How quickly the onset of action should occur
Restraint or behavioral characteristics of the patient
The nature of the condition being treated

The routes of administration of drugs to animal patients are discussed next.

ORAL

A common method of administering drugs in veterinary medicine is the oral route. Medications given by this route may be placed directly in the mouth or given via a tube passed through the nasal passages (nasogastric tube) or through the mouth (orogastric tube). The mucosa of the digestive tract is a large absorptive surface area with a rich blood supply. Drugs given by this route, however, are not absorbed as quickly as drugs administered by injection, and their effects are subject to species (e.g., ruminants versus animals with a simple stomach) and individual differences. Many factors may influence the absorption of drugs from the digestive tract, including the pH of the drug; the solubility (fat versus water); the size and shape of the molecule; the presence or absence of food in the digestive tract; the degree of gastrointestinal (GI) motility; and disease processes. *This route is not suitable for animals with vomiting or diarrhea.* Drugs given by this route generally produce a longer-lasting effect than those given by injection.

PARENTERAL

Drugs that are given by injection are called **parenteral** drugs. There are many different routes for injection of a drug:

1. Intravenous (IV)
2. Intramuscular (IM)
3. Subcutaneous (SC)
4. Intradermal (ID)
5. Intraperitoneal (IP)
6. Intraarterial (IA)
7. Intraarticular
8. Intracardiac
9. Intramedullary
10. Epidural/subdural

Drugs given by the intravenous route produce the most rapid onset of action, accompanied by the shortest duration. Medications irritating to tissue are generally given by this route because of the diluting effect of the blood. Intravenous medications should also be administered slowly to lessen the possibility of a toxic or allergic reaction. Unless a product is specifically labeled for intravenous use, it should never be given by this route. Oil-based drugs and those with suspended particles (i.e., those that look cloudy or thick) should generally not be given intravenously because of the possibility of an embolism. Special care should be taken to ensure that irritating drugs are injected into the vein and not around it to avoid causing phlebitis.

The intramuscular route of administration produces a slower onset of action than the intravenous route, but usually provides a longer duration of action. The onset of action by this route can be relatively fast with a water-based form (aqueous) or slower with other diluents (vehicles), such as oil— or forms, such as microfine crystals. When an injectable drug is placed in a substance that delays its absorption, it may be referred to as a *depot* preparation. Altering the molecule of the drug itself can also influence the onset or duration of its action. The onset of action is usually inversely related to the duration of action. Irritating drugs should not be given by the intramuscular route, and back pressure should always be applied to the syringe plunger before intramuscular administration of a drug to ensure that the injection is not into a blood vessel.

The subcutaneous route has been called *hypodermoclysis* in some texts. It produces a slower onset of action than the intramuscular route but also produces a slightly longer duration. Irritating or hyperosmotic solutions (i.e., those with more suspended particles than body fluid) should not be given by this route.

Quantities of medication that are appropriate for the species or individual being treated should be used to prevent possible dissection of the skin from the underlying tissue, which could lead to death and loss (sloughing) of surface skin. Adding an enzyme called *hyaluronidase* to a drug given subcutaneously may speed its absorption.

The intradermal route involves injecting a drug into the skin. This route is used in veterinary medicine primarily for testing for tuberculosis and allergic conditions.

The intraperitoneal route is used to deliver drugs into the abdominal cavity. The onset and duration of action of drugs given by this route are variable. This route is used to administer fluids, blood, and other medications when the normal routes are not available or are not practical. Problems such as adhesions of abdominal organs and puncture of abdominal organs may result from using this method.

The intraarterial route involves injecting a drug directly into an artery. This route is seldom used intentionally, but may happen by mistake. Administration of drugs into the jugular vein of a horse must be made with caution to avoid injection into the underlying carotid artery. Intracarotid injection into an animal results in a high concentration of the drug delivered directly to the brain, and seizures or death could result.

The intraarticular route consists of injecting a drug directly into a joint. This method is used primarily to treat inflammatory conditions of the joint. Extreme care must be exercised to ensure that sterile technique is used when performing an intraarticular injection. Technicians do not normally use this route.

The intracardiac route is used to inject drugs through the chest wall directly into the chambers of the heart. This provides immediate access to the bloodstream and ensures that the drug is delivered quickly to all tissue in the body. This method is often used in cases of cardiopulmonary resuscitation and in euthanasia.

The intramedullary route is another seldom-used route in veterinary medicine. It involves injection of the substance directly into the bone marrow. The bones usually used are the femur and the humerus. The intramedullary route is used most often to provide blood or fluids to animals with very small or damaged veins or for animals with very low blood pressure.

When producing spinal anesthesia, the drugs may be injected in the epidural or subdural space. The epidural space is outside the dura mater (meninges) but inside the spinal canal. The subdural space is inside the dura mater. Injection of drugs into the subdural space (cerebrospinal fluid) is also called the *intrathecal route*. A veterinarian usually carries out these methods of drug delivery.

INHALATION

Medications may be delivered to a patient in inspired air by converting a liquid form into a gaseous form through the use of a vaporizer or nebulizer. Examples of drugs that may be given by this route include anesthetics, antibiotics, and bronchodilators.

TOPICAL

Drugs that are topically administered are placed on the skin or on mucous membranes. Drugs are generally absorbed more slowly through the skin than through other body membranes. The rate of absorption may be increased or facilitated by placing the drug in a vehicle such as dimethyl sulfoxide (DMSO). Medication may also be applied to the mucosa of the oral cavity (sublingual), the rectum (suppositories), the uterus, the vagina, the mammary glands, the eyes, and the ears. In horses, caustic materials may be applied topically to inhibit the growth of exuberant granulation tissue (proud flesh).

Transdermal drug administration is a form of topical administration that involves using a patch applied to the skin to deliver a drug through the intact skin directly into the blood. This method is most commonly used to provide an analgesic in a slow, continuous manner.

Drug Absorption

Before drugs can reach their site of action, they must pass across a series of cellular membranes that make up the absorptive surfaces of the sites of administration. The degree to which a drug is absorbed and reaches the general circulation is called *bioavailability*.

The **manufacturing** process can have a significant effect on physical and chemical characteristics of drug molecules that influence their bioavailability. Because of manufacturing differences, the generic form of a drug may differ somewhat from a trademark form in overall efficacy. Bioavailability is often demonstrated by the use of a blood level curve (Figure 1-3). Some of the factors that affect the absorption process include the following (Upson, 1988; Boothe, 2001):

> The mechanism of absorption
> The pH and ionization status of the drug
> The absorptive surface area
> The blood supply to the area
> Solubility of the drug
> The dosage form
> The status of the GI tract (motility, permeability, and thickness of the mucosal epithelium)
> Interaction with other medications

Drugs pass across cellular membranes by three common methods. Passive absorption (transport) occurs by simple diffusion of a drug molecule from an area of high concentration of the drug on one side of the membrane to an area of lower concentration on the other side. This method requires no expenditure of energy by the cell. The drug may pass through small pores in the cell membrane or

may dissolve into the cell membrane on one side, pass through the membrane, and exit the other side. For example, a disintegrated tablet or capsule results in a high concentration of the drug in the gastrointestinal (GI) tract. This concentration then passes through the cellular membranes of the intestinal villi and adjacent capillaries into the lesser concentration in the bloodstream. Alternatively, a drug may passively cross a membrane through the help of a carrier.

Some small drug molecules, such as electrolytes, may simply move with fluid through pores in cell membranes. Active transport of drugs across cell membranes moves molecules from an area of lower concentration to an area of higher concentration and requires that the cell use energy. This is the usual mechanism for the absorption of sodium, potassium, and other electrolytes. In pinocytosis, a third method of passive transport, cells engulf drug molecules by invaginating their cell membrane to form a vesicle that then breaks off from the membrane in the interior of the cell. The method of absorption that occurs in a particular situation depends on whether the drug is fat-soluble or water-soluble; the size and shape of the drug molecule; and the degree of ionization of the drug.

Many drugs can pass through a cell membrane only if they are nonionized (i.e., not positively or negatively charged). Most drugs exist in the body in a state that has both ionized and nonionized forms. The pH of a drug and the pH of the area in which the drug is located can determine the degree to which a drug becomes ionized and thus absorbed. Weakly acidic drugs in an acidic environment do not ionize readily and therefore are absorbed well. The absorption of basic drugs is more favorable in an alkaline environment. If a drug is placed in an environment in which it readily ionizes, such as a mildly acidic drug in an alkaline environment or a mildly alkaline drug in an acidic environment, it does not diffuse and may become trapped in that environment.

The greater the absorptive surface of the area of drug placement, the greater the absorption. One of the largest absorptive surfaces in the body is found in the small intestine because the efficient design of the villi maximizes the surface area.

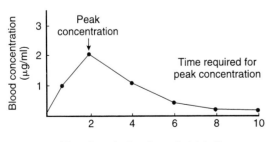

FIGURE 1-3
The blood level of a drug varies with the passage of time.

At any site of drug administration, the greater the blood supply to the area, the faster the absorption of the drug. Drugs are absorbed from an intramuscular site at a faster rate than from a subcutaneous site because of the proportionately larger blood supply to the muscle. Initiating the fight-or-flight response increases blood flow to the muscle but decreases blood flow to the intestines. Heat and massage also increase blood flow to an area. Poor circulation, which may occur in shock or cardiac failure, decreases blood flow—as does cooling or elevation of a body part. These factors can then positively or negatively influence drug absorption.

Another important factor that determines the rate at which drugs pass across cell membranes is the solubility of the drug. The lipid (fat) solubility of a drug tends to be directly proportional to the degree of drug nonionization. As previously stated, the nonionized form is the one that usually is absorbed. The degree of lipid solubility of a drug is often expressed as its lipid **partition coefficient.** A high lipid partition coefficient indicates enhanced drug absorption.

Drug absorption rates often depend on the formulation of the drug. Various inert ingredients—such as carriers (vehicles), binding agents, and coatings—are used to prepare dosage forms. These substances have major roles in the rate at which the formulations dissolve. *Depot* and *spansule* are terms that are associated with prolonged- or sustained-release formulations in veterinary medicine. Subcutaneous implants containing growth stimulants that break down slowly and release their products for prolonged periods are used in some situations.

When drugs are given orally, the condition of the GI tract can have a major influence on the rate and extent of drug absorption. Factors such as the degree of intestinal motility; the emptying time of the stomach; irritation or inflammation of the mucosa (e.g., gastritis or enteritis); damage or loss of villi (e.g., viral diseases); the composition and amount of food material; and a change in intestinal microorganisms can affect the rate and extent of absorbing medications. Another consideration concerning drugs that are absorbed from the GI tract is the first-pass effect (see Figure 1-6). This refers to

the fact that substances are absorbed from the GI tract into the portal venous system, which delivers the drug to the liver before it enters the general circulation. In some instances, a drug is then metabolized in the liver to altered forms, which may make it inactive or less active.

Combining some drugs with other drugs or with certain foods can negatively affect drug absorption. The availability of tetracycline is reduced if it is administered with milk or milk products. Antacids may reduce the absorption of phenylbutazone or iron products. Technicians should always consult appropriate references about potential interactions before administering new drugs.

Drug Distribution

Drug distribution is the process by which a drug is carried from its site of absorption to its site of action. Drugs move from the absorption site into the plasma of the bloodstream; out of the plasma into the interstitial fluid surrounding cells; and from the interstitial fluid into the cells, where they combine with cellular receptors to create an action. Equilibrium is soon established between these three compartments while the drug moves out of the blood into the tissue and then out of the tissue back into the blood (Figure 1-4). How well a drug is dis-

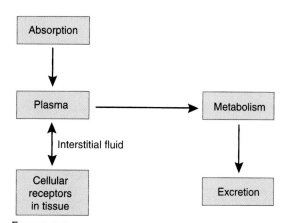

FIGURE 1-4
Drug distribution establishes an equilibrium between the amount of drug at the site of absorption, the amount in the plasma, and the amount at the cellular receptor sites.

tributed throughout the body depends on several factors.

The rate of movement of drug molecules from one of the previously listed compartments to the other is proportional to the difference between the amount of drug in each of the areas. The difference between the amount of drug in two compartments is called the *concentration gradient*, and the greater the gradient (difference), the greater the tendency of the drug to move from the area of higher concentration to the area of lower concentration.

A drug in the plasma comes into contact with various proteins (e.g., albumin) and either binds with these proteins or remains free. When a drug is bound to a protein, it becomes inactive and is unavailable for binding with cell receptors or for metabolism. A bound drug may be considered as a storage site of a drug because a bound drug eventually frees itself from the protein. Low levels of plasma proteins may occur in malnutrition, or in certain diseases, and reduce plasma binding.

Drugs that are highly lipid-soluble tend to move readily out of the plasma and into the interstitial fluid. Drugs in the nonionized form follow a similar pattern. Once a drug is in a tissue, it may become bound or stored there. Tissue—such as fat, liver, kidney, and bone—may act as storage sites for drugs, such as barbiturates, inhalation anesthetics, and others. When a drug moves out of the storage tissue back into the blood, and additional doses are given, it may produce an exaggerated or prolonged result because of the additive effect.

Barriers that exist in particular tissue tend to retard the movement of all or certain classes of drugs into them. The exact nature of these barriers has not been well explained in the literature. The placenta acts as a barrier to some drugs that could be toxic to a fetus and permits the passage of others. Anesthetics that do not excessively depress a fetus must be chosen when a cesarean section is performed. The so-called blood-brain barrier is generally less permeable to all drugs, although it becomes relatively permeable to many antibiotics upon inflammation. The eye also has a barrier that impedes some drugs from diffusing into its tissue.

Disease processes can interfere with drug distribution. Antibiotics usually do not diffuse well into abscesses or exudates. Heart failure and shock can reduce normal blood flow to tissue and thus impede drug distribution. Kidney failure (uremia) can alter the plasma binding of some drugs, such as furosemide and phenylbutazone. Liver failure can cause a reduction in the amount of protein (albumin) available for protein binding.

Reptiles have a renal-portal system that can distribute potentially toxic levels of a drug to the kidney if the drug is injected into the posterior one third of the body.

Biotransformation

Biotransformation, or **metabolism,** is the body's ability to change a drug chemically from the form in which it was administered into a form that can be eliminated from the body. Most biotransformation occurs in the liver because of the action of microsomal enzymes found in liver cells. These enzymes induce chemical reactions that render a drug water-soluble, allowing its subsequent elimination in the urine. Once a drug has been biotransformed, it is called a *metabolite*. Metabolites are usually inactive but in some cases may be more active. A few highly lipid-soluble drugs are incorporated into bile and eliminated through the biliary system. Some biotransformation does occur in other tissue, such as the kidney, lung, and nervous system.

The four chemical reactions induced by microsomal enzymes in the liver to biotransform drugs are:

Oxidation—a loss of electrons
Reduction—a gain of electrons
Hydrolysis—splitting of the drug molecule with the addition of a water molecule to each of the split portions
Conjugation—the addition of glucuronic acid to the drug molecule; when glucuronic acid is attached to a drug molecule, the drug becomes much more water-soluble

Many factors can alter drug metabolism, including species, age, nutritional status, tissue storage, and health status. Cats have limited ability to metabolize aspirin, narcotics, and barbiturates because of reduced ability to form glucuronic acid.

Young animals usually have poor ability to bio-transform drugs because their liver enzyme systems are not fully developed. Old animals have a decreased capacity to biotransform because they have impaired ability to synthesize the needed liver enzymes. Malnourished animals have fewer protein raw materials available to manufacture enzymes for biotransformation, and animals with liver disease are not able to process the raw materials available for enzyme production. Drugs in storage compartments, such as fat or plasma proteins, are not available to be metabolized.

Drug Excretion

Most drugs are metabolized by the liver and then eliminated from the body by the kidneys via the urine. They can be excreted, however, by the liver (bile), mammary glands, lungs, intestinal tract, sweat glands, salivary glands, and skin. It is very important to know the route of excretion of drugs because alterations or diseases of that organ can cause a reduced capacity to excrete the drug, and toxic accumulations may result. For example, the anesthetic agent ketamine can cause serious central nervous system depression in cats with urinary obstruction because the kidneys excrete this drug.

The kidneys excrete drugs by two principal mechanisms. The first method is called *glomerular filtration*. A glomerulus and its corresponding tubule make up the individual functional unit of the kidney, called a *nephron*. A glomerulus acts like a sieve to filter drug molecules (metabolites) out of the blood into the glomerular filtrate, which is then eliminated as urine (Figure 1-5). The second mechanism that the kidneys use to excrete drugs is called *tubular secretion*. Kidney tubule cells secrete metabolites out of the capillaries surrounding the tubule and into the glomerular filtrate, which

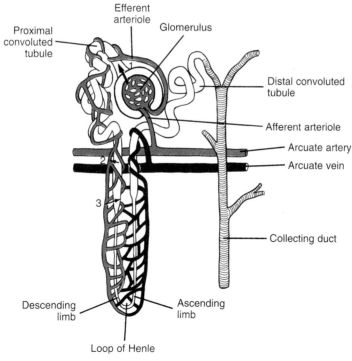

FIGURE 1-5
The kidneys eliminate or conserve drug metabolites by glomerular filtration (*1*), tubular reabsorption (*2*), and tubular secretion (*3*).

becomes urine as it exits the kidneys. In some instances, drug molecules may be reabsorbed out of the glomerular filtrate and back into the blood by *tubular reabsorption*.

It is important that the nephrons (glomerulus and corresponding tubule) be healthy and have an adequate blood supply to do an effective job of excreting metabolites. The lower urinary tract (bladder and urethra) must also be functioning normally to eliminate the filtered or secreted metabolites. If any part of this system from the glomerulus to the urethra is compromised or diseased, toxic levels of a drug may accumulate.

The liver excretes drugs by first incorporating them into bile, which is eliminated into the small intestine. In the small intestine, the drug may then become a part of the feces and be eliminated from the body, or it may be reabsorbed into the bloodstream (Figure 1-6).

Some drugs or their metabolites may pass directly out of the blood and into the milk via the mammary glands. This is an important consideration because of the potential effects of the drug on the nursing of offspring or the effects of the drug on people who drink the milk. Quantities of drug remaining in animal products when consumed are called **residues.** Residues found in milk, eggs, or meat products are potentially dangerous to people because of the following:

People may be allergic to the drug.
Prolonged exposure to antibiotic residues can result in resistant strains of bacteria.
Residue of some drugs may cause cancer in humans.

Drugs that convert readily between a liquid and a gaseous state (gas anesthetics) may be eliminated from the blood via the lungs. These gas molecules move out of the blood and into the alveoli of the lungs to be eliminated in expired air.

Drugs that are given orally and are not absorbed readily out of the intestinal tract may pass through the tract and be eliminated through feces. As

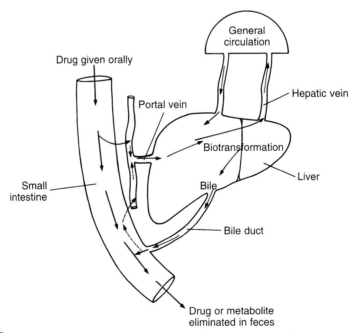

FIGURE 1-6
Drugs or their metabolites in the intestine may be eliminated in the feces or absorbed/reabsorbed for a pass through the liver.

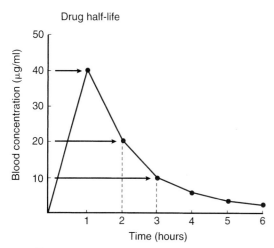

Drug half-life

FIGURE 1-7
This graph illustrates a drug half-life of 1 hour.

mentioned previously, some drugs are excreted through the bile into the intestinal tract, and a few may be actively secreted across the intestinal mucosa into the intestine for elimination.

Some drugs are eliminated through sweat and saliva, although these routes usually are not clinically important. The rate of drug loss from the body can be estimated by calculating the drug's **half-life.** The half-life is the time required for the amount of the drug in the body to be reduced by one half (Figure 1-7).

PHARMACODYNAMICS

Pharmacodynamics is the study of the mechanisms by which drugs produce physiologic changes in the body. Drugs may enhance or depress the physiologic activity of a cell or tissue. Drug molecules combine with components of the cell membrane or with internal components of the cell to cause alterations in cell function. The way in which drugs combine with structures (receptors) on or in a cell can be compared with a lock-and-key model. The geometric match of a drug molecule and a cellular receptor must be exact for the appropriate action to occur (Figure 1-8). The tendency of a drug to combine

with a receptor is called *affinity,* and the degree to which the drug binds with its receptor helps to determine drug efficacy. A drug with a high level of affinity and efficacy causes a specific action and is an **agonist.** A drug with less affinity and efficacy is a partial agonist. A drug that blocks another drug from combining with a receptor is an **antagonist.** The combining of a drug and its receptor causes a particular drug action, and the result of this interaction produces a particular drug effect. Examples of drug effect include stimulation, depression, irritation, and cell death. Sometimes a drug replaces a substance that is missing or is in short supply in the body.

A dose-response curve displays the relationship between the dose of a drug and the body's response. The dose-response curve shows that as a dose increases, an increase in response occurs until achievement of a maximum response or plateau. *No drug produces a single effect.* Low doses of a narcotic may be used to treat diarrhea. Higher doses may be used for pain relief, and even higher doses may depress the respiratory system. The *potency* of a drug is described as the amount of a drug needed to produce a desired response and is represented by a position along the dose-response curve.

The **efficacy** of a drug represents the degree to which a drug produces its desired response in a patient. Once the efficacy level of a drug is reached, increasing the dose does not improve the effect.

The *therapeutic index* is the relationship between a drug's ability to achieve the desired effect compared with its tendency to produce toxic effects. The therapeutic index is expressed as the ratio between the LD_{50} and the ED_{50} and quantitates the drug's margin of safety. The LD_{50} is the dose of a drug that is lethal to 50% of the animals in a dose-related trial. The ED_{50} is the dose of a drug that produces the desired effect in 50% of the animals in a dose-related trial. The index is calculated as follows: Therapeutic index = LD_{50}/ED_{50}.

The larger the number produced by dividing the LD_{50} by the ED_{50}, the greater the safety. Drugs with a narrow margin of safety (low therapeutic index) must be administered with caution to prevent toxic or fatal effects. The drugs used to treat cancer often have a low therapeutic index.

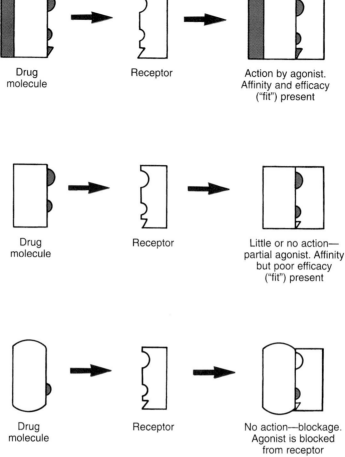

FIGURE 1-8

Drug molecules must combine with specific cellular receptors to exert their effects.

An **adverse drug reaction** is an undesirable response to a drug and can range from mild to life threatening. Adverse reactions can be related to the characteristics of the drug itself, the quality or purity of the drug, and the amount of the drug. Phenobarbital is potentially toxic to the liver, and amphotericin B may damage the kidneys. Drugs can have carriers or vehicles that are toxic to some individuals. Some adverse reactions are allergic and can cause a range of reactions from dermatitis to anaphylactic shock. Drugs can cause changes in the skin that make it very sensitive to sunlight. This type of reaction is called *photosensitivity*.

Other types of adverse responses include abortion, liver or kidney damage, infertility, vomiting or diarrhea, and cancer. An unusual or unexpected reaction is called an *idiosyncratic drug reaction*. All adverse reactions should be reported to the drug manufacturer or the FDA. If the report is made to the drug company, the company is obligated to report the incident to the FDA.

DRUG INTERACTIONS

An altered pharmacologic response to a drug caused by the presence of a second drug is called a *drug interaction*. The normal response may be increased or decreased as a consequence of the interaction. The interaction may be beneficial or harmful to the patient.

Drug interactions can be classified as pharmacokinetic, pharmacodynamic, or pharmaceutic. A pharmacokinetic interaction is one in which plasma or tissue levels of a drug are altered by the presence of another. This alteration may be due to changes in absorption, distribution, metabolism, or excretion of the other drug. Metoclopramide hastens gastric emptying and increases the delivery of a drug to the small intestine for absorption. When calcium and tetracycline are administered at the same time orally, calcium binds the tetracycline and the complex is not absorbed. Displacement of albumin-bound drugs by other drugs with a greater binding affinity may result in an increase in the free drug, leading to an increased response. Many drugs are metabolized by the cytochrome P-450 found in the liver and several drugs can alter the activity (increase or decrease) of the P-450 system causing drug interaction.

A pharmacodynamic interaction is one in which the action or effect on one drug is altered by another. These reactions occur at the site of drug action. These actions may be antagonistic (reversal of an alpha agonist with yohimbine), additive (CNS depression with combinations of preanesthetics), and synergistic (sulfonamide-trimethoprim combinations).

A pharmaceutic interaction occurs when physical or chemical reactions take place as a result of mixing drugs in a syringe or other container. Amphotericin B may form a precipitate when mixed with electrolyte solutions rather than 5% dextrose. Diazepam may precipitate if mixed with certain drugs. Ampicillin and furosemide may be chemically inactivated if mixed with an acid media (Ahrens, 1996).

Drug interactions are described as involving an object drug (the one being acted upon) and a precipitant drug (the one influencing the other) (Mealey, 2002). Table 1-1 lists selected drug combinations that may have undesired consequences.

Table 1-1 Drug Combinations That May Have Undesired Consequences

Precipitant Drug	Object Drug	Consequences
Antacids	Tetracycline	Reduced absorption of tetracycline
Ketoconazole	Digoxin, cyclosporine, tricyclic antidepressants	Decreased metabolism of object drugs
Sucralfate	Fluoroquinolones	Decreased metabolism of fluoroquinolones
Fluoroquinolones	Theophylline	Decreased metabolism of theophylline
Omeprazole	Ketoconazole/itraconazole	Decreased oral absorption of object drugs
Phenobarbital	Theophylline, doxycycline, beta blockers	Increased metabolism of object drugs (cytochrome P-450 induction)
Cimetidine	Diazepam and theophylline	Decreased metabolism of object drugs (cytochrome P-450 inhibition)
MAO Inhibitors	Amitraz, selective serotonin reuptake inhibitors, tricyclic antidepressants, other MAOs	Dangerous accumulation of biogenic amines leading to serotonin syndrome or hypertensive state
Tetracyclines	Penicillins	Tetracyclines slow bacterial growth and inhibit penicillins that are most effective against rapidly growing bacteria

---

Technician's Notes

1. It is generally recommended that the mixing of drugs in the same syringe or fluid administration system be avoided unless the drugs are known to be compatible.
2. When giving two drugs metabolized by the liver, anticipate drug interaction.
3. Concurrent use of drugs from the "behavior modifying" category can cause serious problems such as serotonin syndrome or hypertensive reactions.

DRUG NAMES

During the course of its testing, development, and marketing, a drug may have several names assigned. These multiple names can be a source of confusion. For practical purposes, drugs are given the following names:

1. Chemical—the name that describes the molecular structure of a drug. These names are scientifically very accurate, but complex, and are impractical to use in clinical settings.
2. Code or laboratory—the name given to a drug by the research and development investigators. It is used for communications between the research teams. It includes abbreviations and code numbers.
3. Compendial—the name listed in the *United States Pharmacopoeia (USP)*. The USP is the legally accepted compendium that lists drugs and standards for their quality and purity.
4. Official—usually the same as the compendial or generic name.
5. Proprietary or trade—the name chosen by the manufacturing company. When it is registered, it is the exclusive property of the company. A name that is short and easily recalled is usually picked for the proprietary name. Federal copyright and trademark laws protect this name. On drug container labels, in package inserts, and in drug references, the proprietary name can be distinguished by a superscript R with a circle around it after the name.

6. Generic—the common name chosen by the company. It is not the exclusive right of the company. It may be the same as the official or compendial name. These are drugs with patents that have expired or were never patented.

The following illustration points out the use of the name categories. Ketaset, Ketaject, Ketavet, and Vetalar are proprietary names for ketamine, which is the generic and compendial name for 2-(*o*-chlorophenyl)-2-methyl-aminocyclohexanone (chemical name). Code or laboratory names for this drug include Cl-581 and Cl-369 (Webb and Aeschbacher, 1993).

In textbooks and other scholarly works, generic names begin with a lowercase letter, and proprietary names begin with a capital letter. This practice is followed throughout this text; for example: ketamine (Ketaset).

DRUG LABELS

The Center for Veterinary Medicine of the FDA requires that drug container labels list the following items (Webb and Aeschbacher, 1993):

Drug names (both generic and trade names)
Drug concentration and quantity
Name and address of the manufacturer
The controlled substance status
The manufacturer's control or lot number
The drug's expiration date

The labeling is also required to list instructions for use of the drug and warnings of possible adverse effects of the drug. Because the label on the container usually has limited space, many manufacturers list this added information in an insert. An insert is a small folder that is placed in the box with the drug container or provided as a tear-off portion of the label.

The trade name is usually placed first on a drug label and is scripted in bold letters (Figure 1-9). The generic name typically follows the trade name in smaller print. The label must display the

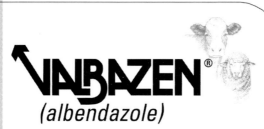

VALBAZEN®
(albendazole)

Broad-Spectrum Dewormer

Oral Suspension for Use in Cattle and Sheep

Controls:

Stomach Worms
including 4th stage inhibited larvae of *Ostertagia ostertagi*

Intestinal Worms

Lungworms

Tapeworms

Mature Liver Fluke

1 L/33.8 fl oz (1 qt 1.8 fl oz)

NADA #110-048, Approved by FDA

989 85-8784-05

Pfizer

VALBAZEN® (albendazole)

Broad-Spectrum Dewormer
Oral Suspension for Use in Cattle and Sheep
For removal and control of liver flukes, tapeworms, stomach worms, intestinal worms, lungworms

Active Ingredient:
Albendazole. 11.36%
(Equivalent to 113.6 mg/mL)

Indications: Valbazen is a broad-spectrum anthelmintic effective in the removal and control of the following internal parasites in cattle and sheep:

Parasite	Cattle	Sheep
Adult Liver Flukes	*Fasciola hepatica*	*Fasciola hepatica, Fascioloides magna*
Heads and Segments of Tapeworms	*Moniezia benedeni, M. expansa*	Common Tapeworms *(Moniezia expansa)*, Fringed Tapeworms *(Thysanosoma actinioides)*
Adult and 4th Stage Larvae of Stomach Worms	Brown Stomach Worms, including 4th stage inhibited larvae *(Ostertagia ostertagi)*, Barberpole Worm *(Haemonchus contortus, H. placeii)*, Small Stomach Worm *(Trichostrongylus axei)*	Brown Stomach Worms *(Ostertagia circumcincta, Marshallagia marshalli)*, Barberpole Worm *(Haemonchus contortus)*, Small Stomach Worm *(Trichostrongylus axei)*
Adult and 4th Stage Larvae of Intestinal Worms	Thread-necked Intestinal Worm *(Nematodirus spathiger, N. helvetianus)*, Small Intestinal Worm *(Cooperia punctata, C. oncophora)*	Thread-necked Intestinal Worm *(Nematodirus spathiger, N. filicollis)*, Cooper's Worms *(Cooperia opcophora)*, Bankrupt Worm *(Trichostrongylus colubriformis)*, Nodular Worm *(Oesophagostomum columbianum)*, Large-mouth Bowel Worm *(Chabertia ovina)*
Adult Stages of Intestinal Worms	Hookworm *(Bunostomum phlebotomum)*, Bankrupt Worm *(Trichostrongylus colubriformis)*, Nodular Worm *(Oesophagostomum radiatum)*	
Adult and 4th Stage Larvae of Lungworms	*Dictyocaulus viviparus*	
Adult and Larval Stages of Lungworms		*Dictyocaulus filaria*

Dosage and Administration: Valbazen Suspension should be administered to cattle at the recommended rate of 4 mL/100 lb of body weight (equivalent to 4.54 mg of albendazole/lb, 10 mg/kg) and to sheep at the recommended rate of 0.75 mL/25 lb of body weight (equivalent to 3.4 mg of albendazole/lb, 7.5 mg/kg). The following table indicates recommended dosing schedules.

Cattle				Sheep			
Body Weight	Dosage	Body Weight	Dosage	Body Weight	Dosage	Body Weight	Dosage
250 lb	10 mL	1000 lb	40 mL	25 lb	0.75 mL	100 lb	3.0 mL
500 lb	20 mL	1250 lb	50 mL	50 lb	1.5 mL	200 lb	6.0 mL
750 lb	30 mL	1500 lb	60 mL	75 lb	2.25 mL	300 lb	9.0 mL

Cattle: 1 liter of Valbazen 11.36% Suspension will treat 50 animals weighing 500 lb.
Sheep: 1 liter of Valbazen 11.36% Suspension will treat 664 animals weighing 50 lb.
Valbazen 11.36% Suspension should be given orally using any type of standard dosing gun or dose syringe.
Important: Accurate estimates of the weight of the cattle and sheep to be treated are essential for most effective results with this product. Animals constantly exposed to internal parasites should be retreated as necessary.

Warnings: Cattle must not be slaughtered within 27 days following last treatment. Sheep must not be slaughtered within 7 days following last treatment. Because a withdrawal time in milk has not been established, do not use in female dairy cattle of breeding age.

Caution: Do not administer to female cattle during first 45 days of pregnancy or for 45 days after removal of bulls. Do not administer to ewes during the first 30 days of pregnancy or for 30 days after removal of rams. Consult your veterinarian for assistance in the diagnosis, treatment, and control of parasitism.

Keep This and All Medication Out of Reach of Children
Shake Well Before Using
For Use in Animals Only
Store at Controlled Room Temperature 15°–30°C (59°–86°F)
Protect From Freezing
U.S. Patent Nos. 3,915,986 and 3,956,499
989 80-8784-05
Made in USA

TAKE TIME OBSERVE LABEL DIRECTIONS

Distributed by:
Pfizer Animal Health
Exton, PA 19341, USA
Div. of Pfizer Inc
NY, NY 10017

0 87219 01421 9

FIGURE 1-9
A label showing the components of a drug as required by the FDA. (Courtesy Pfizer Animal Health, Exton, Pa.)

concentration (strength) of a drug and the total quantity in the container. Drug strength is often expressed as milligrams or units per dosage unit (mg/ml, mg/capsule, and so forth). Some drugs are sold in different concentrations with similar labels, and underdosing or overdosing can result. When the same drug is marketed in different strengths with similar labels, some companies use different sizes of bottles for the different strengths and display the concentration in bold print. Atropine and xylazine are examples of drugs marketed in different concentrations for large and small animals.

The label must include the name and address of the manufacturer of the drug. This is important to be able to know who to contact if adverse drug reactions occur or if other problems with the drug arise.

Drugs that have potential for abuse by humans are controlled under the Comprehensive Drug Abuse Prevention and Control Act of 1970. The Drug Enforcement Administration places drugs into categories or schedules according to their potential for abuse and requires that the label of a container for a controlled substance be identified with a capital C followed by a Roman numeral identifying which of the five categories is appropriate. This labeling must be placed in the upper right side of the container label.

Drug labels are required to list an expiration date for the product. This is to ensure that dispensed drugs have the intended safety and efficacy. Drugs are tested during development to determine the effective shelf life and the proper storage conditions. Some drugs must be stored in refrigeration, and others must be stored in light-resistant (amber) containers to make sure that the shelf life is not shortened. *Storage instructions on the label should be followed carefully to validate the expiration date.*

All drugs must have a lot or batch number on the label. The purpose of the lot number is to allow the manufacturer to know the exact time and date of production of the product and the quality and quantity of the ingredients. The lot number is determined by the manufacturer and may consist of numbers, or numbers and letters.

Another feature often found on a drug label, but not required by the FDA, is the national drug code (NDC) number. The NDC is a 10-digit number that identifies the manufacturer or distributor, the drug formulation, and the package size.

Drugs intended for animals that may be consumed by humans must have the appropriate **withdrawal time** listed on the insert or label.

DEVELOPMENT AND APPROVAL OF NEW DRUGS

The federal government requires that before any new animal health product can be marketed, its safety and efficacy must be proved through rigorous testing. This testing requires the expenditure of much time and money. It has been estimated that on average 7 to 10 years of testing are required at a cost of $15 million to $20 million to the manufacturer to get a new animal drug on the market. The steps in this process are outlined in Figure 1-10.

The development of new animal health products begins in the research and development department of the manufacturing company. The company wants to ensure that the drug is not only safe and effective for animals but also is safe for the environment and the people who will consume products from animals treated with the drug. The company wants to be certain a market is available for the product, that it will be able to produce it at a cost reasonable for consumers, and that it will be profitable.

Regulatory Agencies

The three agencies of the U.S. government that regulate animal health products are the FDA, the Environmental Protection Agency (EPA), and the U.S. Department of Agriculture (USDA). The FDA regulates the development and approval of animal drugs and feed additives through its Center for Veterinary Medicine. The EPA regulates the development and approval of animal topical pesticides, and the USDA regulates the development and approval of biologics (vaccines, serums, antitoxins, and similar products).

THE FOOD ANIMAL RESIDUE AVOIDANCE DATABANK

The Food Animal Residue Avoidance Databank (FARAD) is a project sponsored by the USDA Extension Service and serves as a repository of residue

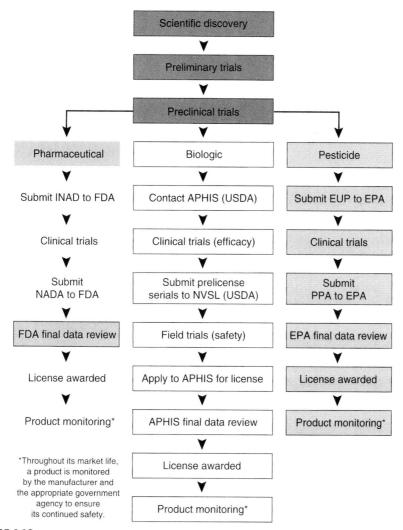

FIGURE 1-10

A flow chart of the animal health product approval process: Investigational New Animal Drug (INAD); Food and Drug Administration (FDA); Animal and Plant Health Inspection Service (APHIS); National Veterinary Services Laboratory (NVSL); United States Department of Agriculture (USDA); Experimental Use Permit (EUP); Environmental Protection Agency (EPA); Pesticide Permit Application (PPA). (From Etchison K, editor: The path to approval: how research discoveries become federally licensed products, Top Vet Med 4[1]:13, 1993.)

avoidance information and educational materials. FARAD provides expert advice concerning the avoidance of drug residues in an effort to achieve its goal of producing "safe foods of animal origin." FARAD produces a compendium of FDA-approved drugs and provides information about withholding times for milk and preslaughter withdrawal times for meat. The information in this compendium is avail-

able online (www.farad.org), and additional direct telephone access is provided for situations in which the online information is not sufficient.

Steps in the Development of a New Drug
PRELIMINARY TRIALS

When a new drug or product shows potential for development by a company, it is first subjected to a series of preliminary trials. The company wants to know whether the product will actually perform as expected, whether it has potential harmful side effects, and whether it will be profitable to market. If these concerns are satisfactorily answered, testing begins. First the product is tested on simple organisms, such as bacteria, yeasts, or molds in a laboratory. Computer models may also be used to simulate animal models at this time.

PRECLINICAL (ANIMAL SAFETY) TRIALS

If the preliminary trials prove satisfactory, the next step involves preclinical trials. These trials are usually carried out using laboratory animals to determine information about appropriate doses of the drug. A few target (intended species) animals may be used as well. If the results of the preclinical trials are satisfactory, the company then notifies the appropriate government agency that a new drug is under investigation. It does this by filing an Investigational New Animal Drug (INAD) application with the FDA. If the product is a pesticide, it files for an Experimental Use Permit (EUP) with the EPA. If a biologic is involved, the company contacts the Animal and Plant Health Inspection Service of the USDA.

CLINICAL TRIALS

By this time, the manufacturer has compiled enough information to decide whether the product should be tested in the target species. The tests must prove that the drug is safe and effective. Potential toxic and adverse side effects must be determined. Tissue residue and withdrawal time information must be accumulated if the product will be used in food-producing animals. Possible toxic effects on pregnant animals is determined, along with information about the potential for birth defects (teratogenesis). Shelf life studies must also be conducted to establish expiration date data. Results of the studies are validated through the use of statistical analysis.

SUBMISSION OF A NEW ANIMAL DRUG APPLICATION

If the manufacturing company decides to market the drug, it then must file a New Animal Drug

Application (NADA) with the FDA. Procedures for pesticides and biologics are similar.

FINAL REVIEW BY THE FDA

Volumes of research are submitted to the FDA, EPA, or USDA for review. Approval and a license for manufacture are granted if the appropriate agency validates the information.

PRODUCT MONITORING

As long as a product is marketed, it is constantly monitored by the company and the government to ensure its continuing safety and efficacy.

THE GREEN BOOK

The *Green Book* is a list of all animal drug products that have been approved by the FDA for safety and effectiveness. This list was first published in 1989 as a cooperative, nonprofit effort between the USDA and Virginia Polytechnic Institute and State University. It is funded through an interagency agreement between the USDA and the FDA. Monthly updates are made to the list, and the entire list is published each January. The *Green Book* is available electronically at the FDA-CVM World Wide Web site (http://www.fda.gov/cvm/greenbook/greenbook.html).

FEDERAL LAWS RELATING TO DRUG DEVELOPMENT AND USE

In 1906 Congress passed the first legislation regulating the manufacture, use, and sale of drugs. Table 1-2 provides a list of the major acts of legislation passed before the 1990s and the significance of each.

The Animal Medicinal Use Clarification Act

In 1994 Congress passed the Animal Medicinal Drug Use Clarification Act (AMDUCA). This legislation made extralabel use of approved veterinary drugs legal under certain well-defined conditions. The act came about because of lobbying efforts by the American Veterinary Medical Association and other groups in response to the FDA, tightening its policies concerning extralabel use of veterinary

Table 1-2 Federal Laws Regulating the Use of Pharmaceutics

Date	Legislation	Summary
1958	Food additives amendment	Regulation of substances added to food for human consumption. Delaney clause provided that no additive may be added if it causes cancer in humans or animals.
1962	Kefauver-Harris amendment	Provided for safety and effectiveness of drugs by strict control of manufacturing for new animal drugs.
1968	Animal drug amendment	Provided regulations for new animal drugs.
1970	Comprehensive drug abuse and control act	Placed controlled substances into schedules according to their potential for abuse. Called for registration of veterinarians.

drugs. Previously, veterinarians had been permitted to use any drug as long as it could be legally obtained, used according to sound professional practice, and left no residue in food products (Coppoc, 2003). However, public concerns over food safety issues related to residues of substances such as diethylstilbestrol, chloramphenicol, and antibiotics caused the FDA to issue compliance policy guidelines (CPGs) that made extralabel use illegal. Even though the FDA would not routinely prosecute veterinarians for extralabel use after the issuance of the CPGs, practitioners were nonetheless placed in the position of breaking federal law to meet their obligations to animals and their owners. AMDUCA allows veterinarians to legally select the most efficacious drug for their patients. The AVMA issued an AMDUCA *Guidance Brochure* in 1998. The brochure outlines requirements of the act and provides and algorithm for determining when extralabel use is appropriate.

A section of the AMCUDA provides that the FDA may prohibit an extralabel use in animals if the agency finds that such use presents a risk to the public health. The following drugs and substances are prohibited for extralabel use in all food-producing animals:

Chloramphenicol
Clenbuterol
Diethylstilbestrol
Dimetridazole
Ipronidazole

Other nitroimidazoles
Furazolidone
Sulfonamide drugs in lactating dairy cattle
Sulfadimethoxine, sulfabromomethazine, and sulfaethoxypyridazine
Fluoroquinolones
Glycopeptides
Phenylbutazone in dairy cattle 20 months of age and older

Compounding of Veterinary Drugs

FDA-approved drugs are labeled for specific therapeutic uses in defined species. Since veterinarians must treat a variety of animal species that may vary greatly in size, it is not always possible to use an approved drug for every clinical situation, therefore veterinarians may need to dilute or combine (compound) existing medications. For example, it may be in the best interest of a horse to combine more than one drug in a single syringe to minimize the number of injections. It also may be essential to dilute an injectable agent to obtain an appropriate concentration for a bird or mouse or to prepare an antidote (e.g., sodium sulfate) that is not commercially available. None of these activities would be permitted under a strict interpretation of FDA regulations, which traditionally have not distinguished the act of diluting or combining drugs from manufacturing. Any alteration of a drug by a veterinarian or his or her employee that changes the concentration of the active ingredient, the preservatives, or the vehicles results in a new animal drug subject to the FDA approval process (Davidson, 1997). Recognizing the difficulties imposed by these regulations, the FDA issued a CPG (608.400) in 1996 to better define the conditions permitting compounding. Those conditions include, but may not be limited to: (1) the identification of a legitimate veterinary medical need; (2) a need for an appropriate regimen for a particular species, size, gender, or medical condition of the patient; (3) no approved animal or human drug that when used as labeled will treat the condition; and (4) too long a time interval for securing the drug to treat the condition.

The Veterinary Feed Directive

Congress established the Veterinary Feed Directive (VFD) as a part of the Animal Drug Availability Act of 1996. The VFD established a new category of drugs "as an alternative to prescription status" for certain antimicrobial animal feed additives. Before this directive, all commercially available animal drugs for use in medicated feeds were available on an over-the-counter basis. The VFD therefore provides the FDA Center for Veterinary Medicine (CVM) greater control over the use of some new animal feed additives. The use of VFD drugs requires a valid veterinarian-patient-client relationship and the issuance of a VFD form by a veterinarian. The animal producer must secure the VFD form from the veterinarian and present it to a feed mill to receive the medicated feed.

The Minor Use and Minor Species Animal Health Act

There is a shortage in the United States of approved animal drugs intended for use in less common animal species or those with less common conditions. The drugs that do exist may not be used legally in the animals that need the treatment. The Minor Use and Minor Species Animal Health Act of 2001 is intended as a mechanism to provide FDA-authorized drugs for those less common species and indications. It is similar to the human Orphan Drug Act of 1983. This act specifically determines the provision of labeled drugs for minor species including sheep, goats, game birds, emus, ranched deer, alpacas, llamas, deer, elk, rabbits,

guinea pigs, pet birds, reptiles, ornamental and other fish, shellfish, wildlife, zoo, and aquarium animals. The MUMS act is also designed to provide major species (cats, dogs, horses, cattle, swine, turkeys, and chickens) with needed drugs for uncommon indications (minor uses).

DISPENSING VERSUS PRESCRIBING DRUGS

Although most physicians prescribe drugs, most veterinarians dispense them. The primary reason why veterinarians maintain a pharmacy in their hospitals is that drug sales represent an important source of income. Food animal practitioners in particular use profit from drug sales to supplement their income because it may be difficult for them to charge sufficiently for their time. Another reason veterinarians dispense drugs from their hospitals is that human pharmacies usually do not stock veterinary drugs. A few drugs are available only from human pharmacies, and others are used so infrequently that veterinarians find it more practical and economical to write a prescription for them.

MARKETING OF DRUGS

Pharmaceutic products are purchased by veterinarians from various sources. Some products are purchased directly from the manufacturer by telephone or mail, and others are obtained from sales representatives (detail persons) who call on the veterinary clinics. Distributors (wholesalers) are companies that buy products from many different manufacturers and then resell the products to veterinarians through sales representatives or by phone. Generic drug companies sell generic products under their own label, usually by mail order.

Most of the pharmaceutic manufacturers are large companies that have separate divisions. One division sells products to veterinarians only, and the other sells over-the-counter products. It should be noted that the statement "sold to graduate veterinarians only" on a drug label does not mean that the product is a prescription drug. It only indicates a sales policy of the company. In a few instances, the same product is sold under different labels to veterinarians only and to over-the-counter markets. Some feed stores and cooperatives are able to sell over-the-counter products (similar to products sold by veterinarians) to consumers at prices lower than veterinarians can charge because of the quantity purchasing power of the stores. This can be a source of tension between veterinarians and the retail markets.

A more recent controversy has arisen over the practices of "rogue Internet pharmacies" (Anonymous, 2001). The primary concern is that some Internet pharmacies are supplying prescription drugs to consumers without the authorization of a veterinarian with a veterinarian-client-patient-relationship. The prescription is often issued by an out-of-state veterinarian, who responds to client questionnaire information rather than by actual patient and client contact. Dealing with these problems may be difficult because the FDA regulates the drug products themselves, not the practice of the pharmacy. The board of pharmacy in the individual states where the Internet pharmacy is located and registered regulates the practice of pharmacy. The board of pharmacy in the states where the consumers receive prescriptions enforces requirements for out-of-state pharmacies. Another related issue is the sale of "ethical products" by these Internet companies. These are products for which the manufacturer has voluntarily limited their sale to veterinarians as a marketing decision. Some flea and tick control products are ethical products registered with the EPA or FDA in the over-the-counter category. Improper sale of these ethical products may then be an ethical rather than a legal issue.

REFERENCES

Ahrens AA: Pharmacology, the national veterinary medical series for independent study, Philadelphia, 1996, Lippincott Williams & Wilkins.

Anonymous (2001): White paper: rogue internet pharmacies, http://www.avma.org/noah/members/scientific/prescribing/white_paper.asp

Boothe DM: Principles of drug therapy. In Boothe DM: Small animal clinical pharmacology, Philadelphia, 2001, WB Saunders Co.

Coppoc GL: Drug residue avoidance. In class notes for BMS 513: http://www.vet.purdue.edu/bms/courses/bms513/scavma97.htm, 2003.

Davidson G: Pharmacy update: new FDA policy gives clear guidance for compounding, Vet Tech 18(3):195-201, 1997.

Mealey KL: Clinically significant drug interactions, Compend Contin Educ Proc Pract Vet 24(1):10-22, 2002.

Upson DW: General principles. In Upson DW, editor: Handbook of clinical veterinary pharmacology, Manhattan, Kan, 1988, Dan Upson Enterprises.

Webb AI and Aeschbacher G: Animal drug container labels: a guide to the reader, JAVMA 202:1591-1599, 1993.

Williams BR and Baer C: Introduction to pharmacology. In Williams BR and Baer C, editors: Essentials of clinical pharmacology in nursing, Springhouse, Pa, 1990, Springhouse Corp.

REVIEW QUESTIONS

1. Define the following terms:
   a. Agonist _____
   b. Contraindication _____
   c. Efficacy _____
   d. Over-the-counter drug _____
   e. Prescription drug _____
   f. Receptor _____
   g. Therapeutic index _____
   h. Withdrawal time _____
   i. Veterinarian-client-patient relationship

   _____

2. List four sources of drugs used in veterinary medicine. _____
3. What are four components of a drug regimen?

   _____

4. Discuss the conditions that must be met before a valid veterinarian-client-patient relationship can be shown to exist.

   _____

5. Discuss the responsibilities of a veterinary technician in the administration of drug orders. _____
6. Describe the sequence of events that a drug undergoes from administration to excretion.

   _____

7. List 11 possible routes for administering a drug to a patient and discuss the advantages and/or disadvantages of each. _____
8. List some of the factors that influence drug absorption. _____
9. Most biotransformation of drugs occurs in which of the following?
   a. Kidney
   b. Liver
   c. Spleen
   d. Pancreas
10. Most drug excretion occurs via which of the following?
    a. Kidneys
    b. Liver

c. Spleen
d. Intestine

11. Drugs usually produce their effects by combining with specific cellular

    _____

12. The drug name that is chosen by the manufacturer and that is the exclusive property of that company is called

    _____.

13. What are six items that must be on a drug label? _____
14. What are three government agencies that regulate the development, approval, and use of animal health products?

    _____

15. Why do many veterinary clinics dispense rather than prescribe most of the drugs that they use? _____
16. Describe the marketing of animal health products. _____
17. All FDA-approved veterinary drugs are listed in the publication entitled _____.
18. What is the purpose of FARAD?

    _____

19. Extralabel veterinary drug use was made legal (under prescribed circumstances) by what act of Congress? _____
20. Define compounding. _____
21. What are the potential dangers of residues in animal products? _____
22. List three classes of drug interactions.
    1. _____
    2. _____
    3. _____
23. Drug interaction can be anticipated when giving two drugs both metabolized by the

    _____

24. Define "ethical product". _____.
25. Once a drug has been biotransformed it is called a _____.

INTRODUCTION
DOSAGE FORMS
DRUG PRESERVATIVES AND
  SOLVENTS
DRUG ADMINISTRATION
  Oral Medications
  Parenteral Medications
  Inhalation Medications
  Topical Medications
MEDICATION ORDERS
CONTROLLED SUBSTANCES
CLIENT EDUCATION

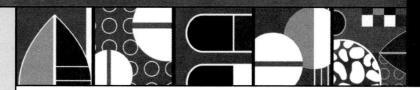

CHAPTER *2*

Routes and Techniques of Drug Administration

LEARNING OBJECTIVES

After studying this chapter, you should be able to:

1. Be familiar with the many types of drug forms available
2. Know and understand the five rights for administering medication
3. Recognize available types of syringes and needles, and know their common uses
4. Correctly read doses in a syringe
5. Know the techniques for administering medications, the routes commonly used, and how to document the treatment
6. Know what is involved in preparing a prescription and how the prescription is posted to the medical record
7. Understand the U.S. Drug Enforcement Administration (DEA) requirements for keeping inventory and dispensing controlled substances

KEY TERMS

COUNTERIRRITANT An agent that produces superficial irritation intended to relieve some other irritation.

CERUMEN A waxy secretion of the glands of the external ear canal.

CREAM A semisolid preparation of oil, water, and a medicinal agent.

ELIXIR A hydroalcoholic liquid containing sweeteners, flavoring, and a medicinal agent.

EMULSION A medicinal agent consisting of oily substances dispersed in an aqueous medium with an additive to stabilize the dispersion.

LINIMENT A medicine in an oily, soapy, or alcoholic vehicle to be rubbed on the skin to relieve pain or to act as a counterirritant.

OINTMENT A semisolid preparation containing medicinal agents for application to the skin or eyes.

PARENTERAL Administration by a route other than the alimentary canal (e.g., intramuscular, subcutaneous, intravenous).

SPECULUM An instrument for dilating a body orifice or cavity to allow visual inspection.

SUSPENSION A preparation of solid particles dispersed in a liquid but not dissolved in it.

INTRODUCTION

In a busy veterinary practice, a veterinary technician often administers treatments ordered by the doctor. Proper techniques should be used along with proper documentation on the medical record. Additionally, a veterinary technician must be knowledgeable about dosage forms, syringe construction, and hatch marks; have the ability to obtain correct amounts of medication within a syringe; know the five rights of drug administration; be capable of administering medication by all available routes; be knowledgeable in the area of client education concerning drugs; and know how to properly handle controlled substances. Proper documentation of administered treatments is of utmost importance and ensures that the same treatment is not repeated by other veterinary personnel. Knowledge of adverse reactions that animals may have to particular medications is also crucial. The veterinary technician is the veterinarian's "right hand" in a busy practice full of hospitalized patients receiving treatment one to three times a day. Through observation of the patient during treatments, the technician is able to provide the veterinarian with information regarding the patient's response. The doctor, thus informed, can easily reach decisions concerning adjustment of treatment regimen. The technician who recognizes the importance of administering the proper treatment to the patient and uses observation skills in assessing the response of that treatment is an invaluable employee.

DOSAGE FORMS

Pharmaceutic companies manufacture drugs in various forms. Some drugs are available in a variety of forms, while others may be available for administration in only one form. Most pharmaceutic companies endeavor to provide comfort to the patient and ease of administration when formulating their drugs. Some common drug preparations include oral administration, parenteral injection, inhalation, and topical medications. The most common type of preparation is a drug administered orally. Oral preparations are usually easy to administer, have extended expiration dates, and are manufactured uniformly with respect to the drug's content.

Tablets are the most commonly used oral form (Figure 2-1). A tablet may be scored or unscored. A scored tablet has indentions made into its surface, allowing it to be broken into halves or quarters. Therefore a scored tablet provides a way of administering a smaller dose to the patient. A tablet that is unscored may also be cut into a smaller size. However, scored tablets break more readily and are less likely to fragment. Some tablets containing a drug type that may be irritating to the

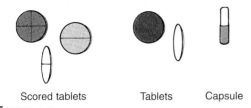

Scored tablets   Tablets   Capsule

FIGURE 2-1
Tablets and capsules are the most common forms of oral medications.

gastrointestinal tract may be enteric-coated. Capsules are containers that house medication. The capsule itself may be made of gelatin and glycerin. The contents of a capsule may contain a powder form or sometimes a liquid. Capsules may be advantageous to use because they allow a patient to be treated without an unpalatable taste coming into contact with the oral mucosa. Unfortunately, capsules cannot be broken down like a scored tablet to provide a smaller dose. Boluses are large rectangular tablets which may be scored or unscored. Boluses are used in the treatment of large animals (e.g., cattle, horses, and sheep). Boluses are usually administered to bovines with the aid of a special instrument called a balling gun.

Liquid preparations for oral administration may be purchased in several different forms (e.g., mixtures, emulsions, syrups, and elixirs). Mixtures are aqueous (i.e., water) solutions or suspensions for oral administration. A **suspension** will usually separate after long periods of shelf life and must be shaken well before use to provide a uniform dose. Syrups are often used as cough remedies and contain the drug and a flavoring in a concentrated solution of sugar water or other aqueous liquid. In veterinary medicine, an antitussive (e.g., Torbugesic) may be mixed with a liquid vitamin (e.g., Lixotinic) to ensure a more palatable taste for the patient. **Elixirs** usually are a hydroalcoholic liquid containing sweeteners, flavoring, and a medicinal agent. **Emulsions** consist of oily substances dispersed in an aqueous medium with an additive stabilizing the mixture. All liquid oral medications should be administered slowly to allow the patient to swallow before more liquid is given. Rapid

administration of oral medication can cause the liquid to be aspirated into the lungs, causing pulmonary problems.

Technician's Notes

Rapid administration of oral medication can cause the liquid to be aspirated into the lungs, causing pulmonary problems.

Two types of parenteral injection forms are available: injections and implants.

Two types of parenteral injection forms are available: injections and implants. Injections are available as single-dose vials, multidose vials, ampules, or large-volume bottles, which may be used to administer intravenous infusions (Figure 2-2). A vial is a bottle that is sealed with a rubber diaphragm. A vial may be either single or multidose. A single-dose vial must be discarded after one use (dose). Multidose vials usually contain preservatives enabling them to have a longer shelf life and thus they may be used for more than one dose. Ampules contain a single dose of medication in a small glass container with a thin neck, which is usually scored so that it can be snapped off easily. Some drugs may be unstable in solution and will need reconstitution with sterile water or other diluent and used immediately for injection (Procedure 2-1).

Technician's Notes

It is a good idea to place a paper towel over the neck of an ampule before breaking the neck, in order to protect fingers from glass cuts.

Syringes and needles are used for parenteral administration of drugs (Box 2-1). This equipment must be sterile and needles must be sharp. Drugs should never be stored in syringes for long amounts of time before administration occurs because some drugs may be absorbed into the plastic make-up of the syringe, resulting in an inadequate dose.

Text continued on p. 33

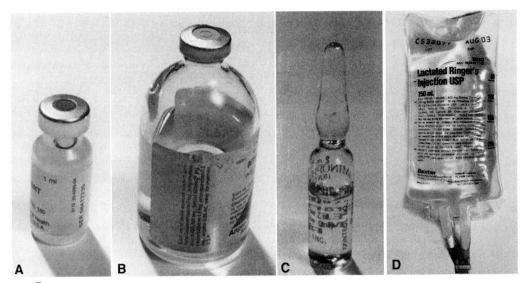

FIGURE 2-2
Parenteral medications are supplied in single-dose vials **(A),** multidose vials **(B),** ampules **(C),** and large-volume bottles or bags used for intravenous administration **(D).**

Table 2-1 Animal and Commonly Used Needle Gauges

Animal	Needle Gauge
Swine	16, 18
Cattle	16, 18
Horses	16, 18, 20
Dogs	20, 21, 22, 25
Cats	22, 25
Small exotics	23, 25, 27

PROCEDURE 2-1

Reconstitution of a Medication

Materials Needed
Syringe of adequate size for the amount of diluent
  with a needle attached
70% isopropyl alcohol
Cotton swab

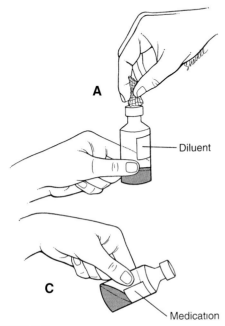

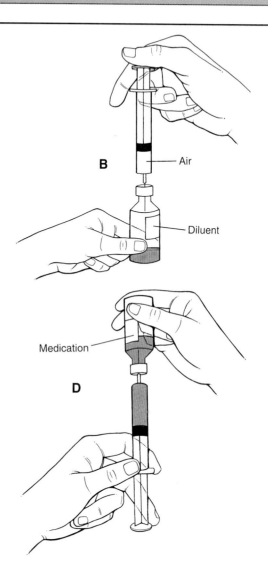

FIGURE 2-3

Procedure
1. Clean the rubber diaphragm of the medication vial and the diluent vial with an alcohol swab (Figure 2-3, *A*).
2. Remove the needle cap and pull back on the plunger to fill the barrel with air equal to the desired amount of diluent. Inject the air into the vial of diluent to create positive pressure and to ease withdrawal (Figure 2-3, *B*). Invert the diluent vial and withdraw the desired amount of diluent.
3. Inject the diluent into the medication vial and withdraw the syringe and needle. Shake the vial to mix well (Figure 2-3, *C*).

4. Positive pressure may be created in the freshly mixed medication vial before withdrawing the desired amount of medication. Once the medication has been withdrawn (Figure 2-3, *D*), label the syringe if needed, or administer the drug to the patient. After withdrawing the patient's medication, dispose of the vial or store it according to the label.

BOX 2-1 Syringes and Needles

Syringes

Syringes are available in various sizes and styles. The most commonly used sizes are 3 ml, 6 ml, 12 ml, 20 ml, 35 ml, and 60 ml. Syringes may be ordered from the manufacturer either with or without an attached needle. The tip of the syringe, where the needle attaches, can be one of four types: Luer-Lok tip (Figure 2-4, A), slip tip (Figure 2-4, B), eccentric tip (Figure 2-4, C), or catheter tip (Figure 2-4, D). Each type of tip has its own advantages and disadvantages and is often chosen because of personal preference. A complete syringe consists of a plunger, barrel, hub, needle, and dead space (Figure 2-5). The area in which fluid remains when the plunger is completely depressed is called dead space.

Tuberculin Syringe

A tuberculin syringe (Figure 2-6) holds up to 1 ml of medication. It usually is available with a 25-gauge or

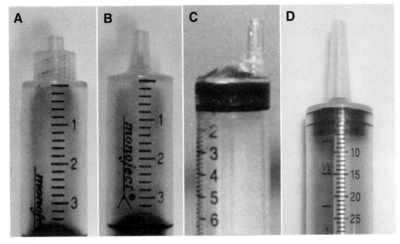

FIGURE 2-4
Syringes are available with different tips, such as Luer-Lok tip **(A)**, slip tip **(B)**, eccentric tip **(C)**, and catheter tip **(D)**. (Courtesy Sherwood Medical, St. Louis)

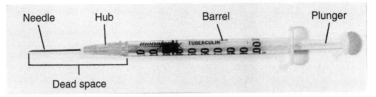

FIGURE 2-5
The parts of a needle and syringe. (Courtesy Sherwood Medical, St. Louis)

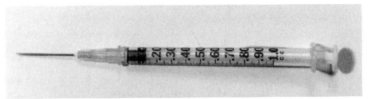

FIGURE 2-6
A tuberculin syringe with needle attached. (Courtesy Sherwood Medical, St. Louis)

BOX 2-1 Syringes and Needles—cont'd

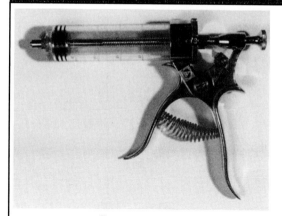

FIGURE 2-7
A multidose syringe.

smaller attached needle. This syringe is commonly used for injections of less than 1 ml.

Multidose Syringe
A multidose syringe (Figure 2-7) is commonly used for large animals when several animals require the same injection. It allows the user to set the dose and give repeated injections until the barrel is empty of medication. This type of syringe may be disassembled and disinfected for reuse.

Insulin Syringe
An insulin syringe (Figure 2-8) is usually supplied with a 25-gauge needle and, unlike other syringes, it has no dead space. The syringe is divided into units instead of milliliters and should be used only for insulin injection.

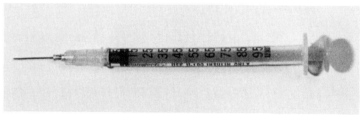

FIGURE 2-8
An insulin syringe with needle attached. (Courtesy Sherwood Medical, St. Louis)

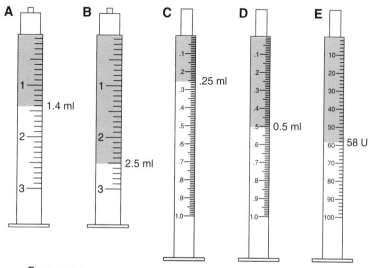

FIGURE 2-9
Examples of how to read amounts of medication contained in a syringe.

Continued

BOX 2-1 Syringes and Needles—cont'd

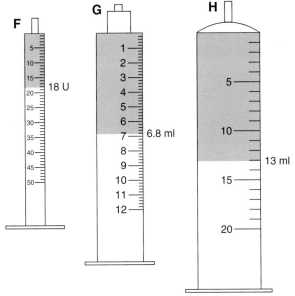

FIGURE 2-9—cont'd

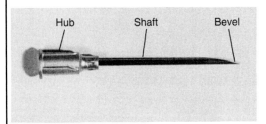

FIGURE 2-10
A needle consists of three parts: hub, shaft, and bevel.

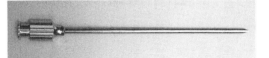

FIGURE 2-11
A 3-inch stainless steel bleeding needle.

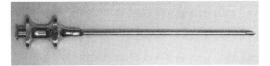

FIGURE 2-12
A stainless steel biopsy needle.

Figure 2-9 illustrates the importance of being familiar with the different types of syringes and the units of measurement found on each. This is necessary in order to be able to draw up an accurate amount of medication.

Needles
Needles are available in various sizes and styles, but all needles have the following three parts: hub, shaft, and bevel (Figure 2-10). Needle sizes vary by gauge and by length. The gauge refers to the inside diameter of the shaft; the larger the gauge number, the smaller the diameter. The length of the needle is measured from the tip of the hub to the end of the shaft. Lengths longer than 1 inch are usually used in large animals and occasionally for biopsy. The bevel is the angle of the opening at the needle tip. It is often helpful when performing venipuncture to have the beveled side of the needle facing up before inserting the needle into the patient.

Bleeding needles (Figure 2-11) may be up to 3 inches long, are large gauge (14 to 16 gauge), and are usually used for obtaining blood from cattle and swine. These needles are made of stainless steel and are reusable following proper cleaning and disinfecting. Biopsy needles (Figure 2-12) are used for obtaining bone marrow, or soft tissue and organ specimens. These needles vary in size and styles.

Implants are very hard sterile pellets that contain a chemical or hormonal agent. Implants are inserted subcutaneously and are absorbed by the body over an extended period of time. Growth hormones are commonly manufactured in this form for use in cattle and are implanted in the subcutaneous dorsal aspect of the ear.

Topical medications are available in several forms. **Liniments** are medicinal preparations for use on the skin as a **counterirritant** or to relieve pain. Lotions are liquid suspensions or solutions with soothing substances that may be applied to the skin. An **ointment** is a semisolid preparation of oil and water, plus a medicinal agent. The water in an ointment evaporates after application and leaves the drug behind on the skin's surface. Dusting powders (e.g., flea powder) are mixtures of drugs in a powder form for topical application. Additionally, powders may have adsorbent (cornstarch) or lubricant (talcum) properties. Aerosols are drugs incorporated in a suitable solvent and packaged under pressure with a propellant. Dusting powders and aerosols are common forms for some topical insecticides and wound dressings.

Microencapsulation is a drug form that stabilizes substances commonly considered unstable. Microencapsulation may also be used for drugs intended to be released slowly over a period of time (e.g., moxidectin [Proheart injection]). When the drug's active ingredients are microencapsulated, a protective environment is formed against harmful substances and improves the stability of the product. Microencapsulation completely masks the flavor of a drug and allows oral treatments to be administered with greater ease since the patient is unable to taste or smell the ingredients.

DRUG PRESERVATIVES AND SOLVENTS

In addition to the active ingredient, many drugs contain organic or inorganic agents as additives or pharmaceutic aids. These inactive (or inert) ingredients facilitate tablet administration, improve solubility, or increase stability. Although the amount of inert ingredients is usually small, they can cause adverse effects or a patient may be sensitive to the ingredients or may smell the ingredients.

Parenterally administered drugs often contain chemical preservatives to prevent destruction and loss of potency through oxidation or hydrolysis. The amount of preservative in the formulation of parenterally administered drugs is an optimal concentration and the reconstituted medication should be used immediately to prevent the possibility of fungal or bacterial growth. Dilution of the drug reduces the effectiveness of the preservatives. Most drugs are water-soluble, although some may need additives to increase solubility. Glycols are one example of additives used to increase solubility. Generally, propylene glycol and polyethylene glycols are preferred.

DRUG ADMINISTRATION

A veterinarian initiates administration of drugs for therapeutic purposes. (It is unlawful for a veterinary technician to prescribe drugs for an animal patient.) The role of the technician is to administer drugs to the patient on the order of a veterinarian. When doing this, a technician must always follow the "five rights":

1. Right patient
2. Right drug—check label three times before administering the drug
3. Right dose
4. Right route
5. Right time and frequency

By following these rules, a technician will efficiently and effectively medicate a patient.

Oral Medications

The most common forms of drug therapy are tablets and capsules. These are easily administered (Procedure 2-2) and are sometimes used in conjunction with other drug forms.

PROCEDURE 2-2

Oral Administration of Tablets or Capsules for Dogs and Cats

Materials Needed
Medication in tablet or capsule form
Pilling gun (optional) (Figure 2-13)

Procedure
1. Hold the animal's upper jaw with one hand and apply pressure against the upper premolars to cause the mouth to open.
2. Push the medication over the tongue of the animal with the other hand or the pilling gun (Figure 2-14).
3. Close the animal's mouth.
4. Initiate swallowing by blowing into the animal's nose and/or rubbing its throat (Figure 2-15).

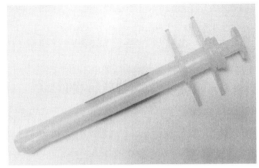

FIGURE 2-13
Example of a small-animal pilling gun.

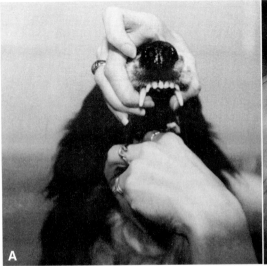
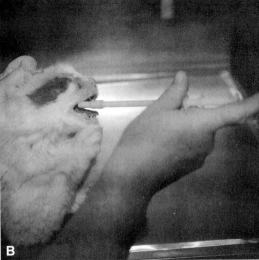

FIGURE 2-14

PROCEDURE 2-2

Oral Administration of Tablets or Capsules for Dogs and Cats–cont'd

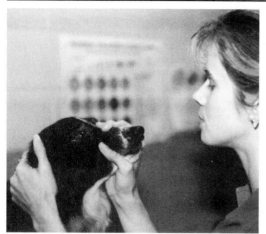

FIGURE 2-15

Technician's Notes
Coating the tablet or capsule with a palatable substance, such as Cat Lax, peanut butter, or canned food, may help in pilling difficult animals.

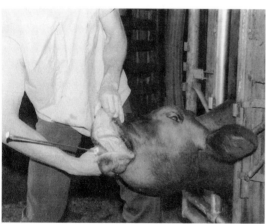

FIGURE 2-16
A balling gun used to administer a bolus to large animals.

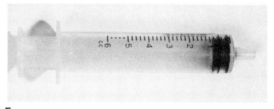

FIGURE 2-17
A syringe without a needle may be used to administer oral liquid medication.

commonly used in exotics and may be administered through the drinking water or an orogastric tube. In large animals, a stomach tube is usually used for administering oral liquid medications (Figure 2-18). In cattle, the stomach tube is passed through a Frick **speculum** (Figure 2-19).

In large animals, a balling gun (Figure 2-16) is used to administer boluses. With proper restraint, this is usually not too difficult.

Liquid oral medications may be administered to small animals through a syringe with the needle removed (Procedure 2-3 and Figure 2-17) or in some instances through an orogastric or nasogastric tube. Most liquid medications are made palatable to ease administration. Oral liquid medications are

Technician's Notes
Oral Medications:
1. Remember when administering oral medications, that it takes longer for a drug to be absorbed into the blood stream by this route as compared with parenteral injection.
2. Do not use oral administration in animals that are vomiting.

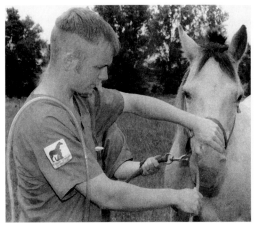

FIGURE 2-18
A large-animal stomach tube may be used to administer liquid medications to cattle or horses.

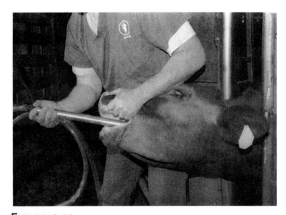

FIGURE 2-19
A Frick speculum can be used to facilitate passage of the stomach tube through the mouth of cattle.

PROCEDURE 2-3

Oral Administration of Oral Liquid Medication with a Syringe for Dogs and Cats

Materials Needed
Syringe with the needle removed or oral dose syringe
Oral medication in liquid form

Procedure
1. Fill syringe with the calculated amount of medication.
2. Tilt the animal's head up slightly.
3. Insert the tip of the syringe into the animal's cheek pouch (Figure 2-20).
4. Administer the medication slowly.

Technician's Notes
Attachment of a J-12 Teat Infusion Cannula (Jorgenson Laboratories) is handy for administering oral liquid medications.

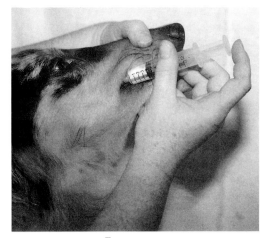

FIGURE 2-20

Parenteral Medications

Parenteral administration (i.e., injection) of liquid medications may be used alone or in conjunction with other forms of medication. Some conditions are unfavorable for oral administration (e.g., in vomiting patients) and some drugs are available only for parenteral administration.

There are approximately 10 common routes for parenteral administration of drugs, the most common being intramuscular, subcutaneous, and intravenous (Figures 2-21 to 2-23). A veterinary technician must be aware of the proper route of administration for each drug. If in doubt, the route of administration is usually listed on the drug label

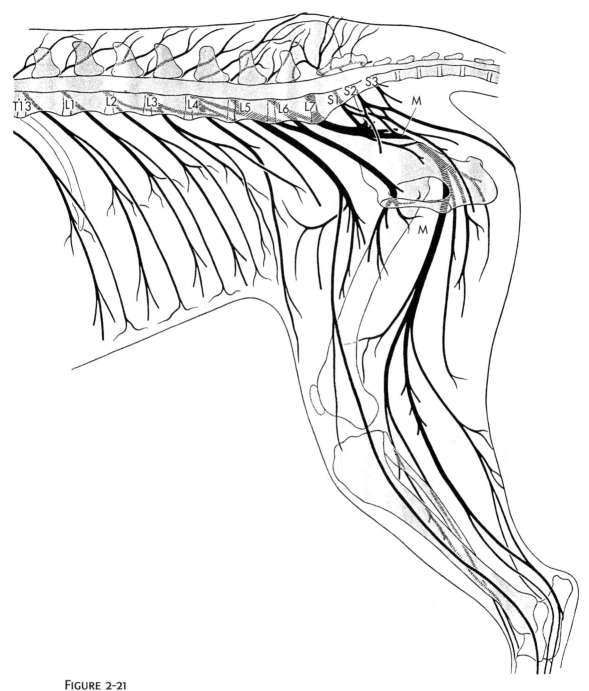

FIGURE 2-21

Intramuscular injections in the pelvic limb should be given in an area that avoids the large sciatic nerve, labeled as M.

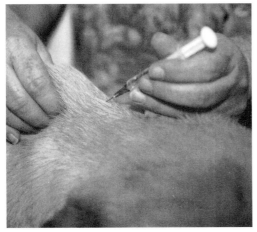

FIGURE 2-22
Subcutaneous injection.

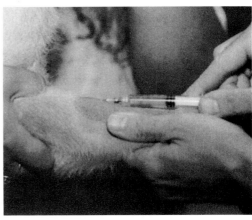

FIGURE 2-23
Intravenous injection.

or package insert. Sometimes complications may result after parenteral administration of a drug. Some common complications include irritation, necrosis, or infection of the injection site. Sometimes allergic reactions to medications may occur. Some clinical signs of an allergic reaction after a parenteral drug has been administered include swelling around the face or extremities, raised "bumps" or swellings on the skin's surface, edema, and salivation. If any complications are observed, they should be immediately reported to the veterinarian. Care should be exercised when administering an intramuscular injection to avoid nerve damage or accidental injection into a vein or artery. The syringe's plunger should have negative pressure applied before an intramuscular (or subcutaneous) injection is made. Should any blood be observed in the hub of the needle, redirect or remove the needle. Care should also be exercised when intraperitoneal injections are made so that peritonitis does not develop or damage does not occur to the abdominal viscera. Proper administration involves knowing what equipment is needed, how to calculate the dose, and the proper method for withdrawing and administering medication (Procedure 2-4).

Intravenous (IV) administration allows the most rapid and effective drug administration (Procedure 2-5). The most common uses of IV therapy are maintaining and restoring fluid and electrolyte balance, administering drugs, transfusing blood, and delivering parenteral nutrition. IV administration is also used when the medication is contraindicated for other routes of administration. Sites for IV administration include the cephalic vein, the jugular vein, the lateral saphenous vein, and sometimes the femoral veins. Long-term IV therapy is best achieved with the cephalic or jugular veins.

In some cases, an animal may need repeated IV injections. The veterinarian may order the placement of an indwelling IV catheter in an effort to lessen vein damage and pain for the animal (Procedures 2-6 and 2-7).

Technician's Notes

An IV catheter must be removed after 72 hours and replaced with a new one. Time can be accounted for by writing (e.g., use a permanent marker) placement time on the adhesive bandage that secures the IV catheter in the animal's vein. Additionally, IV tubing should be changed after a 24- to 48-hour period.

Text continued on p. 43

PROCEDURE 2-4

Parenteral Administration of Medications—Intramuscular or Subcutaneous

Materials Needed
Syringe and needle (Figure 2-24)
Parenteral medication
Cotton swabs
70% isopropyl alcohol

Procedure
1. If the syringe is not supplied ready-to-use, firmly attach the needle to the syringe.
2. Swab the bottle's rubber diaphragm with cotton that is saturated with alcohol.
3. Remove the needle cap, insert the needle at an angle into the rubber diaphragm, and withdraw the calculated amount.

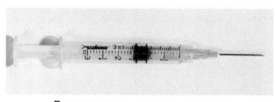

FIGURE 2-24
(Courtesy Sherwood Medical, St. Louis)

4. Hold the syringe with the needle pointing upward and remove the large air bubbles by briskly tapping the barrel of the syringe.
5. Release the air bubbles by slightly pushing on the syringe plunger. Carefully replace the needle cap if the medication is not to be given immediately. Avoid contamination.
6. Swab the injection site with another cotton swab that is saturated with alcohol.
7. Insert the needle into the appropriate site and pull slightly on the plunger. If no blood is seen, inject the medication and remove the needle from the site. Blood indicates that a vessel has been entered. Withdraw the needle and continue with the same procedure at a different site.
8. Massage the injection site to aid distribution and decrease pain.
9. Properly dispose of the syringe and needle.

Technician's Notes
Injecting multidose vials with air sometimes allows easier withdrawal of the medication.

◼◼ PROCEDURE 2-5

Parenteral Administration of Medication—Intravenous Direct Bolus

Materials Needed

Syringe containing calculated dose with needle attached

Cotton swabs

70% isopropyl alcohol or surgical scrub

Butterfly catheter (scalp vein needle, Figure 2-25)—optional

Syringe containing 3 ml of flushing solution (e.g., heparinized saline: 500 IU sodium heparin in 250 ml of normal saline)

Tape (optional)

Procedure Without Catheter

1. Clip the area over the venipuncture site, if desired.
2. Prepare the area with alcohol swabs or surgical scrub.
3. Have the restraint person hold pressure on the vein or use a tourniquet.
4. Perform venipuncture with the medication syringe and needle. If blood enters the hub of the needle, the venipuncture is successful.
5. Release pressure from the vein and proceed to inject the medication over the recommended time interval.
6. Remove the needle and apply pressure to the site to stop bleeding.

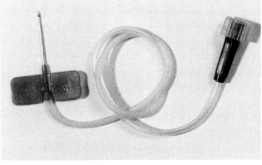

FIGURE 2-25
Butterfly catheter.

7. A bandage made of tape and cotton may be applied if needed.

Procedure With A Butterfly Catheter

Proceed with steps 1 through 3 described in the previous section (McCurnin DM and Bassert JM: Clinical textbook for veterinary technicians, ed 5, Philadelphia, 2002, WB Saunders).

1. Remove the cap from the catheter tubing and needle cover.
2. Perform venipuncture with the catheter. If it is successful, blood will return into the catheter tubing.
3. Release pressure from the vein, and allow the blood to fill the catheter tubing.
4. Remove the needle from the medication syringe and attach the syringe hub to the catheter tubing.
5. Administer the medication at the recommended time interval.
6. Remove the needle from the syringe containing the flushing solution. Remove the medication syringe from the catheter and attach the syringe containing the flushing solution.
7. Flush the catheter with 1 to 2 ml of solution to ensure administration of all medication.
8. Remove the catheter and apply pressure to the site to stop the bleeding.
9. A bandage may be applied as described earlier.
10. Properly dispose of all syringes and needles in an approved sharps container.

Technician's Notes

Watch for swelling at the injection site. Swelling may signal extravascular injection. Notify the veterinarian immediately if this occurs.

■ PROCEDURE 2-6

Administration by Bolus with an Indwelling Intravenous Catheter

Materials Needed
Syringe containing flushing solution (about 3 ml)
70% isopropyl alcohol
Cotton swabs
Syringe with medication and attached needle

Procedure
1. Clean the cap of the indwelling catheter with an alcohol swab.
2. Insert the needle of the syringe containing the flushing solution into the catheter cap. (Use the smallest gauge needle possible to help prevent a leak in the catheter cap.)
3. Gently aspirate to determine correct placement of the catheter (blood entering the hub shows proper placement).
4. Inject half the flushing solution into the catheter. Observe the area over the vein for swelling.
5. Remove the syringe and needle, and carefully replace the cap to prevent contamination.
6. Insert the needle of the syringe containing the medication into the catheter cap, and inject the medication over the recommended time interval.
7. Remove the syringe and needle from the catheter.
8. Flush the catheter with the remaining flushing solution.
9. Observe the area for swelling and look for signs of discomfort. Report any abnormal observations to the veterinarian.
10. Properly dispose of syringes and needles.

Technician's Notes

Some hospitals may require using two syringes with flushing solution instead of using the same syringe and needle for both flushes. Keep additional male adapter plugs (catheter caps) (Figure 2-26) in stock to replace a leaky cap.

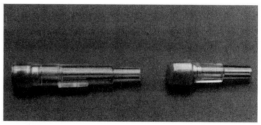

FIGURE 2-26
Examples of a male adapter plug. (Manufactured by Abbott Laboratories.)

■ PROCEDURE 2-7

Administration of Intravenous Fluids

Materials Needed

Indwelling catheter (Figure 2-27)
Tape
70% isopropyl alcohol or surgical scrub
Infusion set
IV fluids
Clippers

Procedure

1. Remove the IV tubing from the container and the protective covering from the medication bottle or bag.
2. Remove the covering of the diaphragm of the medication bag or bottle.
3. Close the clamp on the IV tubing. Remove the cap of the IV tubing spike and insert it into the diaphragm of the medication bag or bottle.
4. Squeeze the drip chamber to allow fluid to collect in the chamber. Fill to the designated line or about half full.
5. Remove the protective cap from the end of the IV tubing and slowly open the roller clamp to allow the fluid to clear the tubing of air. Replace the protective cap and hang the medication bag or bottle on the IV pole near the patient.
6. Clip and scrub the chosen site for catheter placement.
7. After successful catheter placement, cap the catheter, wipe away any blood, and quickly tape in place. Record time of placement on the adhesive tape using a permanent marker.
8. Remove the catheter cap and the protective cap of the IV tubing and insert the end of the tubing directly into the end of the catheter. Or, if desired, a needle may be placed on the end of the tubing and inserted into the catheter cap.
9. Open the clamp to begin a slow drip and lower the medication bag or bottle below the IV site to confirm correct placement.
10. Return the bottle or bag to the IV pole and set at desired flow rate.
11. Tape the tubing to the patient at the catheter site.

Technician's Notes

1. Mark the fluid level and time on tape placed on the bag with a permanent marker (tape can be used on bottles). Use this procedure each time the patient is checked.
2. If any medications are added to the fluids, write the medication, time, and amount on the medication bag or tape.
3. Tape the catheter cap to the bag or bottle so that it will be ready when needed.

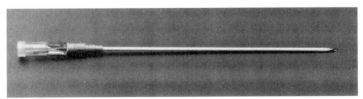

FIGURE 2-27
A 14-gauge indwelling catheter. (ABBOCATH is a registered trademark of Abbott Laboratories.)

◼ PROCEDURE 2-8

Administration by Bolus Using the Y Injection Site

Materials Needed
Syringe with medication and the needle attached
Cotton swabs
70% isopropyl alcohol

Procedure
1. Close the clamp on the infusion set.
2. Clean the Y-injection site (Figure 2-28) with an alcohol swab.

3. Insert the needle of the medication syringe into the Y-injection site.
4. Inject the medication over the recommended time interval.
5. Remove the medication syringe and needle.
6. Open the clamp on the infusion set. Allow enough fluid to flow through the infusion set to ensure that all medication is received. Then return to the desired flow rate.
7. Properly dispose of the syringe and needle.
8. NOTE: No flushing solution is required for this procedure.

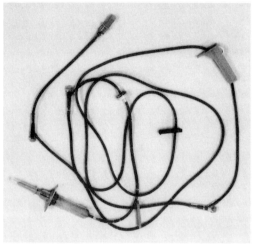

FIGURE 2-28
Intravenous set with Cair clamp and Y injection site.

Technician's Notes

To check for proper placement of the IV catheter, remove the bag of fluids from the IV pole and hold the bag and tubing below the level of the catheter (do not close the clamp on the infusion set). If blood returns into the tubing, the catheter is properly placed. Return the bag to the IV pole and continue fluid administration.

If the patient is receiving IV fluids, the Y-injection site (Figure 2-28)—located on the IV tubing—may be used to administer medications by direct bolus (Procedure 2-8). When medications are to be administered continuously and for long periods of time, the IV tubing needs to be changed after a 24- to 48-hour period. Once the medication bottle or bag is emptied, replacement is necessary to facilitate care of the patient. An indwelling catheter must be removed after 72 hours and replaced with a new one in a different vein location. (McCurnin, 2002). If the IV catheter is not used continuously, it should be flushed with heparinized saline every 8 to 12 hours.

A simplex (i.e., gravity set) IV set is used to administer medications or fluids intravenously to large animals (Figure 2-29). This administration set may be disinfected and reused. Disposable IV sets and large volume fluid bags are available for large animals requiring continuous IV therapy.

In pediatric patients and small exotics, IV medications may be administered by intraosseous cannulation. This route may also be used in larger patients when rapid administration of fluids or drugs

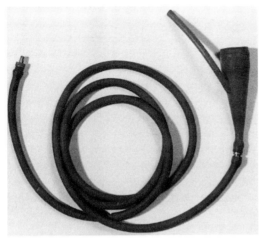

FIGURE 2-29
A large-animal intravenous set.

is necessary and a vein is not readily available. If needed, large volumes of fluid may be administered in this manner.

In some veterinary hospitals, using an infusion pump may facilitate continuous IV administration. Once the necessary flow rate is known (the rate is ordered by the veterinarian), the technician can set the infusion pump to deliver a constant amount of solution per minute or hour. To determine the pump settings, the technician considers the total amount of solution to be given and the time interval for infusion. The operating instructions for the infusion pump should be followed because each model may operate in a slightly different manner.

Technician's Notes

It should be remembered that any patient on IV fluid therapy should be monitored every 15 to 30 minutes.

Monitoring includes evaluation of drip rate; ensuring the IV catheter is still properly placed in the vein; making sure the patient has not moved around in the cage to such an extent the IV tubing has become kinked; and, most importantly, to ensure the patient has not chewed the IV catheter out. Animals can do surprising things, and it is up to the technician to provide an excellent level of nursing to ensure no harm comes to the patient.

Technician's Notes

Parenteral Medications

1. Some liquid medications for parenteral administration may "settle out" or precipitate (e.g., penicillin, Vetalog). Therefore these medications should be shaken gently to mix the solution before it is injected into the patient.
2. Drugs that may cause tissue irritation are administered by the intravenous route (e.g., pentothal, vincristine). Therefore be sure to check the drug's package insert to determine the correct way to administer the drug.

Intramuscular Injections

1. Ketaset can be administered by intramuscular injection. Ketaset has a tendency to "burn" upon injection, and careful restraint methods should be employed along with rapid injection of this drug in cats.
2. Upon insertion of the needle in the chosen muscle, always apply negative pressure to the syringe's plunger to be certain the needle has not entered a blood vessel. If blood is seen in the hub of the syringe, remove and redirect the needle.

Subcutaneous Injections

1. Most vaccines can be administered subcutaneously. However, the intrascapular area should always be avoided when giving subcutaneous injections.

Inhalation Medications

In veterinary medicine, inhalation is primarily used to produce anesthesia. The inhalant gas is placed into the anesthetic machine in liquid form and is then vaporized through the machine and delivered to the patient via an endotracheal tube, anesthetic gas mask, or induction chamber (Figures 2-30 to 2-32). Medications may occasionally be nebulized to treat an upper respiratory tract (URT) problem, and

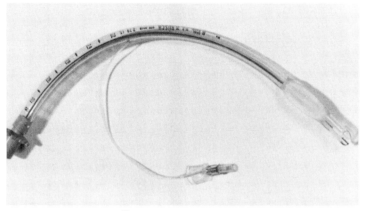

FIGURE 2-30
Endotracheal tube with cuff.

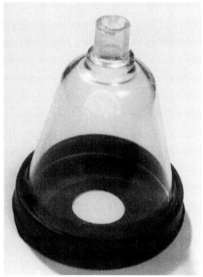

FIGURE 2-31
A small-animal anesthetic mask.

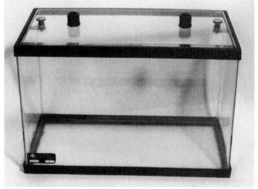

FIGURE 2-32
A small-animal induction chamber.

oxygen may be delivered to a patient with dyspnea using inhalation techniques.

Topical Medications

Topical administration of medicine involves applying drugs (**creams**, ointment, and drops) to the body's surface. Topical preparations usually provide local effects instead of systemic ones. Clipping hair from the affected area will provide better visualiza-

tion during treatment, and makes application easier and absorption faster. The technician should observe the area after treatment and report adverse reactions to the veterinarian. The technician should provide client education regarding skin medications, including information regarding frequency and amount of applications. Many clients may apply too much medication, which is not only unnecessary but can be quite costly with some medications.

Ophthalmic drugs are supplied either as an ointment or solution. The eyes have the ability to remove foreign substances rapidly. Therefore these preparations are usually applied several times a day.

Application frequency depends on the disease or disorder, the drug, and the type of formulation. When applying ophthalmic preparations, the hand holding the medication should rest on the animal's head above the affected eye (Figure 2-33). Drops should be placed at the inner canthus of the eye. If application of ointment is necessary, apply a small strip along the lower palpebral border making sure the applicator tip does not come into contact with the eye or conjunctiva. When demonstrating to a client how to apply eye medications, point out that the applicators have blunt tips. Therefore should the applicator tip inadvertently touch the eye, no harm should occur.

Drugs applied topically to the ears are for local effect to soften **cerumen** and ease its removal, or to treat a superficial infection or ear mites. Cleaning the ears before applying otic medication will aid the effectiveness of the treatment. The veterinary technician should provide instruction to the client regarding the correct way to clean ears and to apply ear medication. By explaining the ear's anatomy, the technician can assure the client that it is difficult to reach the animal's eardrum when swabbing the ear clean.

MEDICATION ORDERS

In a veterinary hospital, most medication orders are written or verbal. A written order may be in prescription form or noted in the medical record. Verbal orders are given directly to the technician by the veterinarian. When filling a prescription, the technician must be familiar with abbreviations frequently applied to the medical record describing drug therapy. Appendix A lists common abbreviations used in veterinary medicine. The technician must know the patient being treated, the route of administration, and the frequency of administration. This information is described by the medication order. After the medication is administered to the patient, a notation should be made in the medical record describing when, what, how, and by whom the medication was administered. Observations of the patient's progress should be noted in the medical record (Figure 2-34). If the medication order is a prescription (Figure 2-35) to be filled, the order should be dated and noted in the medical record (Figure 2-36). If the owner picks up the prescription at the veterinary hospital, the medical record should be retrieved and presented to the vet-

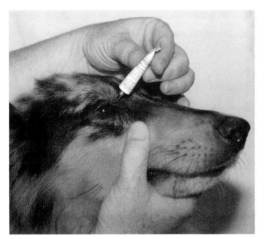

FIGURE 2-33
Ointment is applied to the dog's eye on the lower palpebral border.

6-18-95   9:30 AM patient B&A

T-102°

250 mg Amoxi PO, flushed IV catheter with

heparinized saline, continue IV LR at

15 gtt/min   C. Smith, LVMT

FIGURE 2-34
After administering a medication to a patient, a notation should be made in the patient's medical record.

```
┌─────────────────────────────────────────────────────────┐
│          PET CARE ANIMAL HOSPITAL                        │
│                                                          │
│               1554 Straight Road                         │
│              Anytown, USA 12345                          │
│                455-555-1222                              │
│    Patient  Tuffy Fox                Date   8/28/98      │
│                   Sporanox                               │
│            1 capsule po bid x 3 wks                      │
│                give with food                            │
│                                                          │
│                                                          │
│     Sarah Jones, DVM  D.V.M.                             │
│     DISPENSE AS WRITTEN                                  │
│                                                          │
│                                                          │
│     _____ D.V.M.            0   Refills      │
│       SUBSTITUTION ALLOWED                               │
│     _____ DEA #                               │
└─────────────────────────────────────────────────────────┘
```

FIGURE 2-35
Sample prescription order.

4-10-95   Rx per Dr. Smith
             Amoxi 250 mg 1 tab po bid x 10 days
             Bute 100 mg 2 tab po sid x 3 days
             give c̄ food   K. Jones, LVMT

FIGURE 2-36
Prescriptions should be written in the patient's medical record.

erinarian for approval of the refill. The same format as described earlier should be followed for dispensing medication.

CONTROLLED SUBSTANCES

Substances that have the ability to become habit-forming for humans are labeled as controlled substances. The DEA requires the upper right corner of the original container to show a code containing a capital C (controlled), followed by a Roman numeral indicating one of the five schedules that are defined by the *Code of Federal Regulations*. Since some of these drugs have potential for misuse, the DEA requires that they be kept in an unmovable locked area and an inventory log be kept reporting amounts used and on hand (Figure 2-37). Each time a controlled drug is administered or dispensed to a patient, it must be reported in the controlled substance inventory log in addition to the patient's medical record. This documentation should include

Drug: diazepam

Patient		Owner		Beginning		Administered		On hand		Initials
Toby	:	Smith	:	5 ml	:	0.2 ml	:	4.8 ml	:	BD/JC
Prissy	:	Potts	:	4.8 ml	:	0.15 ml	:	4.65 ml	:	LW/RW
Gilbert	:	Pettes	:	4.65 ml	:	0.5 ml	:	4.15	:	LW/RW
T.J.	:	Curtis	:	4.15 ml	:	0.2 ml	:	3.95	:	BD/JC

FIGURE 2-37
Example of a controlled substance inventory log.

the following: (1) date, (2) owner's name, (3) patient's name, (4) drug name, (5) amount administered or dispensed, and (6) the names of veterinary personnel dispensing the drug. If dispensed, the label must bear the following warning: "Caution: Federal law prohibits the transfer of this drug to any person other than the patient for whom it was prescribed" (Webb and Aeschbacher, 1993). A list of the most common controlled substances used in veterinary medicine is available in Appendix D.

Technician's Notes
Drug Storage
1. The manufacturer's instructions should be followed closely in order to facilitate safe storage.
2. Some drugs are sensitive to light and humidity.
3. The location of the pharmacy in a veterinary hospital should not be accessible to the public.

CLIENT EDUCATION

Veterinary technicians should be familiar with all administered and dispensed drugs. Often it is the technician's duty to educate clients about how a medication should be administered, why it has been prescribed, and any adverse reaction that may occur. The technician should consult the veterinarian to provide information about any questions that he or she cannot answer. If needed, written information about the medication should be available for the client's reference.

REFERENCES
Lane DR and Cooper VN, editors: Veterinary nursing, ed 3, Oxford, 2003, Butterworth-Heinemann.
McCurnin DM and Bassert JM, editors: Clinical textbook for veterinary technicians, ed 5, Philadelphia, 2002, WB Saunders Co.
Webb AI and Aeschbacher G: Animal drug container labels: a guide to the reader, JAVMA 202:10, 1993.

REVIEW QUESTIONS

1. Name four common drug preparations.
   _____
2. Boluses are used in the treatment of
   _____ animals and are
   administered with a
   _____.
3. Name two types of parenteral injection forms.
   _____
4. Vials may be either _____
   dose or _____ dose.
5. All used needles should be discarded in a
   _____.
6. Name the five rights of drug administration.
   _____.
7. Oral drugs should never be administered in
   animals that are _____.
8. Intravenous administration of drugs allows the
   most _____ and effective
   drug administration.

9. An indwelling catheter should be replaced
   with a new one every
   _____ hours.
10. A simplex (i.e., gravity set) IV system is used
    to administer fluids to
    _____ animals.
11. Name six items that should be recorded in the
    controlled substance log.
12. Why should drugs given by injection not be
    stored in syringes for any length of time before
    administration? _____.
13. List four types of syringe tips available for use.
    _____.
14. A tuberculin syringe holds up to
    _____ ml of medication.
15. What type of syringe is divided into units
    rather than milliliters?

INTRODUCTION
MATHEMATICS FUNDAMENTALS
SYSTEMS OF MEASUREMENT
    The Metric System
    Conversion between Metric Units
    The Apothecary and Household
       Systems
DOSAGE CALCULATIONS
SOLUTIONS
PERCENT CONCENTRATIONS
    Calculations Involving Concentrations
MILLIEQUIVALENTS
CALCULATIONS INVOLVING IV
  FLUID ADMINISTRATION
    Calculations for Constant Rate Infusion
      Problems

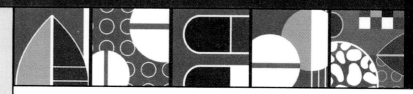

CHAPTER **3**

Practical Calculations in Pharmacology

LEARNING OBJECTIVES

After studying this chapter, you should be able to:

1. Develop an understanding of the systems of measurement
2. Understand how to perform conversions using the metric system and other systems of measurement
3. Know how to perform dosage calculations
4. Understand how to prepare percent concentrations

KEY TERMS

EQUIVALENT WEIGHT 1 g molecular weight (from periodic chart) divided by the total positive valence of the material.

MILLIEQUIVALENT 1/1000 of an equivalent weight. A term used to express the concentration of electrolytes in a solution.

INTRODUCTION

Veterinary technicians are often called on to prepare and administer medications to animal patients. A veterinarian's orders may call for administration of a specific number of milligrams or units of the medication (dose). The technician must then determine the quantity (in milliliters, tablets, and so forth) of the preparation that contains the appropriate dose. In other instances, the technician may be called on to calculate the dose based on a dosage rate (found in the insert or in reference books) and the animal's weight. In either case, an error in calculation can seriously affect the health of a patient. This chapter deals with the background information and applications necessary to accurately carry out a veterinarian's medication orders.

MATHEMATICS FUNDAMENTALS

It is assumed that the student using this text has a basic understanding of fractions and decimals. With these fundamentals as a background, the concepts of percent, ratio, and proportion should be reviewed before moving to the practice problems.

Percent is defined as parts per hundred. Percent is a fraction with the percent as the numerator and 100 the denominator (e.g., 5% = 5/100). Percents may be written as decimals, fractions, or whole numbers.

Example 1: Decimal: 0.3%
(three-tenths percent [3/10 ÷ 100])
Fraction: 1/5%
(one-fifth percent [1/5 ÷ 100])
Whole number: 5%
(five percent [5 ÷ 100])

Percent may be changed to fractions or decimals.

Example 2: Change to a fraction:
5% = 5/100 = 1/20
Change to a decimal:
$$5\% = 5/100 = 100 \times \frac{.05}{5.00} = 0.05$$

Note that a percent can be changed to a decimal quickly by dropping the percent sign and moving the decimal two places to the left.

Example 3: 5% = 0.05

A *ratio* is a way of expressing the relationship between a number, quantity, substance, or degree between two components. In reality, ratios are fractions with the first number in the ratio the numerator and the second number the denominator. The numbers may be placed side by side and separated by a colon or set up as a numerator/denominator (e.g., 1:5 or 1/5). In mathematics, a ratio may be expressed as a quotient, a fraction, or a decimal per the following:

Example 4: $1 \div 5$, $1/5$, $5\overline{)1.0} = 0.2$

A *proportion* shows the relationship between two ratios. When setting up a proportion, the two ratios are usually separated by an = (equal) sign.

Example 5: 8:16   1:2 or $\dfrac{8}{16} = \dfrac{1}{2}$

The proportions above read 8 is to 16 as 1 is to 2. The two inner numbers in the first example (16 and 1) are called the means, and the two outer numbers (8 and 2) are called the extremes. In a true proportion, the product of the means equals the product of the extremes ($16 \times 1 = 16$; $8 \times 2 = 16$). This fact makes the proportion a useful mathematical tool. When a part of the problem is unknown, X can be substituted for the unknown part in the proportion and the equation solved for X. Care must be used to ensure that the proportion is set up correctly and that the same units of measure are on both sides of the equation.

Example 6: $8:16 = 1:X$ or $\dfrac{8}{16} = \dfrac{1}{X}$

$$8X = 16$$
$$X = 2$$

Example 7: To convert 0.2 g to milligrams:

$$1000\,mg:1\,g = X\,mg:0.2\,g \text{ or } \frac{1000\,mg}{1\,g} = \frac{X\,mg}{0.2\,g}$$
$$X = 200(1000 \times 0.2)$$

SYSTEMS OF MEASUREMENT

The first step in the successful calculation of doses is to develop an understanding of the units of measurement used to carry out the calculations. These units are components of the following three separate systems:

1. The metric system
2. The apothecary system
3. The household system

All three systems are expressed in the fundamental units of weight, volume, and length. Technicians should be able to convert values within each system and between the three systems.

The Metric System

The fundamental units of measurement in the metric system are the gram (weight), the liter (volume), and the meter (length). Gram is abbreviated g or gm, liter is abbreviated L or l, and meter is abbreviated m. The utility of the metric system is that all units are powers of the fundamental units. Prefixes are used in combination with the fundamental units to denote smaller or larger quantities. Table 3-1 illustrates the units of measurement for the biologic sciences.

The units that are used most commonly in dosage calculations include the gram, the kilogram (kg, 1000 g), the milligram (mg, 1/1000 g), and the milliliter (ml, 1/1000 L). It should be noted that a milliliter is equivalent to the quantity of water contained in 1 cubic centimeter (cc), which is also equivalent to 1 g of weight. Therefore we may say that for practical purposes, 1 ml = 1 cc = 1 g.

On occasion, the microgram (μg) may be used. (It should be noted that this unit may also be abbreviated as mcg.) Care should be taken to differentiate this abbreviation from mg, which looks very similar when written orders are used.

Conversion between Metric Units

The most fundamental way to convert between metric units is to multiply the units given by the

Table 3-1 Units of Measure for the Biologic Sciences

Weight	Volume	Length	Multiple Power of 10
Gram (g)	Liter (L)	Meter (m)	1
Kilogram (kg)	Kiloliter (kl)	Kilometer (km)	1000
Decigram (dg)	Deciliter (dl)	Decimeter (dm)	1/10
Centigram (cg)	Centiliter (cl)	Centimeter (cm)	1/100
Milligram (mg)	Milliliter (ml)	Millimeter (mm)	1/1000
Microgram (μg)	Microliter (μl)	Micrometer (μm)	1/1,000,000
Nanogram (ng)	Nanoliter (nl)	Nanometer (nm)	1/1,000,000,000
Picogram (pg)	Picoliter (pl)	Picometer (pm)	1/1,000,000,000,000

conversion factor involving the units desired. If the desired conversion is from milligrams (mg) to grams (g), the number of milligrams given should be multiplied by the factor 1 g/1000 mg since 1 g = 1000 mg. The steps involved in this conversion would be:

1. Write down the number of milligrams to be converted to grams.
2. To the right of that number, write down the number of milligrams in 1 g, with the milligrams as the denominator. (The numerator should always contain the unit to which you want to convert.)
3. Multiply the two numbers together.

Example 1: Convert 3000 mg to grams.

1. 3000 mg

2. $3000 \text{ mg} \dfrac{1 \text{ g}}{1000 \text{ mg}}$

3. $3000 \text{ mg} \times \dfrac{1 \text{ g}}{1000 \text{ mg}} = 3 \text{ g}$

Figure 3-1 illustrates the stairstep method to convert from one unit to another within the metric system. When converting measurements in the metric system by using the stairstep method, divide by 10 for each step up to the desired measurement and multiply by 10 for each step down to the desired measurement.

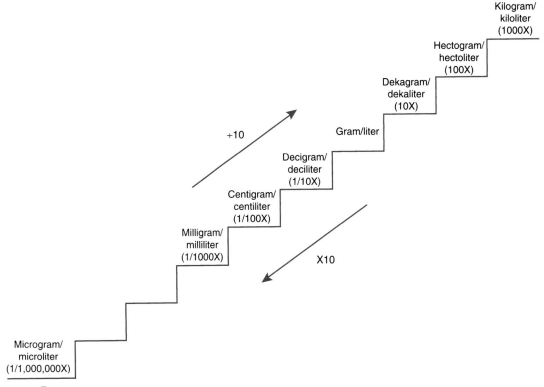

FIGURE 3-1
The stairstep method for converting within the metric system. For each step up the stairs, divide the given amount by 10. For each step down the stairs, multiply the given amount by 10.

You may also think of converting measurements with this method by remembering that for each step up, the decimal point is moved to the left one place. For each step down, the decimal point is moved to the right one place.

Example 2: 500 ml = _____ L

To convert milliliters to liters requires three steps upward. Therefore divide 500 by 10 three times (or 500 ÷ 1000). This moves the decimal point to the left three places, and the answer is 500 ml = 0.5 L.

Example 3: 2 g = _____ mg

To convert grams to milligrams, go down three steps. Multiply 2 by 10 three times (or 2 × 1000). This moves the decimal point to the right three places, and the answer is 2 g = 2000 mg.

A second method for making conversions in the metric system can be called the "arrow" method. When using this method, it is paramount to remember which units of measure are larger. Conversions between the commonly used units of kilogram, grams, milligrams, and micrograms are illustrated in the following text.

A kilogram is 1000 times larger than a gram (g), a gram is 1000 times larger than a milligram (mg), and a milligram is 1000 times larger than a microgram (mcg). This relationship can be abbreviated using the greater than symbol (>):

$$kg > g > mg > mcg$$

Many times the technician will have to calculate the amount of a drug to give when the supply on hand is not in the same units as the order. For example, the order is for 0.3 g of drug A and the supply on hand is 150-mg tablets. Before we can determine how many tablets to give, we must convert 0.3 g to milligrams. Since we know that 1 g = 1000 mg, we could change 0.3 g to milligrams by multiplying 0.3 g by 1000 mg/g (0.3 × 1000 = 300 mg). The decimal point is moved three places to the right (0.3 → 3↑ 0↑ 0↑).
　　　　　　　　　　　　　　　　　　　　1　　2　　3

The conversion could have been made very quickly by simply moving the decimal point three places to the right. To know which direction to move the decimal, determine which way the arrow is pointing (e.g., kg > g > mg > mcg).

Any time the conversion is between two adjacent units in the relationship of kg > g > mg > mcg, the decimal point will be moved three places.

The steps for converting grams to milligrams using this method are as follows:

1. Write down the order first, using the units called for (**0.3 g**).
2. Write down the equivalent units (on hand) needed next to the order units (0.3 g = __ mg).
3. Place an arrow between the two units with the closed part of the arrow pointing toward the smaller unit (**g > mg**).
4. Move the decimal point three places in the direction the arrow points (0.3 g → .3↑0↑0↑).
　　　　　　　　　　　　　　　　　　　　　　　1　2　3

In the previous problem, it would take two of the 150-mg tablets to fill the 300-mg order.

If the order had been for 300,000 mcg of drug A and the supply on hand had been 150 mg tablets, we would need to convert micrograms to milligrams by using the following steps:

1. Write the order (300,000 **mcg**).
2. Write down the equivalent units needed next to the order units (300,000 mcg = ___ mg).
3. Place an arrow between the two units with the closed part of the arrow pointing toward the smaller units (**mcg < mg**).
4. Move the decimal three places in the direction the arrow points (300 mg ←300↑0↑0↑0. mcg)
　　　　　　　　　　　　　　　　　　　　　3　2　1

In this problem, it would take two of the 150-mg (150,000 mcg) tablets to provide the 300,000-mcg order.

More problems for converting within the metric system are provided at the end of this chapter.

The Apothecary and Household Systems

The apothecary and household systems of measurement are older systems than the metric system. The apothecary system is seldom used, but the household system is used in giving clients instructions about dosage.

The units most often encountered in the apothecary system are the minim, abbreviated *m* or *min*; the dram, abbreviated *dr*; the ounce, abbreviated *oz*; and the grain, abbreviated *gr*. A minim is equal to 1 drop, a dram is equal to 4 ml, an ounce is equal to 30 ml, and a grain is equal to 65 mg (64.8, sometimes rounded off to 65). When writing quantities relating to grains, the symbol *gr* should be placed before the number, and common fractions are used when appropriate (e.g., gr 1/50). The apothecary pound (12 oz) is not used when calculating doses. Instead, use the avoirdupois pound (16 oz).

The units commonly used in the household system include the drop, abbreviated *gtt*; the tablespoon, abbreviated *T* or *Tbsp*; and the teaspoon, abbreviated *t* or *tsp*. One drop is equivalent to 1 min, 1 Tbsp is equivalent to 15 ml, and 1 tsp is equivalent to 5 ml. The pint, quart, and gallon are other units sometimes encountered. Boxes 3-1 and 3-2 illustrate equivalent values useful in dosage cal-

BOX 3-1 Weight Equivalents

1 kg = 1000 g = 2.2 lb
1 g = 1000 mg
1 mg = 1000 µg = 0.001 g
65 mg = 1 g
1 µg = 0.001 mg = 0.000001 g
1 lb = 453.6 g = 0.4536 kg = 16 oz
1 oz = 28.35 g

Box 3-2 Volume Equivalents

1 L = 1000 ml = 1 qt (946.4 ml)
500 ml = 1 pt (473 ml) = 2 cups (equivalent to 1 lb of water)
15 ml = 1 Tbsp
5 ml = 1 tsp
30 ml = 1 oz
240 ml = 1 cup/glass
4 ml = 1 dram
1 ml = 15 gtt/min*

*The number of drops/minims in 1 ml depends on the size of the dropper. With a standard-size dropper, 1 ml equals 15 drops.

culations. Problems converting within and between the apothecary and household systems are found at the end of the chapter.

DOSAGE CALCULATIONS

The quantity of drug to be delivered to a patient is called the *dose*. A dosage rate expressed in milligrams per kilogram (or milligrams per pound) is multiplied by the animal's weight in kilograms (or pounds) to determine the dose. The dose is then divided by the amount (concentration) of the drug in the pharmaceutic form (tablet, solution, and so forth) to determine the actual amount of the pharmaceutic form to administer. The formula for dosage calculation, which should be committed to memory, is:

$$Dose = \frac{Animal's\ weight \times dosage\ rate}{Concentration\ of\ drug}$$

Example 1: If a 20-kg dog is to be given amoxicillin at the rate of 10 mg/kg and injectable amoxicillin with a concentration of 100 mg/ml is available, the dosage calculation would be as follows:

$$Dose = \frac{20\ kg \times 10\ mg/kg}{100\ mg/ml} = \frac{200\ mg}{100\ mg/ml} = 2\ ml$$

Note that in the first step of the calculation, kilograms cancel out to leave only milligrams in the numerator. In the second step, milligrams cancel out to leave milliliters. If 100-mg amoxicillin tablets are available, the formula becomes:

$$Dose = \frac{20\ kg \times 10\ mg/kg}{100\ mg/tablet} = \frac{200\ mg}{100\ mg/tablet} = 2\ tablets$$

Because most scales used to weigh animals for drug dosage calculation provide the weight in pounds, a conversion must be made from pounds to kilograms. To do this, divide the weight in pounds by 2.2.

Example 2: The dog in the previous problem weighed 44 lb, and 44 divided by 2.2 equals 20 kg.

To convert kilograms to pounds (if the dose is provided in milligrams per pound), multiply the weight in kilograms by 2.2 (e.g., $20\,kg \times 2.2 = 44\,lb$).

If the order to the technician is to "give a dog 300 mg of amoxicillin," then the ordered amount is simply divided by the concentration of the drug to determine the amount to administer.

Example 3: If the order is to give a dog 300 mg of amoxicillin (concentration 100 mg/ml), the calculation would be:

$$\frac{300\,mg}{100\,mg/ml} = 3\,ml$$

It should be noted that the dose of most drugs used to treat neoplasms is calculated according to the total body surface area of the patient. Body surface area is correlated with the weight of the animal. A table is available in Chapter 16 (Table 16-2) for converting an animal's weight to surface area in square meters (sq M or m^2). In these cases, the formula for dosage calculation becomes:

$$Dose = mg/m^2 \text{ (from insert)} \times m^2 \text{ (from table)}$$

Dosage calculation problems are provided at the end of this chapter.

SOLUTIONS

To understand dosage calculation problems and how to prepare dilutions of substances (e.g., formalin and dextrose), a technician must have a basic understanding of solutions. *Solutions* are mixtures of substances that are not usually chemically combined with each other. Solutions are made up of a dissolving substance, called the *solvent*, and a dissolved substance, called the *solute*. Not all substances form solutions with each other. Those that form solutions are called *miscible*, and those that do not are called *immiscible*. A solution is termed *saturated* if it contains the maximum amount of solute at a particular temperature and pressure. Under some circumstances, a solution can become supersaturated. Mixtures of substances in which the solute is made up of very large particles are called *suspensions*. The particles in suspensions settle upon standing, and the mixture must be agitated before it is administered. True solutions do not settle out and remain mixed without agitation. All parts of solutions contain equal parts of the solute.

When dealing with solutions, it is important to know the amount of solute in the solvent or to be able to measure it. The amount of solute dissolved in the solvent is referred to as the *concentration* of the substance. Concentrations may be expressed in a number of ways, including the following:

1. Parts
2. Weight per volume (w/v) for liquids
3. Volume per volume (v/v) for liquids
4. Weight per weight (w/w) for solids

Solutions can be described in terms of parts without any reference to units of measurement. The parts simply refer to the relationship between the solvent and the solute. For example, instructions may call for a 1-to-30 (1:30) dilution of a disinfectant.

One unit that describes the relationship of parts is called *parts per million* (ppm). Parts per million is equal to 1 mg of a solute in a kilogram or liter of solvent. One part per million is also equivalent to 1 μg in a gram or milliliter. Upson (1988) reports that 1 ppm is equivalent to 1 minute in approximately 2 years or 1 oz of sand in approximately 31 tons of cement. Parts per billion is a unit that is occasionally used. It is equivalent to 1 μg in a kilogram or liter or 1 nanogram in a gram or milliliter.

The most common way of expressing drug concentrations when the solute is a solid and the solvent is a liquid is weight per volume (w/v). For example, the concentration of most pharmaceutic preparations is expressed as milligrams per milliliter (mg/ml); the concentration for Ketaset is 100 mg/ml. The weight-per-weight (w/w) and the volume-per-volume (v/v) solutions are not used as often in veterinary pharmaceutic preparations as the w/v preparations.

PERCENT CONCENTRATIONS

The term *percent concentration* may be used when describing w/v, w/w, or v/v concentrations. Percent (percentage) means parts of solute per 100 parts of the solution. Percent w/v means the number of grams of solute in 100 ml of solution; percent w/w describes the number of grams of solute in 100 g of solution; and v/v expresses the number of milliliters of solute in 100 ml of the solution.

A 100% solution (w/v) contains 100 g of solute per 100 ml of solution. Another way to say this is that it contains 1 g (1000 mg) of solute per 1 ml of solution (1000 mg/ml). To convert from a percent solution to mg/ml, multiply the percentage by 10 (e.g., a 5% Lasix solution contains 50 mg/ml). To convert milligrams per milliliter to a percent, divide the milligrams per milliliter by 10 (e.g., a Lasix solution containing 50 mg/ml is a 5% solution). Sometimes the term called *milligrams percent* (mg%) is encountered. This term is used to refer to the number of milligrams in 100 ml of solution. It is an expression of concentration, but not of percent concentration (g/100 ml). A more accurate description is mg% would be milligrams per deciliter (mg/dl), because a deciliter is equal to 100 ml.

A 100% solution (w/w) contains 100 g of solute in 100 g of solution. A 5% solution (w/w) of sodium chloride would contain 5 g of sodium in 100 g of the solution. To make this preparation, weigh out 5 g of sodium chloride and mix it with 95 g of water.

A 100% solution (v/v) would simply be pure drug or chemical. A 10% solution would contain 10 ml of the chemical in 100 ml of solution. When preparing a w/v solution or v/v solution, the desired amount of solute is added to a container and enough solvent is added to create the desired volume. This process is called *diluting up*, or it may be said that you *q.s.* to the desired volume. The abbreviation *q.s.* means to add a "quantity sufficient" to arrive at the desired volume. For example, to make 100 ml of a 10% formalin solution, place 10 ml of formaldehyde (100% formalin) in a container and q.s. to 100 ml (10 ml formalin, 90 ml distilled water).

Calculations Involving Concentrations

To determine the amount of solute needed to make a desired amount of solution, you may use the following formula:

Grams of solute to q.s. to desired volume

$$= \frac{\% \times \text{desired volume}}{100}$$

Example 1: How many grams of sodium chloride are needed to make 1 L of 0.9% sodium chloride?

Answer: $\text{Grams needed} = \dfrac{0.9 \times 1000\,\text{ml}}{100} = 9\,\text{g}$

Nine grams of sodium chloride would be added to a container and diluted up to 1000 ml.

When the amount of solute and the volume of solution are known, the percent solution may be found as follows:

$$\text{Percent solution} = \frac{\text{grams of solute} \times 100}{\text{volume of solution}}$$

Example 2: What percentage is a solution containing 9 g of sodium chloride?

Answer: $\text{Percent solution} = \dfrac{9 \times 100}{1000} = \dfrac{900}{1000} = 0.9\%$

To solve problems involving a change in concentration of the solution, the following formula may be used:

$$\text{Volume one} \times \text{concentration one}$$
$$= \text{volume two} \times \text{concentration two}$$

Example 3: How would you prepare 100 ml of a 5% dextrose solution from a 50% dextrose solution?

Answer: $V1 \times C1 = V2 \times C2$
$100 \times 5 = V2 \times 50$
$500 = 50V2$
$10 = V2$

This formula demonstrates that you would take 10 ml of the 50% dextrose solution and add q.s. to 100 ml to prepare the 5% solution.

Another formula that may be used to solve problems in which a change in concentration is involved is as follows:

$$\frac{\text{Desired strength}}{\text{Available strength}} = \frac{\text{amount to use}}{\text{amount to make}}$$

Example 4: In solving the foregoing problem, the desired strength is 5%, the available strength is 50%, the amount to make is 100 ml, and the amount to use is the unknown.

Answer:
$$\frac{5}{50} = \frac{X}{100}$$
$$50\,X = 500$$
$$X = 10\,\text{ml}$$

MILLIEQUIVALENTS

When electrolytes are involved, the concentration of a solution is often expressed in terms of **milliequivalents** (mEq). One milliequivalent is equal to 1/1000 of an equivalent. An equivalent is equal to (for practical applications) 1 g molecular weight divided by the total positive valence of the material in question (Blankenship and Campbell, 1976). The concentration of an electrolyte solution is expressed as milliequivalents per liter (mEq/L), which can be calculated when the concentration of the solution is known by using the following formula:

$$\text{mEq/L} = \frac{\text{mg/dl} \times 10}{\text{eq wt}}$$

Example 1: How many milliequivalents per liter are found in a sodium chloride solution that contains 700 mg/dl?

Answer: $\text{mEq/L} = \dfrac{700 \times 10}{58.5} = 119.66$

The number of milligrams per deciliter can also be calculated when the number of milliequivalents per liter is known by manipulating the previous formula as follows:

$$\text{mg/dl} = \frac{\text{mEq/L} \times \text{eq wt}}{10}$$

Example 2: How many milligrams per deciliter are contained in a solution that has 119.66 mEq/L?

Answer: $\text{mg/dl} = \dfrac{119.66 \times 58.5}{10} = \dfrac{7000}{10} = 700\,\text{mg/dl}$

CALCULATIONS INVOLVING IV FLUID ADMINISTRATION

Calculations for determining the volume of fluid to administer are covered in Chapter 15. The rate to run intravenous fluids (in drops per minute) can be determined by dividing the volume of fluids to be given by the time in minutes during administration and then multiplying that number by the drops per milliliter delivered by the administration set.

$$\frac{\text{Volume of infusion (ml)}}{\text{Time of infusion (min)}} \times \text{drop factor (gtt/ml)}$$
$$= \text{drops per minute}$$

The drip rate in drops per minute can be divided by 60 to determine the rate in drops per second, a number that is easier to work with when actually adjusting the flow.

Example 1: Give 480 ml of lactated Ringer's solution to Dog A over a 4-hour period using a standard 15 gtt/ml administration set.

$$\frac{480\,\text{ml}}{240\,\text{min}} = \frac{2\,\text{ml}}{\text{min}} \times \frac{15\,\text{gtt}}{\text{ml}} = \frac{30\,\text{gtt}}{\text{min}} \times \frac{1\,\text{min}}{60\,\text{sec}} = \frac{1\,\text{gtt}}{2\,\text{sec}}$$

Giving one drop every 2 seconds will deliver 30 drops in a minute.

Calculations for Constant Rate Infusion Problems

Sometimes medications given by intravenous infusion need to be administered at a dose delivered at a constant rate over a period of time. The dosage is often ordered in micrograms per kilogram per minute. The following example problem illustrates a method for solving these problems. Short-cut formulas are used by some clinicians.

Example 1: A 44 lb dog in acute heart failure is ordered to receive 10 mcg/kg/min of dopamine. You will add a 200-mg vial of dopamine to a 1 L bag of D5W solution (0.2 mg/ml). At what rate in drops per minute will you administer this solution to deliver the correct dosage?

Step 1: Convert to the same units. The dose is expressed in mcg/kg so the patient's weight must be converted from pounds to kilograms, and the drug concentration must be expressed in mcg/ml.

$$44 \text{ lbs} \times \frac{1 \text{ kg}}{2.2 \text{ lbs}} = \frac{44 \text{ kg}}{2.2} = 20 \text{ kg}$$

$$\frac{0.2 \text{ mg}}{1 \text{ ml}} \times \frac{1000 \text{ mcg}}{1 \text{ mg}} = \frac{200 \text{ mcg}}{1 \text{ ml}}$$

Step 2: Determine the number of mcg/min.

$$20 \text{ kg} \times \frac{10 \text{ mcg}}{\text{kg/min}} = \frac{200 \text{ mcg}}{\text{min}}$$

Step 3: Determine the number of ml per minute.

$$\frac{200 \text{ mcg}}{1 \text{ min}} \times \frac{1 \text{ ml}}{200 \text{ mcg}} = \frac{1 \text{ ml}}{1 \text{ min}}$$

Step 4: Determine the number of drops per minute using a minidrip (60 gtt/ml) administration set.

$$\frac{1 \text{ ml}}{\text{min}} \times \frac{60 \text{ gtt}}{1 \text{ ml}} = \frac{60 \text{ gtt}}{1 \text{ min}} \text{ or } 1 \text{ gtt/sec}$$

REFERENCES

Blankenship J and Campbell JB: Solutions. In Blankenship J and Campbell JB, editors: Laboratory mathematics: medical and biological applications, St. Louis, 1976, Mosby.

Upson DW: General principles. In Upson DW, editor: Handbook of clinical veterinary pharmacology, ed 3, Manhattan, Kan, 1988, Dan Upson Enterprises.

REVIEW QUESTIONS

PROBLEMS USING RATIOS AND PROPORTIONS

Ratios

1. Express 1/4 as a ratio and as a decimal.
2. Express 0.75 as a ratio and as a fraction.
3. Express 0.004 as a ratio and as a fraction.
4. Express 1:80 as a fraction and as a decimal.
5. Express 9/1000 as a ratio and as a decimal.
6. Express 1:32 as a fraction and as a decimal.

Proportions (Solve for X)

1. $25:X = 5:10$
2. $\dfrac{4}{5} = \dfrac{X}{10}$
3. $1/2:100 = X:500$
4. $\dfrac{1/4}{X} = \dfrac{20}{400}$
5. Convert 0.2 g to milligrams using a proportion.

$$\frac{1000\,mg}{1\,g} = \frac{X\,mg}{0.2\,g}$$

6. If a drug concentration is labeled 5 ml = 250 mg, how many mg are in three fourths of a ml?

$$\frac{250\,mg}{5\,ml} = \frac{X}{^3/_4\,ml}$$

7. How much bleach would you use to prepare 1000 ml of a 1:32 solution?

$$1:32 = X:1000$$

8. How much bleach would you use to prepare 1 gallon (3784 ml) of a 1:32 solution?

$$1:32 = X:3784$$

9. If you were to give a horse 1 ml per 250 lb of body weight of an anthelmintic, how many ml would you give to a horse that weighs 1250 lb?

$$\frac{1}{250} = \frac{X}{1250}$$

10. If a 10-lb dog gets one fourth of a tablet of an antibiotic, how many tablets will a 50-lb dog get?

$$1/4:10 = X:50$$

PROBLEMS USING THE METRIC SYSTEM

1. 150 mg = _____ g
2. 2 L = _____ ml
3. 2250 mg = _____ g
4. 5 g = _____ mg
5. 3000 ml = _____ L
6. 2 kg = _____ g
7. 0.5 kg = _____ g
8. 5000 mg = _____ kg
9. 1.25 mg = _____ g
10. 0.004 g = _____ mg
11. 2050 μg = _____ mg
12. How many grams would you administer if the veterinarian ordered 10 mg of acepromazine? _____
13. If the medical order is 0.5 L of sodium chloride 0.9%, how many milliliters would be administered? _____
14. How many liters would you give to the patient if the order called for 750 ml to be administered? _____
15. If the veterinarian orders 300 μg of vitamin B_{12}, how much is this in milligrams? _____
16. If the order is 2.5 mg of vitamin B_{12}, how many micrograms are administered? _____

PROBLEMS USING THE APOTHECARY AND HOUSEHOLD SYSTEMS

1. 1.5 qt = _____ pt
2. 12 pt = _____ gal
3. 3 tsp = _____ Tbsp
4. 3 qt = _____ cups
5. 12 cups = _____ pt
6. 2 oz = _____ Tbsp
7. 1 gal = _____ oz
8. 1 pt = _____ oz
9. 6 pt = _____ qt

PROBLEMS COMBINING BOTH SYSTEMS

1. 1 pt = _____ ml
2. 2 Tbsp = _____ ml
3. 15 ml = _____ cc
4. 2 cups = _____ oz
5. 6.5 ml = _____ pt
6. 125 ml = _____ tsp
7. 1.5 oz = _____ ml
8. 15 kg = _____ lb
9. 250 ml = _____ pt
10. 5 oz = _____ ml
11. 35 lb = _____ kg

PROBLEMS MEASURING ORAL MEDICATIONS

1. The order is 500 mg of amoxicillin, and tablets on hand are 250 mg. How many tablets will be administered? _____
2. The order is 15 mg of prednisone, and 10-mg (scored) tablets are on hand. How many tablets will be administered?

   _____

3. The order is 960 mg of SMZ-TMP. Tablets on hand are 240 mg. How many tablets will be administered? _____
4. The order is 0.5 mg of Centrine, and 0.2-mg tablets are on hand. How many tablets will be administered? _____
5. The veterinarian prescribes 15 mg of prednisone every other day for 10 days. The tablets on hand are 10 mg. How many tablets will be administered? How many tablets will be dispensed? _____
6. The veterinarian prescribes 100 mg of cephalexin twice a day (b.i.d.) for 10 days.

You have 100-mg tablets on hand. How many will be dispensed? _____

7. The veterinarian prescribes Albon for *Coccidia*. Your patient is a puppy weighing 8 lb and needing treatment for 21 days. The dose for Albon is 25 mg/lb loading dose and 12.5 mg/lb maintenance dose to be given once daily (s.i.d.) The drug is supplied at 250 mg/5 ml. How many milligrams does your patient need for a loading dose? _____
   A maintenance dose?

   _____

   How many mg/ml are there in Albon?

   _____

   How many milliliters does your patient need for a loading dose? _____
   A maintenance dose?

   _____

   How many milliliters will be dispensed?

   _____

8. The veterinarian prescribes 250-mg phenylbutazone b.i.d. for 5 days for your patient. Tablets on hand are 100 mg (scored). How many tablets will be administered?

   _____

   How many tablets will be dispensed?

   _____

9. The veterinarian prescribes chloramphenicol, 250 mg three times daily (t.i.d.) for 7 days, for your patient. The tablets on hand are 1 g (scored). How many tablets will be given?

   _____

   How many will be dispensed?

   _____

10. The veterinarian prescribes 2.5 mg of acepromazine t.i.d. for 3 days, and tablets on hand are 5 mg (scored). How many tablets will be administered? _____
    How many will be dispensed?

    _____

11. The veterinarian prescribes aminophylline to be given three times daily for 14 days to a 15-lb dog. The dose for aminophylline is 10 mg/kg. How many kg does your patient weigh?

    _____

    How many milligrams need to be administered to your patient? _____

Because the tablets on hand are 100 mg (scored), how many tablets will you give to the patient? _____

How many tablets will be dispensed? _____

12. The veterinarian orders mebendazole and Combot to deworm a 1000-lb horse via a nasogastric tube. The dose for mebendazole is 30 ml/250 lb body weight, and the dose for Combot is 0.5 oz/100 lb body weight. How many milliliters of mebendazole and Combot are needed? _____

13. A farmer has 10 calves weighing approximately 100 lb each. A microscopic fecal examination reveals *Coccidia*. The veterinarian chooses to treat all 10 calves with Corid powder (20% amprolium) by drenching daily for 10 days. To make a drench solution, mix 3 oz of Corid powder in 1 qt of water (1 oz of powder = 3.5 Tbsp). The dose of Corid for drenching is 1 oz of solution per 100 lb of body weight. How much solution should be mixed to drench these 10 calves for 10 days?

_____

14. Doxycycline has been chosen as a treatment for a 1-kg Amazon parrot at the rate of 25 mg/kg b.i.d. for 7 days. The tablets on hand are 50 mg (scored). How many tablets will be given for each treatment?

_____

How many tablets will be dispensed?

_____

15. The veterinarian orders doxylamine succinate to treat a 200-lb foal. The dosage to be administered is 1 mg/lb/day, divided into three doses and given orally. The vial is labeled 11.36 mg/ml. How many milligrams will be given at each treatment?

_____

How many milliliters of medication will be needed for treatment for 1 day?

_____

PROBLEMS MEASURING PARENTERAL MEDICATIONS

1. The veterinarian orders prednisone, 20 mg intramuscularly (IM). The vial is labeled 50 mg/ml. How many milliliters will be administered? _____

2. The veterinarian orders Cortisate-20 at 2 mg/lb to be administered intravenously. Your patient weighs 37 lb. The vial of Cortisate-20 is labeled 20 mg/ml. How many milliliters will be administered? _____

3. The veterinarian orders phenylbutazone to be administered to a 1500-lb horse at a dose of 5 mg/kg intravenously. The vial is labeled 200 mg/ml. How many milliliters will be administered? _____

4. The veterinarian orders penicillin G procaine for a 25-lb dog to be administered at a dose of 40,000 U/kg IM. The vial is labeled 300,000 U/ml. How many milliliters will be administered? _____

5. The veterinarian orders cephalothin sodium to be administered every 8 hours IM to a 23-lb dog. The dosage to be given is 50 mg/kg/day. The vial is labeled 1 g/10 ml. How many milligrams will be administered for the day?

_____

How many milliliters will be administered at each treatment? _____

6. A 78-lb dog is to be administered ampicillin trihydrate at a dose of 5 mg/lb subcutaneously. The antibiotic has been reconstituted, and the concentration is 200 mg/ml. How many milliliters will be administered to the patient?

_____

7. A microscopic fecal examination reveals a *Giardia* infection in a 500-g African gray parrot. The veterinarian chooses to treat the infection with metronidazole, injectable at a dosage of 30 mg/kg daily for 3 days. How many milligrams will the parrot receive at each treatment? _____

8. A 45-lb dog is to be treated for lymphosarcoma with vincristine sulfate, 1 mg/ml. The dose is 0.5 mg/m². How many square meters of body surface area does this patient have? _____

How many milligrams will be given to the patient? _____

How many milliliters?

_____

9. The veterinarian orders lincomycin HCl for a 500-lb Yorkshire boar. The dosage to be administered is 5 mg/lb/day IM for 5 days. The medication on hand is 100 mg/ml in a 50-ml multidose vial. How many milligrams will the boar be administered each day?

_____

How many milliliters will the boar be administered each day?

_____

How many bottles of medication does the owner need to purchase to treat the boar for 5 days? _____

10. A cat weighing 8 lb, which has a small laceration on its left hip, is to be administered ketamine HCl to produce anesthesia. The veterinarian orders 15 mg/kg IM. The vial is labeled 100 mg/ml. How many milligrams will be administered to the cat?

_____

How many milliliters will be administered?

_____

11. The veterinarian orders 7 mEq of potassium chloride to be added into the IV fluids. The vial is labeled 20 mEq in 10 ml. How many milliliters will be added to the fluids?

_____

12. The veterinarian orders 4 U of regular insulin to be administered to a diabetic cat. The regular insulin is labeled 40 U/ml. How many milliliters will be administered?

_____

13. The veterinarian orders testosterone propionate for a 475-lb Landrace boar. The dose to be administered is 1 mg/10 lb. The label on the vial is 25 mg/ml. How many milligrams will be administered?

_____

How many milliliters will be administered?

_____

14. The veterinarian orders dexamethasone, 60 mg IV, to be given to a patient. The vial is labeled 2 mg/ml. How many milliliters will be administered? _____

15. The veterinarian orders 15 mg of vitamin K_1. The vial is labeled 10 mg/ml. How many milliliters will be administered?

_____

INJECTION PROBLEMS

Order	Stock	Give
1.	0.5 g IM	250 mg/ml
2.	20 mEq IV	40 mEq/10 ml
3.	0.75 mg IM	0.50 mg/ml
4.	150 mg IM	0.2 g/5 ml
5.	25 mg IM	100 mg/ml
6.	0.5 mg IM	0.5 mg/2 ml
7.	0.3 mg IV	0.4 mg/ml
8.	300,000 U SC	40,000 U/ml
9.	0.3 mg IM	0.5 mg/ml
10.	55 mg SC	250 mg/ml

PREPARING SOLUTIONS

1. Order: 100 ml of 10% formalin solution
   On hand: formaldehyde 37% (considered as 100% formalin) and water
   Amount needed: _____

2. Order: 1000 ml 0.9% NaCl and 5% dextrose
   On hand: 1000 ml 0.9% NaCl and 500 ml D$_{50}$W
   Amount of each needed:

   _____

3. Order: 100 ml D$_{50}$W
   On hand: 500 ml D$_{50}$W and 250 ml sterile water for injection
   Amount needed: _____

4. Order: 500 ml 0.45% NaCl and 5% dextrose
   On hand: 500 ml 0.9% NaCl and 500 ml D$_5$W
   Amount of each needed:

   _____

5. Order: 2000 ml lactated Ringer's solution and 2.5% dextrose
   On hand: 2 containers of 1000 ml lactated Ringer's solution and 250 ml D$_{50}$W
   Amount of each needed:

   _____

6. Order: 50 ml D$_5$W
   On hand: 1000 ml sterile water for injection and 250 ml D$_{50}$W

Amount of each needed:

_____

7. Order: 500 ml 2.5% dextrose and 0.45% NaCl
   On hand: 1000 ml 0.45% NaCl and 500 ml D$_{50}$W
   Amount of each needed:

   _____

8. Order: 1000 ml of 10% glyceryl guaiacolate solution
   On hand: packets containing 50 g guaifenesin (GG) powder and 1000 ml sterile water for injection
   Amount of each needed:

   _____

9. Order: 8% thiamylal sodium solution
   On hand: One 5-g vial of powder and sterile water for injection
   Amount of sterile water needed:

   _____

10. Order: 5 ml of 2% cyclosporine ophthalmic solution
    On hand: 50 ml Sandimmune Oral Solution (cyclosporine) 100 mg/ml and 16 oz of extra virgin olive oil
    Amount of each needed:

    _____

11. Order: 50 ml of 2% formalin for Knott's heartworm test
    On hand: 37% formaldehyde and water
    Amount of each needed:

    _____

PROBLEMS CALCULATING IV DRIP RATES

1. What drip rate will you use to administer 500 ml of lactated Ringer's solution over a 3-hour period with a standard (15 gtt/ml) administration set?

2. What drip rate would you use to deliver 120 ml 0.9% NaCl over a 2-hour period using a microdrip (60 gtt/ml) administration set?

3. What drip rate would you use to deliver 1.2 L of Normosol over a 10-hour period using a standard (15 gtt/ml) administration set?

4. What drip rate would you use to deliver 8 mcg/kg/min of drug C (500 mg/250 ml) to a 83-lb dog using a microdrip (60 gtt/ml) administration set?

5. What drip rate would you use to deliver 10 mcg/kg/min of dopamine (0.2 mg/ml) to a 22-lb dog using the microdrip (60 gtt/ml) administration set?

INTRODUCTION
ANATOMY AND PHYSIOLOGY
AUTONOMIC NERVOUS SYSTEM
　How Drugs Affect the Autonomic
　　Nervous System
CLASSES OF AUTONOMIC NERVOUS
　SYSTEM AGENTS
Cholinergic Agents
　Direct-Acting Cholinergics
　Indirect-Acting Cholinergics
　　(Anticholinesterase) Agents
Cholinergic Blocking Agents
　(Anticholinergic)
Adrenergic (Sympathomimetic) Agents
Adrenergic Blocking Agents
CENTRAL NERVOUS SYSTEM
Tranquilizers
　Phenothiazine Derivatives
　Benzodiazepine Derivatives
　Xylazine Hydrochloride
　Detomidine Hydrochloride
　Medetomidine
Barbiturates
　Long-Acting Barbiturates
　Short-Acting Barbiturates
　Ultrashort-Acting Barbiturates
Dissociative Agents
Opioid Agonists
　Naturally Occurring Narcotics
　Synthetic Narcotics
Opioid Antagonists
Neuroleptanalgesics
Drugs to Prevent or Control Seizures
Inhalant Anesthetics
Miscellaneous Central Nervous System
　Drugs
　Propofol
　Glyceryl Guaiacolate or Guaifenesin
　　(Guailaxin, Gecolate)
　Chloral Hydrate/Magnesium Sulfate
Central Nervous System Stimulants
　Doxapram
　Pentylenetetrazol (Metrazol)
Caffeine
Amphetamines
Neuromuscular Blocking Drugs
BEHAVIORAL PHARMACOTHERAPY
　Pharmacotherapeutic Agents
Antianxiety Medications
　Benzodiazepines
　Azapirones
Antidepressants
　Tricyclics
　Serotonin Reuptake Inhibitors
　Monoamine Oxidase-B Inhibitors
　Synthetic Progestins
Euthanasia Agents

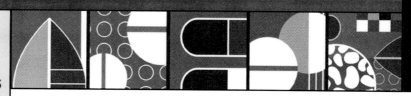

CHAPTER **4**

Drugs Used in Nervous System Disorders

LEARNING OBJECTIVES

After studying this chapter, you should be able to:

1. Define terms related to the pharmacology of the nervous system
2. Develop a basic understanding of the anatomy and physiology of the nervous system
3. Describe the subdivisions, functions, and primary neurotransmitters of the autonomic nervous system (ANS)
4. Describe how drugs affect the ANS
5. List the different classes of ANS drugs
6. List the two major classification schemes of barbiturates
7. List indications and precautions for the use of the barbiturates
8. Describe dissociative anesthesia, and list three dissociative agents
9. List the opiate receptors and the basic function of each
10. List the indications for the use of the narcotics
11. List potential side effects of narcotic use or overdose
12. Describe how opioid antagonists exert their effect, and list three examples of this category of drug
13. Define neuroleptanalgesic and give an example
14. List examples of drugs used to control seizures
15. List the commonly used inhalant anesthetic agents and compare their characteristics
16. Describe the primary use of the central nervous system (CNS) stimulants
17. List drugs used in behavioral pharmacotherapy
18. Describe the characteristics of a good euthanasia agent

67

KEY TERMS

ACETYLCHOLINE A neurotransmitter that allows a nerve impulse to cross the synaptic junction (gap) between two nerve fibers or between a nerve fiber and an organ (e.g., muscle, gland).

ACETYLCHOLINESTERASE An enzyme that brings about the breakdown of acetylcholine in the synaptic gap.

ADRENERGIC A term used to describe an action or a receptor that is activated by epinephrine or norepinephrine.

ANALGESIA Loss of pain sensation (other sensations may be present).

ANESTHESIA The loss of all sensations. May be described as local (affecting a small area), regional, or surgical (accompanied by unconsciousness).

AUTONOMIC NERVOUS SYSTEM That portion of the nervous system that controls involuntary activities.

CATALEPSY A state of involuntary muscle rigidity that is accompanied by immobility, amnesia, and variable amounts of analgesia. Some reflexes may be preserved.

CATECHOLAMINE The class of neurotransmitters that includes dopamine, epinephrine, and norepinephrine. When given therapeutically, catecholamines mimic the effect of stimulating the sympathetic nervous system.

CHOLINERGIC A term used to describe an action or receptor that is activated by acetylcholine.

EFFECTOR A gland, organ, or tissue that responds to nerve stimulation with a specific action.

GANGLIONIC SYNAPSE The site of the synapse between neuron one and neuron two of the autonomic nervous system.

MUSCARINIC RECEPTORS Receptors activated by acetylcholine and muscarine that are found in glands, the heart, and smooth muscle. An acronym for remembering muscarinic effects is "SLUD." S = salivation; L = lacrimation; U = urination; D = defecation.

NICOTINIC RECEPTORS Receptors activated by acetylcholine and nicotine found at the neuromuscular junction of the skeletal muscle and at the ganglionic synapses.

PARASYMPATHETIC NERVOUS SYSTEM That portion of the autonomic nervous system that arises from the craniosacral portion of the spinal cord, is mediated by the neurotransmitter acetylcholine, and is primarily concerned with conserving and restoring a steady state in the body.

PARASYMPATHOMIMETIC A drug that mimics the effects of stimulating the parasympathetic nervous system.

SYMPATHETIC NERVOUS SYSTEM That portion of the autonomic nervous system that arises from the thoracolumbar spinal cord, is mediated by catecholamines, and is concerned with the fight-or-flight response.

SYMPATHOMIMETIC A drug that mimics the effects of stimulating the sympathetic nervous system.

INTRODUCTION

The nervous system is the body's primary communication and control center. It functions in harmony with the endocrine system to allow an animal to respond and adapt to its environment and to maintain a relatively constant internal environment (homeostasis) through control of the many internal organ systems. In broad terms, the nervous system serves three functions: (1) sensory, (2) integrative (analysis), and (3) motor (action). It senses changes within the environment and within the body, interprets the information, and responds to the interpretation by bringing about an appropriate action. The nervous system carries out this complex activity very rapidly by sending electric-like messages over a network of nerve fibers. The endocrine system works much more slowly by sending chemical messengers (hormones) through the bloodstream to target structures. The two systems are very closely interrelated functionally and anatomically. The nervous system exerts control over the endocrine system through the influence of the hypothalamus (brain) on the pituitary gland.

ANATOMY AND PHYSIOLOGY

The nervous system has two main divisions, the CNS and the peripheral nervous system, and their related subdivisions (Figure 4-1). The CNS is composed of the brain and spinal cord and serves as the control center of the entire nervous system. All sensory information must be relayed to the CNS before it can be interpreted and acted on. Most impulses that stimulate glands to act and muscles to contract originate in the CNS.

The nerve processes that connect the CNS with the various glands, muscles, and receptors in the body make up the peripheral nervous system. Functionally, the peripheral nervous system is divided into afferent and efferent portions. The afferent portion is composed of nerve cells that carry information from receptors in the periphery of the body to the CNS. The efferent system consists of nerve cells that carry impulses from the CNS to muscles and glands. Anatomically, the peripheral nervous system is composed of cranial nerves and spinal nerves.

The peripheral nervous system is also subdivided into a somatic nervous system and an **autonomic nervous system.** The somatic nervous system

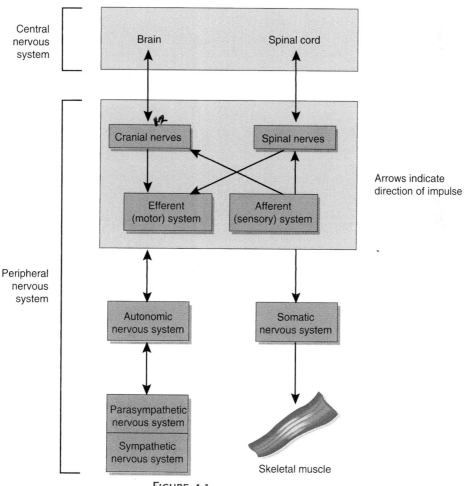

FIGURE 4-1
Organization of the nervous system.

consists of efferent nerves that carry impulses from the CNS to skeletal muscle tissue. It is under conscious control and is therefore called *voluntary*. The ANS consists of efferent nerve cells that carry information from the CNS to cardiac muscle, glands, and smooth muscle. It is under unconscious control and is called *involuntary*. The ANS has two subdivisions, the **sympathetic nervous system** and the **parasympathetic nervous system.** Most tissues innervated by the ANS receive both sympathetic and parasympathetic fibers. In general, one division stimulates an activity by a receptor and the other inhibits the activity to serve as a method of checks and balances.

The fundamental unit of all branches and divisions of the nervous system is the neuron (nerve cell). Neurons have the amazing ability to transmit information from point to point. The second point may be nearby or at a great distance. Like all cells in the body, neurons have a nucleus surrounded by cytoplasm. Unlike other cells, however, neurons have cellular extensions or processes called *axons* and *dendrites*. The axons carry electric-like messages away from the nerve cell, and the dendrites carry electric-like messages toward the nerve cell (Figure 4-2). Transmission of these messages along nerve fibers occurs through a wave of charge reversal moving down the fiber (Figure 4-3). The resting (polarized) fiber has positive charges lined up on the outside of its membrane and negative charges lined up on the inside of its membrane. When a stimulus of sufficient magnitude reaches the fiber, depolarization or charge reversal (positive in, negative out) occurs in a progressive wave down the fiber toward the synapse. Repolarization is the

movement of the charges back to their original positions.

Axons may be short or long (up to 4 feet in humans), and they end, or terminate, in as many as 10,000 nerve endings called *telodendra* (Snyder, 1986). The large number of nerve endings allows

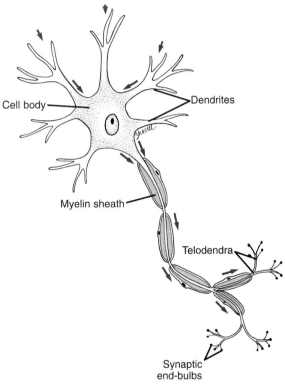

FIGURE 4-2
Impulse transmission through the neuron.

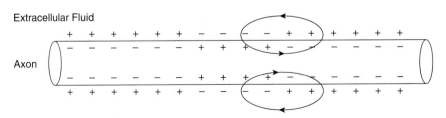

FIGURE 4-3
Electrical impulse transmission along a nerve fiber.

for a great variety in the number and type of connections made with other neurons. The synaptic end bulbs of the telodendra pass nerve impulses to an adjacent structure (another neuron, gland, or muscle) by emitting a chemical messenger called a *neurotransmitter* into the gap or junction (synapse) between the nerve ending and the adjacent structure (Figure 4-4). Neurotransmitters then combine with receptors on the dendritic side of the synapse and cause a stimulatory or inhibitory effect. Dendrites may respond to neurotransmitters by generating a nerve impulse, which is conducted via the axon to the adjacent structure (neuron, gland, or muscle). Neurotransmitters can be mimicked or blocked by the use of appropriate drugs (Figure 4-5).

Nerve fibers (nerves) may have a large diameter (A fibers), medium diameter (B fibers), or small diameter (C fibers) (Boothe, 2001). Fibers with large diameters conduct nerve impulses faster than those with small diameters. Fibers that are surrounded by the insulating substance called *myelin* also transmit impulses faster than nonmyelinated fibers. Type A and B fibers are generally myelinated fibers.

The most basic impulse conduction system through the nervous system is the reflex arc (Figure 4-6). The reflex arc is composed of the following:

1. A receptor
2. A sensory neuron
3. A center in the CNS for a synapse

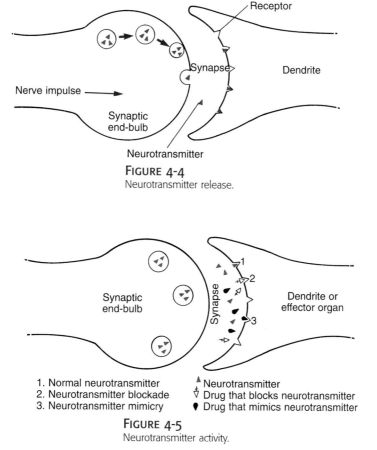

FIGURE 4-4
Neurotransmitter release.

1. Normal neurotransmitter
2. Neurotransmitter blockade
3. Neurotransmitter mimicry

▲ Neurotransmitter
▽ Drug that blocks neurotransmitter
● Drug that mimics neurotransmitter

FIGURE 4-5
Neurotransmitter activity.

4. A motor neuron
5. An effector

The receptor of the reflex arc may be located in a peripheral site—such as the skin—or a central area, such as a muscle, tendon, or visceral organ. The sensory neuron carries the impulse from the receptor to the CNS. In the CNS, the sensory neuron synapses with interneurons in the spinal cord. These interneurons send the impulse to the brain for interpretation or send the impulse to a motor neuron. The motor neuron carries the message to an effector organ. If the impulse travels around the arc without going to the brain for analysis, the sequence of events is called a *spinal reflex* (see Figure 4-6). A spinal reflex can occur even if the spinal cord is completely severed. For example: a hemostat applied to the toe of a dog with a severed cord can cause the dog to withdraw its leg by means of the spinal reflex.

Areas of the brain that have importance to an understanding of the pharmacology of the CNS are illustrated in Figure 4-7. The cerebrum is responsible for higher functions of the brain, such as

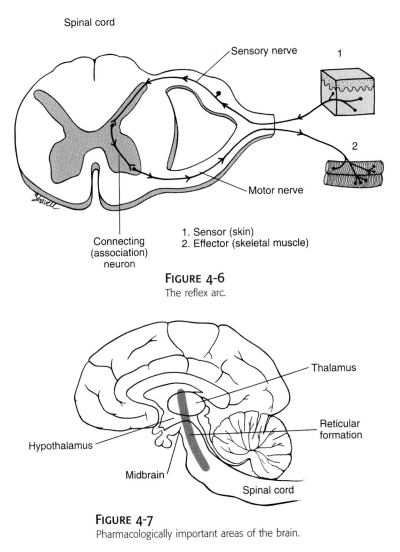

Spinal cord

Sensory nerve

1

Motor nerve

Connecting
(association)
neuron

1. Sensor (skin)
2. Effector (skeletal muscle)

2

FIGURE 4-6
The reflex arc.

Thalamus

Reticular
formation

Hypothalamus

Midbrain

Spinal cord

FIGURE 4-7
Pharmacologically important areas of the brain.

learning, memory, and interpretation of sensory input (vision, pain recognition, and so forth). The thalamus serves as a relay center for sensory impulses from the spinal cord, brain stem, and cerebellum to the cerebrum. The thalamus may also be involved in pain interpretation. The hypothalamus serves as the primary mediator between the nervous system and the endocrine system through its control of the pituitary gland. The hypothalamus also controls and regulates the ANS. The medulla carries both sensory and motor impulses between the spinal cord and the brain. It also contains centers that control vital physiologic activities, such as breathing, heartbeat, blood pressure, vomiting, swallowing, coughing, body temperature, hunger, thirst, and others. The reticular formation is a network of nerve cells scattered through bundles of fibers that begin in the medulla and extend upward through the brain stem. The reticular activating system is a part of the reticular formation, which functions to arouse the cerebral cortex and is responsible for consciousness, sleep, and wakefulness (DeLahunta, 1983).

In summary, nerve activity is usually described as the generation of nerve impulses occurring in a dendrite or cell body and then traveling down an axon by electric-like activity, which is similar to the passage of an electric current down a wire. When this current reaches a synapse, a chemical "bridge" or neurotransmitter allows the message to be passed to one or as many as thousands of other neurons. Neurotransmitter substances include acetylcholine, norepinephrine, dopamine, serotonin, and gamma-aminobutyric acid (GABA). These other neurons then carry the message to an interpretation center or a structure that takes appropriate action. CNS drugs act by mimicking or blocking the effect of neurotransmitters.

AUTONOMIC NERVOUS SYSTEM

The ANS is that portion of the nervous system that controls unconscious body activities. ANS fibers innervate smooth muscle, heart muscle, salivary glands, and other viscera. This system operates automatically and involuntarily to control visceral functions, such as gastrointestinal (GI) motility, rate and force of the heartbeat, secretion by glands, sizes of the pupils, and various other involuntary functions. Unlike the somatic nervous system, the ANS has two subdivisions: the parasympathetic (cholinergic) and the sympathetic (adrenergic). The sympathetic division regulates energy-expending activities (fight-or-flight responses), and the parasympathetic division regulates energy-conserving activities.

The ANS has two neurons carrying impulses to target structures (unlike the somatic nervous system, which has only one). The cell body of the first neuron arises in the CNS: in the thoracolumbar cord for the sympathetic nervous system and craniosacral cord for the parasympathetic nervous system (Figure 4-8). The axon of the first neuron leaves the CNS and travels to a ganglion, where it synapses with dendrites of the second neuron. This second neuron then travels to the target structure (Figure 4-9). Axons of the first neuron are called *preganglionic,* and those of the second are called *postganglionic.*

Preganglionic fibers of the sympathetic nervous system are short. They end in ganglia adjacent to the spinal cord. The only exception is the preganglionic fiber to the adrenal medulla. The adrenal medulla itself is analogous to a postganglionic fiber because it releases epinephrine and norepinephrine directly into the bloodstream when stimulated by preganglionic fibers. Postganglionic sympathetic fibers are long.

Preganglionic fibers of the parasympathetic nervous system are generally long. They travel to ganglia located in the wall of the target organ. Postganglionic fibers are consequently short.

Normally, target sites of the ANS have both sympathetic and parasympathetic innervation. The physiologic functions of the two systems usually oppose each other and thereby bring about a state of balance. When this balance is disrupted, drug therapy may be indicated to restore the balance. The adrenal medulla, sweat glands, and hair follicles have only sympathetic fibers.

Stimulation of the sympathetic nervous system causes an increase in heart rate and respiratory rate, a decrease in GI activity, dilation of the pupils, con-

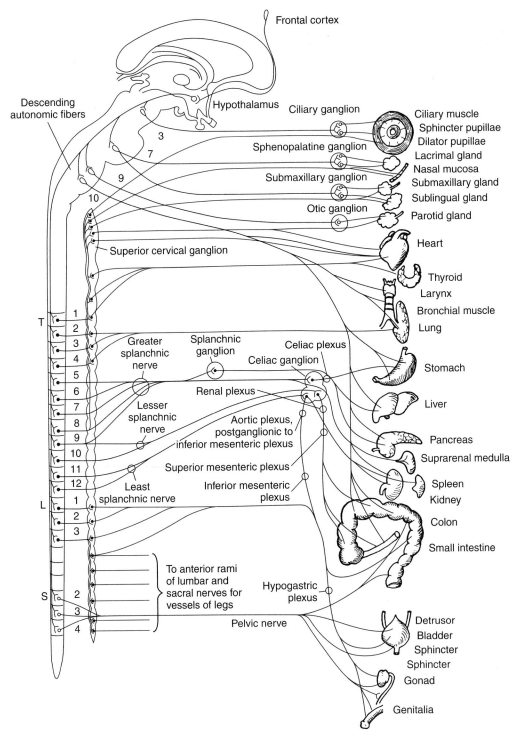

FIGURE 4-8

Schematic of the autonomic nervous system. (From Thibodeau JA: Anatomy and physiology, St. Louis, 1987, Mosby.)

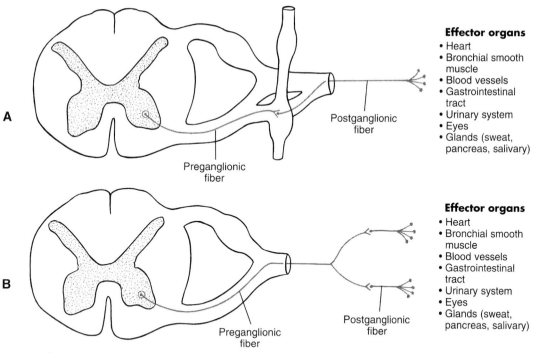

Effector organs
- Heart
- Bronchial smooth muscle
- Blood vessels
- Gastrointestinal tract
- Urinary system
- Eyes
- Glands (sweat, pancreas, salivary)

Postganglionic fiber

Preganglionic fiber

Effector organs
- Heart
- Bronchial smooth muscle
- Blood vessels
- Gastrointestinal tract
- Urinary system
- Eyes
- Glands (sweat, pancreas, salivary)

Preganglionic fiber

Postganglionic fiber

FIGURE 4-9
Preganglionic and postganglionic fibers of the autonomic nervous system. **A,** Sympathetic. **B,** Parasympathetic.

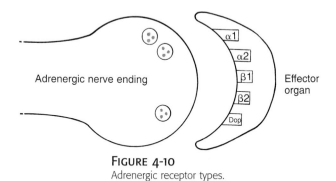

FIGURE 4-10
Adrenergic receptor types.

striction of blood vessels in smooth muscle, dilation of blood vessels in skeletal muscle, dilation of bronchioles, and an increase in blood glucose levels. These actions prepare an animal to fight or to flee. On the other hand, stimulation of the parasympathetic nervous system causes a decrease in heart rate and respiratory rate, an increase in GI activity, constriction of the pupils, and constriction of the bronchioles.

Receptors of the sympathetic (adrenergic) nervous system are subdivided as follows (Figure 4-10):

1. Alpha-1
2. Alpha-2
3. Beta-1
4. Beta-2
5. Dopaminergic

Generally, alpha receptors are stimulatory and beta receptors are inhibitory (Table 4-1). The parasympathetic (cholinergic) nervous system has **nicotinic** and muscarinic receptors. **Effector** organs have one or a combination of these receptors. A drug's effect is determined by the number of receptors in the effector and the drug's specificity for the receptor (Williams and Baer, 1990).

The primary neurotransmitters for adrenergic sites are norepinephrine, epinephrine, and dopamine. Epinephrine equally stimulates both alpha and beta receptors and is therefore a potent stimulator of the heart and an equally powerful dilator of bronchioles. Acetylcholine is the neurotransmitter at sympathetic postganglionic fibers to sweat glands and the smooth muscle of blood vessels (**muscarinic** sites).

The neurotransmitter for cholinergic sites is **acetylcholine.** Acetylcholine combines with both nicotinic and muscarinic receptors.

Cholinergic sites are found in both the sympathetic and parasympathetic nervous systems. Nicotinic receptors are found in all autonomic ganglia, in the adrenal medulla, and at the neuromuscular junction of the somatic nervous system. Muscarinic receptors are found at the synapse of postganglionic fibers of the parasympathetic nervous system and at a few of the sympathetic postganglionic fibers.

How Drugs Affect the Autonomic Nervous System

Autonomic drugs bring about their effects by influencing the sequence of events involving neurotransmitters. Most autonomic drugs bring about this alteration of events by the following:

1. Mimicking neurotransmitters
2. Interfering with neurotransmitter release
3. Blocking the attachment of neurotransmitters to receptors
4. Interfering with the breakdown or reuptake of neurotransmitters at the synapse

CLASSES OF AUTONOMIC NERVOUS SYSTEM AGENTS

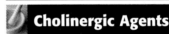

Cholinergic Agents

Cholinergic agents are drugs that stimulate receptor sites mediated by acetylcholine. They achieve these effects by mimicking the action of acetylcholine (direct acting) or by inhibiting its breakdown (indirect acting). Cholinergic agents are also called **parasympathomimetic** because their effects resemble those produced by stimulating parasympathetic nerves.

Clinical Uses. Cholinergic agents do the following:

1. Aid in the diagnosis of myasthenia gravis
2. Reduce the intraocular pressure of glaucoma
3. Stimulate GI motility
4. Treat urinary retention
5. Control vomiting
6. Act as an antidote for neuromuscular blockers

Table 4-1 Adrenergic Receptor Responses

Receptor	Target Organ	Response
Alpha-1	Arterioles	Constriction
	Urethra	Increased tone
	Eye	Dilation of pupil
Alpha-2	Skeletal muscle	Constriction
Beta-1	Heart	Increased rate, conduction, and contractility
	Kidneys	Renin release
Beta-2	Skeletal blood vessels	Dilation
	Bronchioles	Dilation
Dopaminergic	Kidneys	Dilation of blood vessels
	Heart	Dilation of coronary vessels
	Mesenteric blood vessels	Dilation

Direct-Acting Cholinergics

1. Acetylcholine. Acetylcholine is seldom used clinically because it is broken down so rapidly by **acetylcholinesterase**.
2. Carbamylcholine. This product has been used to treat atony of the GI tract and to stimulate uterine contractions in swine.
3. Bethanechol (Urecholine). Bethanechol is used to treat GI and urinary tract atony.
4. Pilocarpine (Isopto Carpine, Akarpine, Pilocar). Pilocarpine reduces intraocular pressure associated with glaucoma.
5. Metoclopramide (Reglan). Metoclopramide is used to control vomiting and to promote gastric tract emptying.

Indirect-Acting Cholinergics (Anticholinesterase) Agents

1. Edrophonium (Tensilon). Edrophonium is used to diagnose myasthenia gravis.
2. Neostigmine (Prostigmine, Stiglyn). These products are used to treat urine retention and GI atony and as an antidote to neuromuscular blocking agents.
3. Physostigmine (Antilirium, Eserine). Uses of this product are similar to those of neostigmine.
4. Organophosphate compounds. These are commonly used as insecticide dips and may result in toxicity if used inappropriately. See pralidoxime below.
5. Demecarium (Humorsol). This drug is used in the preventive management of glaucoma.
6. Pyridostigmine (Mestinon). This drug is used for the treatment of myasthenia gravis.

Adverse Side Effects. Adverse side effects of the cholinergic drugs may include bradycardia, hypotension, heart block, lacrimation, diarrhea, vomiting, increased intestinal activity, intestinal rupture, and increased bronchial secretions.

Cholinergic Blocking Agents (Anticholinergic)

Cholinergic blocking agents are drugs that block the action of acetylcholine at muscarinic receptors of the parasympathetic nervous system.

Clinical Uses. Clinical uses of these drugs are as follows:

1. Treatment of diarrhea and vomiting by decreasing GI motility
2. As a preanesthetic to dry secretions and prevent bradycardia
3. To dilate the pupils for ophthalmic examination
4. To relieve ciliary spasm of the eye
5. To treat sinus bradycardia

The belladonna alkaloids of the deadly nightshade family of plants have been used as drugs for centuries and represent the prototype for this category of agents.

Dosage Forms

1. Atropine. Numerous generic and trade name products are available for parenteral or ophthalmic administration. Atropine is used as a preanesthetic to dry secretions and to prevent bradycardia; as an antidote to organophosphate poisoning; to dilate the pupils for ophthalmic examination; to control ciliary spasms of the eye; to treat sinus bradycardia; and to slow a hypermotile gut.
2. Scopolamine. This is used in antidiarrheal medications.
3. Methscopolamine is an ingredient of Biosol-M. Methscopolamine is used to control diarrhea.
4. Glycopyrrolate (Robinul-V). Glycopyrrolate is a quaternary ammonium compound, with actions similar to atropine. It provides longer action than atropine and is used primarily as a preanesthetic.
5. Aminopentamide (Centrine). Aminopentamide is used to control vomiting and diarrhea in dogs and cats.
6. Propantheline (Pro-Banthine). Propantheline is used to treat diarrhea, urinary incontinence, and bradycardia, and to reduce colonic peristalsis in horses to allow rectal examination. Propantheline, like glycopyrrolate, is a quaternary ammonium compound.
7. Pralidoxime (Protopam, 2-PAM). A cholinesterase reactivator used to treat organophosphate intoxication.

Adverse Side Effects. Adverse side effects of the cholinergic blockers are dose related. Overdose can cause drowsiness, disorientation, tachycardia, photophobia, constipation, anxiety, and burning at the injection site.

Technician's Notes

1. Atropine administered as a preanesthetic causes dilation of the pupils. It dries secretions and prevents bradycardia.
2. Atropine is packaged in small-animal and large-animal concentrations. Care should be taken not to confuse the two preparations.

Adrenergic (Sympathomimetic) Agents

Adrenergic **(sympathomimetic)** agents bring about action at receptors mediated by epinephrine or norepinephrine. Adrenergic agents may be classified as **catecholamines** or noncatecholamines, and either category can also be classified according to the specific receptor types (alpha-1, alpha-2, beta-1, beta-2) activated. In most cases, alpha receptor activity causes an excitatory response (except in the GI tract), and beta stimulation causes an inhibitory response (except in the heart). Adrenergic activity is a complex subject, and more advanced texts should be consulted for a thorough explanation.

Clinical Uses. Adrenergic agents are used for the following purposes:

1. To stimulate the heart to beat during cardiac arrest
2. To reverse the hypotension and bronchoconstriction of anaphylactic shock
3. To strengthen the heart during congestive heart failure
4. To correct hypotension through vasoconstriction
5. To reduce capillary bleeding through vasoconstriction
6. To treat urinary incontinence
7. To reduce mucous membrane congestion (vasoconstriction) in allergic conditions
8. To prolong the effects of local anesthetic agents by causing vasoconstriction of blood vessels at the injection site, thereby prolonging their absorption
9. To treat glaucoma (alpha stimulation increases the outflow of and beta stimulation decreases the production of aqueous humor)

Dosage Forms
1. Epinephrine (Adrenalin). Epinephrine stimulates all receptors to cause an increase in heart rate and cardiac output, constriction of the blood vessels in the skin, dilation of the blood vessels in muscle, dilation of the bronchioles, and an increase in metabolic rate.
2. Norepinephrine (Levophed, Noradrenalin). Norepinephrine is mostly an alpha stimulator with some beta stimulation. Its primary influence is that of a vasopressor (to raise blood pressure).
3. Isoproterenol (Isuprel). Isoproterenol is a pure beta stimulator. Its primary use is for bronchodilation.
4. Phenylephrine (Neo-Synephrine). Phenylephrine is an alpha stimulator used as a nasal vasoconstrictor.
5. Dopamine (Intropin). Dopamine is a precursor of epinephrine and norepinephrine. Its action is dose dependent. It is used to treat shock and congestive heart failure and to increase renal perfusion.
6. Phenylpropanolamine (Ornade, Prolamine, Dexatrim). Phenylpropanolamine is used to treat urinary incontinence in dogs.
7. Dobutamine (Dobutrex). Dobutamine is a beta-1 agonist that is used for short-term treatment of heart failure.
8. Ephedrine (Vatronol), terbutaline (Brethine), and albuterol (Proventil). These products are beta agonists and their main use is bronchodilation.
9. Xylazine (Rompun, AnaSed). Xylazine is an alpha-2 agonist with analgesic and sedative properties.

Adverse Side Effects. These may include tachycardia, hypertension, nervousness, and cardiac arrhythmias. Hypertension, arrhythmia, and pulmonary edema may occur with an overdose.

Adrenergic Blocking Agents

Adrenergic blocking agents are used to disrupt the activity of the sympathetic nervous system. They are classified according to the site of their action as an alpha blocker, beta blocker, or ganglionic blocker. Drugs usually block only one category of receptor.

Alpha Blockers. Alpha blockers have had limited use in veterinary medicine. Phenoxybenzamine has been advocated by some clinicians for the treatment of laminitis in horses and urethral obstruction in cats. Yohimbine is used for xylazine antagonism.

Clinical Uses. See Dosage Forms.

Dosage Forms
1. Phenoxybenzamine (Dibenzyline). Phenoxybenzamine is a hypotensive (vasodilator) agent.
2. Tranquilizers (acepromazine, droperidol). These tranquilizers act as alpha blockers and cause vasodilation.
3. Prazosin (Minipress). Prazosin is a hypotensive agent.
4. Yohimbine (Yobine). Yohimbine is used as an antidote for xylazine toxicity.
5. Atipamezole (Antisedan). Atipamezole is a reversal agent for medetomidine.

Adverse Side Effects. Adverse side effects may include hypotension (phenoxybenzamine, tranquilizers, prazosin), tachycardia (phenoxybenzamine),

muscle tremors (yohimbine), and seizures (acepromazine).

Beta Blockers. Beta blockers are used to treat glaucoma, arrhythmias, and hypertrophic cardiomyopathy.

Clinical Uses. See Dosage Forms.

Dosage Forms
1. Propranolol (Inderal). Propranolol is used to treat cardiac arrhythmias and hypertrophic cardiomyopathy.
2. Timolol (Timoptic). Timolol is an ophthalmic preparation used to treat glaucoma.
3. Atenolol. Used in a similar way to propranolol.

Adverse Side Effects. These include bradycardia, hypotension, worsening of heart failure, bronchoconstriction, heart block, and syncope.

Ganglionic Blockers. Ganglionic blockers are seldom used in veterinary medicine.

CENTRAL NERVOUS SYSTEM

CNS drugs have various uses in veterinary medicine. Depressant drugs are used to tranquilize or sedate animals to facilitate restraint or anesthetic procedures. They are also used to control pain, to induce **anesthesia,** and to prevent or control seizures. CNS drugs are also available to antagonize (reverse) the effects of some depressant drugs. Another group of CNS agents is used to stimulate the CNS to treat cardiac or respiratory depression or arrest. The euthanasia drugs allow veterinarians to provide a quick and painless end to hopeless medical situations.

Drugs affecting the CNS generally cause either depression or stimulation. They are thought to generate these changes by altering nerve impulse transmissions between the spinal cord and the brain or within the brain itself. Altering impulse transmissions within the thalamus could prevent messages regarding painful stimuli from reaching the interpretation centers within the cerebrum. Interfering with impulses within the reticular activating system could alter levels of consciousness or wakefulness (Ganong, 2003). The changes that occur in the transmission of nerve impulses as a result of administration of CNS drugs are probably brought about by altered neurotransmitter activity.

The categories of CNS drugs that are covered in this chapter include the following:

1. Tranquilizers
2. Barbiturates
3. Dissociatives
4. Opioid/antagonists
5. Neuroleptanalgesics/antagonists
6. Drugs to prevent or control seizures
7. Inhalants
8. Miscellaneous CNS drugs
9. CNS stimulants
10. Euthanasia agents

 ## Tranquilizers

Phenothiazine Derivatives

The mechanism of action of the phenothiazine derivatives on the CNS is not well understood. However, it has been proposed that they are dopamine blockers (Muir and Hubbell, 2000). The effects on the cardiovascular system are a result of alpha-adrenergic blockade.

The phenothiazine derivative tranquilizers produce sedation and allay fear and anxiety without producing significant **analgesia.** Sudden painful stimuli arouse the animal. Phenothiazine derivative tranquilizers produce an antiemetic effect by depressing the chemoreceptor trigger zone in the brain and have a mild antipruritic effect. These agents also reduce the tendency of epinephrine to induce cardiac arrhythmias.

Clinical Uses. Phenothiazine derivatives are used for prevention or treatment of vomiting, relief of mild pruritus, and sedation/tranquilization.

Dosage Forms

1. Acepromazine maleate (Acepromazine, Promace)
2. Chlorpromazine hydrochloride (Thorazine)
3. Promazine HCl (Sparine)
4. Prochlorperazine/isopropamide   (Darbazine, Compazine)

Adverse Side Effects. The phenothiazine derivative tranquilizers can cause hypotension and hypothermia because of their vasodilator effect (alpha blockade). They also can induce seizures (by lowering the seizure threshold) in epileptic animals.

Technician's Notes

1. Phenothiazine derivatives should not be used within 1 month of worming with an organophosphate anthelmintic.
2. The tranquilizing effect may be reduced in an excited animal.

The phenothiazine derivative tranquilizers are approved for use in a wide variety of animals and for administration by almost any route. They generally are relatively safe drugs to use when administered appropriately. They should be given with care when used with other CNS depressants because of the additive effect. Most phenothiazine derivative tranquilizers are metabolized by the liver and excreted by the kidneys.

Benzodiazepine Derivatives

The mechanism of action of diazepam is through depression of the thalamic and hypothalamic areas of the brain. This drug produces sedation, muscle relaxation, appetite stimulation (especially in cats), and anticonvulsant activity. Diazepam also produces minimal depression of the cardiovascular and respiratory systems when compared with other CNS depressants. It is sometimes used in combination with ketamine to induce short-term anesthesia. Diazepam is very useful for treating seizures in progress.

Several potential drug interactions can occur when administering diazepam simultaneously with other drugs, and appropriate references should be consulted.

Clinical Uses. Clinical uses include sedation, relief of anxiety and behavioral disorders, treatment of seizures, and appetite stimulation. Diazepam can be used as an injectable anesthetic.

Dosage Form
1. Diazepam (Valium, Vazepam)
2. Midazolam (Versed)

Adverse Side Effects. These are limited when used as directed. Dogs can exhibit excitement. Overdose may cause excessive CNS depression.

Technician's Notes
1. Diazepam should be stored at room temperature and protected from light.
2. Diazepam should not be stored in plastic syringes or in solution bags because it can be absorbed into the plastic.
3. The manufacturers recommend that it not be mixed with other medications or solutions.
4. Diazepam is metabolized by the liver and eliminated by the kidneys.

Xylazine Hydrochloride

Xylazine is an alpha-2 agonist with sedative, analgesic, and muscle relaxant properties. It is approved for use in dogs, cats, horses, deer, and elk. This agent causes vomiting in a large percentage of cats and in some dogs. Xylazine is antagonized by yohimbine. It produces effective analgesia in horses and is often used for treating the pain associated with colic and for sedation for minor procedures. It is also used in combination with ketamine for short-term field procedures in horses, such as castration and suturing of extensive wounds, because this combination usually produces 15 to 20 minutes of recumbency. Extralabel use of xylazine for cesarean sections in cattle and other surgical procedures is common. Xylazine is used in cats and dogs as a tranquilizer and in combination with other injectable agents for surgical procedures.

Clinical Uses. Clinical uses include sedation, analgesia, short-term anesthesia (when combined with other agents), and induction of vomiting.

Dosage Forms
1. Rompun
2. AnaSed
3. Gemini
4. Sedazine

Adverse Side Effects. These include bradycardia, hypotension, respiratory depression, and increased sensitivity to epinephrine, resulting in cardiac arrhythmias. An overdose increases the potential for these effects.

Technician's Notes
1. Because of the potential of xylazine to cause bradycardia or heart block in dogs, atropine should be used as a premedicant in this species.
2. Xylazine is used in cattle at one tenth of the equine dose.
3. Horses may appear heavily sedated with xylazine and still respond to painful stimuli by kicking.
4. Small-animal (20 mg/ml) and large-animal (100 mg/ml) concentrations are available. Care should be taken not to confuse them when administering a drug dose to an animal.

Detomidine Hydrochloride

Detomidine, like xylazine, is an alpha-2 agonist. It is approved as a sedative/analgesic for horses, and clinicians often report excellent analgesic properties in their patients when using this product. It is used for procedures in horses when sedation and analgesia are needed and reportedly produces better analgesia of the rear limbs than does xylazine.

Clinical Uses. Detomidine is used for sedation and analgesia in horses.

Dosage Form
Dormosedan

Adverse Side Effects. These may include sweating, muscle tremors, penile prolapse, bradycardia, and heart block.

Technician's Notes
The manufacturer warns that detomidine should be used very carefully with other sedative drugs and that it should not be used with the potentiated sulfa drugs such as trimethoprim/sulfa.

Medetomidine

Medetomidine is an alpha-2–adrenergic agonist labeled for use as a sedative and analgesic in dogs more than 12 weeks of age. Atipamezole (Antisedan) is the reversal agent for this drug.

Clinical Uses. Uses include facilitating clinical examination, minor surgical procedures, and minor dental procedures that do not require intubation.

Dosage Form
Domitor

Adverse Side Effects. Side effects include bradycardia (product insert states that hemodynamics are maintained), AV heart block, decreased respirations, hypothermia, urination, vomiting, hyperglycemia, and pain at the injection site.

Technician's Notes
1. Treatment of medetomidine-induced bradycardia with anticholinergic drugs (atropine or glycopyrrolate) is not recommended because of the potential for more serious arrhythmias.
2. Antisedan is recommended for treatment of medetomidine-induced effects.
3. Before attempting the use of medetomidine in combination with other sedatives, references should be consulted for potential side effects and dosages.

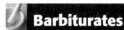

Barbiturates

The barbiturates are one of the oldest categories of CNS depressants used in veterinary medicine. They are derived from the parent compound barbituric acid and cause various responses ranging from sedation to death, depending on the dose and the circumstances of use. Barbiturates are used in veterinary medicine as sedatives, anticonvulsants, general anesthetics, and euthanasia agents. They are easy and cheap to administer. But they have much potential for complications because of their potent depressing effects on the cardiac and pulmonary systems (especially in cats) and because they are nonreversible and must be metabolized by the liver before elimination can occur. Individual patients with poor liver function, little body fat, or preexisting illnesses that cause acidosis may be at risk when receiving barbiturates. Because of their alkalinity, the ultrashort-acting barbiturates can cause necrosis of the tissue if administered outside the vein in the subcutaneous space. The barbiturates are metabolized by the liver and are potent depressors of the respiratory system.

Barbiturates are classified according to their duration of action as long-acting, short-acting, and ultrashort-acting. Or they are classified according to the chemical side chain on the barbituric acid molecule as an oxybarbiturate or a thiobarbiturate (Table 4-2). The long- and short-acting barbiturates have a side chain connected by oxygen and are therefore called *oxybarbiturates*. The thiobarbiturates have a side chain connected by a sulfur. The thiobarbiturates are very soluble in fat and tend to move rapidly out of the CNS into the fat stores of the body, thus accounting for their ultrashort activity.

Clinical Uses. Clinical uses include the prevention and treatment of seizures, and for sedation, anesthesia, and euthanasia.

Long-Acting Barbiturates (Oxybarbiturates, 8 to 12 Hours)
Phenobarbital. Numerous proprietary and generic products exist. Phenobarbital is used primarily as an

Table 4-2 Barbiturate Classifications

Generic Name	Proprietary Name	Classification	Duration of Action
Phenobarbital	Luminal	Long-acting oxybarbiturate	4-8 hours
Penobarbital	Nembutal	Short-acting oxybarbiturate	½-2 hours
Thiopental	Pentothal	Ultrashort-acting thiobarbiturate	10-30 minutes

anticonvulsant to prevent epileptic seizures. It is administered by the oral route. Phenobarbital is a Class IV controlled substance.

Short-Acting Barbiturates (Oxybarbiturates, 45 Minutes to 1.5 Hours)

Pentobarbital sodium (Nembutal and numerous generic products). Pentobarbital is given by intravenous injection (the intraperitoneal route may also be used) and provides 1 to 2 hours of general anesthesia. In the earlier days of veterinary anesthesia, it was the routine general anesthetic used in dogs. Today, pentobarbital is used primarily to control seizures in progress and as a euthanasia agent. Intravenous administration of glucose or concurrent use of chloramphenicol may prolong the recovery period. Pentobarbital is a Class II controlled substance.

Ultrashort-Acting Barbiturates (Thiobarbiturates, 5 to 30 Minutes)

The thiobarbiturates are very alkaline (especially at the higher concentrations) and must be given intravenously to avoid necrosis and subsequent sloughing of tissue. The thiobarbiturates are rapidly redistributed into the fat stores of the body within 5 to 30 minutes.

Extreme care should be taken when administering a thiobarbiturate to a thin animal because of the lack of fat stores. The thiobarbiturates are prepared as a sterile powder in vials for dilution up to the desired concentration. They are stable for long periods in the undiluted form. Sterile water for injection should be used as the diluent because solutions with electrolytes hasten precipitate formation. Solutions should not be administered if precipitates are present.

The thiobarbiturates can cause a period of apnea when they are rapidly administered intravenously. If spontaneous respirations do not resume in a short time, controlled respirations should be started. The barbiturates can also cause a period of CNS excitement when administered intravenously if they are given too slowly. It is often recommended to give one third to one half of the calculated dose rapidly to avoid the excitement phase. The remainder of the dose is administered in increments until the desired effect is achieved.

Dosage Forms

1. Thiopental (Pentothal). Thiopental is used as an intravenous agent to induce general anesthesia.
2. Methohexital (Brevane). Methohexital is an ultrashort-acting barbiturate that produces 5 to 10 minutes of anesthesia. It has been recommended for use in sight hounds because of its rapid redistribution and metabolism by the liver.

Adverse Side Effects. These include excessive CNS depression, paradoxical CNS excitement, severe respiratory depression, and cardiovascular depression. Tissue irritation may occur when the barbiturates are injected perivascularly.

Technician's Notes

1. Recovery from pentobarbital is often prolonged, and dogs exhibit padding limb movements during this time.
2. Thiobarbiturates should not be used in sight hounds or in any very thin animal.
3. Giving additional doses of thiobarbiturates may prolong recovery.
4. Barbiturates are potent depressors of the respiratory system.

Dissociative Agents

The dissociative agents belong to the cyclohexylamine family, which includes phencyclidine, ketamine, and tiletamine. Involuntary muscle rigidity (catalepsy), amnesia, and analgesia characterize dissociative anesthesia. Pharyngeal/laryngeal reflexes are maintained, and muscle tone is increased. Because deep abdominal pain is not eliminated (surgical stage III is not usually reached) with dissociative anesthesia, it is recommended only for restraint, diagnostic procedures, and minor surgery. Dissociative agents are often combined with other agents for abdominal surgery, however. Dissociative drugs produce minor cardiac stimulation, and respiratory depression can occur at the higher doses. These agents act by altering neurotransmitter activity, causing depression of the thalamus and cerebral cortex, and activation of the limbic system (Plumb, 2002).

Some species are often ataxic and hyperresponsive during induction and recovery with dissociative agents (Muir and Hubbell, 2000). Tremors, spasticity, and convulsions can occur at the higher doses. Hallucinations have been reported in humans and are suspected in cats.

Clinical Uses. Dissociative agents are used for sedation, restraint, and anesthesia.

Dosage Forms
1. Ketamine HCl (Ketaset, Vetalar, Ketalar). Ketamine is approved for use in humans, primates, and cats but has extralabel uses in various species including dogs, horses, birds, small ruminants, and reptiles. Tranquilizers, such as acepromazine, xylazine, and diazepam, are often used concurrently with ketamine to increase muscle relaxation and to deepen the level of anesthesia. Oral, ocular, and laryngeal reflexes are maintained when ketamine is used alone (except at the high doses). Occasional spastic jerking movements can occur in cats that are administered ketamine. Ketamine produces good somatic analgesia but poor visceral analgesia.

Increased salivation may accompany administration of this drug and can be controlled or prevented with the use of atropine or glycopyrrolate. An ophthalmic lubricant should be used because cats' eyes remain open after the administration of ketamine. Ketamine is a class III controlled substance.
2. Tiletamine HCl (Telazol—tiletamine plus zolazepam HCl). Telazol is an injectable anesthetic and consists of a combination of tiletamine (chemically related to ketamine) and zolazepam (a tranquilizer). Telazol is approved for use in dogs and cats. The pharmacokinetics and pharmacotherapeutics of tiletamine are similar to those of ketamine. Because of the zolazepam in this product, additional agents are not needed for muscle relaxation. Ocular lubrication should be used in cats receiving Telazol. Telazol is a Class III controlled substance.
3. Phencyclidine (Sernylan). This dissociative agent is no longer available. It was originally used as an immobilizing agent for nonhuman primates. Its street name is "PCP" or "angel dust" (Upson, 1988).

Adverse Side Effects. These are usually associated with high doses and include spastic jerking movement, convulsions, respiratory depression, burning at the intramuscular injection site, and drying of the cornea.

> ## Technician's Notes
> 1. Both ketamine and tiletamine may cause burning at the injection site. Adequate restraint should be used to ensure injection of all the medication.
> 2. The metabolites of the dissociative agents are excreted through the kidneys. These drugs may be contraindicated in animals with compromised kidney function.

Opioid Agonists

An opioid is any compound derived from opium poppy alkaloids and the synthetic drugs with similar pharmacologic properties. These drugs produce analgesia and sedation (hypnosis) while reducing anxiety and fear. Narcotic effects are produced in combination with opiate receptors at the deep levels of the brain (e.g., thalamus, hypothalamus, and limbic system). The opioid receptors are grouped into the following four classes (Paddleford, 1999):

1. Mu—found in pain-regulating areas of the brain; contribute to analgesia, euphoria, respiratory depression, physical dependence, and hypothermic actions
2. Kappa—found in the cerebral cortex and spinal cord; contribute to analgesia, sedation, and miosis
3. Sigma—may be responsible for struggling, whining, hallucinations, and mydriatic effects
4. Delta—modify mu receptor activity

The opioids are used as preanesthetics or postanesthetics because of their sedative and analgesic properties. Sedation is more pronounced at the higher doses. They are sometimes used alone or in combination with tranquilizers as anesthetics for surgical procedures, for relief of colic pain in horses, and for restraint/capture of wild/zoo animals. At low doses, the opioids have antitussive (cough suppression) properties owing to depression of the cough center in the brain and antidiarrheal action because they cause a reduction in peristalsis or segmental contractions. Several potential adverse side effects are associated with the narcotics. Opioids are potent respiratory depressants. Because they affect the thermoregulatory centers in the brain (the body's thermostat), they may cause panting, defecation, flatulence, and vomiting. Sound sensitivity may also occur. Excitement may occur in dogs if the narcotic is rapidly given intravenously. Cats and horses are reported to be sensitive to the opioids and may exhibit excitatory effects at high doses. Because opioids cross the placenta fairly slowly and their effects can be antagonized, they can be useful when performing cesarean sections. The liver metabolizes opioids, and the resulting metabolites are eliminated in the urine. Most of the opioid

preparations are class II controlled substances, and the narcotic antagonists can antagonize them.

Clinical Uses. Opioid agonists are used for analgesia, sedation, restraint, anesthetics, treatment of coughing, and treatment of diarrhea.

Naturally Occurring Narcotics

1. Opium (laudanum—10% opium), paregoric. Opium is derived from the seed capsule of the opium poppy. Paregoric, also called *camphorated tincture of opium*, has been used for more than 100 years for the treatment of diarrhea. It has been used in veterinary medicine for treating diarrhea primarily in calves and foals.
2. Morphine sulfate (Duramorph). Morphine is an opium derivative used to treat severe pain. Occasionally, it is used as a preanesthetic or anesthetic agent (e.g., cesarean section in dogs). It is also used to relieve the anxiety associated with acute congestive heart failure. It exerts its effects primarily on mu receptors. Morphine is a Class II controlled substance that should be used under strict supervision because of its potential for abuse. It is the standard opioid with which all others are compared in terms of analgesic effect.

Synthetic Narcotics

1. Meperidine (Demerol). Meperidine is a mu agonist that is approximately one eighth as potent an analgesic as morphine. It is used for relief of acute pain, such as that occurring after orthopedic procedures. It also may be combined with a tranquilizer for use as an anesthetic agent (neuroleptanalgesic). No meperidine products carry a veterinary label. However, the human products often have extralabel uses in animals. Naloxone is the preferred antagonist.
2. Oxymorphone (Numorphan). Oxymorphone is a semisynthetic opioid that is a mu agonist. It is approximately 10 times more potent an analgesic than morphine. This drug is used primarily in dogs for restraint, for diagnostic procedures, and for minor surgical procedures. It (locked away in a safe)

may be combined with tranquilizers to produce neuroleptanalgesia; naloxone is the antagonist.

3. Butorphanol tartrate (Torbutrol, Torbugesic). Butorphanol is a synthetic, partial opioid agonist. Its narcotic activity is exerted on kappa and sigma receptors. It is a class IV controlled substance. Butorphanol has 4 to 7 times the analgesic properties of morphine and significant antitussive effect (Plumb, 2002). Torbutrol is a product that is approved as an antitussive agent in dogs. It is also used in dogs and cats as an analgesic and preanesthetic. Torbugesic is approved for the treatment of the pain associated with colic in horses. It is also used in combination with other sedatives/tranquilizers in horses, dogs, and cats as a preanesthetic or for minor surgical procedures.

4. Fentanyl (Sublimaze). Fentanyl is an opioid agonist that is found in the neuroleptanalgesic Innovar-Vet. It has approximately 100 times the analgesic properties of morphine. Fentanyl is a class II controlled substance. Fentanyl transdermal patches are sometimes used in animals to control chronic pain (see Chapter 14).

5. Hydrocodone bitartrate (Hycodan, Tussigon). Hydrocodone is an opioid agonist that is used as an antitussive agent in dogs. It is a Class III controlled substance.

6. Etorphine (M-99). Etorphine is an opioid that produces analgesic effects 1000 times those of morphine. It is restricted to use by veterinarians in zoo or exotic animal practice (Upson, 1988). It is lethal to people who accidentally inject themselves (it also can be absorbed through intact skin) if the antagonist (diprenorphine) is not administered immediately. Etorphine is a Class II controlled substance.

7. Pentazocine (Talwin, Talwin-V). Pentazocine is a partial opioid agonist that is approved for pain relief in horses and dogs. It is a Class IV controlled substance.

8. Diphenoxylate (Lomotil). Diphenoxylate is a synthetic opioid agonist that is combined with atropine for use as an antidiarrheal agent. This drug is a Class V controlled substance.

9. Apomorphine—generic labeling. Apomorphine is an opioid with the principal effect of inducing vomiting by stimulating the chemoreceptor trigger zone in the brain. This drug is often administered by placing a portion of a tablet in the conjunctival sac for absorption (see Chapter 8). (put in eye)

10. Methadone (Dolophine). Methadone is a synthetic opioid that was developed as a treatment for morphine and heroin addiction in humans. Its primary use in veterinary medicine is in the treatment of colic pain in horses. Methadone is a Class II controlled substance.

11. Codeine—generic labeling or in combination. Codeine is an opioid that is available in human-label products for use as an antitussive in dogs.

12. Carfentanil (Wildnil). Carfentanil is used to induce wildlife anesthesia. It has 10,000 times the potency of morphine.

13. Buprenorphine (Buprenex). Buprenorphine is a human label, partial mu agonist-antagonist. It is a potent analgesic with potential for use in cats.

Adverse Side Effects. These can include respiratory depression, excitement (cats and horses), nausea, vomiting, diarrhea, defecation, panting, and convulsions. Overdose causes profound respiratory depression.

Opioid Antagonists

Opioid antagonists block the effects of opioids by binding with opiate receptors, displacing narcotic molecules already present, and preventing further narcotic binding at the sites. These antagonists are classified as pure antagonists or as partial antagonists. The partial antagonists may have some agonist activity (analgesic and respiratory depressant effects).

These drugs are usually administered by the intravenous route and exert their effects very rapidly (15 to 60 seconds).

Clinical Uses. Opioid antagonists are used to antagonize the effects of the opioid agonists.

Dosage Forms

1. Naloxone (naloxone HCl injection, Narcan). Naloxone is a pure opioid antagonist chemically similar to oxymorphone, with high affinity for mu receptors. It has no agonist activity.
2. Nalorphine (Nalline). Nalorphine is a partial antagonist that may produce untoward analgesic and respiratory depressant effects.

Adverse Side Effects. Nalorphine and levallorphan may induce respiratory depression. Naloxone usually has few adverse effects if given in the correct dose.

Neuroleptanalgesics

A neuroleptanalgesic agent consists of an opioid and a tranquilizer. Animals receiving neuroleptanalgesics may or may not remain conscious (Muir and Hubbell, 2000). They often defecate and are highly responsive to sound stimuli. The opioid effects of the neuroleptanalgesics can be antagonized with the opioid antagonists.

Clinical Uses. Neuroleptanalgesics are used for sedation, restraint, and to produce anesthesia.

Dosage Forms

1. Fentanyl and droperidol (Innovar-Vet). Innovar-Vet is the only commercially available neuroleptanalgesic. It may be used for restraint, for diagnostic procedures, as a preanesthetic, and for minor surgical procedures.
2. Other neuroleptanalgesics may be prepared by a clinician and include the following:
   Acepromazine and morphine
   Acepromazine and oxymorphone
   Xylazine and butorphanol

Adverse Side Effects. These can include panting, flatulence, personality changes, increased sound sensitivity, and bradycardia. Overdose may cause severe depression of the CNS, respiratory system, and cardiovascular system.

Drugs to Prevent or Control Seizures

Seizures occur in animals for various reasons, which include but are not limited to unknown (idiopathic), infectious (postdistemper), traumatic (head injury), toxicity (strychnine poisoning), and metabolic (heatstroke) factors. Prolonged seizures in progress require emergency action with intravenous therapy. Periodic, recurring seizures require preventive oral medication. Oral preventive therapy often must be titrated to the individual patient and reviewed regularly for the appropriate dose adjustment that controls the seizure activity.

Clinical Uses. These drugs are used to prevent seizures or to control seizures in progress.

Dosage Forms

1. Diazepam (Valium). Diazepam is a tranquilizer with potent antiseizure properties. It is administered intravenously and has a 3- to 4-hour duration of action.
2. Pentobarbital—generic products. Pentobarbital is a short-acting barbiturate that is effective for controlling seizures. It is administered intravenously and has a 1- to 3-hour duration.
3. Phenobarbital (Luminal, Solfoton, generic formulations). Phenobarbital is an effective antiseizure drug and is available in oral and parenteral formulations. The oral route is the usual means of administering this drug to dogs and cats. The injectable form is used in horses (foals) by some clinicians. Drowsiness is a potential side effect of phenobarbital. Phenobarbital is a class IV controlled substance.
4. Primidone (Mylepsin). Primidone is similar chemically to phenobarbital, and a portion of the primidone dose is metabolized to phenobarbital by the liver. It is administered orally to dogs and cats, although its use in cats is controversial. Adverse side effects may include agitation, anxiety, polyuria, polydipsia, and dermatitis.
5. Phenytoin sodium (Dilantin). The use of phenytoin has declined considerably through the years because of its variable pharmacokinetics in dogs

and cats (Plumb, 2002). It may occasionally be used in combination with other antiseizure medications.

6. Bromide is an old anticonvulsant that has sparked renewed interest, mainly as an adjunct to phenobarbital or primidone therapy.
7. Clorazepate
8. Felbamate

Adverse Side Effects. These may include drowsiness, CNS depression, anxiety, agitation, polyuria, polydipsia, and hepatotoxicity (phenobarbital and primidone). Consult product inserts or appropriate references for specific effects.

Technician's Notes

1. Inadequate client compliance is a frequent cause of the failure of anticonvulsant therapy. Clients should be advised about the importance of following medication instructions carefully.
2. Reserpine and phenothiazine drugs should not be given to epileptic animals.

 Inhalant Anesthetics

Inhalant anesthetic agents are used to produce general anesthesia. They are converted from a liquid to a gaseous phase by an anesthetic vaporizer and delivered to the lungs using an oxygen source and a patient breathing circuit. From the alveoli of the lungs they are absorbed into the bloodstream and delivered to the central nervous system where they produce unconsciousness, analgesia, and muscle relaxation through mechanisms not fully understood.

Inhalants generally require little biotransformation for elimination from the body. Since they enter and exit the body through the lungs, this facilitates a rapid induction and recovery from the effects of the agent compared with the injectable anesthetic agents. It also permits a quicker alteration of the depth of anesthesia.

The amount (partial pressure) of inhalant anesthetic in the brain is proportionate to the alveolar concentration of the agent. Alveolar concentration depends upon the amount of agent delivered to the lungs compared with the amount removed from the lungs. Delivery of the agent to the lungs can be increased by increasing the vaporizer setting, increasing the fresh gas (oxygen) flow, increasing minute ventilation, or by decreasing mechanical and physiologic dead space. Factors that influence the removal of the agent from the lungs include the solubility (blood-gas partition coefficient) of the agent, the molecular weight of the agent, the partial pressure difference between the agent in the alveolus and the agent in the blood, the amount of alveolar surface available for exchange (absence of lung pathology), and cardiac output.

The uptake by tissue of an anesthetic agent depends mainly upon the degree of tissue perfusion and the solubility of the agent in the tissue. The vessel-rich tissue (brain, heart, lungs, liver, kidneys, intestine, and endocrine glands) receives the greatest percentage of cardiac output and is consequently the first to reach equilibrium during uptake of an anesthetic gas and the first to download an agent. Lipid-rich cells, like brain cells, absorb more agent than lipid-poor cells.

Characteristics important to the understanding of inhalant agents include MAC (minimum alveolar concentration), partition coefficient, and vapor pressure (Table 4-3). The MAC value of an anesthetic agent is a measure of potency and is the alveolar concentration that prevents gross purposeful movement in 50% of the patients in response to a standardized painful stimulus. Lower numbers indicate more potent agents, and the values may vary slightly between species. The partition coefficient is the ratio of the number of molecules of an anesthetic gas existing in two phases (blood/gas). It indicates the solubility of an agent in a tissue like blood and correlates with the speed of induction and recovery. Lower numbers indicate faster agents. Vapor pressure of an agent indicates how volatile it is and the maximum concentration that can be achieved. Higher numbers indicate more volatility and the requirement of a precision vaporizer.

Exposure to anesthetic waste gases can pose a health hazard to the veterinary technician if improper scavenging of the waste is not carried out.

Table 4-3 Physical Properties of Currently Used Inhalation Anesthetics

Property	Sevoflurane	Desflurane	Isoflurane	Halothane	Methoxyflurane	Nitrous Oxide
Formula	*(chemical structure)*	*(chemical structure)*	*(chemical structure)*	*(chemical structure)*	*(chemical structure)*	*(chemical structure)*
Molecular weight	200	168	184.5	197.4	165.3	44
Specific gravity (20° C)	1.52	1.47	1.49	1.86	1.41	—
Boiling point (° C)	59	23.5	48.5	50.2	104.7	—
Vapor pressure at 20° C (mm Hg)	160	664	239.5	244.1	22.8	—
mL Vapor/mL liquid at 20° C	182.7	209.7	194.7	227	207	—
Preservative	None	None	None	0.01% thymol	0.01% butyl hydroxytoluene	None
Stability						
Soda lime	No?	Stable	Stable	Decomposes	Decomposes	Stable
UV light	—	—	Stable	Decomposes	Decomposes	—

From Paddleford RR: Manual of small animal anesthesia, ed 2, Philadelphia, 1999, WB Saunders Co.

Reproductive, hepatic, and renal effects have been noted. Toxicity is likely due to the biotransformation of by-products of the agents. The inhalant agents are biodegraded to various degrees (methoxyflurane, 50%; halothane, 25%; isoflurane, <0.2%; sevoflurane, 3%; nitrous oxide, 0.0004%).

Clinical Uses. Inhalant anesthetics are used to induce and maintain general anesthesia in animal patients.

Dosage Forms. The inhalant agents discussed in this section include isoflurane, sevoflurane, halothane, methoxyflurane, and nitrous oxide.

1. Isoflurane (Forane, Isoflo). Isoflurane was synthesized in 1968 and used clinically in people in 1970. Isoflurane is a colorless liquid with a pungent odor. It is stable and does not require a preservative. A halogenated ether, it is one of the least soluble of the inhalant agents. It is less potent than halothane and methoxyflurane but has very rapid induction and recovery times. Isoflurane allows a stable heart rhythm and does not decrease cardiac output at clinically used levels. It is metabolized at a very low rate (<0.2%). This agent is used in a wide variety of species.
2. Sevoflurane (SevoFlo). Sevoflurane is a halogenated ether with little odor, which makes it a good choice for mask induction. This agent is characterized by very rapid induction and recovery times. The cardiovascular and respiratory effects are similar to those of isoflurane. Sevoflurane is often used in high-risk, small animal patients because of its safety and rapid, smooth induction. Only 3% of sevoflurane is metabolized. The disadvantage of the use of this agent is its cost compared with isoflurane.
3. Halothane (Halothane). Halothane is a halogenated hydrocarbon that was first used clinically in human anesthesia in 1956. Halothane decomposes when exposed to ultraviolet light and for this reason has thymol added as an antioxidant. Halothane sensitizes the heart to the catecholamines, which may result in cardiac dysrhythmias. Like isoflurane and sevoflurane, halothane has a high vapor pressure and must be used in precision vaporizers. "Halothane hepatitis" has been reported in humans but is a very rare occurrence. This agent is metabolized at the rate of 25%, a considerably higher rate than the previous two agents.

4. Methoxyflurane (Metofane). Methoxyflurane has been used since 1959. It is a methyl-ethyl-ether that is very soluble in blood and other tissues. It consequently has a very slow induction and recovery time. Methoxyflurane is the most potent (MAC = 0.23%–0.27%) of the agents considered in this section. It has a relatively low vapor pressure making 3% the maximum level that can be vaporized. Also, because of this low vapor pressure, it can be used in nonprecison, in-circuit vaporizers or precision, out-of-circuit vaporizers. Methoxyflurane undergoes the most biotransformation (50%) of any of the inhalants. It has been associated with renal toxicity in human patients.
5. Nitrous Oxide. Nitrous oxide is a colorless inorganic gas. It was discovered to have anesthetic properties in the late 1700s. Nitrous oxide may be used as an adjunct to the more potent agents during mask induction to speed the induction of anesthesia. General anesthesia cannot be produced using nitrous oxide alone. It is compressed to form a liquid and is supplied in blue cylinders. It has the lowest solubility coefficient of any of the inhalants, which means that it enters and exits the blood and tissue rapidly. Since nitrous oxide is 30 times more soluble than nitrogen, it displaces nitrogen from the alveoli, blood, and gas-filled cavities in the body. This means it will diffuse into and potentially cause distention of the intestines and other gas-filled areas (e.g., the pneumothorax). Nitrous oxide is delivered through a flowmeter and must always be given with oxygen to prevent hypoxia. Oxygen should always be administered for several minutes after the nitrous oxide is turned off to prevent diffusion hypoxia. (The rapid exit of nitrous oxide from the blood will dilute the oxygen in the alveoli).

Miscellaneous Central Nervous System Drugs

Propofol

Propofol is a short-acting hypnotic unrelated to other general anesthetic agents. Its mechanism of action is not well understood. Chemically it is an alkylphenol derivative. The product that is commercially available is an emulsion, which contains soybean oil, glycerol, and egg lecithin. Because of its white color, some clinicians have called this product "milk of amnesia." Propofol produces a rapid and smooth induction in dogs when given slowly intravenously. It produces sedation, restraint, or unconsciousness depending on the dose. A single bolus lasts 2 to 5 minutes, making it particularly useful when rapid recovery is important.

Clinical Uses. Propofol is useful for anesthetic induction before administration of an inhalant anesthetic, for outpatient procedures, as a substitute for barbiturates in sight hounds, and for patients with preexisting cardiac arrhythmias.

Dosage Forms
1. Rapinovet
2. PropoFlo
3. Diprivan (human label)

Adverse Side Effects. Apnea may occur if propofol is given too rapidly intravenously. Occasional seizure-like signs may be seen. Prolonged recoveries and/or Heinz body production may be seen in cats with repeated use.

Technician's Notes

Propofol is an expensive agent that contains no preservatives. It is recommended that unused portions be discarded because bacteria may grow in the opened container.

Glyceryl Guaiacolate or Guaifenesin (Guailaxin, Gecolate)

Guaifenesin is a skeletal muscle relaxant that exerts its effects on the connecting neurons of the spinal cord and brain stem (Plumb, 2002). It is used primarily in equine medicine to induce general anesthesia or to extend the anesthetic activity of other injectable field anesthetics (i.e., ketamine and xylazine). It may be used as a 5% or 10% solution in 5% dextrose. Some clinicians add an ultrashort-acting barbiturate to the solution before administering it intravenously. Relatively large amounts are required to induce general anesthesia, and small increments are given to maintain or extend the anesthetic effects of other agents.

Clinical Uses. These include induction or prolongation of general anesthesia in large animals and occasional use as an expectorant.

Dosage Forms
1. Guailaxin
2. Gecolate

Adverse Side Effects. Adverse side effects are limited. Hemolysis has been reported when greater than 5% solutions are used.

Technician's Notes

1. Guaifenesin is packaged as a soluble powder. It may be difficult to dissolve when the diluent is added. Warming the 5% dextrose before mixing may aid solution preparation. It should be mixed only immediately before use because a precipitate forms if the solution is allowed to stand for several hours.
2. When administering increments of guaifenesin to maintain or extend anesthesia, communicate thoroughly with the veterinarian to understand the quantity of this drug to administer.

Chloral Hydrate/Magnesium Sulfate

This combination has been used as an intravenous agent to produce anesthesia in large animals.

Because of the potential for severe irritation of tissue if administered outside of the vein, and because of the advent of more efficacious agents, this combination is seldom used.

Central Nervous System Stimulants

The primary medical use of the CNS stimulants is for treatment of respiratory depression or arrest. Many of the other uses of CNS stimulants are illegal or unethical (e.g., to enhance athletic performance).

Doxapram

Doxapram activates the respiratory system by stimulating respiratory centers in the medulla. It is labeled for use in dogs, cats, and horses. Its main indications are to stimulate respirations during or after general anesthesia, in newborns, and in cases of cardiopulmonary arrest. It is labeled for intravenous use, but it may be administered under the tongue (1 to 2 drops) or into the umbilical vein of newborns.

Clinical Uses. These include stimulation of respiration in newborns, and during or after anesthesia.

Dosage Forms
1. Dopram-V
2. Dopram. Approved for use in humans.

Adverse Side Effects. Adverse side effects are rare and usually associated with overdose. Hypertension, seizures, and hyperventilation may occur.

Technician's Notes
One to two drops of doxapram may be placed under the tongue or injected into the umbilical vein of newborns to stimulate respirations.

Pentylenetetrazol (Metrazol)
Pentylenetetrazol is a generalized stimulant of the CNS that has been used to stimulate respirations

and to hasten recovery from anesthesia. It has limited use in veterinary medicine.

Caffeine

Caffeine is a general CNS stimulant that increases wakefulness.

Amphetamines

Amphetamines, which are potent stimulants of the cerebral cortex, are similar chemically to epinephrine. They have no legitimate medical indications in veterinary medicine.

Neuromuscular Blocking Drugs

Neuromuscular blocking drugs, sometimes called muscle relaxants, interfere with neuromuscular transmission of impulses and are used as an adjunct to general anesthesia. These drugs provide no analgesia or sedation. However, they do stop ventilation and that makes ventilation and constant patient monitoring necessary (Muir and Hubbell, 2000).

Neuromuscular blocking drugs are classified as either depolarizing agents or nondepolarizing agents. Depolarizing agents act in a way similar to acetylcholine at the neuromuscular synapse, but the effect lasts longer leading to muscle paralysis (Phase I block). These drugs are not broken down by acetylcholinesterase and have no antagonist. Nondepolarizing agents prevent (competitive inhibition) acetylcholine from binding to receptor sites (Phase II block). These drugs are not degraded by cholinesterase, but they can be antagonized by edrophonium or neostigmine.

Clinical Uses. Neuromuscular blocking agents are used as an adjunct to general anesthesia (e.g., ophthalmic/orthopedic) and to facilitate endotracheal intubation.

Dosage forms

Depolarizing
1. Succinylcholine chloride (Sucostrin, Anectine)
2. Decamethonium (Syncurine)

Nondepolarizing
1. d-Tubocurarine chloride (Curare)
2. Gallamine (Flaxedil)
3. Pancuronium bromide (Pavulon)
4. Vecuronium bromide (Norcuron)
5. Atracurium (Tracrium)

BEHAVIORAL PHARMACOTHERAPY

The use of drugs to treat behavioral problems in animals is a relatively new, but rapidly growing area of veterinary medicine. Behavior problems—such as separation anxiety, fears and phobia, unruliness, hyperactivity, compulsive disorders, cognitive dysfunction in older dogs, and inappropriate elimination in cats—are being diagnosed in increasing numbers. Many animals with behavioral disorders are taken in desperation to animal shelters, but a growing number of clients are willing to attempt to correct the conditions with environmental management, behavior modification, and/or pharmacotherapy.

Informed consent should be obtained from the client before these drugs are used (Shull, 1998) because many of the drugs used in behavioral pharmacotherapy are human psychiatric drugs that have not been approved for use in animals. The technician or veterinarian should explain to the animal owner the extralabel status of the drug, possible side effects or precautions, and the medical effects to be expected in the pet. Owners should also be aware that pharmacotherapy may not be a cure-all for problems of behavior and that the problems may return after discontinuing therapy.

All drugs used in psychotherapy are thought to produce their effects through altering neurotransmitter activity in the brain (Simpson, 1996a,b). The five neurotransmitters of clinical importance in behavioral pharmacotherapy are acetylcholine, dopamine, norepinephrine, serotonin, and gamma-aminobutyric acid (GABA).

Dopamine, norepinephrine, and serotonin are called *monoamine neurotransmitters* since they have similar chemical structures. Monoamines are found in large quantities in areas of the brain often associated with the expression and control of emotions. The primary method by which monoamines are inactivated is by their reuptake from the synapse back into synaptic vesicles in nerve endings (see Figure 4-4). Drugs that block or inhibit their reuptake increase their activity. Acetylcholine is the most widely distributed neurotransmitter in the body. It is associated with a variety of behavioral effects and inactivated by cholinesterase at the synapse. Some of the most common side effects of drugs used in behavioral psychotherapy are related to their anticholinergic effects, such as dry mouth, increased heart rate, urine retention, and constipation. Gamma-aminobutyric acid is considered to be an inhibitory neurotransmitter and is widely distributed in the brain.

Pharmacotherapeutic Agents

The most commonly used drugs in treating behavioral problems in veterinary medicine are the antianxiety medications, the antidepressants, and miscellaneous agents—such as the synthetic progestins. All the drugs listed in the following carry a human label, except those otherwise indicated.

 Antianxiety Medications

Benzodiazepines

The benzodiazepines most commonly used in veterinary medicine include diazepam, alprazolam, and lorazepam. All the benzodiazepines are similar in structure and mechanism of action. They are thought to bind with and promote GABA activity in both the cerebral cortex and in subcortical areas, such as the limbic system.

Clinical Uses. Behavioral uses of benzodiazepines include the treatment of fears and phobias, separation anxiety, fear, aggression, anxiety-induced stereotypes, urine marking in cats, and appetite stimulation.

Dosage Forms

1. Diazepam (Valium)
2. Alprazolam (Xanax)
3. Lorazepam (Ativan)

Adverse Side Effects. These may include lethargy, ataxia, polyuria and polydipsia (PUPD), hyperexcitability, and hepatic necrosis (cats).

Azapirones

Buspirone is the azapirone agent used in behavioral pharmacotherapy. Unlike the benzodiazepines, it possesses no muscle relaxant, anticonvulsant, or sedative effects. Its antianxiety effect is thought to be a result of blocking serotonin receptors.

Clinical Uses. Veterinary uses include the control of urine spraying/marking and the control of fearfulness and anxiety.

Dosage Form

Buspirone (BuSpar)

Adverse Side Effects. Few serious side effects appear to exist.

 Antidepressants

Tricyclics

The tricyclics used commonly in veterinary medicine include amitriptyline, imipramine, and clomipramine. These drugs are thought to exert their effects by preventing the reuptake of norepinephrine and serotonin. Clomipramine is apparently a selective inhibitor of serotonin reuptake. The tricyclic group is often used on a long-term basis and may take several weeks of use to become effective. Some of the tricyclics are available in the generic form and are relatively inexpensive to use.

Clinical Uses. Uses include the treatment of separation anxiety, obsessive disorders (e.g., lick granuloma, tail chasing), fearful aggression, hyperactivity, hypervocalization, and urine marking.

Dosage Forms

1. Amitriptyline (Elavil, generic forms)
2. Imipramine (Tofranil)
3. Clomipramine (Anafranil, Clomicalm [veterinary label])

Adverse Side Effects. Side effects may include sedation, tachycardia, heart block, mydriasis, dry mouth, reduced tear production, urine retention, and constipation.

Serotonin Reuptake Inhibitors

The serotonin reuptake inhibitors include fluoxetine, sertraline, paroxetine, and fluvoxamine. As their name indicates, these drugs increase the amount of serotonin in the synapse by inhibiting its reuptake back into the nerve terminal. The serotonin reuptake inhibitors have fewer potential side effects than the tricyclics but are usually more expensive.

Clinical Uses. Used for a variety of behavioral syndromes including obsessive disorders, phobias, aggression, and separation anxiety.

Dosage Forms

1. Fluoxetine (Prozac)
2. Sertraline (Zoloft)
3. Paroxetine (Paxil)
4. Fluvoxamine (Luvox)

Adverse Side Effects. Side effects are relatively few but include anorexia, nausea, lethargy, anxiety, and diarrhea.

Monoamine Oxidase-B Inhibitors

The neurotransmitter dopamine is broken down by the enzyme monoamine oxidase-B (MOA-B). Substances such as selegiline (a MOA-B inhibitor) block or inhibit MOA-B and allow dopamine levels to increase. Decreased dopamine levels may be associated with certain types of dementia seen in older dogs (canine cognitive dysfunction). Canine cognitive dysfunction is characterized by disorientation, decreased activity level, abnormal sleep-wake cycles, loss of house training, decreased or altered responsiveness, and decreased or altered greeting behavior.

Clinical Uses. Uses include treatment of old-dog dementia and treatment of canine Cushing's disease.

Dosage Form
Selegiline (Eldepryl, Atapryl, Anipryl [veterinary label])

Adverse Side Effects. Side effects include vomiting, diarrhea, anorexia, restlessness, lethargy, salivation, shaking, and deafness.

Synthetic Progestins
The synthetic progestins are sometimes used to treat behavioral problems through mechanisms associated with changing hormonal levels (reduced gonadotropins) or through some direct effect on the cerebral cortex.

Clinical Uses. Uses include the treatment of urine spraying/marking, intermale aggression, or dominance aggression.

Dosage Forms
1. Megestrol acetate (Megace, Ovaban [veterinary label])
2. Medroxyprogesterone (Depo-Provera)

Side Effects. Transient diabetes mellitus (cats), PUPD, increased weight gain, personality changes, endometritis, endometrial hyperplasia, mammary hypertrophy, mammary tumor, adrenal atrophy, and lactation.

 Euthanasia Agents

Euthanasia agents should have several properties to make them effective medically and aesthetically for this emotion-laden procedure. These drugs should rapidly produce unconsciousness without struggling, vocalizations, or excessive involuntary movements. Death should follow quickly owing to the cessation of all vital functions, such as respiratory and cardiac functions.

The main component of most of the euthanasia agents is pentobarbital. Pentobarbital may also be combined with other agents, such as propylene glycol and alcohol. Pentobarbital alone is a Class II controlled substance, and pentobarbital combinations usually are Class III controlled substances.

Clinical Uses. These agents are used to produce a rapid, humane death.

Dosage Forms
1. Pentobarbital sodium (Sleepaway, pentobarbital generic). These products are Class II controlled substances for intravenous use.
2. Pentobarbital sodium (Beuthanasia-D). This drug is a Class III controlled substance for intravenous use. This product is different from the pentobarbital sodium described above because it contains rhodamine B, a bluish-red dye to help distinguish it from other parenteral pentobarbital solutions, and phenytoin and preservatives.
3. Euthanasia-6. This product contains pentobarbital only.
4. T-61. T-61 is a nonnarcotic, nonbarbiturate agent that contains a general anesthetic, a local anesthetic, and a muscle paralyzer. It is not a controlled substance. It must be administered according to manufacturer instructions (first two thirds slowly) to avoid apparent anxiety or pain.
5. Fatal-Plus. Contains pentobarbital sodium and is available as a sterile powder for dilution or as a prepared solution. The solution contains a stabilizer, a solvent, and a preservative. (use tap water)

Adverse Side Effects. These may include muscle twitching, and death may be delayed if the drug is injected outside the vein.

REFERENCES
Boothe DM: Control of pain in small animals: Opioid agonists and antagonists and other locally and centrally acting analgesics. In Boothe DM, editor: Small animal clinical pharmacology and therapeutics, Philadelphia, 2001, WB Saunders Co.

DeLahunta A: Diencephalon. In DeLahunta A, editor: Veterinary neuroanatomy and clinical neurology, Philadelphia, 1983, WB Saunders Co.

Ganong WF: Review of medical physiology, ed 21, New York, 2003, McGraw-Hill.

Muir WW and Hubbell JA: Handbook of veterinary anesthesia, ed 3, St. Louis, 2000, The CV Mosby Co.

Paddleford RR: Manual of small animal anesthesia, Philadelphia, 1999, WB Saunders Co.

Plumb DC: Veterinary drug handbook, ed 4, Ames, 2002, Iowa State University Press.

Shull EA: Psychopharmacology in veterinary behavioral medicine, Annual Conference for Veterinarians and Technicians, Knoxville, Tenn, 1998, UT-CVM.

Simpson BS and Simpson DM: Behavioral pharmacotherapy part I: antipsychotics and antidepressants, Compend Contin Educ Pract Vet 18(10):1067-1081, 1996.

Simpson BS and Simpson DM: Behavioral pharmacotherapy part II: anxiolytics and mood stabilizers, Compend Contin Educ Proc Vet 18(11):1203-1210, 1996.

Snyder S: Mood modifiers. In Snyder S, editor: Drugs and the brain, New York, 1986, Scientific American Library.

Upson DW: Central nervous system. In Upson DW, editor: Handbook of clinical veterinary pharmacology, ed 3, Manhattan, Kan, 1988, Dan Upson Enterprises.

Williams BR and Baer C: Drugs affecting the autonomic nervous system. In Williams BR and Baer C, editors: Essentials of clinical pharmacology in nursing, Springhouse, Pa, 1990, Springhouse Corp.

REVIEW QUESTIONS

1. Define the difference between an agonist and an opioid antagonist. _____
2. Define neurotransmitter.

   _____
3. The area of the brain that serves to relay information from the spinal cord and brain stem to the interpretation center in the cerebrum is the
   a. Cerebellum
   b. Thalamus
   c. Hypothalamus
   d. Hippocampus
4. Most CNS drugs act by
   _____mimicking_____ or
   _____blocking_____ the effects of neurotransmitters.
5. What are the primary neurotransmitters for adrenergic receptors? _____
6. List the four primary ways in which drugs affect the ANS. _____
7. List five indications for the use of cholinergic agents. _____
8. Atropine, scopolamine, glycopyrrolate, and aminopentamide are examples of what specific drug class? _____
9. What category of drug is used to treat cardiac arrest and anaphylactic shock?

   _____
10. Propranolol is an example of what category of drug?
    a. Alpha agonist
    b. Beta agonist
    c. Alpha blocker
    d. Beta blocker
11. What are some adverse side effects of xylazine, and what drug may be used to antagonize its effects? _____
12. Why would you be concerned about using a thiobarbiturate to induce anesthesia in a very thin dog? _____

13. What are some of the characteristics of a cat anesthetized with ketamine?

    _____
14. List some of the signs of a narcotic overdose.

    _____
15. List two narcotic antagonists.

    _____
16. Why should glyceryl guaiacolate not be mixed until just before use? _____
17. You are assisting in the delivery of a litter of puppies and you deliver one that is not breathing adequately. What drug would the veterinarian instruct to give and by what route? _____
18. Why are euthanasia solutions containing only pentobarbital classified as Class II controlled substances, whereas those containing pentobarbital and other substances are classified as Class III controlled substances?

    _____
19. All psychotherapy drugs are thought to produce their effects by altering

    _____ activity in the brain.
20. Dissociative agents, such as ketamine and tiletamine, may cause _____ at the injection site.
21. A hypnotic (anesthetic) known for its very short duration and its white color is

    _____.
22. An inhibitory neurotransmitter widely distributed in the brain is

    _____.
23. A benzodiazepine used as an antianxiety medication and as an appetite stimulant in cats is _____.
24. An example of a tricyclic antidepressant used in veterinary medicine for separation anxiety in dogs is _____
25. _____ is used to treat old-dog dementia.

INTRODUCTION
RESPIRATORY ANATOMY AND
  PHYSIOLOGY
RESPIRATORY DEFENSE
  MECHANISMS
PRINCIPLES OF RESPIRATORY
  THERAPEUTICS
INHALATION THERAPY FOR
  RESPIRATORY DISEASE
CATEGORIES OF RESPIRATORY
  DRUGS
Expectorants
  Guaifenesin (Glyceryl Guaiacolate)
Mucolytics: Acetylcysteine
Antitussives: Centrally Acting Agents
  Butorphanol Tartrate
  Hydrocodone Bitartrate
  Codeine
  Dextromethorphan
  Temaril-P
Bronchodilators
  Cholinergic Blockers
  Antihistamines
  Beta-2-Adrenergic Agonists
  Methylxanthines
Decongestants
Antihistamines – histamine blocker (allergies)
Corticosteroids – help inflammation
Miscellaneous Respiratory Drugs
  Respiratory Stimulants
    DOXAPRAM HYDROCHLORIDE
    NALOXONE
    YOBINE

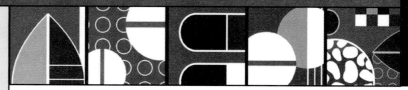

CHAPTER **5**

Drugs Used in Respiratory System Disorders

LEARNING OBJECTIVES

After studying this chapter, you should be able to:

1. Describe the basic anatomy and physiology of the respiratory system
2. List the protective mechanisms of the respiratory system
3. Describe the fundamental principles of treatment of the respiratory system
4. List the difference between the actions of the expectorants, antitussives, and mucolytics
5. Describe the action of the bronchodilators
6. Describe the use of antihistamines and decongestants in respiratory disease
7. List potential uses for respiratory stimulants
8. List the advantages and disadvantages of inhalant therapy

KEY TERMS

AEROSOLIZATION The conversion of a liquid into a fine mist or colloidal suspension in air.

ANTITUSSIVE A drug that inhibits or suppresses the cough reflex.

BRONCHOCONSTRICTION Narrowing of the bronchi and bronchioles, which results in increased airway resistance and decreased airflow.

BRONCHODILATION Widening lumen of bronchi and bronchioles, which results from relaxation of the smooth muscle in the walls of the bronchi and bronchioles. Airway resistance is decreased, and airflow is increased.

DECONGESTANT A substance that reduces the swelling of mucous membranes.

EXPECTORANT A drug that enhances the expulsion of secretions from the respiratory tract.

HUMIDIFICATION Addition of moisture to the air.

IGA The class of antibody produced on mucous membrane surfaces, such as those of the respiratory tract.

INSPISSATED Thickened or dried out.

MUCOLYTIC Having the ability to break down mucus.

NEBULIZATION The process of converting liquid medications into a spray that can be carried into the respiratory system by inhaled air.

NONPRODUCTIVE COUGH A cough that does not result in coughing up of mucus, secretions, or debris (a dry cough).

PRODUCTIVE COUGH A cough that results in coughing up of mucus, secretions, or debris.

REVERSE SNEEZE Aspiration reflex—short periods of noisy inspiratory effort in dogs.

SURFACTANT A mixture of phospholipids secreted by type II alveolar cells that reduces surface tension of pulmonary fluids.

VISCID Sticky.

INTRODUCTION

Veterinary references list a wide variety of diseases of the respiratory system. A partial listing of the general etiologies includes the following:

1. Allergy
2. Aspiration
3. Bacteria
4. Congenital defects
5. Fungi
6. Immunologic factors
7. Neoplasia
8. Neurologic conditions
9. Parasites
10. Trauma
11. Viruses

The respiratory system has a series of defense mechanisms for protecting itself from disease. These natural defenses can be damaged by management practices—such as those that cause a buildup of ammonia in enclosed, poorly ventilated housing. They can also be suppressed by inappro-

priate therapy, such as the use of cough suppressants on a productive cough. Because it is essential that these defense mechanisms function optimally for prompt recovery from respiratory disease, it is very important that technicians have a basic understanding of respiratory anatomy and physiology, respiratory defense mechanisms, and respiratory therapeutics.

RESPIRATORY ANATOMY AND PHYSIOLOGY

The respiratory system consists of the lungs and the passageways that carry air into and out of the lungs (Figure 5-1). These passageways include the nostrils, nasal cavity, pharynx, larynx, trachea, bronchi, and bronchioles.

The passageways leading to the lungs are referred to as the *upper respiratory system*. The upper respiratory system begins with the nostrils, which open into the nasal cavity. The nasal cavity contains turbinates covered with mucous membranes. These turbinates increase the surface area of the nasal

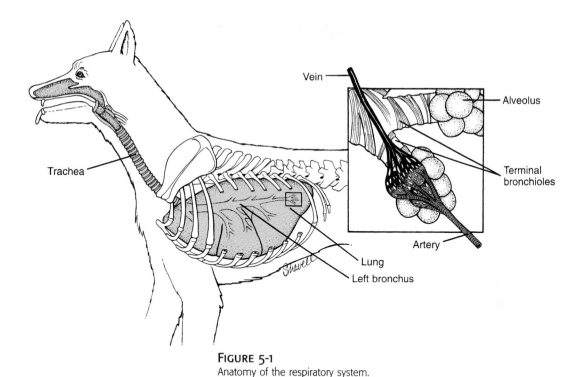

FIGURE 5-1
Anatomy of the respiratory system.

cavity to allow for **humidification** and warming of inspired air. Air passing out of the nasal cavity moves in turn through the pharynx and the larynx into the trachea. The trachea bifurcates into right and left bronchi, which lead to the right and left lungs, respectively. Each bronchus then divides into a series of passageways of decreasing size, called *bronchioles*. Smooth muscle fibers are found in the walls of the bronchioles. Contraction of the smooth muscle fibers decreases the diameter of the bronchioles, and relaxation of the fibers allows the diameter to return to normal size (Figure 5-2).

The upper respiratory tract is lined with ciliated, pseudostratified columnar epithelial cells. Interspersed between the epithelial cells are goblet cells capable of secreting mucus. Mucus is secreted onto the surface of the epithelial cells and is moved toward the pharynx by the movement of the cilia (mucociliary apparatus).

Sympathetic stimulation results in decreased mucus production by the goblet cells and relaxation of the smooth muscle in the walls of the bronchioles, leading to **bronchodilation.**

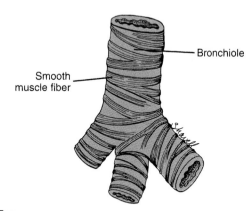

FIGURE 5-2
Smooth muscle fibers in the walls of the bronchioles relax to allow bronchodilation and contract to cause bronchoconstriction.

Parasympathetic stimulation causes increased secretion of mucus and constriction of smooth muscle **(bronchoconstriction)** (Figure 5-3).

The bronchioles terminate in small, saclike structures called *alveoli*. The alveoli are arranged in

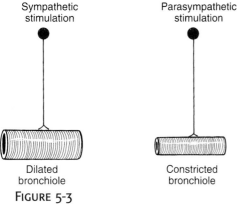

FIGURE 5-3
Effects of autonomic stimulation on bronchioles.

grapelike clusters and are lined with a chemical substance called **surfactant,** which reduces the surface tension of the alveoli and helps to keep them from collapsing. The alveoli are surrounded by capillaries, making it possible for the blood to unload its carbon dioxide into the alveoli and pick up oxygen from the alveoli.

The functions that the respiratory system serves include the following:

1. Oxygen-carbon dioxide exchange
2. Regulation of acid-base balance
3. Body temperature regulation
4. Voice production

The work of the respiratory system can also be divided into the following four parts:

1. Ventilation—the movement of air into and out of the lungs. The inspiratory portion of ventilation is usually an active process, whereas expiration is usually a passive process. Forced inspiration may be associated with upper airway obstruction, and active expiration may be related to intrathoracic airway obstruction (Tilley, 2000).
2. Distribution—the distributing of the inspired gases throughout the lungs.
3. Diffusion—the movement of gases across the alveolar membrane.

4. Perfusion—the supply of blood to the alveoli. The ratio of perfusion to ventilation of the alveoli is normally close to 1:1.

RESPIRATORY DEFENSE MECHANISMS

The respiratory system has several effective methods of defense against disease processes, including the following:

1. Nasal cavity: The turbinates of the nasal cavity provide a large surface area for warming and humidifying inspired air. Hair in the nasal passages also may help to filter out larger particulate matter.
2. Protective reflexes: The cough, sneeze, and perhaps the **reverse sneeze** respond to stimulation of receptors on the surface of the air passageways to expel foreign material forcefully. Laryngospasm and bronchospasm also help to prevent introduction of materials into the lung tissue.
3. Mucociliary clearance: The layer of mucus secreted onto the surface of the epithelial lining of the respiratory tract helps to trap foreign debris that enters the respiratory passages. The wavelike action of the cilia then moves the debris up the passages ("escalator" action) to the pharynx, where it can be swallowed or expelled. Macrophages and immunoglobulins **(IgA)** also contribute to the defensive qualities of the mucociliary apparatus by immobilizing or phagocytizing foreign material.

PRINCIPLES OF RESPIRATORY THERAPEUTICS

It is important that a specific diagnosis be made through radiology, cytology, or appropriate culture before beginning treatment of respiratory disease because the correct treatment for one type of disease may be contraindicated for another. Once the diagnosis has been made, the treatment of respiratory disease is divided into the following three general goals (McKiernan, 1988):

1. Control of secretions: Secretions may be reduced by decreasing their production or increasing their elimination. Removing the cause of the secretions through antibiotic, antifungal, antiparasitic, or other appropriate therapy is of vital concern. Methods are also aimed at making the secretions less **viscid** through the use of expectorants or through **nebulization** of **mucolytics** (aerosol therapy).

2. Control of reflexes: Coughing may be suppressed through the use of antitussives or bronchodilators if the cough is **nonproductive.** Sneezing is controlled by removing the offending agent or through the use of vasoconstrictors. Bronchospasms may be controlled with bronchodilators and corticosteroids.

3. Maintaining normal airflow to the alveoli: Airflow to the alveoli may be maintained by reversing bronchoconstriction, by removing edema or mucus from alveoli and air passages, and by providing oxygen therapy. Intermittent positive-pressure ventilation and other ventilation strategies are often used in humans and may have application in selected animal cases.

INHALATION THERAPY FOR RESPIRATORY DISEASE

While drugs used to treat respiratory diseases are often administered by the oral or parenteral route, inhalant therapy may also be useful. Aerosolization (nebulization) of drugs allows their delivery at high concentrations directly into the airways while minimizing their blood levels, a feature that may reduce the chance of toxic reaction. The efficacy of inhaled drugs depends upon the dose and how well it is distributed in the lungs. Distribution of an aerosol depends upon several factors, such as the size, shape, and pattern of the airways and breathing pattern of the animal. The size of the inhaled particle plays a significant role in its distribution. The optimum particle size for entry into the peripheral airways is 1 to 5 microns (Lavoie, 2001). Particles smaller than 0.5 micron are likely to be exhaled and those larger than 5 microns could be deposited in the upper airways. Airway pathology

(e.g., excessive mucous or exudate) can interfere with distribution of the drug, causing some clinicians to assert that inhalant therapy should always be accompanied by systemic treatment (Boothe, 2001). Concurrent use of a bronchodilator and/or a mucolytic may be helpful adjuncts to inhalant therapy. Relatively inexpensive infant units for inhalation therapy are available for use in small animals (Opti-Chamber, Aero-Chamber) and horses (Aero-Mask).

CATEGORIES OF RESPIRATORY DRUGS

 Expectorants

Expectorants are drugs that liquefy and dilute viscid secretions of the respiratory tract and thereby help in evacuating those secretions. Most expectorants are administered orally, although a few are given by inhalation or parenterally. Expectorants are thought to act directly on the mucus-secreting glands or by reducing the adhesiveness of the mucus. Expectorants are indicated when a **productive cough** is present and are often combined with other substances, such as ammonium chloride, antihistamines, or dextromethorphan.

Guaifenesin (Glyceryl Guaiacolate)

Guaifenesin is found in a few veterinary label products and many human label over-the-counter cough preparations. Guaifenesin is more commonly used in equine practice to induce or maintain general anesthesia.

Clinical Uses. These include relief of cough symptoms related to upper respiratory tract conditions.

Dosage Forms. These are primarily liquid (syrup) and tablet preparations.

1. Antitussive syrup
2. Cough syrup
3. Cough tablets
4. Robitussin-AC
5. Triaminic Expectorant

Adverse Side Effects. Adverse side effects of guaifenesin are rare, although mild drowsiness or nausea may occur.

 ## Mucolytics: Acetylcysteine

Mucolytics, such as acetylcysteine, decrease the viscosity of respiratory secretions by altering the chemical composition of the mucus through the breakdown of chemical (disulfide) bonds. Acetylcysteine is the only mucolytic of clinical significance in veterinary medicine. It is administered by nebulization for pulmonary uses. This drug is also administered orally as an antidote for acetaminophen toxicity.

Clinical Uses. Acetylcysteine is used to break down thick or **inspissated** respiratory mucus or to treat acetaminophen toxicity.

Dosage Forms. Dosage forms (human label) include a 10% solution and a 20% solution in 4-ml, 10-ml, and 30-ml vials.

1. Mucomyst
2. Mucosil-10
3. Mucosil-20

Adverse Side Effects. Adverse side effects are few when acetylcysteine is nebulized. However, the drug may cause nausea or vomiting when administered orally.

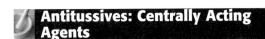 ## Antitussives: Centrally Acting Agents

Antitussives are drugs that inhibit or suppress coughing. Antitussives are classified as centrally acting or peripherally acting (Figure 5-4). Centrally acting agents suppress coughing by depressing the cough center in the brain, whereas peripherally acting agents depress cough receptors in the airways. The peripherally acting antitussives are seldom used in veterinary medicine because they are usually prepared as cough drops or lozenges,

which are not practical to administer to animal patients.

Butorphanol Tartrate

Butorphanol is a synthetic opiate, partial agonist with significant antitussive activity. It is a C-IV controlled substance. It is also used as a preanesthetic and as an analgesic.

Clinical Uses. Butorphanol tartrate is used for the relief of chronic nonproductive cough in dogs and for analgesia and preanesthesia in dogs and cats.

Dosage Forms. Dosage forms include injectable and tablet forms.

1. Butorphanol (Torbutrol) injection (0.5 mg/ml, 10-ml vial). Approved for use in dogs
2. Butorphanol (Torbugesic) injection (10 mg/ml, 50 ml). Approved for use in horses
3. Butorphanol (Torbutrol) tablets (1 mg, 5 mg, and 10 mg; 100/bottle)

Adverse Side Effects. Adverse side effects may include sedation and ataxia.

Hydrocodone Bitartrate

Hydrocodone is a schedule III opiate agonist used for the treatment of nonproductive coughs in dogs.

Clinical Uses. Hydrocodone is primarily used as an antitussive for harsh, nonproductive coughs.

Dosage Forms. Dosage forms include several human label combination products in syrup and tablet form.

1. Hycodan (hydrocodone and homatropine) tablets
2. Tussigon (hydrocodone and homatropine) tablets
3. Hycodan (hydrocodone and homatropine) syrup
4. Hydropane (hydrocodone and homatropine) syrup
5. Codan syrup (hydrocodone and homatropine)
6. Generic hydrocodone syrup

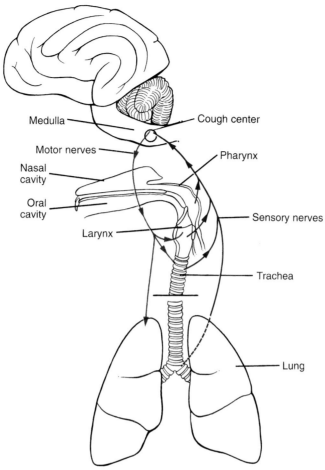

FIGURE 5-4
Antitussives act peripherally on sensory nerve endings or centrally on cough centers.

Adverse Side Effects. These include potential sedation, constipation, and gastrointestinal upset.

Codeine

Codeine is a schedule V opiate agonist that is used as an antitussive in human label combination products.

Clinical Uses. The clinical uses of codeine are similar to those of hydrocodone.

Dosage Forms. These include combination human label products primarily in the syrup form.

1. Codeine phosphate oral tablets, 30 mg and 60 mg
2. Codeine sulfate oral tablets, 15 mg, 30 mg, and 60 mg
3. Codeine phosphate with aspirin (Empirin with codeine)

Adverse Side Effects. Adverse side effects include sedation and constipation.

> **Technician's Notes**
> 1. Codeine only products are Class II (C-II).
> 2. Codeine with aspirin or acetaminophen is C-III.
> 3. Codeine syrups are C-III or C-V (by state).

Dextromethorphan

Dextromethorphan is a nonnarcotic antitussive that is chemically similar to codeine. It has no analgesic or addictive properties. It acts centrally and elevates the cough threshold. Like the two drugs previously mentioned, it is available primarily in human label combination products.

Clinical Uses. Dextromethorphan is used to suppress a nonproductive cough.

Dosage Forms. The primary dosage form is the syrup product.

1. Phenergan with dextromethorphan
2. Dimetapp DM (dextromethorphan, phenylpropanolamine, and brompheniramine)
3. Robitussin DM (dextromethorphan and guaifenesin)

Adverse Side Effects. Adverse side effects are rare when this drug is given in the correct dose but can include drowsiness or gastrointestinal upset.

Technician's Notes

Technicians administering combination products to cats should take special precautions to ensure that the product does not contain acetaminophen.

Temaril-P

Temaril-P is a combination product that contains a centrally acting antitussive (trimeprazine tartrate) and a corticosteroid (prednisolone).

Clinical Uses. Temaril-P is used as an antitussive and as an antipruritic.

Dosage Forms. Dosage forms include tablets.

Temaril-P tablets (5 mg trimeprazine tartrate, 2 mg prednisolone)

Adverse Side Effects. These include sedation, depression, hypotension, and minor central nervous system signs.

Bronchodilators

Contraction of the smooth muscle fibers surrounding the bronchioles results in bronchoconstriction and often a corresponding dyspnea. Contraction of these smooth muscle fibers can result from the following three basic mechanisms (Bill, 1997) (Figure 5-5):

1. Release of acetylcholine at parasympathetic nerve endings or inhibition of acetylcholinesterase. Increased acetylcholine levels also tend to increase the secretions of the respiratory tract, thus reducing airflow and adding to the level of dyspnea.
2. Release of histamine through allergic or inflammatory mechanisms. Histamine combines with H_1 receptors on the smooth muscle fibers to cause bronchoconstriction. Histamine also increases the inflammatory response in the airways, further leading to increased levels of secretions and viscosity.
3. Blockade of beta-2-adrenergic receptors by drugs such as propranolol results in bronchoconstriction. Stimulation of beta-2-adrenergic receptors, however, produces bronchodilation.

Drugs that cause bronchodilation are of four basic categories. Those categories include the cholinergic blockers, the antihistamines, the beta-2 adrenergics, and the methylxanthines (Boothe, 2001).

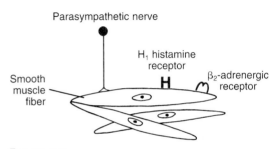

FIGURE 5-5
Bronchoconstriction may result from (*1*) acetylcholine release at parasympathetic nerve endings, (*2*) stimulation of H_1 histamine receptors, (*3*) blockade of beta-2-adrenergic receptors.

Cholinergic Blockers

The cholinergic blockers produce bronchodilation by combining with acetylcholine receptors on the smooth muscle fibers and preventing the bronchoconstricting effects of acetylcholine. Cholinergic blockers such as atropine, aminopentamide (Centrine), and glycopyrrolate (Robinul-V) have limited use in treating bronchoconstriction except in cases of organophosphate or carbamate toxicity. Ipratropium bromide, a synthetic anticholinergic, may be of some value in treating equine pulmonary obstructive disease (Hoffman, 2001).

Antihistamines

The antihistamines are addressed later in this chapter.

Beta-2-Adrenergic Agonists

Beta-2-adrenergic agonists combine with appropriate receptors on the smooth muscle fibers and effect relaxation of those fibers. They also stabilize mast cells and reduce the amount of histamine released (Bill, 1997). It is desirable that these drugs have limited beta-1 activity because beta-1 stimulation can produce tachycardia.

Clinical Uses. Beta-2-adrenergic agonists are used as bronchodilators.

Dosage Forms
1. Epinephrine. This drug is a potent bronchodilator used only in life-threatening situations (e.g., anaphylactic shock) because it also produces significant tachycardia.
2. Isoproterenol (Isuprel). Also causes beta-1 stimulation and has limited use as a bronchodilator in veterinary medicine.
3. Albuterol (Ventolin, Proventil), clenbuterol (Ventipulmin syrup and clenbuterol HCl oral syrup), terbutaline (Brethine), and metaproterenol (Alupent). These are beta-2 agonists that have little stimulatory influence on the heart. Clenbuterol is veterinary approved for horses and is not intended for food. None of the other products carry a veterinary label.
4. Salmeterol (Serevent)

Adverse Side Effects. These include tachycardia and hypertension.

Methylxanthines

The methylxanthine derivatives that are used therapeutically include aminophylline and theophylline. These two products are very similar in their chemistry and pharmacologic effects. Both inhibit an enzyme in smooth muscle cells called phosphodiesterase. When beta-2 receptors are stimulated, a chemical messenger called cyclic adenosine monophosphate (cyclic AMP) released in the smooth muscle cell completes the relaxation response to allow dilation. Phosphodiesterase inhibits cyclic AMP in the cell and thereby tends to promote bronchoconstriction. By inhibiting the inhibitor (phosphodiesterase) and allowing cyclic AMP to accumulate, the methylxanthines tend to promote bronchodilation.

The methylxanthines also cause mild stimulation of the heart and respiratory muscles and minor diuresis.

Caffeine and theobromine (found in chocolate) are methylxanthines.

Aminophylline is an ethylenediamine salt of theophylline. It is available in various human label products. One hundred milligrams of aminophylline contain approximately 79 mg of theophylline (Plumb, 2002). Injectable forms are available, as are immediate- and sustained-release oral forms.

Clinical Uses. Methylxanthines are used for bronchodilation in respiratory and cardiac conditions and for mild heart stimulation (positive ionotropic effect).

Dosage Forms
1. Theo-Dur
2. Slo-bid
3. Choledyl SA
4. Aminophylline (generic)

Adverse Side Effects. These may include gastrointestinal upset, central nervous system stimulation, tachycardia, ataxia, or arrhythmias.

Technician's Notes

Because theophylline may interact adversely with many drugs, including phenobarbital, cimetidine, erythromycin, thiabendazole, clindamycin, and lincomycin, appropriate precautions should be taken before administering this drug.

Decongestants

Decongestants are drugs that reduce the congestion of nasal membranes by reducing the associated swelling. Decongestants may be administered as a spray or as nose drops or may be given orally as a liquid or tablet. These drugs act directly or indirectly (Williams and Baer, 1990) to reduce congestion through vasoconstriction of nasal blood vessels. These products have limited use in veterinary medicine but may be used to treat selected feline upper respiratory tract disease.

Many human label decongestants are available. Those that are given orally and act systemically include ephedrine (Primatene), pseudoephedrine (Sudafed), and phenylpropanolamine (Ornade). Topically applied decongestants include oxymetazoline (Afrin) and phenylephrine (Neo-Synephrine).

Antihistamines

Antihistamines are substances that are used to block the effects of histamine. Histamine is released from mast cells in the allergic response and combines with H_1 receptors on bronchiole smooth muscle to cause bronchoconstriction. Antihistamines may be useful in treating respiratory disease because they prevent mast cell degranulation and they block H_1 receptors on smooth muscle. Antihistamines are thought to be more effective when used preventively because they apparently do not replace histamine that has already combined with receptors (Bill, 1997).

Respiratory conditions that may be treated using antihistamines include "heaves" in horses, pneumonias in cattle, feline asthma, and insect bites.

Generic names for antihistamines are often easily recognized because most end in the suffix -*amine* (e.g., pyrilamine, diphenhydramine, chlorpheniramine).

Veterinary label antihistamines for treating respiratory conditions are available in injectable and oral preparations.

Clinical Uses. Antihistamines are used in the treatment of allergic and respiratory conditions. They may also be used for their antiemetic effect.

Dosage Forms
1. Pyrilamine (Histavet-P)
2. Tripelennamine (Re-Covr)
3. Probahist Syrup
4. Antihistamine Injection
5. Diphenhydramine (Benadryl). Human approved
6. Doxylamine (A-H, injection or tablets)
7. Hydroxyzine (Atarax)
8. Terfenadine (Seldane). Human approved
9. Clemastine (Tavist)
10. Cyproheptadine (Periactin). May be used in cats to block bronchoconstriction.

Adverse Side Effects. These include sedation and, occasionally, gastrointestinal effects.

Corticosteroids

Corticosteroids are used primarily in the treatment of allergic respiratory conditions. They are considered the most effective drugs in treating equine chronic obstructive pulmonary disease (Lavoie, 2001). Corticoteroids prepared for inhalation therapy have strong antiinflammatory effects locally in the lungs and are rapidly biodegraded when absorbed into the general circulation. Oral corticosteroids (prednisone or prednisolone) are considered the drugs of choice in treating chronic airway inflammation in dogs and cats (Dowling, 2001). Corticosteroid therapy controls the signs of respiratory disease, not the cause: good short-term effects often ensue with few residual effects requiring the need for long-term use.

Clinical Uses. Corticosteroids are used in the treatment of equine heaves, feline asthma, acute respiratory distress syndrome, and allergic pneumonia.

Dosage forms
1. Prednisolone sodium succinate (Solu-Delta-Cortef, Delta-Cortef)
2. Prednisolone (Delta Albaplex, Temaril-P, generic forms)
3. Dexamethasone (Dexasone, Dexamethasone Solution, Azium)
4. Beclomethasone dipropionate (Vanceril) (For inhalation)
5. Fluticasone proprionate (Flo Vent) (For inhalation)
6. Triamcinolone (Vetalog, Aristocort)

Adverse Side Effects. Few side effects are noted if the products are used according to recommendations.

 Miscellaneous Respiratory Drugs

Many other drugs are used to treat respiratory disorders. These include antimicrobials, mast cell stabilizers, and diuretics. Antimicrobials are used in cases of bacterial infections of the respiratory tract and may be administered parenterally or by nebulization. Mast cell stabilizers, such as cromolyn, are most effective if used before the inflammatory activation. Diuretics are used to treat respiratory disease in which pulmonary edema is a major problem.

Respiratory Stimulants
DOXAPRAM HYDROCHLORIDE
Doxapram is a general central nervous system stimulant that is used primarily as a stimulant for the respiratory system.

Clinical Uses. Doxapram is used for stimulation of respiration during and after anesthesia and to speed awakening and restoration of reflexes after anes-

thesia. In neonatal animals, doxapram is used to stimulate respiration after dystocia or cesarean section.

Dosage Form
An injectable form is Dopram-V for injection (20 mg/ml, 20-ml vial)

Adverse Side Effects. These include hypertension, arrhythmias, hyperventilation, central nervous system excitation, and seizures. These effects are most likely at high doses (Plumb, 2002). The safety of doxapram in pregnant animals has not been established.

NALOXONE
Naloxone is used to stimulate respirations in narcotic overdose.

YOBINE
Yobine is used to stimulate respirations in xylazine overdose.

REFERENCES
Bill R: Drugs affecting the respiratory system. In Bill R, editor: Pharmacology for veterinary technicians, ed 2, St Louis, 1997, Mosby.

Boothe DM: Drugs affecting the respiratory system. In small animal clinical pharmacology and therapeutics, Philadelphia, 2001, WB Saunders Co.

Dowling PM: Respiratory drugs. Proceedings of the annual meeting of the American Veterinary Medical Association, Boston, 2001.

Hoffman AM: What's new with aerosol medications in the horse. Proceedings of the annual meeting of the American Veterinary Medical Association, Boston, 2001.

Lavoie JP: Inhalation therapy for equine heaves, Comp Contin Educ Prac Vet 23(5):475-477, 2001.

McKiernan B: Respiratory therapeutics. In proceedings of the 17th seminar for veterinary technicians, The Western Veterinary Conference, Las Vegas, 1988.

Plumb DC: Veterinary drug handbook, ed 4, Ames, 2002, Iowa State University Press.

Tilley LP and Smith WK: The 5-minute veterinary consult: canine and feline, ed 2, Baltimore, 2000, Lippincott Williams & Wilkins.

Williams BR and Baer C: Essentials of clinical pharmacology in nursing, Springhouse, Pa, 1990, Springhouse Publishing Corp.

REVIEW QUESTIONS

1. What structures would a molecule of oxygen pass over or through as it travels from the environment to the alveoli?

_____

2. What are the four primary functions of the respiratory system? _____

3. Describe the function of the three basic defense mechanisms of the respiratory system.

_____

4. What are three important principles of respiratory therapeutics?

_____

5. Expectorants are indicated when what type of cough is present? _____

6. Mucolytics decrease the viscosity of respiratory mucus by what mechanism?

_____

7. Acetylcysteine is administered by what method for pulmonary uses?

_____

8. What is the mechanism of action of most antitussives used in veterinary medicine?

_____

9. Codeine is classified in what category of controlled substances?

_____

10. List three mechanisms that can cause smooth muscle contraction in the bronchioles.

_____

11. List two bronchodilators that are beta-2-adrenergic agonists. _____

12. The methylxanthines bring about bronchodilation by inhibiting what cellular enzyme? _____

13. List two potential uses for antihistamines in veterinary medicine. _____

14. What suffix is found at the end of many antihistamine names? _____

15. List two potential uses for dopram.

_____

16. Use your textbook and formulary to answer the following questions.
Maxi Jones is being treated for canine infectious tracheobronchitis. Dr. Ladd has instructed you to dispense Hycodan tablets at 0.22 mg/kg b.i.d. for 7 days. Maxi weighs 50 lb. What dose of Hycodan does Maxi require?

_____

How many tablets will you dispense?

_____

Create a label for this prescription.

_____

17. List two uses of acetylcysteine in veterinary medicine. 1. _____
2. _____

18. Which of the following is *not* an example of a methylxanthine?
   a.   Aminophylline
   b.   Theophylline
   c.   Caffeine
   d.   Theobromine
   e.   These are all examples of methylxanthines

19. What size particle is capable of reaching the alveoli? _____

20. Give an example of a beta-2-adrenergic agonist bronchodilator.

_____.

INTRODUCTION
PHYSIOLOGIC PRINCIPLES
RENAL FAILURE
COMMON DRUGS FOR THE
  TREATMENT OF RENAL
  DYSFUNCTION AND ASSOCIATED
  HYPERTENSION
Diuretic Drugs
  Loop Diuretics
  Osmotic Diuretics
  Thiazide Diuretics
  Potassium-Sparing Diuretics
  Carbonic Anhydrase Inhibitors
Cholinergic Agonists
Anticholinergic Drugs
Adrenergic Antagonists
  Alpha-Adrenergic Antagonists
  Beta-Adrenergic Antagonists
Angiotensin-Converting Enzyme
  Inhibitors
Vasodilators and Calcium Channel
  Blockers
Antidiuretic Hormone
Urinary Acidifiers
Xanthine Oxidase Inhibitors
Urinary Alkalizers
PHARMACOTHERAPY OF RENAL
  FAILURE COMPLICATIONS
PHARMACOTHERAPY OF URINARY
  INCONTINENCE
Miscellaneous Renal Drugs
  Urinary Tract Analgesics
    PHENAZOPYRIDINE
  Tricyclic Antidepressants
    AMITRIPTYLINE
  Glycosaminoglycans
    PENTOSAN POLYSULFATE SODIUM
    (ELMIRON)
TECHNICIAN'S ROLE

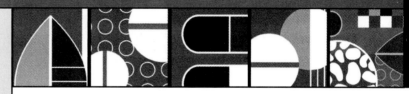

CHAPTER **6**

Drugs Used in Renal and Urinary Tract Disorders

LEARNING OBJECTIVES

After studying this chapter, you should be able to:

1. Identify the anatomic features of the urinary system
2. Discuss the formation of urine through glomerular filtration, tubular reabsorption, and tubular secretion
3. Compare the different classes of drugs and understand the indications for each class
4. Understand how renal dysfunction can affect the metabolizing and excreting of many drugs and their metabolites

KEY TERMS

AGONIST A drug that competes for the same receptor site as another drug or natural substance and enhances or stimulates the receptor's functional properties.

ANTAGONIST A drug that competes for the same receptor site as another drug or natural substance but does not produce a physiologic effect by itself.

ATONY The absence or lack of normal tone or strength.

CATECHOLAMINE A group of sympathomimetic amines including dopamine, norepinephrine, and epinephrine.

DETRUSOR The smooth muscle of the urinary bladder that is mainly responsible for emptying the bladder during urination.

DETRUSOR AREFLEXIA The absence of detrusor contractions.

ENURESIS Involuntary discharge of urine while sleeping.

HEMATURIA Blood in the urine.

HYPERTENSION Persistently high blood pressure.

HYPERTONUS The state characterized by an increased tonicity or tension.

HYPOKALEMIA Abnormally low potassium concentration in the blood.

HYPOTONUS The state characterized by a decreased tonicity or tension.

LOWER MOTOR NEURONS Peripheral neurons whose cell bodies lie in the central gray columns of the spinal cord and whose terminations are in skeletal muscles. A sufficient number of lesions of lower motor neurons causes muscles supplied by the nerve to atrophy, resulting in weak reflexes and flaccid paralysis.

MICTURITION Urination.

NOCTURIA Excessive urination at night.

POLYDIPSIA Excessive thirst.

POLYURIA Excessive urination.

UPPER MOTOR NEURONS Neurons in the cerebral cortex that conduct impulses from the motor cortex to the motor nuclei of the cerebral nerves or to the ventral gray columns of the spinal column. A sufficient number of lesions of upper motor neurons interrupts the inhibitory effect that upper motor neurons have on lower motor neurons, resulting in exaggerated or hyperactive reflexes.

UREMIA Abnormally high concentrations of urea, creatinine, and other nitrogenous end products of protein and amino acid metabolism in the blood.

URINARY INCONTINENCE Lack of voluntary control over the normal excretion of urine.

URINARY TRACT INFECTION Infection of the urinary tract. The infection may be localized or may affect the entire urinary tract.

INTRODUCTION

The urinary system is composed of the kidneys, ureters, bladder, and urethra (Figures 6-1 to 6-4). The urinary system regulates several functions, including water balance, acid-base balance, osmotic pressure, electrolyte levels, and concentrations of many plasma substances. This system is also active in the elimination of many drugs and toxins from the body. Homeostasis may be interrupted by changes in plasma composition, cardiovascular changes (e.g., arterial blood pressure), hormones, the autonomic nervous system, and certain drugs and toxins.

Veterinary technicians should educate clients regarding the importance of nutrition, especially in

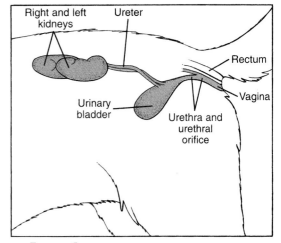

FIGURE 6-1
Side view of the urogenital system of a female dog.

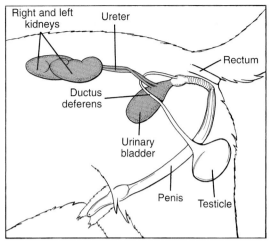

FIGURE 6-2
Side view of the urogenital system of a male dog.

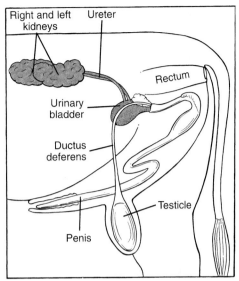

FIGURE 6-4
Side view of the urogenital system of a bull.

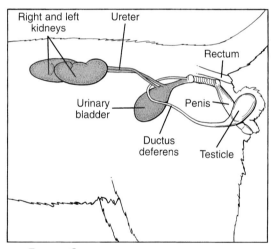

FIGURE 6-3
Side view of the urogenital system of a male cat.

those dog breeds predisposed to developing bladder stones (e.g., Dalmatians, miniature schnauzers, etc.). Fresh water should be available for animals at all times. Companion animals observed straining to urinate or with bloody urine (i.e., **hematuria**) should be presented to the veterinary hospital immediately.

PHYSIOLOGIC PRINCIPLES

The formation of urine is a rather complex process that involves glomerular filtration, tubular reabsorption, and tubular secretion (Figure 6-5). The glomerular filtrate is composed of water and dissolved substances, which pass from the plasma into the glomerular capsule. The formation of glomerular filtrate is controlled by the effective filtration pressure [EFP = arterial blood pressure − (plasma osmotic pressure · capsule pressure)]. The amount of glomerular filtrate is directly proportional to the effective filtration pressure (Figure 6-6). Any changes in blood flow through the glomerulus, glomerular blood pressure, plasma osmotic pressure, or capsule pressure affect glomerular filtration.

The kidney tubules are responsible for the reabsorption, or the secretion, of certain substances. Substances needed by the body are reabsorbed from the filtrate, pass through the tubular cell wall, and reenter the plasma. This process filters needed substances and returns them to the body. Reabsorbed materials include water, glucose, amino acids, urea, and ions such as Na^+, K^+, Ca^{2+}, Cl^-, HCO_3^-, and

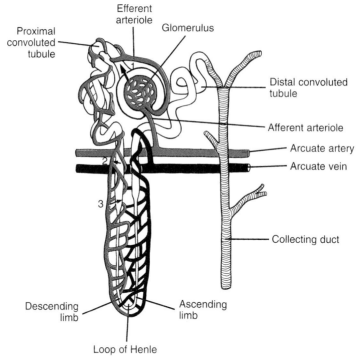

FIGURE 6-5
Shown are the direction and location of glomerular filtration: *1*, tubular reabsorption; *2*, tubular secretion; *3*, as they would occur in the glomerulus and proximal tubule.

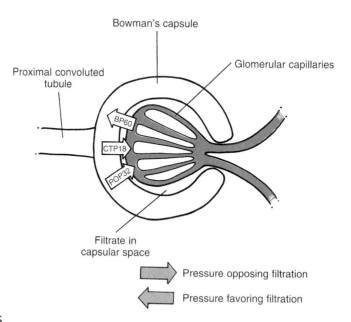

FIGURE 6-6
Filtration occurs through the glomerular membrane within Bowman's capsule. The amount of filtrate produced is determined by the difference between the pressures favoring filtration and those opposing filtration. This diagram shows that filtration occurs because 60 − (32 + 18) = 10 mm Hg. Values greater than or less than 10 mm Hg would correlate with more or less filtration, respectively. Pressure values (60, 32, 18) are measured in mm Hg. *BP,* blood pressure; *CTP,* capsular tissue pressure; *POP,* plasma osmotic pressure.

HPO_4^{2-}. Any excess of these substances, or substances that are not useful, remain in the filtrate and are excreted in the urine.

Tubular secretion occurs when substances are carried to the tubular lumen. This includes the active transport of certain endogenous substances and many exogenous substances. These secreted substances include potassium and hydrogen ions, ammonia, creatinine, and some drugs. The main effects of tubular secretion are to rid the body of certain materials and help control blood pH (Figure 6-7). The kidneys are active in the metabolizing and excreting of many drugs and their metabolites. Therefore, it is very important to remember that these actions may be inhibited in cases of renal failure or dysfunction. Drug therapy in animals with renal dysfunction has increased risks. Renal failure can impair a drug's absorption from an administration site or affect a drug's distribution in the body.

Uremia can increase the sensitivity of some tissues to certain drugs. For example, sensitivity to central nervous system depressants is increased, and therefore the dose of opiates, barbiturates, and tranquilizers should be reduced in uremic patients. Xylazine (Rompun) and ketamine hydrochloride (Ketaset) are contraindicated in uremic patients. Impaired renal excretion or biotransformation causes delayed elimination of many drugs and increases their toxicity and duration of action.

Box 6-1 lists common drugs that may require dosage modification in renal insufficiency. Modification can be made by measuring the plasma concentration of drugs and adjusting the dose accordingly. Since this is usually impractical in

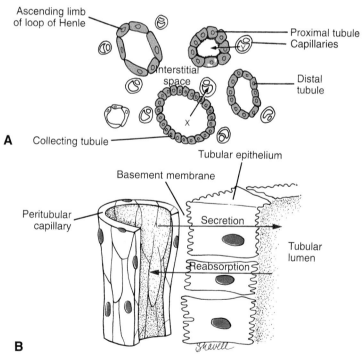

FIGURE 6-7
Tubular reabsorption and secretion. **A,** Cross-section of nephron tubules and peritubular capillaries. Interstitial fluid occupies the interstitial space. Reabsorption is represented by substance X going from tubule to capillary, and secretion is represented by substance Y going from capillary to tubule. **B,** Longitudinal section of nephron tubule. Shown is the relationship among the tubular lumen, epithelial cell, and capillary. (From Reece WO: Physiology of domestic animals, Philadelphia, 1991, Lea & Febiger.)

BOX 6-1 Dosage Modifications in Renal Insufficiency

Drugs that Require Dosage Modification or that are Contraindicated in Renal Insufficiency

Acetazolamide
Antimonials
Aspirin
Atropine
Barbital
Bendroflumethiazide
Cephalothins
Chelating agents
Chlorothiazide
Clindamycin
Colistin and polymyxin
Decamethonium
Digoxin
Erythomycin
Furosemide (increased dose)
Gentamicin
Iodide
Kanamycin
Lincomycin
Mannitol
Mercurials
Methenamine
Methotrexate
Neomycin
Neostigmine
Nitrofurantoin
Ouabain
Penicillins
Phenazopyridine
Procainamide
Spironolactone
Streptomycin
Sulfonamides
Tetracyclines
Tetraethyl-ammonium
Tubocurarine, gallamine
Vancomycin

Drugs that do *not* Require Dosage Modification or that are *not* Contraindicated in Renal Insufficiency

Acetaminophen
Chloramphenicol
Diazepam
Narcotic analgesics
Novobiocin
Pentobarbital
Phenobarbital
Phenothiazine
Phenytoin
Procaine
Propranolol

From Kirk RW: Current veterinary therapy VII: small animal practice, Philadelphia, 1980, WB Saunders Co.

most clinical settings, a veterinarian may use the normal dose but lengthen the time intervals at which it is administered or give a smaller dose at the normal time intervals. Technicians may be responsible for administering anesthesia, and it is important to remember that patients with renal failure are a greater anesthetic risk and require even closer monitoring than patients with normal renal function.

RENAL FAILURE

Renal failure is among the major causes of nonaccidental death in dogs and cats. Although the disease is most common in older animals, it may be diagnosed in younger animals. Renal damage may stem from many causes, including infectious diseases, toxins, neoplasia, congenital disorders, immunologic problems, and amyloidosis. Diets with excessive protein, phosphorus, and sodium are also factors that may cause renal damage. Renal damage may be categorized as prerenal, renal, and postrenal. Renal failure may be differentiated as acute or chronic according to certain parameters common to each condition.

COMMON DRUGS FOR THE TREATMENT OF RENAL DYSFUNCTION AND ASSOCIATED HYPERTENSION

 Diuretic Drugs

Diuretics are used to remove excess extracellular fluid by increasing urine flow and sodium excretion, and reducing **hypertension.** A number of conditions may indicate the need for a diuretic drug. The classifications of commonly used diuretics are loop diuretics, osmotic diuretics, thiazide and thiazide-like diuretics, potassium-sparing diuretics, and carbonic anhydrase inhibitors.

Loop Diuretics
Loop diuretics are highly potent diuretics that inhibit the tubular reabsorption of sodium. Once administered, their actions are generally rapid. Additionally, loop diuretics increase the excretion of chloride, potassium, and water.

Dosage Forms
1. Furosemide (Lasix, Disal, Diuride)
2. Ethacrynic acid (Edecrin—human label)

Adverse Side Effects. These include **hypokalemia** because of the increased excretion of potassium.

> *Technician's Notes*
> To prevent hypokalemia, a potassium supplement is commonly given to patients who are receiving long-term potassium-depleting diuretic therapy.

Osmotic Diuretics
Osmotic diuretics can be administered intravenously to promote diuresis by exerting high osmotic pressure in the kidney tubules and limiting tubular reabsorption. Water is drawn into the glomerular filtrate, reducing the reabsorption and increasing the excretion of water. These drugs may be used to treat oliguric acute renal failure and to reduce intracranial pressure.

Dosage Forms
1. Mannitol 20%
2. Glucose

Adverse Side Effects. These are uncommon.

> *Technician's Notes*
> These drugs are administered over a 10- to 15-minute period.

Thiazide Diuretics
Thiazide diuretics reduce edema by inhibiting reabsorption of sodium, chloride, and water. Their duration of action is longer than that of loop diuretics.

Dosage Forms
1. Chlorothiazide (Diuril—human label)
2. Hydrochlorothiazide (HydroDIURIL—human label)

Adverse Side Effects. These include hypokalemia if therapy is prolonged.

> *Technician's Notes*
> 1. Like loop diuretics, thiazide diuretics cause an increase in potassium excretion. A potassium supplement may be necessary to prevent hypokalemia.
> 2. These drugs will cross the placental border.

Potassium-Sparing Diuretics
Potassium-sparing diuretics have weaker diuretic and antihypertensive effects than other diuretics, but they have the ability to conserve potassium. These agents are also referred to as aldosterone antagonists. They work by antagonizing aldosterone, an adrenal mineralocorticoid. This action increases the excretion of sodium and water and reduces the excretion of potassium. Aldosterone secretion may be a factor in edema associated with heart failure.

Dosage Forms
1. Spironolactone (Aldactone—human label)
2. Triamterene (Diazide, Dyrenium—human label)

Adverse Side Effects. These are uncommon, but hyperkalemia may result if these drugs are administered concurrently with potassium supplements or angiotensin-converting enzyme (ACE) inhibitors, such as captopril or enalapril.

Technician's Notes
These drugs may be used alone or with other diuretic agents.

Carbonic Anhydrase Inhibitors

A carbonic anhydrase inhibitor is a substance that decreases the rate of carbonic acid and H^+ production in the kidney, thereby increasing the excretion of solutes and the rate of urinary output (Mosby, 1998). These drugs also reduce intraocular pressure by reducing the production of aqueous humor and may be used in the treatment of glaucoma.

Dosage Forms
1. Acetazolamide (Diamox—human label)
2. Dichlorphenamide (Daranide—human label)

Adverse Side Effects. These include the ability to cause hypokalemia.

Technician's Notes
Carbonic anhydrase inhibitors have the least efficacy when compared with the other tubular inhibitors and are not commonly used to treat edema.

 ## Cholinergic Agonists

Cholinergic agents act directly or indirectly to promote the function of acetylcholine. The cholinergic agents may also be referred to as *parasympath-* *omimetic agents* because their effects mimic the stimulation of the parasympathetic nervous system. Cholinergic **agonists** mimic the action of natural acetylcholine by directly stimulating cholinergic receptors. Once the cholinergic agonist binds with the receptors on the cell membrane of smooth muscles, the permeability of the cell membrane changes, permitting calcium and sodium to enter into the cells. Depolarization of the cell membrane occurs, and muscle contraction is achieved.

Clinical Uses. Cholinergic agents are used to help void the urinary bladder. Their action increases the tone of the detrusor muscle of the bladder and decreases bladder capacity.

Dosage Form
Bethanechol (Urecholine—human label)

Adverse Side Effects. These include the potential for cholinergic toxicity.

 Technician's Notes
1. Observe the patient for signs of cholinergic toxicity (e.g., vomiting, defecation, dyspnea, and tremors).
2. Atropine is antidotal.

Anticholinergic Drugs

The action of anticholinergic drugs is the opposite of the cholinergic agents. They block the action of acetylcholine at receptor sites in the parasympathetic nervous system. These drugs may also be described as parasympatholytic because of their ability to block the passage of impulses through the parasympathetic nerves. Their action produces muscle relaxation.

Clinical Uses. Anticholinergic drugs can be used for treating urge incontinence by promoting the retention of urine in the urinary bladder.

Dosage Forms
1. Propantheline (Pro-Banthine—human label)
2. Butyl hyoscine (Buscopan)

Adverse Side Effects. These include decreased gastric motility and delayed gastric emptying, which may decrease the absorption of other medications.

 Adrenergic Antagonists

Adrenergic blocking agents disrupt the sympathetic nervous system by blocking impulse transmission at adrenergic neurons, adrenergic receptor sites, or adrenergic ganglia. These agents may also be described as sympatholytic agents because of their ability to block sympathetic nervous system stimulation. The classification of adrenergic **antagonists** is based on their site of action (i.e., alpha blockers, beta blockers, or autonomic ganglionic blockers).

Alpha-Adrenergic Antagonists
Alpha-adrenergic antagonists relax vascular smooth muscle, increase peripheral vasodilation, and decrease blood pressure by interrupting the actions of sympathomimetic agents at alpha-adrenergic receptor sites.

Clinical Uses. In the urinary system, these drugs reduce internal sphincter tone when the urethral sphincter is in **hypertonus.** This action is useful in the treatment of urinary retention because of **detrusor areflexia** or functional urethral obstruction. Prazosin is effective in controlling moderate to severe hypertension, which may be a complicating factor in chronic renal failure.

Dosage Forms
1. Phenoxybenzamine (Dibenzyline—human label)
2. Nicergoline (Sermion)
3. Moxisylyte (Carlytene)
4. Prazosin (Minipress—human label)

Adverse Side Effects. These include rapid decrease of blood pressure, resulting in weakness or syncope

after the first dose of prazosin. This is usually self-limiting.

Technician's Notes
1. Prazosin may be used alone or combined with a diuretic to produce the desired effect.
2. Since alpha-adrenergic antagonists are metabolized by the liver, dosage modification is not necessary in patients with renal dysfunction.

Beta-Adrenergic Antagonists
Beta-adrenergic antagonists inhibit the action of **catecholamines** and other sympathomimetic agents at beta-adrenergic receptor sites and thereby inhibit stimulation of the sympathetic nervous system.

Clinical Uses. These include control of mild to moderate hypertension associated with chronic renal failure.

Dosage Form
Propranolol (Inderal—human label)

Adverse Side Effects. These include decreased cardiac output and the promotion of bronchospasm. Therefore caution should be exercised with their use in patients with cardiac or pulmonary disease (Cowgill, 1991).

Technician's Notes
Combination with a diuretic is common because of beta-adrenergic antagonists' tendency to cause salt and fluid retention.

 Angiotensin-Converting Enzyme Inhibitors

ACE inhibitors block the conversion of angiotensin I to angiotensin II, decrease aldosterone secretion, decrease peripheral arterial resistance, and alleviate vasoconstriction.

Clinical Uses. ACE inhibitors are used to treat nonresponding hypertension or moderate to severe hypertension.

Dosage Forms
1. Benazepril
   a. Fortekor (veterinary)
   b. Lotensin (human)
2. Captopril (Capoten—human label)
3. Enalapril (Enacard)

Adverse Side Effects. These include complications in patients with renal insufficiency because of excretion by the kidneys.

Vasodilators and Calcium Channel Blockers

A vasodilator or calcium channel blocker may be substituted for or used in combination with other medications if previous drug therapy to control hypertension fails.

Clinical Uses. These drugs are used to treat nonresponding hypertension. Dopamine may be used to promote diuresis in patients unresponsive to loop or osmotic diuretics.

Dosage Forms
1. Vasodilators
   a. Hydralazine (Apresoline—human label)
   b. Dopamine (Intropin—human label)
2. Calcium channel blockers
   a. Diltiazem (Cardizem—human label)
   b. Verapamil (Isoptin—human label)

Adverse Side Effects. These include hypotension, edema, conduction disturbances, heart failure, and bradycardia (Cowgill, 1991). Hydralazine is excreted by the kidneys and requires dosage modification when used to treat hypertension in patients with renal failure.

Antidiuretic Hormone

Antidiuretic hormone (ADH) is normally secreted by the posterior pituitary gland. This secretion regulates fluid balance in the body. In some conditions, such as pituitary diabetes insipidus, this hormone fails to be synthesized or excreted properly and **polyuria** and **polydipsia** occur.

Clinical Uses. ADH is used to treat diabetes insipidus.

Dosage Form
Vasopressin (Pitressin—human label)

Adverse Side Effects. These are uncommon.

> *Technician's Notes*
> Chlorpropamide (Diabinese, Glucamide) is a human product used to control type II diabetes mellitus. It potentiates the action of ADH and may be used to treat mild diabetes insipidus.

Urinary Acidifiers

Urinary acidifiers are used to produce acid urine, which assists in dissolving and preventing formation of struvite uroliths. Since the introduction of urinary acidifying diets, urinary acidifiers have not been routinely prescribed.

Dosage Forms
1. Methionine (Methigel, Methio-Tabs)
2. Ammonium chloride (Uroeze)

Adverse Side Effects. These include gastrointestinal disturbance. These products should not be administered to patients with severe liver, kidney, or pancreatic diseases or to those exhibiting acidosis.

Xanthine Oxidase Inhibitors

Xanthine oxidase inhibitors decrease the production of uric acid and are used in combination with a urate calculolytic diet for the dissolution of ammonium acid urate uroliths. Once dissolution occurs, a urine-alkalizing, low-protein, low-purine, low-oxalate diet is usually prescribed to prevent recurrence of the uroliths.

Dosage Form
Allopurinol (Zyloprim—human label)

Adverse Side Effects. These are uncommon, but because excretion occurs via the kidneys, the dosage may be altered in patients with renal insufficiency.

Urinary Alkalizers

Urinary alkalizers may be used in the management of ammonium acid urate, calcium oxalate, and cystine urolithiasis.

Dosage Forms
1. Potassium citrate (Urocit-K—human label)
2. Sodium bicarbonate, administered orally
3. Tiopronin tablets (Thiola—human label)

Adverse Side Effects. These include possible fluid and electrolyte imbalance with the use of sodium bicarbonate.

PHARMACOTHERAPY OF RENAL FAILURE COMPLICATIONS

Since the renal cortex produces erythropoietin, chronic renal failure can cause an absolute or relative deficiency in its production. The resulting complication is normocytic, normochromic anemia. Parenteral androgens, such as nandrolone (Durabolin) and testosterone enanthate, are capable of stimulating the production of red blood cell precursors and may increase the level of erythropoietin. Recombinant human erythropoietin (Epogen) has been shown to correct anemia associated with chronic renal failure (Ettinger, 2000). Vitamin D supplements may be used in the control of renal secondary hyperparathyroidism. Rocaltrol and dihydrotachysterol (Hytakerol) may be used for this purpose. Serum calcium, creatinine, and phosphate levels should be monitored in patients receiving this therapy because hypercalcemia, hyperphosphatemia, or deteriorating renal function can occur (Ettinger, 2000).

PHARMACOTHERAPY OF URINARY INCONTINENCE

Ettinger (2000) states: "pharmacologic agents are selected for management of **urinary incontinence** when **urinary tract infection,** morphologic abnormalities, and mechanical types of excessive outlet resistance have been excluded as possible causes of the problem." Urinary incontinence may be described as a neurogenic disorder or a nonneurogenic disorder. A neurogenic disorder is evidenced by a neurologic lesion that affects either the **upper motor neuron** segments or the **lower motor neuron** segments. When the upper motor neuron segments are affected, the result is a spastic neuropathic bladder.

The **detrusor** muscle contractions are normal, but the bladder and urethral functions are abnormal. Therefore as the bladder fills with urine, contractions will occur more frequently (hypercontractility) and bladder capacity will decrease. Also, the contraction of the detrusor muscle and the relaxation of the urethral sphincter are often not coordinated. This results in interrupted, incomplete, and involuntary urination.

Functional urinary obstruction and urinary retention may also be present. When the lower motor neuron segments are affected, the result is an **atonic,** neuropathic bladder. With this disorder, the detrusor muscle contractions are abnormal and the sensation of fullness is absent when the bladder fills (hypocontractility). This causes the bladder to distend, and eventually bladder capacity increases. Bladder distention may also cause damage to the tight junctions between the smooth muscle fibers. Urination eventually occurs when the pressure inside the bladder exceeds the urethral outlet resistance.

Nonneurogenic disorders occur as a result of some type of anatomic anomaly of the lower urinary tract. In the young dog this is usually a congenital anomaly. A congenital anomaly seen in young female dogs is ectopic ureter, which causes constant dribbling of urine. This occurs when the ureters end in abnormal places rather than at the normal sphincters. In the older dog, acquired anatomic anomalies are usually responsible for nonneurogenic disorders. The conditions that commonly cause such problems include chronic cystitis, chronic urethritis, neoplasia, urolithiasis, and postsurgical adhesions. Other nonneurogenic disorders include functional abnormalities, such as urethral incompetence and partial urethral obstruction. One type of nonneurogenic urethral incompetence is often seen in spayed female dogs and is usually responsive to hormonal therapy. Once the cause of the urinary incontinence is identified, medical or surgical management will begin. If there is a morphologic abnormality that is causing urinary incontinence, surgical correction of the problem will be necessary.

Medical management may include treatment of infection, if present, and treatment for the cause of the urinary incontinence (e.g., urethral incompetence or bladder hypercontractility or hypocontractility). The drugs used in the medical management of urinary incontinence include the previously mentioned cholinergic agonists, anticholinergics, alpha-adrenergic antagonists, smooth muscle relaxants, skeletal muscle relaxants, tranquilizers, alpha-adrenergic agonists, and hormones—such as estrogen and testosterone. Table 6-1 outlines these drugs for easy reference.

Table 6-1 Pharmacotherapy of Urinary Incontinence

Drug	Action	Examples of Indications
Bethanechol (Urecholine)	Cholinergic agonist	Bladder hypocontractility
Propantheline (Pro-Banthine)	Anticholingeric agent	Urge incontinence, bladder hypercontractility
Butyl hyoscine (Buscopan)	Anticholingeric agent	Urge incontinence, bladder hypercontractility
Phenoxybenzamine (Dibenzyline)	Alpha-adrenergic antagonist	Urethral hyperreflexia
Nicergoline (Sermion)	Alpha-adrenergic antagonist	Urethral hyperreflexia
Moxisylyte (Carlytene)	Alpha-adrenergic antagonist	Urethral hyperreflexia
Aminopropazine (Jenotone)	Smooth muscle relaxant	Urge incontinence, bladder hypercontractility
Dantrolene (Dantrium)	Skeletal muscle relaxant	Urethral hyperreflexia
Diazepam (Valium)	Tranquilizer/skeletal muscle relaxant	Urethral hyperreflexia
Phenylporpanolamine	Alpha-adrenergic agonist	Urethral incompetence
Diethylstilbestrol (DES)	Antineoplastic, estrogen (hormone)	Hormone-responsive urethral incompetence
Testosterone cypionate	Hormone	Hormone-responsive urethral incompetence
Testosterone propionate	Hormone	Hormone-responsive urethral incompetence

Miscellaneous Renal Drugs

Urinary Tract Analgesics
PHENAZOPYRIDINE
Phenazopyridine is used in humans as a urinary tract analgesic. It can be bought over-the-counter. It can be used alone or with sulfa drugs. Its use is contraindicated in felines because they are quite susceptible to dose-related methemoglobinemia and oxidative changes in hemoglobin may be irreversible, causing formation of Heinz bodies and anemia (Osborne, 2001).

Tricyclic Antidepressants
AMITRIPTYLINE
Dosage form
Amitriptyline (Elavil)

Amitriptyline has many properties and has been used in treating interstitial cystitis in humans. Its mechanism is not fully understood. Amitriptyline is a tricyclic, antidepressant, and anxiolytic drug with anticholinergic, antihistaminic, antialpha-adrenergic, antiinflammatory, and analgesic properties. It has been used extensively for treatment of interstitial cystitis in humans. Although a popular drug, its exact mechanism of action and therapeutic value in managing patients with interstitial cystitis is unknown. This drug has recently been used for symptomatic therapy of idiopathic feline lower urinary tract disease (LUTD) (Osborne, 2001).

Adverse Side Effects. Many side effects are associated with this drug, such as dry mouth, rapid heart rate, sedation (i.e., antihistamine effects). High doses can cause heart toxicity. Sometimes it may cause cats to be less interested in grooming themselves. Additionally, weight gain may occur (Papich, 2002).

Glycosaminoglycans
Glycosaminoglycans (GAGs) are found covering the transitional epithelium of the urinary tract. These urothelial GAGs have the ability to keep microorganisms and crystals from adhering to the bladder wall and also limit the transepithelial movement of urine proteins and solutes (ionic or nonionic). Defects in surface GAGs and subsequent urothelial permeability are supposed to be a factor in the pathogenesis of feline idiopathic LUTD (Osborne, 2001).

PENTOSAN POLYSULFATE SODIUM (ELMIRON)
Clinical Uses. Often used to manage human interstitial cystitis. Used to reinforce urothelial glycosaminoglycans (GAGs) and reduces transitional cell injury.

Adverse effects. The safety and efficacy of pentosan polysulfate or other GAGs for the treatment of feline LUTD has not been reported. This treatment remains a logical choice, but it is not possible to make recommendations at this time (Osborne, 2001).

TECHNICIAN'S ROLE

Veterinary technicians have a vital role in the care of patients with problems affecting the urinary system. This role includes providing client support and education, carrying out patient nursing care, performing necessary laboratory or radiologic examinations, giving surgical assistance, and understanding the various drugs and diets available for the treatment of renal diseases.

REFERENCES
Anderson KN and Anderson L, editors: Mosby's pocket dictionary of medicine, nursing, and allied health, ed 4, St. Louis, 2002, Mosby.

Cowgill LD: Clinical significance, diagnosis, and management of systemic hypertension in dogs and cats. In Cowgill LD: Managing renal disease and hypertension, 1991, Harmon-Smith.

Ettinger SJ: Textbook of veterinary internal medicine, vol. I and II, ed 5, Philadelphia, 2000, WB Saunders Co.

Giovanoni R and Warren RG: Principles of pharmacology, St. Louis, 1983, Mosby.

Mosby's pocket dictionary of medicine, nursing and allied health, ed 3, St. Louis, 1998, Mosby.

Osborne CA: Idiopathic lower urinary tract diseases: Therapeutic rights and wrongs, Boston, 2001, Proceedings of the annual meeting of the American Veterinary Medical Association.

Papich MG: Saunders handbook of veterinary drugs, Philadelphia, 2002, Saunders.

REVIEW QUESTIONS

1. What structures constitute the urinary system?

   _____

2. Name two drugs contraindicated in uremic patients. _____

3. Renal damage may be categorized as

   _____,

   _____, or

   _____.

4. Explain how diuretics work.

   _____.

5. What supplement may be administered in conjunction with loop diuretics?

   _____.

6. ACE inhibitors block the conversion of angiotensin I to _____.

7. Urinary acidifiers are used to produce acid urine, which assists in dissolving and preventing the formation of

   _____ uroliths.

8. The renal cortex produces

   _____, and thus chronic renal failure can cause an absolute or relative

   _____ in its production.

9. Why is furosemide referred to as a loop diuretic? _____.

10. Where is ADH secreted?

INTRODUCTION
ANATOMY AND PHYSIOLOGY OF THE HEART
COMPENSATORY MECHANISMS OF THE CARDIOVASCULAR SYSTEM
BASIC OBJECTIVES IN THE TREATMENT OF CARDIOVASCULAR DISEASE
CATEGORIES OF CARDIOVASCULAR DRUGS
Positive Inotropic Drugs
   Cardiac Glycosides (Digitalis)
   Catecholamines
      EPINEPHRINE
      ISOPROTERENOL
      DOPAMINE
      DOBUTAMINE
   Bipyridine Derivatives
Antiarrhythmic Drugs
   Class IA
      QUINIDINE
      PROCAINAMIDE
   Class IB
      LIDOCAINE
      TOCAINIDE AND MEXILETINE
   Class IC
   Class II
      PROPRANOLOL
      ATENOLOL
      OTHER BETA BLOCKERS
   Class III
   Class IV
      VERAPAMIL HYDROCHLORIDE
      DILTIAZEM
   Other Class IV Antiarrhythmics
Vasodilator Drugs
   Hydralazine
   Nitroglycerin Ointment
   Prazosin
   Angiotensin-Converting Enzyme Inhibitors
Diuretics
   Furosemide
   Thiazides
   Spironolactone
DIETARY MANAGEMENT OF HEART DISEASE
ANCILLARY TREATMENT OF HEART FAILURE
   Bronchodilators
   Oxygen Therapy
   Sedation
   Aspirin
   Thoracocentesis and Abdominocentesis

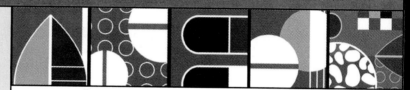

CHAPTER **7**

Drugs Used in Cardiovascular System Disorders

LEARNING OBJECTIVES

After studying this chapter, you should be able to:

1. Describe the basic anatomy and physiology of the cardiovascular system
2. List four compensatory mechanisms of the cardiovascular system
3. List five basic objectives of the treatment of cardiovascular disease
4. Differentiate between an inotropic and a chronotropic drug
5. List and describe the indications, physiologic effects, and toxic side effects of the cardiac glycosides
6. List the four categories of antiarrhythmic drugs and an example in each category
7. List potential adverse side effects of the antiarrhythmic drugs
8. Describe the actions and potential side effects of the vasodilator drugs
9. Describe the actions and potential side effects of the angiotensin-converting enzyme (ACE) inhibitors
10. Describe the actions and potential side effects of the diuretics used to treat cardiovascular disease
11. Describe the purpose of dietary sodium restriction in the therapy of cardiovascular disease
12. List ancillary drugs or procedures that may be used in the treatment of cardiovascular disease

KEY TERMS

AFTERLOAD The resistance (pressure) in arteries that must be overcome to empty blood from the ventricle.

ARRHYTHMIA (DYSRHYTHMIA) A variation from the normal rhythm.

AUTOMATICITY The ability of cardiac muscle to generate impulses.

BRADYARRHYTHMIA Bradycardia associated with an irregularity of heart rhythm.

BRADYCARDIA A slower-than-normal heart rate.

CHRONOTROPIC Affecting the heart rate.

DEPOLARIZATION Neutralizing of the polarity of a cardiac cell by an inflow of sodium ions. Depolarization results in contraction of the cardiac cell and renders it incapable of further contraction until repolarization occurs.

INOTROPIC Affecting the force of cardiac muscle contraction.

PRELOAD The volume of blood in the ventricles at the end of diastole.

PREMATURE VENTRICULAR CONTRACTION (PVC) Contraction of the ventricles without a corresponding contraction of the atria. PVCs arise from an irritable focus or foci in the ventricles.

REPOLARIZATION The return of the cell membrane to its resting polarity after depolarization.

STROKE VOLUME The amount of blood ejected by the left ventricle with each beat.

TACHYARRHYTHMIA Tachycardia associated with an irregularity of normal heart rhythm.

TACHYCARDIA A faster-than-normal heart rate.

INTRODUCTION

Heart disease has a relatively high incidence in veterinary medicine. Studies have found that approximately 11% of all dogs presented to veterinary clinics exhibited some degree of heart disease (Roudebush, et al, 2000). Heart disease may be congenital or acquired. However, the acquired form accounts for most of the cases. The incidence and cause may vary from location to location. Heartworm disease accounts for a large percentage of heart disease in some parts of the country, whereas acquired disease of the atrioventricular valves or myocardium has a more uniform distribution. Acquired disease is encountered more often in older animals, and congenital disease is more prevalent in younger ones.

Whatever the cause, treatment of heart disease is often individualized to the particular patient according to the cause, degree of progression, and owner cooperation. The response to treatment must be carefully monitored and adjusted while the disease progresses and causes poor liver or kidney function or while toxic side effects develop. Some cardiovascular drugs have a narrow margin of safety (i.e., they are potentially toxic at low doses), and failing liver and kidney function may reduce

the body's ability to metabolize or eliminate the drugs.

Because veterinary technicians are often the persons monitoring the progress of hospitalized patients, they must be aware of the signs of cardiovascular disease and of the normal and abnormal responses to the drugs used to treat this disease.

ANATOMY AND PHYSIOLOGY OF THE HEART

The heart is a four-chambered pump that is responsible for moving blood through the vascular system. The two dorsal chambers are called *atria*, and the two ventral chambers are called *ventricles* (Figure 7-1). Each of the chambers is composed primarily of strong muscle tissue called *myocardium*, which contracts to eject the blood. Even though the heart is considered one organ, it is functionally two pumps (Spinelli and Enos, 1978).

The right atrium and ventricle constitute the "right-side pump," and the left atrium and ventricle make up the "left-side pump." Blood from the general circulation returns by way of the vena cava to the right atrium, enters the right ventricle through the right atrioventricular valve (tricuspid

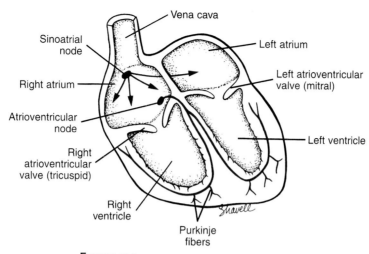

FIGURE 7-1
Schematic of the heart and its conduction system.

valve), and is pumped through the pulmonary artery to the lungs. In the lungs, the blood gives up carbon dioxide and picks up oxygen. The oxygenated blood returns to the heart via the pulmonary veins, where it fills the left atrium, passes through the left atrioventricular valve (mitral valve), and enters the left ventricle. The mitral and tricuspid valves swing open when the atria contract and snap shut when the ventricles contract. The closing of the valves as the ventricles contract prevents blood from flowing back into the atria. The left ventricle then contracts and ejects the oxygenated blood through the aorta out into the branching arteries. These arteries divide into arterioles and end in the thin-walled capillaries throughout the body where carbon dioxide is loaded to the blood and oxygen is unloaded to the tissue. Because the left ventricle must work harder to pump blood throughout the body than the right ventricle must work to pump blood to the lungs, the left ventricular wall is thicker than the right ventricular wall.

The pumping action of the heart is divided into two phases, systole and diastole. Systole is the period of contraction of the chambers, and diastole represents the relaxation phase when the chambers are filling with blood. Because each cell in the heart

is capable of contracting spontaneously, the interaction of these two phases must be carefully coordinated to create an efficient pumping action. Diastolic time must be adequate to allow the atria to fill completely, and atrial systole must occur shortly before ventricular systole to allow the ventricles to fill maximally. Coordination of these two phases is achieved primarily by a wave of electric activity that arises in a specialized group of cells in the right atrium and is then conducted throughout the myocardium by a special conduction system.

The structures that make up the cardiac conduction system (see Figure 7-1) include the sinoatrial node, the atrioventricular node, the bundle of His and its branches, and the Purkinje system. Under abnormal conditions, parts of the myocardium and conduction system are capable of spontaneous discharge. Normally, however, the sinoatrial node discharges most rapidly and spreads a wave of depolarization over the remaining areas of the heart before they can depolarize spontaneously. The rate of discharge of this node therefore controls the heart rate and is called the *cardiac pacemaker*. The impulses generated by the sinoatrial node travel over the atria to the atrioventricular node, face a brief delay (about 0.1 second) in the atrioventricular node, travel down the bundle of

His to its left and right branches, and pass into the ventricular muscle via the Purkinje fibers. Myocardial cells are joined together by structures called *intercalated disks* and by fusing of cell membranes into an interconnected mass of cells called a *syncytium*. The syncytium of cells in the atria is separate and insulated from the syncytium in the ventricles (Ganong, 2003). An electric stimulus from the sinoatrial node is transmitted over the entire atrial mass by the syncytial arrangement of cells. The impulse is not, however, transmitted directly into the ventricular syncytium. The impulse first must be picked up and transmitted by the atrioventricular node through its conduction system to the ventricular syncytium. Stimulation of a single atrial or ventricular muscle fiber causes the entire atrial or ventricular muscle mass to contract as a unit. When situations cause spontaneous depolarization of cardiac muscle or abnormalities of the conduction system, **arrhythmias** may occur.

When a cardiac cell is stimulated by electric activity arising in the sinoatrial node, it undergoes depolarization and contracts. **Depolarization** is characterized by the rapid influx of sodium ions into the cell through channels or "gates," the slower influx of calcium ions, and the outflow of potassium ions (Figure 7-2). Until the sodium, potassium, and calcium ions have returned to the positions they had before depolarization, the cell is in a refractory period (Figure 7-3). A cell in an absolute refractory state cannot normally depolarize. In a relative refractory period, however, a cardiac cell can depolarize again but the stimulus must be stronger than normal (Bill, 1997). A refractory period is essential for a cardiac cell to prevent it from remaining in a constant state of contraction resulting from stimulation by recycling impulses. The return of the ions to their original positions is brought about in part by the sodium-potassium pump and is an essential part of the **repolarization** process. The summed electric activity arising from the contraction of all the heart cells represents the electrocardiogram (Figure 7-4), with each of its waves signifying activity in a particular area.

Even though the heart establishes its own inherent rate of beating, this rate is also subject to outside

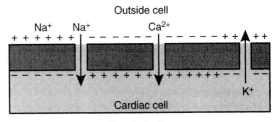

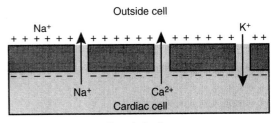

FIGURE 7-2

Depolarization and repolarization of a cardiac cell. Repolarization: The $Na^+ = K^+$ = ATPase pump restores the electrolytes to their resting sites.

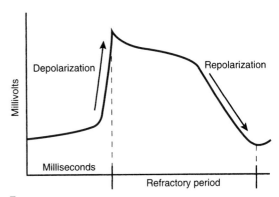

FIGURE 7-3

Schematic of the refractory period of a cardiac cell. After depolarization (contraction), cardiac muscle cells are unable to contract again until they have undergone repolarization. The time while they are unable to contract is the refractory period.

influences through the autonomic nervous system. The sympathetic portion of the autonomic nervous system, through beta-1 receptors, produces positive **chronotropic** and **inotropic** effects on the heart. The parasympathetic branch of the autonomic

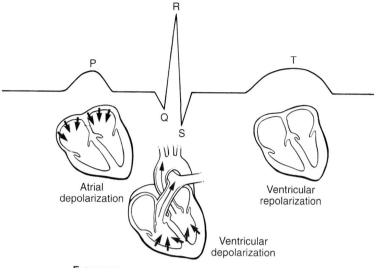

FIGURE 7-4
Cardiac events as depicted on an electrocardiogram.

nervous system causes negative chronotropic effects through cholinergic receptors.

The heart pumps blood through a series of arteries (arterial tree) to deliver it to the tissues. The larger of these arteries have elastic properties, which allow them to stretch and recover when blood is pumped into them—thereby serving as a second pump (Upson, 1988). The smaller arteries are capable of changing their diameter (constricting or dilating) through the action of smooth muscle in their walls to increase or decrease the resistance that the heart must pump against. Stimulation of alpha-1 receptors causes vessels to constrict, and stimulation of beta-2 receptors causes vessels to dilate.

The amount of blood that the heart is capable of pumping per minute is called *cardiac output,* which is calculated by multiplying the heart rate by the stroke volume. The **stroke volume** is determined in part by the amount of blood that fills the ventricle during diastole, called the **preload,** and the arterial resistance that the ventricle must pump against, called the **afterload.**

COMPENSATORY MECHANISMS OF THE CARDIOVASCULAR SYSTEM

The cardiovascular system has a built-in reserve capacity, which allows it to increase its output during times of need (e.g., athletic performance) and to compensate for cardiac disease. The four basic factors of cardiac reserve or compensation are described in the following (Barragry, 1994):

1. Increasing heart rate. Increasing the rate of contraction increases cardiac output up to the point at which the rate is so fast that there is inadequate time for ventricular filling.
2. Increasing the stroke volume. Up to a point, an increased force of contraction results in an increased amount of blood being pumped.
3. Increasing the efficiency of the heart muscle.
4. Physiologic heart enlargement. The heart is composed of muscle that responds to work by increasing its size and becoming stronger.

Many disorders can result in cardiac disease. However, most that respond to pharmacologic therapy fall into one of the following categories:

1. Valvular disease. Valvular insufficiency, a backflow or leakage of blood backward through the valve, is a relatively common acquired heart disorder of dogs. If the tricuspid valve is affected, ascites may occur. If the mitral valve is involved, pulmonary edema may result. Valvular disease may be a result of progressive bacterial endocarditis. Inadequate opening of valves may also occur and cause disease. Either insufficiency or stenosis may be accompanied by a murmur.

2. Cardiac arrhythmias. If a focus of cardiac tissue depolarizes out of sequence with the sinoatrial node, an arrhythmia may result. Various types of arrhythmias may occur, including **tachyarrhythmias** (arrhythmias with a rapid rate) and **bradyarrhythmias** (arrhythmias with a slow rate). Arrhythmias may occur in the atria (supraventricular) or in the ventricles (ventricular). Several categories of drugs predispose the heart to arrhythmias (catecholamines, thiobarbiturates, xylazine, digoxin, and others).

3. Myocardial disease. Cardiomyopathy, a disease of the myocardium, primarily affects dogs and cats. It may be classified as congestive (the myocardium becomes thin and ineffective in its pumping action) or hypertrophic (the myocardium becomes thickened and restricts ventricular filling). Each type is often accompanied by various arrhythmias.

4. Other potential causes of cardiac disease include congenital defects (right to left shunts), abnormalities of cardiac innervation, vascular disease (hypertension), and heartworm disease.

Cardiovascular diseases with the greatest prevalence are mitral disease in dogs, hypertrophic cardiomyopathy in cats, dilated cardiomyopathy in dogs, "Boxer" cardiomyopathy, and heartworms (Hamlin, 2003).

Congestive heart failure (CHF) (Figure 7-5) results when the pumping ability of the heart is

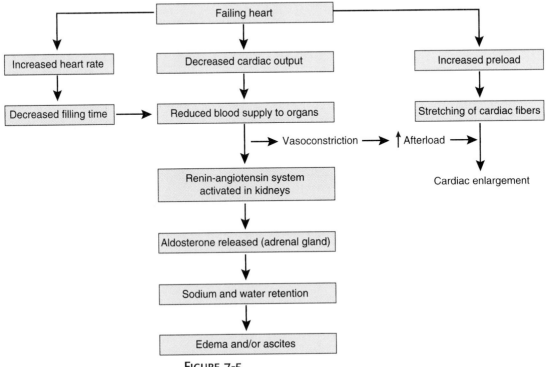

FIGURE 7-5
Pathophysiology of congestive heart failure.

Table 7-1 Stages and Treatment of Cardiac Disease

Stage	Signs	Treatment
I	None/murmur	None
II	Cough	Restricted sodium diet
		Diuretic
		Bronchodilator
III	Cough	Sodium restriction
	Reduced exercise	Digitalis
	tolerance	Diuretic
		Vasodilators
IV	Dyspnea at rest	Oxygen
		Diuretics
		Sedatives
		Vasodilators
		Others

impaired to the extent that sodium and water are retained in an effort to compensate for inadequate cardiac output. It is associated with exercise intolerance, pulmonary edema, and ascites. The heart usually becomes enlarged in this condition.

Cardiac disease has been divided into four phases according to the degree of severity. Table 7-1 lists the phases with corresponding clinical signs and treatments.

BASIC OBJECTIVES IN THE TREATMENT OF CARDIOVASCULAR DISEASE

The basic objectives of the treatment of cardiovascular disease include the following (Ettinger, 2000):

1. Control rhythm disturbances
2. Maintain or increase cardiac output
   a. Increase the strength of contraction
   b. Decrease the afterload
      (1) Arteriolar dilator
   c. Decrease the preload
      (1) Venodilator
3. Relieve fluid accumulations
   a. Diuretics
   b. Dietary salt restriction
4. Increase the oxygenation of the blood
   a. Bronchodilation
5. Ancillary treatment
   a. Narcotics/sedatives
   b. Oxygen

CATEGORIES OF CARDIOVASCULAR DRUGS

 Positive Inotropic Drugs

The general principle of the use of the drugs that improve the strength of contraction is that the heart, even in the presence of disease, has reserve capacity for contraction that can be called on to improve cardiac output. Some clinicians advise cautious use of positive inotropic drugs because these can increase the oxygen demand of cardiac muscle, can potentially damage the contractile apparatus, and can increase the tendency for arrhythmias. Proof of clinical efficacy of the positive inotropic drugs is lacking and their use is controversial (Boothe, 2001). Their popularity has waxed and waned through the years as newer, more effective products have come into use.

Cardiac Glycosides (Digitalis)

The digitalis compounds (digoxin and digitoxin) are obtained from the dried leaves of the plant *Digitalis purpurea*. The beneficial effects of these compounds have been known for hundreds of years and include (1) improved cardiac contractility, (2) a decrease in heart rate, (3) antiarrhythmic effect, and (4) decreased signs of dyspnea.

Digitalis increases the strength of contraction by increasing the level of calcium ions available in the contractile filaments within the cardiac muscle cells. This action occurs as a result of inhibition of sodium-potassium-adenosine triphosphatase (Figure 7-6). The heart rate is slowed by prolonging the atrioventricular conduction time and by increasing parasympathetic, autonomic stimulation. The primary actions of the digitalis drugs are

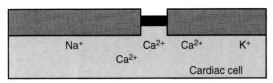

FIGURE 7-6
Effect of digitalis on the $Na^+ = K^+ = ATPase$ pump. Digitalis compounds block the $Na^+ = K^+ = ATPase$ enzyme, reduce the amount of Ca^2 pumped out of the cell during repolarization, and increase the amount of Ca^2 available for depolarization.

to (1) increase force of contraction, (2) decrease rate of contraction, (3) improve baroreceptor function (Hamlin, 2003).

Digitalis use is indicated in patients with cardiac disease that results from impaired cardiac contraction or atrial arrhythmias as suggested by clinical signs, such as exercise intolerance, weak peripheral pulses, pulmonary edema, and coughing—or by electrocardiographic diagnosis.

Clinical Uses. Clinical uses of the digitalis compounds include the treatment of CHF, atrial fibrillation, and supraventricular tachycardia.

Dosage Forms. Dosage forms include tablets and elixirs. Veterinary and human label products are available for digoxin, but digitoxin is no longer marketed.

1. Veterinary approved
   a. Digoxin elixir (Cardoxin LS, 0.05 mg/ml; Cardoxin, 0.15 mg/ml)
   b. Digitoxin—not available
2. Human approved
   a. Digoxin for injection (Lanoxin, 0.25 mg/ml or 0.1 mg/ml in ampules and vials)
   b. Digoxin tablets (Lanoxin, 0.125, 0.25, and 0.5 mg)
   c. Digoxin capsules (Lanoxicaps, 0.05, 0.1, and 0.2 mg)
   d. Digoxin elixir (Lanoxin, 0.05 mg/ml, 60-ml bottle)

Adverse Side Effects. Adverse side effects from the use of the digitalis compounds are often associated with high or toxic serum levels of the drugs and can include anorexia, vomiting, diarrhea, and various arrhythmias. Cats are relatively more sensitive than dogs to toxic effects (Plumb, 2002). Digitalis compounds are adversely affected when given concurrently with many drugs (cimetidine, metoclopramide, diazepam, anticholinergics, and others). Consult appropriate references for suitability.

Technician's Notes

1. The bioavailability of digoxin varies from 60% in tablet form to 75% in the elixir form, and adjustments are probably needed if the dosage form is changed.
2. Clients should be advised to monitor their pets carefully for signs of toxicity and to advise the veterinarian if any arise.

Catecholamines

The catecholamines include a group of sympathomimetic (adrenergic) compounds that (1) increase the force and rate of muscular contraction of the heart (increase in cardiac output), (2) constrict peripheral blood vessels (increase blood pressure), and (3) elevate blood glucose levels. Catecholamines increase cardiac contractility primarily by stimulating beta-1 receptors. Because of their short serum half-lives, catecholamines are used mainly for short-term management of severe heart failure.

EPINEPHRINE

Epinephrine is the preferred drug for providing stimulation for contraction of the heart and for supporting the circulatory system after cardiac arrest. It may be administered by the intracardiac, intratracheal, or intravenous route, and a 1:10,000 solution is preferred. Most products provide a 1:1000 solution. Because epinephrine greatly increases the workload of the heart and increases the tendency for arrhythmias, it is not used for therapy of chronic heart failure.

Clinical Uses. Epinephrine is used in veterinary medicine for cardiac resuscitation and for the treatment of anaphylaxis.

Dosage Forms. Human label forms of epinephrine are used.

1. Epinephrine HCl for injection, 0.1 mg/ml (1:10,000) in 10-ml syringes
2. Epinephrine HCl for injection (Adrenalin Chloride, 1 mg/ml [1:1000] in ampules and vials)

Adverse Side Effects. These include hypertension, arrhythmias, anxiety, and excitability.

> ## Technician's Notes
> A 1:10,000 solution can be prepared from a 1:1000 solution by mixing 1 ml of the drug with 9 ml of sterile water for injection. Alternatively, 0.5 ml of drug can be mixed with 4.5 ml of sterile water for injection.

ISOPROTERENOL

Isoproterenol is seldom used in the treatment of cardiac disease. It is indicated in atropine-resistant **bradycardia.**

DOPAMINE

Dopamine is a biosynthetic precursor of norepinephrine. It stimulates dopaminergic receptors in coronary, mesenteric, renal, and cerebral vascular beds. It also is capable of stimulating alpha- and beta-adrenergic receptors to increase heart contractility, heart rate, and blood pressure. Dopamine use in cardiac cases is mainly limited to heart failure associated with anesthetic emergencies or after cardiac resuscitation.

Clinical Uses. Dopamine is used for adjunctive treatment of acute heart failure and oliguric renal failure and for the supportive treatment of shock.

Dosage Forms
1. Intropin
2. Dopamine HCl
3. Dopamine HCl in 5% dextrose

Adverse Side Effects. These include vomiting, tachycardia, dyspnea, and blood pressure variations (hypotension or hypertension).

DOBUTAMINE

Dobutamine is a synthetic inotropic agent related structurally to dopamine. It causes increased cardiac contractility, as does dopamine, but does not produce dilation of selected vascular beds. Dobutamine is a direct beta-1–adrenergic agent. It produces increased cardiac output with little tendency to cause arrhythmias or increased heart rate. It is available only as a human label product (Dobutrex solution) and is administered in a diluted form by intravenous infusion. Consult the *Veterinary Drug Handbook* (Plumb, 2002) for directions on preparation of the solution for infusion.

Bipyridine Derivatives

Amrinone and milrinone are representatives of a new class of positive inotropic drugs that appear to work by inhibiting enzymes that ultimately lead to an increase in cellular calcium. Amrinone (Inocor) is given intravenously and is limited to short-term inpatient use, whereas milrinone is given orally and has potential for long-term use.

 Antiarrhythmic Drugs

An arrhythmia is a variation from the normal rhythm of the heart. Such a variation may result from an abnormality of impulse generation (increased **automaticity**) or from abnormalities of impulse conduction. Many arrhythmias arise when a local group of cells begins to depolarize faster than the sinoatrial node (pacemaker), causing disruption of the normal depolarization pattern of the heart. The location of this group of cells is called an *ectopic focus* (foci if more than one location is involved). Arrhythmias usually result in reduced cardiac output resulting from poorly coordinated pumping activity. Some arrhythmias may be auscultated by an experienced ear, but arrhythmias more often are diagnosed through their production of abnormal waveforms seen on an electrocardiogram.

Factors that may cause or predispose the heart to arrhythmias include the following:

1. Conditions that cause hypoxia
2. Electrolyte imbalances
3. Increased levels of or increased sensitivity to catecholamines
4. Drugs such as digitalis compounds, thiobarbiturates, inhalant anesthetics (halothane), xylazine, and others
5. Cardiac trauma or disease resulting in altered cardiac cells

Arrhythmias are classified in relation to the heart rate as either tachyarrhythmias or bradyarrhythmias. Tachyarrhythmias are further classified into ventricular or atrial, depending on their location, and can lead to rapid contraction rates of the corresponding chambers. At these rapid rates, pumping efficiency is greatly reduced because of decreased filling time. Rapid, incoordinated activity called *flutter* or *fibrillation* may also result.

Pharmacologists classify antiarrhythmic drugs into the following four basic categories (Boothe, 2001):

1. Class IA includes quinidine, procainamide, and others.
   Class IB includes lidocaine, tocainide, and mexiletine.
   Class IC includes flecainide and encainide.
2. Class II includes the beta-adrenergic blockers (propranolol).
3. Class III includes bretylium and amiodarone.
4. Class IV includes the calcium channel blockers (verapamil, nifedipine, amlodipine, and diltiazem).

Class IA

Drugs in Class IA depress myocardial excitability, prolong the refractory period, decrease automaticity, and increase conduction times. Class IA drugs are used to treat both atrial and ventricular arrhythmias and may be given orally on a long-term basis.

QUINIDINE

Quinidine is an alkaloid obtained from cinchona plants or is prepared from quinine (Plumb, 2002).

Clinical Uses. Quinidine is used to treat ventricular arrhythmias, ventricular tachycardia, and atrial fibrillation.

Dosage Forms. Human label forms are used.
1. Quinidine sulfate
   a. Tablets, 200 and 300 mg (Quinora)
   b. Sustained-release tablets, 300 mg (Quinidex Extentabs)
2. Quinidine gluconate
   a. Sustained-release tablets (Quinaglute Dura-Tabs [324 mg])
   b. Injection, 80 mg/ml
3. Quinidine polygalacturonate
   a. Tablets, 275 mg (Cardioquin)

Adverse Side Effects. These include anorexia, vomiting, diarrhea, weakness, and laminitis (horses).

Technician's Notes
Quinidine doses must be reduced in animals being concurrently treated with digoxin.

PROCAINAMIDE
Procainamide is an antiarrhythmic that is chemically related to procaine.

Clinical Uses. Procainamide is used to treat **premature ventricular contractions (PVC),** ventricular tachycardia, and some forms of atrial tachycardia.

Dosage Forms. Human label procainamide hydrochloride is used.

1. Injection, 100 mg/ml in 10-ml vials and 500 mg/ml in 2-ml vials (Pronestyl)
2. Tablets or capsules, 250, 375, and 500 mg (Pronestyl)

Adverse Side Effects. These include anorexia, vomiting, diarrhea, hypotension, and others. However, these effects are generally dose-related.

Class IB

Drugs in this category exert their influence by stabilizing myocardial cell membranes. By blocking the influx of sodium into the cell, these drugs prevent depolarization and decrease cell automaticity (Figure 7-7). They are used to treat ventricular arrhythmias, but they are not approved by the Food and Drug Administration (FDA) for this use.

LIDOCAINE

Lidocaine is a local anesthetic and antiarrhythmic. It is prepared only in the injectable form, and is administered intravenously. It is frequently used in emergency medicine and acute care.

Clinical Uses. Lidocaine is primarily used for the control of PVCs and for the treatment of ventricular tachycardia.

Dosage Forms. Various veterinary brand name forms are available in 1% and 2% solutions.

Adverse Side Effects. These are rare but may include drowsiness, depression, ataxia, and muscle tremors. Cats are potentially sensitive to the central nervous system effects of lidocaine. They should be monitored carefully when receiving this drug.

Technician's Notes

When administering lidocaine for an arrhythmia, make certain that it is lidocaine without epinephrine. Epinephrine (a catecholamine) predisposes the heart to arrhythmia.

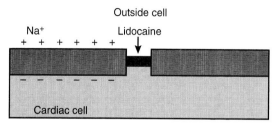

FIGURE 7-7
Effect of lidocaine on sodium channels. Lidocaine blocks sodium channels and reduces the automaticity of the cardiac cells.

TOCAINIDE AND MEXILETINE

Tocainide and mexiletine are other class IB agents that may be given orally.

Class IC

Class IC agents are seldom used in veterinary medicine.

Class II

Class II antiarrhythmics are the beta-adrenergic blockers. Propranolol has been the most widely used agent in this class for veterinary therapeutics, although atenolol and other examples are now used as well. Beta blockers may block only beta-1 receptors, or only beta-2 receptors (selective), or both types (nonselective). They are also thought to "upregulate" or increase adrenergic receptors to improve cardiac efficiency (Hamlin, 2003). These drugs may be used to treat atrial or ventricular arrhythmias, decrease cardiac conduction, reduce cardiac output, and decrease blood pressure.

PROPRANOLOL

Propranolol reduces automaticity of cardiac conduction cells by blocking both beta-1 and beta-2 receptor sites. Myocardial oxygen demand is reduced by propranolol. Reducing the myocardial oxygen demand reduces the tendency for ischemia, in turn reducing automaticity (Williams and Baer, 1990). Propranolol reduces the heart rate, cardiac output, and blood pressure. It also may improve cardiac performance in animals with hypertrophic cardiomyopathy.

Clinical Uses. In veterinary medicine, propranolol is used to treat hypertrophic cardiomyopathy and various atrial and ventricular arrhythmias. It is used in cats to treat systemic hypertension and hyperthyroidism (Plumb, 2002).

Dosage Forms
1. Propranolol HCl tablets, 10, 20, 40, 60, 80, and 90 mg (Inderal)
2. Propranolol HCl extended-release capsules, 60, 80, 120, and 160 mg (Inderal LA)
3. Propranolol for injection, 1 mg/ml in 1-ml ampules or vials (Inderal)

4. Propranolol oral solution, 4, 8, and 80 mg/ml concentrate (Intensol)

Adverse Side Effects. These include bradycardia, hypotension, worsening of heart failure, lethargy, bronchospasm, and depression.

Technician's Notes

1. Propranolol is contraindicated in patients with overt heart failure, greater than first-degree heart block, and sinus bradycardia (Plumb, 2002).
2. Do not discontinue therapy abruptly because tachycardia or hypertension may occur.

ATENOLOL

Atenolol is a selective beta-1 blocker (Papich, 2002). Atenolol decreases heart rate, slows cardiac conduction, decreases myocardial oxygen demand, reduces blood pressure, and diminishes cardiac output. Because of its selective beta-1 effect, atenolol may be safer to use in animals prone to bronchospasm.

Clinical Uses. Atenolol is used in the treatment of supraventricular tachyarrhythmias, premature ventricular contractions, hypertension, and cardiomyopathy.

Dosage Forms.
1. Atenolol tablets, 25, 50, and 100 mg (Tenormin)
2. Atenolol injection, 5 mg/ml (Tenormin)
3. Atenolol (Tenormin)
4. Atenolol (Anselol)

Adverse Side Effects
Bradycardia, lethargy and depression, hypotension, syncope, or heart failure is most commonly reported in older animals.

OTHER BETA BLOCKERS
1. Carvedilol (Dilatrend)
2. Sotalol (Betapace, Cardol). Nonselective with action similar to propranolol. This drug is replac-

ing quinidine as the antiarrhythmic of choice by some clinicians.
3. Esmolol (Brevibloc). Selective beta-1 blocker for short term use.
4. Metoprolol (Lopressor, Betaloc). Beta-1 blocker otherwise similar to propranolol.
5. Pindolol (Barbioc)

Class III
The class III antiarrhythmics bretylium (Bretylol) and amiodarone (Cordarone) are not in common use in veterinary medicine. Some clinicians have reported that Bretylol has promise for treating ventricular fibrillation in the absence of a defibrillation unit. These drugs are used in human medicine to treat ventricular arrhythmias.

Class IV
Class IV antiarrhythmic drugs work by blocking the channels that permit entry of calcium ions through the cardiac cell membrane. This effect causes depression of the contractile mechanism in myocardial and smooth muscle cells and depresses automaticity and impulse transmission (Williams and Baer, 1990).

VERAPAMIL HYDROCHLORIDE
Verapamil is a channel blocking agent and is available in oral and injectable forms. It has had limited use in veterinary medicine.

Clinical Uses. Verapamil is used to treat supraventricular tachycardia, atrial flutter, or atrial fibrillation.

Dosage Forms. Human label products are used.
1. Verapamil HCl tablets, 40, 80 and 120 mg (Calan, Isoptin)
2. Verapamil HCl sustained-release tablets, 120, 180, 240, and 360 mg (Calan SR, Isoptin SR)
3. Verapamil HCl for injection, 5 mg/2 ml in ampules, vials, and syringes (Isoptin)

Adverse Side Effects. These include hypotension, bradycardia, tachycardia, pulmonary edema, and worsening of CHF.

DILTIAZEM

Diltiazem is a channel blocking agent similar in action to verapamil.

Clinical Uses. Diltiazem is used in dogs and cats for supraventricular tachyarrhythmias and for hypertrophic cardiomyopathy in cats.

Dosage Forms

1. Diltiazem tablets, 30, 60, 90, and 120 mg (Cardizem)
2. Diltiazem oral capsules extended/sustained release, 60, 90, 120, 180, 240, 300, 360, and 420 mg (Cardizem SR, Cardiazen CD, Dilacor XR)

Other Class IV Antiarrhythmics

Other channel blockers include nifedipine (Adalat) and amlodipine (Norvasc). These agents are used primarily for the treatment of hypertension rather than as antiarrhythmics.

Vasodilator Drugs

When heart failure occurs, cardiac output is reduced, resulting in hypotension and poor perfusion of tissue. As a reaction to this poor perfusion of tissue, the body activates compensatory mechanisms to increase the blood pressure and to improve blood supply to tissue. The first compensatory activity is stimulation of the sympathetic nervous system to increase the heart rate and to cause constriction of small arteries, which in turn raises the blood pressure. Next, the renin-angiotensin system is activated by the release of renin from the poorly perfused kidneys (Figure 7-8). Renin causes angiotensinogen to be converted to angiotensin I. Angiotensin I is then converted by ACE to angiotensin II. Angiotensin II causes further vasoconstriction and stimulates the adrenal glands to release aldosterone. Aldosterone acts on the kidney

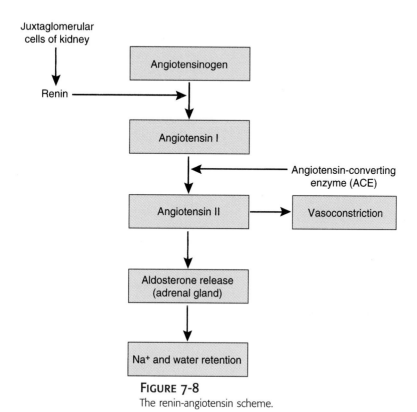

FIGURE 7-8
The renin-angiotensin scheme.

tubules to cause reabsorption of sodium ions and osmotic retention of water. The water that is retained helps to expand the circulating blood volume to improve tissue perfusion.

In the short term, these compensatory mechanisms are beneficial. In the long term, however, they become harmful because the heart must work harder to pump blood through vessels constricted by sympathetic nervous stimulation and by the effects of angiotensin II (increased afterload). The ever-increasing blood volume (increased preload) caused by aldosterone release and water retention also necessitates more strenuous activity by the heart, which in a weakened state initiates the preceding chain of events.

Vasodilator drugs act by dilating arteries (arteriolar dilator), veins (venodilator), or both (combined vasodilator). Dilatory activity may be brought about by direct action on vessel smooth muscle, through blockage of sympathetic stimulation, or by preventing conversion of angiotensin I to angiotensin II. Dilation of constricted arteries tends to decrease the afterload and improve cardiac output. Preload is also reduced because of pooling of blood in dilated veins.

Many forms of CHF are improved by the use of vasodilators, which can be used in conjunction with other heart medications.

Hydralazine

Hydralazine is primarily an arteriolar dilator. It acts directly on smooth muscle in the arterial wall by interfering with calcium movements and inhibiting the contractile state (Plumb, 2002). The net result is that peripheral resistance is reduced and cardiac output is often greatly improved in animals with CHF. Some clinicians recommend that hydralazine be used with a diuretic because it may activate the renin-angiotensin system and cause water retention (Bill, 1997).

Clinical Uses. Hydralazine is used for afterload reduction associated with CHF, especially CHF caused by mitral valve insufficiency.

Dosage Forms. Human forms are used.
1. Hydralazine HCl tablets, 10, 25, 50, and 100 mg (Apresoline)

2. Hydralazine for injection, 20 mg/ml in ampules or vials (Apresoline)

Adverse Side Effects. Adverse side effects in small animals include hypotension, vomiting, diarrhea, sodium and water retention, and tachycardia.

Nitroglycerin Ointment

Nitroglycerin is primarily a venodilator that reduces preload resulting from the pooling of blood in peripheral vessels and decreased venous return to the heart. Some arteriolar dilation may occur at the higher doses. Nitroglycerin is applied topically in hairless areas of small animal patients. The medical vehicle of nitroglycerin causes it not to be explosive.

Clinical Uses. In small-animal medicine, nitroglycerin is used as a vasodilator to improve cardiac output and reduce associated pulmonary edema. In equine medicine nitroglycerin is used as a leg sweat to reduce swelling and to treat laminitis.

Dosage Forms. Human forms are used, such as nitroglycerin topical ointment, 2% in 20-, 30-, and 60-g tubes (Nitro-Bid, Nitrol).

Adverse Side Effects. Adverse side effects are minimal and may include rashes at the application site and hypotension.

Technician's Notes

1. Gloves should be worn when applying nitroglycerin.
2. Rotate application sites.
3. Do not pet animals at application sites.
4. The dose is measured in inches by application of a strip of ointment to measuring paper that is supplied with the product.
5. The veterinarian should be contacted if a rash appears at the application site.

Prazosin

Prazosin is a combined vasodilator. It reduces blood pressure and peripheral vasoconstriction by blocking alpha-1–adrenergic receptor sites. Prazosin apparently does not activate the renin-angiotensin system.

Clinical Uses. Prazosin is used for adjunctive treatment of CHF, dilated cardiomyopathy in dogs, systemic hypertension, and pulmonary hypertension.

Dosage Forms. Human forms are used; prazosin capsules, 1, 2, and 5 mg (Minipress).

Adverse Side Effects. These include hypotension, syncope, vomiting, and diarrhea.

Angiotensin-Converting Enzyme Inhibitors

Captopril and enalapril are combined vasodilators that exert their effects on blood vessels by preventing formation of the potent vasoconstrictor angiotensin II. They prevent the conversion of angiotensin I to angiotensin II by inhibiting ACE. Drugs in this category are sometimes called ACE inhibitors. Both products may be administered with cardiac glycosides and furosemide.

Clinical Uses. ACE inhibitors act as vasodilators in the treatment of class II, III, and IV heart failure.

Dosage Forms.
1. Veterinary approved: enalapril tablets, 1, 2.5, 5, 10, and 20 mg (Enacard)
2. Human approved: captopril tablets, 12.5, 25, 50, and 100 mg (Capoten)
3. Human approved: Vasotec tablets, 2.5, 5, 10, and 20 mg
4. Human approved: Vasotec injection for IV use, 1.25 mg/ml

Adverse Side Effects. These include hypotension, azotemia, vomiting, diarrhea, hyperkalemia, and others. The safety of enalapril in breeding dogs has not been established.

Technician's Notes

1. Care should be taken when administering captopril or enalapril with other vasodilators and certain diuretics because of potential hypotension.
2. Concurrent use of nonsteroidal antiinflammatory drugs may reduce the effectiveness of captopril.
3. Captopril may cause a false-positive urine acetone finding.

 Diuretics

Diuretics have been some of the most commonly used drugs in the treatment of heart failure because of their ability to promote the reduction of preload through diuresis. The diuretics reduce the harmful effects of CHF (pulmonary edema, ascites, and increased cardiac work) by reducing the plasma volume through various mechanisms.

Many different diuretics are available, and most work by inhibiting reabsorption of sodium and water in the loop of Henle or the distal tubules. If sodium ions remain in the tubules, they exert an increased osmotic "pull" on water molecules to cause them to remain in the tubules and be excreted as urine. The diuretics used most in veterinary medicine include furosemide, the thiazides, and spironolactone.

Furosemide

Furosemide is very powerful and is the most important and efficacious diuretic for removing edema from animals with heart failure (Hamlin, 2003). Furosemide may be administered intravenously, intramuscularly, subcutaneously, or orally and works rapidly to reduce pulmonary edema and other signs of CHF. It causes diuresis by reducing reabsorption of sodium and other electrolytes in the kidney tubules. Because much of the reabsorption occurs in the loop of Henle, furosemide is sometimes called a *loop diuretic*.

Clinical Uses. Furosemide is used for diuretic therapy (in CHF and other conditions) in all species.

Dosage Forms. Injectable and oral (solution, tablet, and bolus) human label products are used.

1. Lasix
   a. Tablets, 12.5 and 50 mg
   b. Bolus, 2 g
   c. Oral solution, 10 mg/ml
   d. Injection, 5% (50 mg/ml)
2. Furosemide injection, generic 5%
3. Furosemide tablets, generic, 12.5 and 50 mg

Adverse Side Effects. These include low blood potassium (hypokalemia), dehydration, low blood sodium (hyponatremia), ototoxicity (cats), weakness, and shock.

Technician's Notes

1. Furosemide should be administered carefully to animals that are dehydrated or in shock.
2. Furosemide can cause hypokalemia that can increase the chances of digitalis toxicity (anorexia increases the chances of hypokalemia).
3. Animals who are receiving diuretics such as furosemide should always have free access to water.
4. Administer the dose at convenient times for the client because urination follows within 20 to 30 minutes.

Thiazides

Thiazide diuretics such as (chlorothiazide) Diuril act on the Henle's loop and distal tubules to inhibit reabsorption of sodium. The thiazides are seldom used in veterinary medicine.

Spironolactone

Spironolactone is a potassium-sparing diuretic (it does not normally cause hypokalemia) and is an antagonist of aldosterone. By inhibiting aldosterone, it reduces the amount of sodium reabsorbed from the kidney tubules. Spironolactone (Aldactone) is usually not used alone but is combined with a loop diuretic or a thiazide (Plumb, 2002). Like the thiazides, it has limited use in veterinary medicine.

DIETARY MANAGEMENT OF HEART DISEASE

Dietary management is an important part of the overall treatment of patients with heart disease. Dietary measures are often instituted early in the pathogenesis of heart disease (before clinical signs are observed or drug therapy is begun). Two of the primary goals of dietary management of heart disease are sodium restriction, and maintenance of good body weight and condition (reduction of obesity or cachexia). Specific nutrient deficiencies (taurine or carnitine), concurrent disease (chronic renal failure), and electrolyte disorders may also need to be addressed (Roudebush, et al, 2000).

Sodium restriction has long been recognized as an important part of the management of CHF. As previously mentioned, increased sodium levels in the body lead to water retention, increased plasma volume, and exacerbation of the clinical signs of heart failure. The primary source of sodium is food. However, water and treats must also be considered when limiting dietary intake. Prescription diets (Hill's and Purina) provide sodium-restricted nutrition for dogs and cats. These diets may also be restricted in chloride and phosphorus. They may have added taurine and/or carnitine, B-complex vitamins, and normal or added levels of potassium. Sometimes it is difficult to get an animal to accept a sodium-reduced diet because of palatability issues. These foods may be made more palatable by adding flavor enhancers or warming the food.

Because heart failure may impair other internal organs, such as the kidneys, gastrointestinal tract, and liver, cardiac diets should be highly digestible and easily metabolized. They are balanced with adequate (but not excessive) levels of high-biologic-value protein to address potential renal failure. The energy level may need to decrease or increase based upon the individual animal and its cardiac condition. Improvements in cachexia in dogs with congestive failure have been seen with dietary supplementation of fish oils, which are high in omega-3 fatty acids (Ware, 2002).

> ### Technician's Notes
> Clients should be instructed not to supplement their pet's diet with treats, human foods, or vitamin-mineral supplements when the animal is receiving a prescription sodium-restricted diet.

ANCILLARY TREATMENT OF HEART FAILURE

Various ancillary drugs and procedures are used in the treatment of heart failure. The following section provides a partial list of these therapies.

Bronchodilators

Bronchodilators, such as aminophylline and theophylline, are sometimes used in the treatment of heart failure. These agents increase the size of lung passageways to allow more efficient oxygenation of blood, exert a mild positive ionotropic effect on heart muscle, and provide a mild diuretic effect.

Oxygen Therapy

Oxygen therapy can be crucial in treating animals in the advanced stages of CHF. Animals with pulmonary edema benefit greatly from the administration of 40% to 50% oxygen via cage, mask, or nasal cannula.

Sedation

Animals with pulmonary edema resulting from heart failure often experience a great deal of anxiety because of the dyspnea that they encounter. This anxiety often leads to hyperventilation and even more oxygen demand and anxiety. To break the cycle and calm the animal, sedative drugs are often administered. The clinician may chose morphine, meperidine, diazepam, or other drugs.

Aspirin

Aspirin is known for its ability to reduce pain and inflammation, fever, and platelet aggregation. It is sometimes used in heart disease when clot formation may be a potential problem. It is used by some veterinarians to reduce the tendency for clot for-

mation in heartworm treatment and for the same purpose in congestive cardiomyopathy in cats.

Thoracocentesis and Abdominocentesis

When heart failure is accompanied by excessive fluid (effusion) in the thoracic cavity, drawing the fluid from the cavity may be lifesaving. Removal of ascitic fluid is controversial but may relieve pressure on the diaphragm and improve ventilation.

REFERENCES

Bill R: Drugs affecting the cardiovascular system. In Barragry TB: Cardiac disease: veterinary drug therapy, Philadelphia, 1994, Lea and Febiger.

Bill R, editor: Pharmacology for veterinary technicians, ed 2, St Louis, 1997, Mosby.

Boothe DM: Therapy of cardiovascular diseases: small animal clinical pharmacology and therapeutics, Philadelphia, 2001, WB Saunders Co.

Ettinger S: Therapy of heart failure. In Ettinger S, editor: Textbook of veterinary internal medicine, ed 5, Philadelphia, 2000, WB Saunders Co.

Ganong W: Origin of the heartbeat and the electrical activity of the heart. In Ganong W, editor: Review of medical physiology, ed 21, New York, 2003, McGraw-Hill.

Giovanoni R and Warren RC: Cardiovascular drugs. In Giovanoni R and Warren RC, editors: Principles of pharmacology, St. Louis, 1983, Mosby.

Hamlin RL: Cardiovascular system, introduction. Proceedings of Music City Veterinary Conference, Nashville, Tenn, 2003.

Papich MG: Handbook of veterinary drugs, Philadelphia, 2002, WB Saunders Co.

Plumb DC: Veterinary drug handbook, ed 4, Ames, Iowa, 2002, Iowa State University Press.

Roudebush P, Keene BW and Mizelle HL: Cardiovascular disease. In Hand MS, Thatcher CD, Remillard RL and Roudebush PR, editors: Small animal clinical nutrition, ed 4, Topeka, Kan, 2000, Mark Morris Institute.

Spinelli JS and Enos LR: Drugs for treatment of cardiovascular disorders. In Spinelli JS and Enos LR, editors: Drugs in veterinary practice, St. Louis, 1978, Mosby.

Upson DW: Cardiovascular system. In Upson DW, editor: Handbook of clinical veterinary pharmacology, ed 3, Manhattan, Kan, 1988, Dan Upson Enterprises.

Ware WA: Problems in chronic heart failure management, Proceedings of AVMA annual conference, Nashville, Tenn, 2002.

Williams BR and Baer C: Antiarrhythmic agents. In Williams BR and Baer C, editors: Essentials of clinical pharmacology in nursing, Springhouse, Pa, 1990, Springhouse Publishing Co.

REVIEW QUESTIONS

1. Why is the heart considered to be two pumps functionally? _____
2. Cardiac cells are connected by intercalated disks and a fusion of cell membranes to form a _____.
3. Depolarization of cardiac cells is characterized by a rapid influx of _____ ions, a slower influx of _____ ions, and the outflow of _____ ions.
4. A relatively long _____ is important to cardiac cells to prevent a constant state of contraction from recycling impulses.
5. Define chronotropic and inotropic effects in relation to the heart. _____
6. Define preload and afterload in relation to the pumping mechanism of the heart. _____
7. List the four basic compensatory mechanisms of the cardiovascular system. _____
8. List five objectives of the treatment of heart failure. _____
9. List four beneficial effects and one potential toxic effect of the use of the cardiac glycosides. _____
10. Catecholamines, such as epinephrine, are used in veterinary cardiology primarily for _____.
11. List five factors that may predispose the heart to arrhythmias. _____
12. List six categories of antiarrhythmic drugs and an example of each. _____
13. List four vasodilator drugs and classify each as arteriodilator, venodilator, or mixed. _____

14. Why is Lasix sometimes called a loop diuretic? _____
15. The use of many diuretics can lead to a dangerous loss of what electrolyte? _____
16. List five ancillary methods of the treatment of cardiovascular disease. _____
17. _____ is characterized by the rapid influx of sodium ions into the cell through channels, the slower influx of calcium ions, and the outflow of potassium ions.
18. The amount of blood that the heart is capable of pumping per minute is called _____.
19. _____ results when the pumping ability of the heart is impaired to the extent that sodium and water are retained in an effort to compensate for inadequate cardiac output.
20. ACE causes the conversion of _____ to _____.
21. Nitroglycerin is supplied as an ointment. List the precautions that should be taken when applying. _____
22. What is the most common diuretic used in the treatment of heart failure? _____
23. What is hypokalemia? _____
24. What are the primary goals of the dietary management of heart disease? _____
25. List three effects of the administration of catecholamines.
    1. _____
    2. _____
    3. _____

INTRODUCTION
ANATOMY AND PHYSIOLOGY
REGULATION OF THE
  GASTROINTESTINAL SYSTEM
VOMITING
Emetics
    Centrally Acting Emetics
        APOMORPHINE
        XYLAZINE
    Locally Acting Emetics
        SYRUP OF IPECAC
Antiemetics
    Phenothiazine Derivatives
        CHLORPROMAZINE
        PROCHLORPERAZINE
    Procainamide Derivatives:
        Metoclopramide
    Antihistamines
    Anticholinergics
        AMINOPENTAMIDE HYDROGEN SULFATE
        PROPANTHELINE
    Butyrophenones
Antiulcer Medications
    H₂ Receptor Antagonists
        CIMETIDINE
        RANITIDINE
        FAMOTIDINE
        NIZATIDINE
    Proton Pump Inhibitors
    Antacids
    Gastromucosal Protectants
    Prostaglandin E-1 Analogs
DIARRHEA
Antidiarrheal Medications
    Narcotic Analgesics
    Anticholinergics/Antispasmodics
    Protectants/Adsorbents
Laxatives
    Saline/Hyperosmotic Agents
    Bulk-Producing Agents
    Lubricants
    Surfactants/Stool Softeners
    Irritants
Gastrointestinal Prokinetics/Stimulants
    Dopaminergic Antagonists
    Serotonergic Drugs
    Motilin-Like Drugs
    Direct Cholinergics
    Acetylcholinesterase Inhibitors
Digestive Enzymes
Miscellaneous Gastrointestinal Drugs
    Antibiotics
        METRONIDAZOLE
    Antiinflammatory Agents
    Antifoaming Agents
Oral Products
    Dentifrice and Cleansing Products
    Fluoride Products
    Perioceutic Agents
    Polishing Paste
    Disclosing Solution

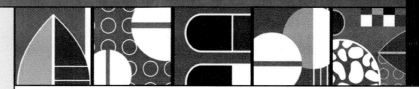

CHAPTER **8**

Drugs Used in Gastrointestinal System Disorders

LEARNING OBJECTIVES

After studying this chapter, you should be able to:

1. Develop a basic understanding of the anatomy and physiology of the gastrointestinal (GI) system
2. Become familiar with the various mechanisms of control of the GI system
3. Understand the difference between vomiting and diarrhea
4. Develop a working knowledge of drugs that induce vomiting and those that inhibit it
5. Become familiar with antiulcer medications used in veterinary medicine
6. Develop a knowledge of the pathophysiology of diarrhea and the medications used to control this condition
7. List the different categories of laxatives and their respective mechanisms of action
8. List the two basic categories of GI prokinetics and stimulants
9. Understand the reasons for using digestive enzymes
10. Become acquainted with the use of antibiotics and antiinflammatory agents in GI disease
11. List the categories of oral products and an example of each category

143

KEY TERMS

ADSORBENT A drug that inhibits GI absorption of drugs, toxins, or chemicals by attracting and holding them to its surface.

ANTICHOLINERGIC Blocking nerve impulse transmission through the parasympathetic nervous system; also called parasympatholytic. Anticholinergic drugs may be used for the treatment of diarrhea or vomiting.

CHEMORECEPTOR TRIGGER ZONE (CRTZ) An area found in the brain that activates the vomiting center when stimulated by certain toxic substances in the blood.

CHOLINERGIC Activated by or transmitted through acetylcholine; also called parasympathomimetic. Cholinergic drugs increase activity in the GI tract.

DENTIFRICE A preparation for cleansing teeth available in a powder, paste, or liquid.

EMESIS The act of vomiting.

HEMATEMESIS Vomiting of blood (the character of the vomitus often resembles coffee grounds).

MELENA Dark or black stools resulting from blood staining. The bleeding has occurred in the anterior part of the GI tract.

MOTILIN A hormone secreted by cells in the duodenal mucosa that causes contraction of intestinal smooth muscle.

PARIETAL CELL A cell located in the gastric mucosa that secretes hydrochloric acid.

PERISTALSIS A wave of smooth muscle contraction passing along a tubular structure (GI or other) that moves the contents of that structure forward.

REGURGITATION Casting up of undigested or semidigested (ruminant) foodstuff from the esophagus or rumen.

SEGMENTATION Periodic constrictions of segments of the intestine without movement backward or forward; a mixing rather than a propulsive movement.

VOMITING CENTER An area found in the medulla that may be stimulated by the CRTZ, the cerebrum, or peripheral receptors to induce vomiting.

INTRODUCTION

Problems of the GI system are common reasons for visits to a veterinary practice. These problems include **regurgitation**, vomiting, diarrhea, weight loss, colic, bloat, flatulence, abnormal stools, and constipation. Because veterinary technicians are expected to answer clients' questions about the GI tract, administer therapeutic GI medications, and monitor the response to GI medications, they must be knowledgeable about this system. They should have a basic knowledge of GI anatomy, physiology, pathophysiology, therapeutic principles, and medications.

ANATOMY AND PHYSIOLOGY

The anatomic and physiologic differences between the GI systems of different animal species are greater than for any other organ system (Bill, 1997). Despite these differences, the functions are basically the same in each species: (1) taking food and fluid into the body, (2) absorption of nutrients and fluid, and (3) excretion of waste products. A discussion of the anatomy and physiology of the GI tract with an emphasis on the similarities and differences between the species follows.

The basic structures of the GI tract include (depending on the species) the mouth, teeth, tongue, salivary glands, esophagus, outpocketings of the esophagus (crop, reticulum, rumen, and omasum), stomach, liver, pancreas, duodenum, jejunum, ileum, cecum, colon, rectum, and anus.

Carnivorous or omnivorous species (cats, dogs, and primates) are often described as monogastric or simple-stomach animals because they have no outpocketings or forestomachs arising from the basic configuration (Figure 8-1). The function of the stomach in these monogastric animals is primarily to store ingested material and to begin some enzymatic breakdown of protein. The salivary glands begin enzymatic digestion by producing enzymes that break down starch into simpler carbohydrates.

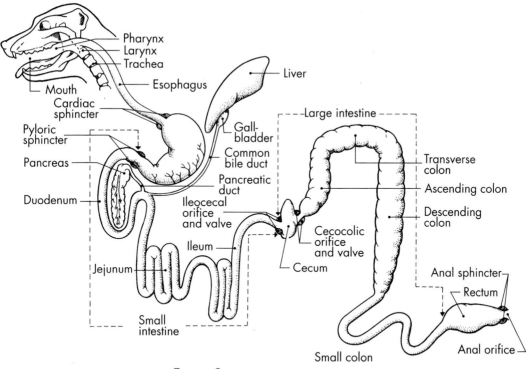

FIGURE 8-1
The monogastric gastrointestinal system.

Pancreatic enzymes delivered to the duodenum break down fats, carbohydrates, and proteins, and sodium bicarbonate from the pancreas neutralizes hydrochloric acid from the stomach. Bile salts, produced in the liver and delivered to the duodenum, aid in digestion by emulsifying fats. Bile is stored in the gallbladder, which is absent in some animals (horses and rats). Digestion and its control mechanisms are complex, and students should consult an appropriate text for further information.

Ruminant animals are herbivorous and have a GI system characterized by three forestomachs, the reticulum, rumen, omasum, and a "true" stomach—the abomasum (Figure 8-2). The reticulum receives ingested material and passes it to the rumen, where it is mixed and acted on by microorganisms to digest cellulose and other coarse plant material (roughage). Some refer to the rumen as a "fermentation vat," where microorganisms break down coarse feeds into forms that can be used by the

simple stomach portion of the GI system in ruminants. Partially digested material (cud) in the rumen is regurgitated and remasticated to further facilitate digestion. In an immature ruminant, an esophageal groove allows milk to bypass the rumen and flow directly into the abomasum, and the rumen gains full function only after several months.

Equines, rabbits, and some rodents are chiefly herbivorous animals that have a monogastric GI configuration. They possess, however, a large cecum, which is capable of limited roughage digestion (hindgut fermentation) (Figure 8-3).

Birds have an outpocketing of the esophagus called the crop, which is used for food storage. They also have a ventriculus, or gizzard, which serves to grind coarse food material (Figure 8-4).

The small intestine comprises three sections: the duodenum, which has a sharp bend and in which the pancreas is located; the long and highly coiled jejunum; and the short ileum, which connects to

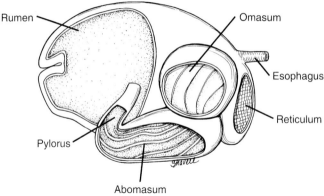

FIGURE 8-2
Compartments of the ruminant forestomach.

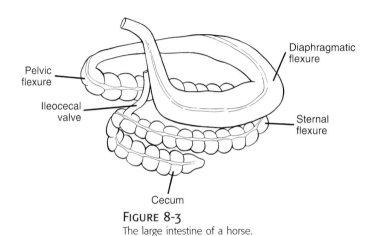

FIGURE 8-3
The large intestine of a horse.

the large intestine. In the small intestine, contents passing from the stomach are mixed with intestinal secretions, pancreatic juice, and bile. The digestive process that began in the mouth and stomach is completed in the small intestine. The products of this process are absorbed together with most of the vitamins and a great deal of fluid. Villi and microvilli protrude from the mucosal surface into the lumen of the small intestine and greatly enhance the absorptive process.

The movements of the small intestine mix the intestinal contents, called chyme, and move them toward the large intestine. Normal intestinal motility includes two different patterns—peristalsis and segmentation (Figure 8-5). Peristalsis is a wave of contractions that propels contents along the digestive tract. Segmentation is a periodic, repeating pattern of intestinal constrictions that serves to mix and churn the contents.

The colon has a considerably larger diameter than the small intestine. The colon is connected to both the ileum and the cecum through the ileocecocolic valve. The surface of the colon may exhibit one or more longitudinal bands (depending on the species) called tenias. The wall of the colon may also form outpocketings called haustra. The colon of monogastric animals has an ascending portion, a transverse portion, and a descending portion

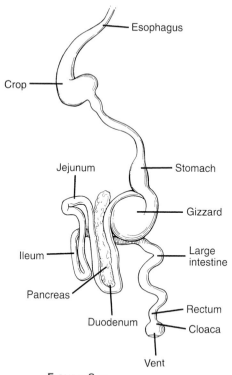

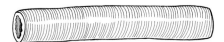

1. A section of intestine exhibiting no activity

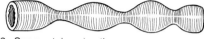

2. Segmental contractions

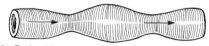

3. Peristaltic

FIGURE 8-4
The digestive system of a bird.

FIGURE 8-5
Peristalsis and segmentation.

leading into the rectum. The functions of the colon include the absorption of water, the synthesis of certain vitamins, and the storage of waste material.

The movements of the colon include peristalsis and segmentation (like the small intestine) and a third type called mass action contraction (Ganong, 2003). Mass action contraction is a result of simultaneous contraction of smooth muscle over a large area and serves to move fecal material from one portion of the colon to another and from the colon into the rectum.

REGULATION OF THE GASTROINTESTINAL SYSTEM

Regulation of GI system activity is complex but can be said to be under the influence of the following three basic control systems:

1. The autonomic nervous system (ANS).
   a. Stimulation of the parasympathetic portion of the ANS increases intestinal motility and tone, increases intestinal secretions, and stimulates relaxation of sphincters. Drugs that mimic parasympathetic stimulation (cholinergic or parasympathomimetic) cause similar results. Anticholinergic, or parasympatholytic, drugs inhibit these ANS actions.
   b. Stimulation of the sympathetic branch of the ANS decreases intestinal motility and tone, decreases intestinal secretions, and inhibits sphincters.
   c. Stimulation of various intrinsic receptors in the GI tract, such as the myenteric plexus (stretch receptor), also may increase peristaltic activity. Some physiologists consider the intrinsic receptors (myenteric plexus and Meissner's plexus) to be a third portion of the ANS called the enteric nervous system (Ganong, 2003).
2. GI hormones, such as gastrin, secretin, and cholecystokinin released from intestinal cells exert control over many functions, such as gastric secretions, emptying of the gallbladder, and gastric emptying.

3. Substances, such as histamine, serotonin, and prostaglandin, are released from specialized cells of the GI tract. Histamine attaches to H_2 receptors in gastric parietal cells to cause the increased release of hydrochloric acid in the stomach. The influences of serotonin and prostaglandin are not as well-defined.

Another factor that can have a major influence on GI activity is the presence of bacterial endotoxins. Endotoxins are components of the bacterial cell wall of certain bacteria (often gram-negative bacteria) that may increase the permeability of intestinal blood vessels and cause increased fluid loss and fever.

VOMITING

Vomiting is forceful ejection of the contents of the stomach, and sometimes the contents of the proximal small intestine, through the mouth. Vomiting is initiated by activation of the vomiting (emetic) center in the medulla of the brain. The vomiting center is connected by nerve pathways to the chemoreceptor trigger zone (CRTZ); the cerebral cortex; and peripheral receptors in the pharynx, GI tract, urinary system, and heart. Impulses from any of these areas activate the vomiting reflex, which requires a coordinated effort of the GI, musculoskeletal, respiratory, and nervous systems (Figure 8-6). Impulses may be generated by: (1) pain, excitement, or fear (cortex); (2) disturbances of the inner ear (CRTZ); (3) drugs, such as apomorphine and digoxin (CRTZ); (4) metabolic conditions, such as uremia, ketonemia, or endotoxemia (CRTZ); and (5) irritation of peripheral receptors.

Occasional vomiting by a dog or cat is considered normal. However, persistent vomiting is not normal. Horses and rats do not normally vomit. Persistent vomiting can cause serious problems because of resulting dehydration, electrolyte disturbances, and acid-base imbalances. Sizable amounts of sodium, potassium, and chloride are lost in vomit. However, potassium loss is usually the most significant abnormality.

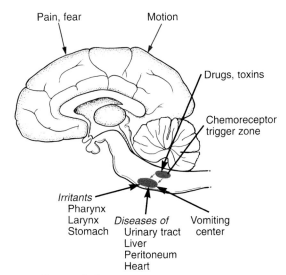

FIGURE 8-6
The vomiting center/chemoreceptor trigger zone.

Emetics

Emetics are drugs that induce vomiting. Emetics are administered to animals that have ingested toxins, but they must be used carefully to avoid serious complications. Emetics should not be used in animals that (1) are comatose or having a seizure; (2) have depressed pharyngeal reflexes; (3) are in shock or dyspnea; or (4) have ingested strong acids, alkali, or other caustic substances. Obviously, emetics should not be given to animals that do not normally vomit, such as rabbits, some rodents, and horses. Emetics usually remove about 80% of the stomach contents. Therefore the animal should still be closely monitored for signs of toxicity after induced vomiting (Plumb, 2002).

Emetics are classified according to the site of their action. Those acting on the CRTZ are called centrally acting, and those that act on peripheral receptors are called locally acting.

Centrally Acting Emetics
APOMORPHINE
Apomorphine is a morphine derivative that stimulates dopamine receptors in the CRTZ, which then

activates the vomiting center. This drug is poorly absorbed after oral administration and is therefore usually administered topically in the conjunctival sac or parenterally. Vomiting follows rapidly after intravenous administration, 5 to 10 minutes after intramuscular injection, and variably (10 to 20 minutes) after conjunctival administration.

Clinical Uses. Apomorphine is primarily used for induction of vomiting in dogs. It is considered by many to be the emetic of choice for dogs. Its use in cats is controversial and possibly contraindicated. Xylazine, which is safer than apomorphine, is effective as an emetic in most cats.

Dosage Form
Apomorphine HCl soluble tablets, 6 mg (human label), are commonly used. Apomorphine is a Class II controlled substance.

Adverse Side Effects. These include protracted vomiting, restlessness, and depression.

```
Technician's Notes
1. Whole or divided apomorphine tablets may be
   placed in the conjunctival sac of the eye. The
   tablets or portions can also be crushed, dissolved
   in saline, and placed in the conjunctiva. Once
   vomiting has occurred, the remaining apomor-
   phine should be rinsed out of the conjunctiva to
   prevent protracted vomiting.
2. Naloxone may be used to treat an overdose or
   toxicity.
```

XYLAZINE
Although xylazine is not classified as an emetic, the label indicates that it induces vomiting in 3 to 5 minutes in cats and occasionally in dogs. Some clinicians consider xylazine to be the agent of choice to induce vomiting in cats. Normal precautions should be followed for the administration of this product.

Locally Acting Emetics
Syrup of ipecac is the primary agent. Other locally acting emetics that have been used with various degrees of effectiveness include mustard and water, hydrogen peroxide, and warm salt water.

SYRUP OF IPECAC
Ipecac is obtained from plant roots and contains alkaloids that irritate the gastric mucosa and induce vomiting within 10 to 30 minutes. Some stimulation of the CRTZ is thought to occur also. This agent may be used in dogs and cats. Some veterinarians question the efficacy of this emetic.

Clinical Uses. Ipecac is used to induce emesis in dogs and cats.

Dosage Form
Ipecac oral syrup in 15- and 30-ml, pint, and gallon bottles (generic) is an over-the-counter product.

Adverse Side Effects. These include cardiotoxicity (high doses), lacrimation, and salivation.

```
Technician's Notes
1. Ipecac should be administered with caution to
   animals with an existing heart condition. It is a car-
   diotoxic drug in high doses.
2. Extract of ipecac should never be substituted for
   syrup of ipecac because it is several times more
   potent than the syrup.
```

 Antiemetics

Antiemetics are drugs used to prevent or control vomiting. The use of antiemetics is a form of symptomatic treatment because these drugs do not necessarily correct the underlying cause of the vomiting. Many cases of vomiting in small animals are self-limiting or can be controlled by withholding food and water for 24 to 48 hours. Other cases are more difficult to control and necessitate the use of antiemetic agents and careful attention to determining the underlying cause. Antiemetics are usually given parenterally because vomiting precludes use of the oral route.

Phenothiazine Derivatives

Phenothiazine derivative antiemetics act centrally by blocking dopamine receptors in the CRTZ and possibly by direct inhibition of the vomiting center. These agents are in widespread use. They are very useful in preventing motion sickness in dogs and cats but may be less effective against irritant emetics (Upson, 1988). Common side effects include hypotension and sedation.

CHLORPROMAZINE

Chlorpromazine is a phenothiazine derivative tranquilizer that has little popularity as a tranquilizer in veterinary medicine but is more often used as an antiemetic.

Clinical Uses. Chlorpromazine is used as an antiemetic in dogs and cats. It is more effective in dogs than in cats.

Dosage Forms
1. Chlorpromazine tablets (Thorazine), various sizes
2. Chlorpromazine extended-release capsules (Thorazine Spansule), various sizes
3. Chlorpromazine oral solution (Thorazine), 2 mg/ml, 30 mg/ml, and 100 mg/ml
4. Rectal suppositories (Thorazine), 25 and 100 mg
5. Chlorpromazine injection (Thorazine), 25 mg/ml in ampules and vials

Adverse Side Effects. These are primarily limited to sedation, ataxia, or hypotension.

Technician's Notes
1. Chlorpromazine is incompatible when mixed with several other injectable agents. Check the label before administering.
2. Chlorpromazine may interact adversely when given concurrently with several other drugs. Read the label before administering to determine whether the combination is compatible.

PROCHLORPERAZINE

Prochlorperazine is a phenothiazine derivative agent with moderate sedative effects and strong antiemetic effects. The approved form of this drug is a combination product that contains an anticholinergic agent (Darbazine). Prochlorperazine is available singly as Compazine (human label).

Clinical Uses. These include control of vomiting (prochlorperazine alone) in dogs and cats and treatment of vomiting, gastroenteritis, diarrhea, spastic colitis, and motion sickness (combination product).

Dosage Forms
1. Prochlorperazine. Injection, oral syrup, sustained-release capsules, and suppositories (Compazine)
2. Prochlorperazine/isopropamide. Injectable and capsule (Darbazine)

Adverse Side Effects. These are similar to those of chlorpromazine, but they may also include dry mucous membranes, dilated pupils, and urinary retention because of the effects of the anticholinergic in the combination product.

Procainamide Derivatives: Metoclopramide

Metoclopramide is a derivative of procainamide that has both central and peripheral antiemetic activities. Centrally, it blocks the dopamine receptors in the CRTZ, whereas peripherally it increases gastric contraction, speeds gastric emptying, and strengthens cardiac sphincter tone. Metoclopramide has a limited influence on GI secretions. This drug has a short half-life and may have to be administered often or in a continuous drip in severe cases of vomiting (Plumb, 2002).

Clinical Uses
1. As an antiemetic (especially for parvoviral enteritis, uremic vomiting, and vomiting associated with chemotherapy)
2. For the treatment of gastric motility disorders

Dosage Forms
1. Metoclopramide HCl tablets (Reglan), 5 and 10 mg
2. Metoclopramide HCl oral solution (Reglan), 1 mg/ml in containers of various sizes
3. Metoclopramide HCl injection (Reglan), 5 mg/ml

Adverse Side Effects. The most common side effects in horses, dogs, and cats are behavioral or other disorders associated with the central nervous system (CNS). Constipation may also occur.

Technician's Notes
1. Reglan is contraindicated if GI obstruction is suspected.
2. Atropine and the opioid analgesics may antagonize the action of metoclopramide.

Antihistamines

Antihistamines are most effective as antiemetics in dogs and cats when the vomiting is a result of motion sickness or inner ear abnormalities. Antihistamines block vomiting at the level of the CRTZ. All antihistamines may cause sedation.

Dosage Forms
1. Trimethobenzamide HCl (Tigan). Trimethobenzamide is an antiemetic for use in dogs only.
2. Dimenhydrinate (Dramamine). Dimenhydrinate is an antihistamine labeled for treatment of motion sickness in dogs and cats. It is available in tablet, liquid, and injectable forms.
3. Diphenhydramine (Benadryl). Diphenhydramine is used in veterinary medicine as an antiemetic and for the treatment of motion sickness, pruritus, and allergic reactions. It is available in tablet, capsule, oral elixir, and injectable forms.
4. Meclizine (Antivert). Meclizine is mainly used in small animals for the treatment of motion sickness.
5. Promethazine (Phenergan)

Anticholinergics

Anticholinergic or parasympatholytic drugs block the effects of acetylcholine at parasympathetic nerve endings. The result is reduction of GI spasms, intestinal motility, and intestinal secretions. These drugs act peripherally—except for atropine sulfate and aminopentamide, which have some capacity to cross the blood-brain barrier and block the CRTZ. Many clinicians believe that these drugs have a limited ability to reduce vomiting. Gastric emptying is slowed by anticholinergics, which may actually increase the tendency for vomiting.

AMINOPENTAMIDE HYDROGEN SULFATE

Aminopentamide is an anticholinergic, antispasmodic agent for use in dogs and cats.

Clinical Uses. These include the treatment of acute abdominal spasm and associated nausea, vomiting, and diarrhea.

Dosage Forms
1. Aminopentamide hydrogen sulfate tablets (Centrine), 0.2 mg
2. Aminopentamide hydrogen sulfate injection (Centrine), 0.5 mg/ml, 10-ml vials

Adverse Side Effects. These include dry mucous membranes and urinary retention.

PROPANTHELINE

Propantheline is a quaternary ammonium compound with anticholinergic activity similar to that of atropine.

Clinical Uses. The antispasmodic and antisecretory activity of propantheline is useful in the treatment of vomiting and diarrhea.

Dosage Form
Propantheline bromide tablets, 7.5 and 15 mg (Pro-Banthine)

Adverse Side Effects. These are similar to those of atropine and include dry mucous membranes, tachycardia, urinary retention, and constipation.

Butyrophenones

The butyrophenones are a group of tranquilizers that are capable of blocking both the CRTZ and the vomiting center. These drugs are relatively effective antiemetics but are seldom used for this purpose in veterinary medicine. Domperidone has been used in Europe but has seldom been used as an antiemetic in the United States.

Dosage Forms

1. Droperidol/fentanyl (Innovar-Vet)
2. Haloperidol (Haldol)
3. Pimozide (Orap)

SEROTONIN RECEPTOR ANTAGONISTS

Serotonin receptors are found on vagal nerve terminals and in the CRTZ (Plumb, 2002). Blockade of these receptors has antiemetic activity.

Dosage Form

Ondansetron (Zofran). Zofran is used mainly as an antiemetic during chemotherapy and is noted for special effectiveness during this application.

 Antiulcer Medications

Gastric ulcers may occur in animals for various reasons including stress, metabolic disease, gastric hyperacidity, and drug therapy (corticosteroids or nonsteroidal antiinflammatory agents) (Hall, 2001). Anorexia, hematemesis, pain, and melena are common signs of gastric ulcers. Most cases of gastric ulceration involve increased gastric acid production, and require treatment of the underlying cause and symptomatic therapy. Five classes of drugs are most commonly used to treat gastric ulcers: (1) H_2 receptor antagonists, (2) proton pump inhibitors, (3) antacids, (4) gastromucosal protectants, and (5) prostaglandin E-1 analogs.

H_2 Receptor Antagonists

One of the primary stimuli for secretion of hydrochloric acid by gastric parietal cells is activation of H_2 receptors by histamine. By blocking H_2 receptors, H_2 receptor antagonists reduce the release of hydrochloric acid, thus decreasing irritation of the eroded mucosa and promoting healing (Figure 8-7). H_2 blockers in current use include cimetidine, ranitidine, famotidine, and nizatidine. They are all available as over-the-counter products.

CIMETIDINE

Cimetidine competitively inhibits histamine at H_2 receptors of gastric parietal cells, thereby reducing hydrochloric acid secretion by these cells. Cimetidine is the least potent of the H2 receptors and must be given 3 to 4 times daily to be effective (DeNovo, 2002).

Clinical Uses. Cimetidine is used for treatment or prevention of gastric, abomasal, or duodenal ulcers; hypersecretory conditions of the stomach; esophagitis; gastric reflux; and experimentally as an immunomodulator.

Dosage Forms. Products approved for use in humans are also used in animals.

1. Cimetidine tablets (Tagamet), 100, 200, 300, 400, and 800 mg
2. Cimetidine oral solution (Tagamet), 60 mg/ml
3. Cimetidine HCl for injection (Tagamet)

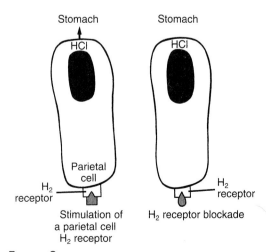

FIGURE 8-7
H_2 receptor blockade (parietal cell). HCl, hydrochloric acid.

Adverse Side Effects. These are rare in animals; however, cimetidine does inhibit microsomal enzymes in the liver and thus may alter the rate of metabolism of other drugs.

> ## Technician's Notes
> 1. Because of its inhibition of liver microsomal enzymes, cimetidine may prolong the effects of drugs that are highly metabolized by the liver (lidocaine, propranolol, metronidazole, diazepam, and others). References should be checked before using cimetidine in combination with other drugs.
> 2. If using cimetidine with antacids, metoclopramide, digoxin, sucralfate, or ketoconazole, separate the doses by at least 2 hours.

RANITIDINE

Ranitidine is also an H_2 receptor antagonist that competitively inhibits histamine at parietal cell receptors and reduces hydrochloric acid secretion. Ranitidine has little effect on hepatic microenzymes and is unlikely to cause drug interactions. Rantidine is the preferred H_2 receptor antagonist by many clinicians because of its greater potency (five times that of cimetidine) and duration of action. Rantidine also has prokinetic activity in that it promotes gastric emptying (DeNovo, 2002).

Clinical Uses. Clinical uses are identical to those of cimetidine.

Dosage Forms
1. Ranitidine HCl tablets (Zantac), 75, 150 and 300 mg
2. Ranitidine HCl oral syrup (Zantac), 15 mg/ml
3. Ranitidine injection (Zantac), 25 mg/ml

Adverse Side Effects. Adverse side effects are rare in animals.

> ## Technician's Notes
> A practical advantage of ranitidine over cimetidine is its reduced frequency of dosing (twice a day rather than three or four times).

FAMOTIDINE

Famotidine is an H_2 receptor antagonist that is considerably more potent than cimetidine. It is administered once a day and may have fewer drug interactions than cimetidine or ranitidine.

Clinical Uses. The clinical uses are similar to cimetidine and ranitidine.

Dosage Forms
1. Famotidine film coated tablets (Pepcid or Pepcid AC), 10, 20, and 40 mg
2. Famotidine oral powder (Pepcid)
3. Famotidine injection (Pepcid IV)

Adverse Side Effects. Because of limited use, side effects have not been determined.

NIZATIDINE

Nizatidine is an H_2 receptor antagonist that also has prokinetic activity like ranitidine.

Clinical Uses. Even though nizatidine is a H_2 receptor blocker, it is used primarily in small animal medicine as a prokinetic agent for the treatment of constipation and delayed gastric emptying (Plumb, 2002).

Dosage Forms
1. Axid tablets.
2. Axid capsules.

Proton Pump Inhibitors

Omeprazole and lansoprazole are benzimidazoles that act as proton pump inhibitors. These agents bind irreversibly at the secretory surface of the parietal cell to the enzyme Na-K ATPase. This enzyme is responsible for "pumping" hydrogen ions into the stomach against a concentration gradient. When bound in this way the enzyme is inactivated and the cell is unable to secrete acid until a new enzyme is synthesized.

Clinical Uses. These agents are used to treat gastric or duodenal ulcers and esophagitis and may be useful in treating parietal hypersecretion associated with gastrinomas and mastocytosis (DeNovo,

2002). Omeprazole has a veterinary approved label for the treatment and prevention of recurrence of gastric ulcers in horses and foals (Foushee, 2000).

Dosage Forms

1. Omeprazole oral sustained release capsules (Prilosec), 10 and 20 mg
2. Omeprazole (Losec) (Canada)
3. Omeprazole Oral Paste
4. Gastrogard (Equine product)
5. Lansoprazole (Prevacid)

Adverse Side Effects. These are constipation, sedation, ileus, pancreatitis, and CNS effects.

Antacids

Antacids used in veterinary medicine are (relatively) nonabsorbable salts of aluminium, calcium, or magnesium. Antacids are used to decrease the hydrochloric acid levels in the stomach as an aid in the treatment of gastric ulcers. In ruminants, antacids—such as magnesium hydroxide—are used to treat rumen acidosis (rumen overload syndrome) and are used as a laxative. Antacids may also be used in patients with renal failure to bind with (chelate) intestinal phosphorus and reduce hyperphosphatemia.

Clinical Uses. These include treatment of gastric ulcers, gastritis, esophagitis, and hyperphosphatemia in small animals. In ruminants, they are used to treat rumen overload.

Dosage Forms

1. Human label
   a. Aluminum/magnesium hydroxide (Maalox, Mylanta, WinGel)
   b. Aluminum carbonate (Basaljel)
   c. Aluminum hydroxide (Amphojel)
   d. Magnesium hydroxide (milk of magnesia)
2. Veterinary label: magnesium hydroxide (Magnalax, Rulax II)

Adverse Side Effects. Adverse side effects in monogastric animals include constipation (with aluminium- and calcium-containing products) and diarrhea (with magnesium-containing products).

Gastromucosal Protectants

Sucralfate is the only gastromucosal protectant in common use in veterinary medicine. This drug is a disaccharide that, when administered orally, forms a pastelike substance in the stomach which binds to the surface of gastric ulcers. This pastelike material forms a barrier over the ulcer to protect it from further damage and to allow healing. Because sucralfate binds better to ulcers in an acidic environment, it should be administered 30 minutes to 1 hour before H_2 receptor antagonists. It may also reduce the availability of some other drugs.

Clinical Uses. Sucralfate is used in the treatment of oral, esophageal, gastric, and duodenal ulcers.

Dosage Form

Sucralfate (Carafate), 1 g tablets

Adverse Side Effects. These are usually limited to constipation. However, there can be notable drug interactions.

Prostaglandin E-1 Analogs

Misoprostol is a prostaglandin E-1 analog that directly inhibits the parietal cell from secreting hydrogen ions into the stomach. It also protects the gastric mucosa by increasing the production of mucus and bicarbonate.

Clinical Uses. Prostaglandin E-1 analogs are used primarily to prevent or treat gastric ulcers associated with the use of NSAIDs.

Dosage Form

Misoprostol oral tablets (Cytotec), 100 and 200 g

Adverse Side Effects. Side effects include diarrhea, vomiting, flatulence, and abdominal pain.

Technician's Notes

Misprostol will cause abortions and should not be used in pregnant animals.

DIARRHEA

Diarrhea is the passage of loose or liquid stools, often with increased frequency. Diarrhea can result from primary disease of the intestinal tract or may accompany non-GI disease. Explanation of the pathophysiology of diarrhea is beyond the scope of this text. However, categories of mechanisms described in veterinary references include hypersecretion, increased permeability, osmotic overload, and altered intestinal motility. Parasitism is a common cause of diarrhea in all domestic animal species and causes diarrhea because of a combination of the previously described mechanisms. Parasitism should always be ruled out when determining a diagnosis.

Increased secretion of fluid from the intestine may result from the action of bacterial endotoxins from microorganisms, such as *Escherichia coli*, *Clostridium perfringens*, *Clostridium difficile*, *Campylobacter jejuni*, and *Helicobacter*. Intestinal epithelium damaged by viruses or other organisms may lose fluid as a result of increased permeability. Osmotic overload may occur as a result of poorly digestible foods, a rapid change in diet, or maldigestion or malabsorption. Although diarrhea has often been associated with hypermotility of the GI tract, the current belief is that most patients with diarrhea actually have hypomotility.

Decreased segmental contractions (hypomotility) increase the lumen diameter and allow more rapid passage of contents, resulting in diarrhea. Normal segmental constrictions narrow the diameter of the intestinal lumen and actually slow the passage of contents.

Diarrhea, if not controlled, can result in substantial fluid and electrolyte (sodium, chloride, potassium, and bicarbonate) losses. Dehydration, acidosis, weakness, and anorexia may follow.

Acute diarrhea, like acute vomiting, in dogs and cats often responds to dietary management and conservative treatment. In cases that do not respond to conservative management, symptomatic and specific treatments are essential. A discussion of the medications used in the treatment of diarrhea follows.

 Antidiarrheal Medications

Narcotic Analgesics

Narcotic analgesics (opiates) are effective agents in the control of diarrhea because of their ability to (1) increase segmental contractions, (2) decrease intestinal secretions, and (3) increase intestinal absorption. Many clinicians consider opiates to be the drugs of choice for the control of diarrhea in dogs. They are also used for the treatment of diarrhea in calves, but their use in cats and horses is controversial because of a tendency to cause CNS stimulation. Narcotic agents are sometimes prepared as combination products with other classes of antidiarrheals.

Clinical Uses. The opiates are used in GI therapy for the control of diarrhea.

Dosage Forms

1. Diphenoxylate (Lomotil). Diphenoxylate is a synthetic narcotic agent (Class V) that is structurally similar to meperidine. Atropine sulfate is added to commercial preparations to discourage substance abuse.
2. Loperamide (Imodium). Loperamide is a synthetic narcotic and is available in a non-prescription preparation. Loperamide poorly penetrates the CNS in cats and is acceptable in this species (Willard, 1998).
3. Paregoric/kaolin/pectin (Parepectolin)
4. Opium/kaolin/pectin/anticholinergics (Donnagel)

Adverse Side Effects. Adverse side effects of all the opiates include constipation, ileus, sedation, and CNS excitement (cats and horses).

Anticholinergics/Antispasmodics

The anticholinergics and antispasmodics have been widely used in veterinary medicine for the treatment of diarrhea. Because hypomotility rather than hypermotility is now considered to be associated with most cases of diarrhea, anticholinergics and antispasmodics should be used with caution for the treatment of diarrhea. A few commercial antidiarrheal preparations contain an anticholinergic plus a CNS depressant.

Clinical Uses. Anticholinergics/antispasmodics are used for the treatment of diarrhea.

Dosage Forms

1. Aminopentamide (Centrine)
2. Methscopolamine (Pamine)
3. Hyoscyamine (Levsin)
4. Propantheline (Pro-Banthine)
5. Clidinium/chlordiazepoxide (Librax)
6. Hyoscyamine/phenobarbital (Donnatal)

Adverse Side Effects. Adverse side effects are addressed in the antiemetic section.

Protectants/Adsorbents

Products in this category may have protectant or adsorbent qualities in the GI tract. The coating action of these drugs protects inflamed mucosa from further irritation. Their adsorbent activity binds bacteria or their toxins to protect against the harmful effects of these organisms. Kaolin and pectin are two ingredients often used in protectant compounds. The ability of protectants to control diarrhea has been questioned by some clinicians.

Bismuth subsalicylate is a compound found in products such as Corrective Suspension and Pepto-Bismol. Bismuth subsalicylate is converted to bismuth carbonate and salicylate in the small intestine. The bismuth has a coating and antibacterial effect, and the salicylate (an aspirin-like compound) has an antiinflammatory effect and reduces secretion by inhibiting prostaglandins (Boothe, 2001).

Activated charcoal is an adsorbent that is used primarily to treat poisoning.

Clinical Uses. These agents are used to control diarrhea and act as an adsorbent.

Dosage Forms

1. Bismuth subsalicylate
   a. Corrective Mixture (veterinary approved)
   b. Pepto-Bismol (human label)
2. Kaolin/pectin
   a. Kaopectolin
   b. Kao-Forte
   c. K-Pek
3. Activated charcoal
   a. Toxiban Suspension and Granules
   b. SuperChar-Vet Powder and Liquid

Adverse Side Effects. Adverse side effects are rare and are usually limited to constipation.

Technician's Notes

1. Bismuth subsalicylate compounds should be used with caution in cats because of the conversion to aspirin.
2. Bismuth may appear opaque on radiographs.
3. Administration of bismuth subsalicylate can result in black stools that resemble melena.

Laxatives

Laxatives are substances that loosen the bowel contents and encourage their evacuation. Laxatives with a strong or harsh effect are called cathartics, or purgatives. Categories of laxatives include saline/hyperosmotic agents, bulk-producing agents, lubricants, surfactants/stool softeners, irritants, and miscellaneous agents.

Saline/Hyperosmotic Agents

Saline or hyperosmotic laxatives contain magnesium or phosphate anions that are very poorly absorbed from the GI tract. It is generally held that these anions hold water in the tract osmotically. The increased water in the GI tract then softens the stool and stimulates stretch receptors in the gut wall to enhance peristalsis.

Clinical Uses. These agents are used for the relief of constipation.

Dosage Forms. Dosage forms include suspensions, crystals, powders, and boluses.

1. Lactulose (Cephulac, Constulose, or Enulose). Lactulose also reduces blood ammonia levels in certain hepatic diseases.
2. Magnesium hydroxide
   a. Milk of magnesia is a suspension for use in dogs and cats.
   b. Carmilax-Powder and Bolets is for use in cattle (laxative/antacid).
   c. Magnalax Bolus and Powder is for use in cattle.
   d. Poly Ox II Bolus is for use in cattle.
3. Magnesium sulfate
   a. Epsom salts has been used in horses and birds.
4. Sodium phosphate salts
   a. Fleet enema is for use in dogs and foals.
   b. Gent-L-Tip Enema is for dog and foal use.

Adverse Side Effects. These are rare but may include cramping or nausea. Overdose or overuse may result in hyperphosphatemia or hypocalcemia. Cats are especially susceptible to these electrolyte imbalances.

Technician's Notes

Phosphate enemas should not be used in cats because cats are especially sensitive to the electrolyte imbalances that may occur.

Bulk-Producing Agents

Bulk-producing agents are often indigestible plant materials (cellulose or hemicellulose) that act by absorbing water and swelling to increase the bulk of the intestinal contents—thereby stimulating peristalsis.

Clinical Uses. Bulk-producing agents are used for relief of constipation and for relief of certain types of impaction (sand primarily) in horses.

Dosage Forms. Dosage forms are primarily psyllium preparations. Psyllium is obtained from the ripe seed of a species of *Plantago* (Plumb, 2002).

1. Metamucil
2. Equine Psyllium
3. Equi-Phar Sweet Psyllium
4. Equine Laxative
5. Bran—a bulk-producing agent often used in horses (bran mash)

Adverse Side Effects. Adverse side effects are rare.

Lubricants

Lubricants are typically oils or other hydrocarbon derivatives (petrolatum) that soften the fecal mass and make it easier to move through the GI tract.

Clinical Uses. These include treatment of constipation and fecal impaction.

Dosage Forms. Dosage forms are liquids (mineral oil) or a jellylike mass (petrolatum).

1. Mineral oil. Mineral oil is used in horses for the treatment of constipation, colic, and impaction. This substance is also used as a laxative in other species. Heavy mineral oil is preferred over light mineral oil.

2. Petrolatum. This is a jellylike mass that is insoluble in water and only slightly soluble in alcohol. Petrolatum is the principal ingredient in many of the oral laxatives for hairball treatment in cats.
   a. Laxatone
   b. Felaxin
   c. Kat-A-Lax

Adverse Side Effects. These are minimal when used appropriately.

Technician's Notes

When administering mineral oil orally to a patient, care should be taken to avoid aspiration. Mineral oil is very bland and may not readily stimulate a swallowing reflex.

Surfactants/Stool Softeners

Surfactants reduce surface tension and allow water to penetrate the GI contents and thus soften the stool. They may also increase intestinal secretions.

Clinical Uses. Clinical uses include the treatment of hard, dry feces in small animals, impaction in horses, and occasionally digestive upsets in cattle.

Dosage Forms. These products are available in liquid, syrup, capsule, tablet, and enema forms. Docusate sodium, also called dioctyl sodium sulfosuccinate, is the main ingredient.

1. Docusate Sodium (Colase)
2. Docusate Calcium (Surfak)
3. Disposable Enema

Adverse Side Effects. Adverse side effects are rare.

Technician's Notes

Docusate sodium given with mineral oil may result in some absorption of the mineral oil.

Irritants

Irritants act by irritating the gut wall, causing stimulation of GI smooth muscle and increased peristalsis. These drugs are seldom used in veterinary medicine. This category includes several agents that are sometimes used in the treatment of constipation in humans.

1. Bisacodyl (Dulcolax)
2. Castor oil
3. Emodin

Gastrointestinal Prokinetics/Stimulants

Prokinetic/stimulant drugs increase the motility of a part or parts of the gastrointestinal tract and by doing this enhance the transit of material through the tract. Several classes of drugs have the ability to enhance gastrointestinal motility, including the dopaminergic antagonists, the serotonergic drugs, the motilin-like drugs, the direct cholinergics, and the acetylcholinesterase inhibitors. As previously noted, some H_2 receptor antagonists have prokinetic activity (see ranitidine above).

Dopaminergic Antagonists

The dopaminergic antagonists used as prokinetics in veterinary medicine include metoclopramide and domperidone (Hall and Washabau, 1997). These agents stimulate motility of the gastroesophageal sphincter, stomach, and the small intestine. Domperidone has had limited use as a prokinetic in the United States but is approved in Europe for the treatment of nausea, vomiting, and gastric reflux in humans (Parker, 2001).

Clinical Uses. Metoclopramide is used to treat gastroesophageal reflux and delayed gastric emptying, to stimulate the gastrointestinal tract in foals, and for gastrointestinal motility disorders in dogs and cats. Metoclopramide has been shown to increase the gastric emptying of liquids faster than solids. The use of metoclopramide as an antiemetic is discussed in a previous section.

Dosage Forms
1. Metoclopramide (Reglan) tablets, syrup, and injection
2. Domperidone (Motilium, Equidone). Domperidone may have use in regulating gastrointestinal motility in horses, cats, and dogs.

Adverse Side Effects. Side effects include behavioral changes in dogs, cats, and adult horses. Cats have shown frenzied behavior (Plumb, 2002), and adult horses have shown alternating periods of sedation and excitement.

Serotonergic Drugs
Cisapride is the serotonergic prokinetic used frequently in veterinary medicine. Cisapride stimulates motility of the proximal and distal gastrointestinal tract, including the gastroesophageal sphincter, stomach, small intestine, and colon (Boothe, 2001). Cisapride is not effective as an antiemetic but may be better than metoclopramide in treating certain motility disorders and in promoting the gastric emptying of solid material. Cisapride is not currently commercially available. However, compounding pharmacies may be able to make the product available.

Clinical Uses. Uses include the treatment of constipation (along with dietary and/or surgical considerations) in cats; gastroesophageal reflux; and gastrointestinal stasis in dogs, cats, and horses.

Dosage Form
Cisapride (Propulsid), 10 and 20 mg tablets or 1 mg/ml suspension

Adverse Side Effects. Side effects may include diarrhea and abdominal pain.

Motilin-Like Drugs
Erythromycin has been used by veterinarians to treat bacterial and mycoplasmal infections for many years. This drug has also been shown to stimulate gastrointestinal motility by mimicking the effect of the hormone motilin (Hall and Washabau, 2000). Erythromycin stimulates motility in the esophageal sphincter, stomach, and small intestine at microbially ineffective doses.

Clinical Uses. Uses may include increasing the lower esophageal sphincter pressure, accelerating gastric emptying, or facilitating intestinal transit time.

Dosage Form
Erythromycin (Erythro)

Adverse Side Effects. Side effects can include anorexia, vomiting, diarrhea, and abdominal pain.

Direct Cholinergics
Clinical Uses. These include postoperative treatment of ileus—or retention of flatus or feces—and equine colic (without obstruction).

Dosage Forms
1. Veterinary approved: dexpanthenol (d-Panthenol Injectable, d-Panthenol Injection)
2. Human approved: dexpanthenol (Ilopan injection)

Adverse Side Effects. Adverse side effects are rare but can include cramping or diarrhea.

Technician's Notes
Dexpanthenol should not be used within 12 hours of the use of neostigmine, parasympathomimetic agents, or succinylcholine.

Acetylcholinesterase Inhibitors
These drugs increase the amount of acetylcholine available to bind smooth muscle receptors.

Clinical Uses. These agents are used to treat rumen atony, to increase gastric emptying (ranitidine), to stimulate peristalsis, to empty the bladder of large animals, and to aid in the diagnosis of myasthenia gravis (neostigmine) in dogs. They may also be used to treat curare overdose.

Dosage Forms
1. Neostigmine methylsulfate (Stiglyn injection)
2. Ranitidine (Zantac)

Adverse Side Effects. Adverse side effects are cholinergic and can include nausea, vomiting, diarrhea, drooling, sweating, lacrimation, bradycardia, and various others.

Technician's Notes
Ranitidine and nizatidine, H₂ receptor antagonists, increase acetylcholine by inhibiting acetylcholinesterase. The increase in acetylcholine stimulates smooth muscle in the stomach and promotes gastric emptying to reduce vomiting in patients with gastritis and related disorders.

Digestive Enzymes

Pancrelipase is a product containing pancreatic enzymes to aid in the digestion of fats, proteins, and carbohydrates. The powder containing the enzymes is mixed with the animal's food, which is allowed to stand for 15 to 20 minutes before feeding.

Clinical Uses. This product is used to treat pancreatic exocrine insufficiency.

Dosage Form
Pancrelipase (Viokase-V powder, Pancrezyme powder). Both are approved for use in dogs and cats.

Adverse Side Effects. Adverse side effects of high doses include cramping, nausea, and diarrhea.

Technician's Notes
1. Powder spilled on the skin should be washed off to prevent irritation.
2. Inhaled powder can cause nasal irritation or can precipitate an asthma attack.

Miscellaneous Gastrointestinal Drugs

The drugs discussed in this section include the antibiotics, the antiinflammatory agents, and the antifoaming agents.

Antibiotics
Antibiotics are not routinely used in the treatment of GI tract disease in small animals because these agents may destroy the normal inhabitants of the GI tract and allow pathogenic bacteria (*Salmonella* species, *C. jejuni*, *C. perfringens*, *Clostridium difficie*, *Helicobacter*, and others) to grow on the mucosal surface. Bloody diarrhea or signs of sepsis may indicate the need for antibiotic therapy. Antibiotics that are often used for treating bacterial overgrowth and other GI conditions are metronidazole, amoxicillin, clavamox, and tylosin.

METRONIDAZOLE
Metronidazole is a synthetic antibacterial and antiprotozoal agent.

Clinical Uses
1. Treatment of giardiasis, trichomoniasis, balantidiasis, plasmacytic/lymphocytic enteritis, ulcerative colitis, hepatic encephalopathy, and anaerobic infections in dogs
2. Treatment of giardiasis and anaerobic infections in cats
3. Treatment of anaerobic infections in horses

Dosage Form
Metronidazole (Flagyl tablets, Flagyl IV powder for reconstitution, and Flagyl IV RTU injection)

Adverse Side Effects. These include anorexia, hepatotoxicity, neutropenia, vomiting, and diarrhea.

Technician's Notes
1. Metronidazole should not be given to debilitated, pregnant, or nursing animals.
2. Tylosin is a macrolide antibiotic that is sometimes used to treat chronic colitis in animals.

Antiinflammatory Agents

Antiinflammatory agents are used in the treatment of idiopathic inflammatory bowel disease in animals. The increased numbers of lymphocytes, macrophages, plasma cells, or eosinophils in the intestinal wall characterize these diseases. Treatment often involves the use of hypoallergenic diets and antiinflammatory agents.

Dosage Forms. The antiinflammatory agents used in the treatment of inflammatory bowel disease include prednisone, azathioprine, sulfasalazine, and olsalazine.

1. Prednisone. Many generic and trade name products are available.
2. Azathioprine (Imuran). A purine antagonist antimetabolite that may be used in the treatment of inflammatory bowel diseases because of its immunosuppressive effects.
3. Sulfasalazine (Azulfidine). A drug that is converted by intestinal bacteria to a sulfa drug (sulfapyridine) and aspirin (salicylic acid). Aspirin is the active component that has an antiinflammatory effect and is useful in many cases of colitis in dogs and cats. It should be used with care in cats because of their poor ability to metabolize aspirin.
4. Olsalazine (Dipentum). Olsazine is used for treatment of dogs with chronic colitis that cannot tolerate sulfasalazine or respond poorly to the product.

Antifoaming Agents

Antifoaming agents are used to treat frothy bloat in ruminants. In this condition, gas bubbles form and become trapped in the rumen fluid as a result of the consumption of wheat pasture or legumes, such as alfalfa or clover. The trapped bubbles cause a form of bloat that cannot be relieved by usual means.

The antifoaming agents act as surfactants (reduce surface tension) and cause the bubbles to break down so that the gas can be relieved by eructation or stomach tube. These products are given orally.

Clinical Uses. Antifoaming agents are used for the treatment of frothy bloat in ruminants.

Dosage Forms
1. Bloat Guard
2. Bloat Treatment
3. Bloat-Pac
4. Therabloat

Adverse Side Effects. These are rare if the products are given as directed.

Oral Products

An increased emphasis on dentistry in veterinary practice in recent years has fueled a demand for products that promote and maintain oral health. Many of these products help to remove food particles and plaque and assist in the maintenance of pleasant-smelling breath. Some are labeled as a dentifrice, and others may be applied as an oral rinse or with a toothbrush. They are prepared as solutions, gels, and premoistened gauze sponges. Various flavors are available, and also products with fluoride. These products should not be considered a substitute for veterinary dental treatment.

Other oral products include grit impregnated in paste for polishing teeth and smoothing rough surfaces left by scaling, and also disclosing solution to assist in identifying plaque.

Dentifrice and Cleansing Products
1. C.E.T. Dentifrices. Contain various active ingredients and mint, malt, and poultry flavors; should not be rinsed
2. Nolvadent oral cleansing solution. Chlorhexidine acetate is the active ingredient; also contains a peppermint flavor; may be used with a toothbrush or as a rinse
3. Oral Dent. Similar to Nolvadent but made by a different company
4. Oxydent. An effervescent dentifrice with various ingredients
5. VRx Oral Hygiene Pads
6. C.E.T. Oral Hygiene Spray
7. CHx Gel and Solution

8. PetDent
9. Maxi/Guard Oral Cleansing Gel
10. Fresh Mouth Oral Spray
11. C.E.T. Chews
12. Friskies Cheweez
13. C.E.T. Cat Toothbrush
14. Hills t/d Diet
15. Heinz Tartar Check
16. Friskies Dental Diet

Fluoride Products

1. SF04 Stannous Fluoride Gel
2. FluroFom
3. C.E.T. Oral Hygiene Spray with Fluoride

Perioceutic Agents

Doxirobe. This agent is placed in the periodontal pocket after dental cleaning using a cannula. Upon contact with the aqueous environment, the product coagulates and releases doxycycline for several weeks.

Polishing Paste

C.E.T. Prophypaste

Disclosing Solution

Duo 128 Disclosing Solution

REFERENCES

Bill R: Drugs affecting the gastrointestinal system. In Bill R, editor: Pharmacology for veterinary technicians, ed 2, St Louis, 1997, Mosby.

Boothe DM: Gastrointestinal pharmacology. In small animal clinical pharmacology and therapeutics, Philadelphia, 2001, WB Saunders Co.

DeNovo RC: Chronic vomiting in the cat and dog. Proceedings of the annual meeting of the American Veterinary Medical Association, Nashville, Tenn, 2002.

Foushee LL: Omeprazole, Compend Contin Educ Pract Vet 22(8):746-749, 2000.

Ganong W: Regulation of gastrointestinal function. In Ganong W, editor: Review of medical physiology, ed 21, New York, 2003, McGraw-Hill.

Hall JA: Diseases of the stomach. In Ettinger SJ, editor: Pocket companion to textbook of veterinary internal medicine, Philadelphia, 2001, WB Saunders Co.

Hall JA and Washabau RJ: Gastrointestinal prokinetic therapy: dopaminergic antagonist drugs, Compend Contin Pract Vet 19(2):214-219, 1997.

Hall JA and Washabau RJ: Gastrointestinal prokinetic agents. In Kirk's current veterinary therapy XIII: small animal practice, Philadelphia, 2000, WB Saunders Co.

Parker AR: Domperidone, Compend Contin Educ Pract Vet 23(10):906-908, 2001.

Plumb DC: Apomorphine. In Plumb DC, editor: Veterinary drug handbook, ed 4, Ames, Iowa, 2002, Iowa State University Press.

Upson DW: Gastrointestinal system. In Upson DW editor: Handbook of clinical veterinary pharmacology, ed 3, Manhattan, Kan, 1988, Dan Upson Enterprises.

Willard MD: Gastrointestinal drugs. In Boothe DM, editor: The veterinary clinics of North America, small animal practice, Philadelphia, 1998, WB Saunders Co.

REVIEW QUESTIONS

1. List three general functions of the GI tract.
   _____

2. List three examples of monogastric animals.
   _____

3. What is the GI configuration of ruminant animals? _____

4. What is the difference between vomiting and regurgitation? _____

5. Ruminants are animals that use _____ to digest coarse plant material.

6. What are the three basic control mechanisms of the GI tract? _____

7. What is the significance of the presence of bacterial endotoxins in the GI tract?
   _____

8. The CRTZ stimulates vomiting when activated by _____

9. List two examples of centrally acting emetics and two examples of peripherally acting emetics. _____

10. Drugs that inhibit vomiting are called
    _____

11. H₂ receptor antagonists promote the healing of GI ulcers by _____

12. List two H₂ receptor antagonists.
    _____

13. What are the two types of intestinal motility patterns? _____

14. Acute vomiting and diarrhea in dogs and cats often respond to conservative management such as _____

15. List two species that do not vomit.
    _____

16. What is the mechanism of action of saline/hyperosmotic laxatives?
    _____

17. What is the active ingredient of Metamucil?
    _____

18. Direct cholinergic drugs stimulate the GI tract by what mechanism?
    _____

19. A synthetic antibiotic/antiinflammatory agent used to treat giardiasis and anaerobic bacterial infections in animals is called
    _____

20. List four products used as dentifrice/oral cleansing agents. _____

21. What is the difference between peristalsis and segmentation? _____

22. True or False: Stimulation of the parasympathetic portion of the ANS decreases intestinal motility. _____

23. About what percent of the stomach's contents do emetics usually remove?
    _____

24. How does Sucralfate work to treat/prevent gastric ulcers? _____

25. Bismuth subsalicylate compounds should be used with caution in what species?
    _____

INTRODUCTION
ANATOMY AND PHYSIOLOGY
  Pituitary Gland
  Control of the Endocrine System
    FEEDBACK MECHANISM
    NEUROHORMONAL REFLEX
    CONTROL OF THE REPRODUCTIVE
    SYSTEM
HORMONAL DRUGS ASSOCIATED
WITH REPRODUCTION
Gonadotropins and Gonadal Hormones
  Gonadotropins
    GONADORELIN
    CHORIONIC GONADOTROPIN
    FOLLICLE-STIMULATING HORMONE—
    PITUITARY
  Estrogens
  Androgens
    TESTOSTERONE CYPIONATE,
    TESTOSTERONE ENANTHATE, AND
    TESTOSTERONE PROPIONATE
    MIBOLERONE
  Progestins
    MEGESTROL ACETATE
    MEDROXYPROGESTERONE ACETATE
    ALTRENOGEST
    NORGESTOMET
    MELENGESTROL ACETATE
Prostaglandins
  Dinoprost Tromethamine
  Fenprostalene
  Fluprostenol
  Cloprostenol Sodium
Drugs Affecting Uterine Contractility
  Oxytocin
  Ergot
  Prostaglandins
  Corticosteroids
  Miscellaneous Reproductive Drugs
    BROMOCRIPTINE
    LEUPROLIDE
    MELATONIN
    NEUTERSOL
Pheromones
THYROID HORMONES
Drugs Used to Treat Hypothyroidism
  Levothyroxine Sodium (T₄)
  Liothyronine Sodium
  Thyroid-Stimulating Hormone
Drugs Used to Treat Hyperthyroidism
  Methimazole
  Carbimazole
  Ipodate
  Propylthiouracil
  Radioactive Iodine
  Propranolol
Agents for the Treatment of Diabetes
  Mellitus
  Insulin
    INSULIN CLASSIFICATIONS
    USE OF INSULIN PRODUCTS
  Oral Hypoglycemic Agents
Hyperglycemic Agents
HORMONES THAT ACT AS GROWTH
PROMOTERS
Sex Steroids, Synthetic Steroid Analogs,
  and Nonsteroidal Analogs
Growth Hormone: Bovine
  Somatotropin, Bovine Growth
  Hormone
ANABOLIC STEROIDS
  Stanozolol
  Boldenone Undecylenate
  Nandrolone Decanoate

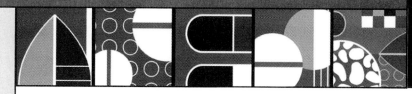

CHAPTER **9**

Drugs Used in Hormonal, Endocrine, and Reproductive Disorders

LEARNING OBJECTIVES

After studying this chapter, you should be able to:

1. Discuss the control mechanisms (physiology) of the endocrine system
2. List the endocrine glands
3. List the reasons why hormones are clinically used
4. Describe the difference between an endogenous and an exogenous hormone
5. Describe the location and functions of the pituitary gland
6. Differentiate between a positive and a negative feedback control mechanism
7. Describe a neurohormonal reflex
8. Discuss the uses and classes of gonadotropins, gonadal hormones, progestins, and prostaglandins used in veterinary medicine
9. Describe the uses and classes of drugs that affect uterine contractility
10. Define pheromone and give an example
11. Describe the location, function, and hormonal products of the thyroid gland
12. Describe the hormonal treatment of hypothyroidism and hyperthyroidism
13. List the endogenous source of insulin and its metabolic effects
14. List the classes of insulin products and their general characteristics
15. Describe the method of action of the growth promoters
16. List the clinical uses for the anabolic steroids

165

KEY TERMS

ANABOLISM The constructive phase of metabolism in which body cells repair and replace tissue.

ANALOG A chemical compound having a structure similar to another but differing from it in some way.

DYSTOCIA Difficult birth.

ENDOMETRIUM The mucous membrane lining of the uterus.

EUTHYROID A normal thyroid gland.

FEED EFFICIENCY The rate at which animals convert feed into tissue. It is expressed as the number of pounds or kilograms of feed needed to produce 1 lb or 1 kg of animal.

FEEDBACK The return of some of the output product of a process as input in a way that controls the process.

GONADOTROPIN A hormone that stimulates the ovaries or testes.

HYPOPHYSEAL PORTAL SYSTEM This is the portal system of the pituitary gland in which venules from the hypothalamus connect with capillaries of the anterior pituitary.

INVOLUTION A return of a reproductive organ to normal size after delivery.

LEVO ISOMER A left-sided arrangement of a molecule that may exist in either a left- or right-sided configuration. Levo and dextro isomers have the same molecular formula.

MYOFIBRIL A muscle fibril composed of numerous myofilaments.

NITROGEN BALANCE The condition of the body as it relates to protein intake and use. Positive nitrogen balance implies a net gain in body protein.

PRIMARY HYPOTHYROIDISM Hypothyroidism resulting from a pathologic condition in the thyroid.

RELEASING FACTOR (RELEASING HORMONE) A hormone produced by the hypothalamus and transported to the anterior pituitary to stimulate the release of trophic hormones.

TROPHIC HORMONE A hormone that results in production of a second hormone in a target gland.

INTRODUCTION

The traditional definition of the endocrine system states that it is composed of organs (glands) or groups of cells that secrete regulatory substances (hormones) directly into the bloodstream. This definition has now been extended to include regulatory substances that are distributed by diffusion across cell membranes.

The endocrine system and the nervous system constitute the two major control mechanisms of the body. These two control mechanisms are linked together through the complex integrating action of the hypothalamus (Figure 9-1). Coordination of these two systems allows an individual to adapt its reproductive and survival strategies to changes in the environment.

Endocrine glands include the pituitary, adrenals, thyroid, ovaries, testicles, pancreas, and kidneys. These glands produce hormones that are carried to target organs, where they influence the physiologic activity of these structures.

Hormones are generally administered to animals for one of two reasons: (1) to correct a deficiency of that hormone or (2) to obtain a desired effect (e.g., to postpone estrus). Hormones that are administered to an animal are called *exogenous* hormones, whereas those produced naturally in the body are *endogenous* hormones.

ANATOMY AND PHYSIOLOGY

Pituitary Gland

The pituitary gland has been called the master gland of the endocrine system because of the control it exerts over the regulation of this system. It is located at the base of the brain just ventral to the hypothalamus and is connected to the brain by a stalk. It is divided into two main lobes—an anterior lobe

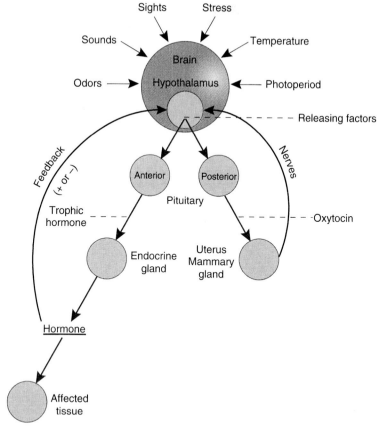

FIGURE 9-1
Hypothalamic integration of endocrine and nervous systems.

(adenohypophysis), which arises from the embryologic pharynx, and a posterior lobe (neurohypophysis), which arises from the brain (Figure 9-2).

The hypothalamus exerts control over the anterior pituitary through the transport of **releasing hormones, or factors,** down the **hypophyseal portal system.** In the anterior pituitary, these releasing factors cause the secretion of **trophic hormones** into the circulation. The trophic hormones produced by the anterior pituitary include the thyroid-stimulating hormone (TSH), adrenocorticotropic hormone (ACTH), luteinizing hormone (LH), follicle-stimulating hormone (FSH), prolactin (LTH), and growth hormone (GH or somatotropin). These trophic hormones are sometimes called *indirect-acting hormones* because

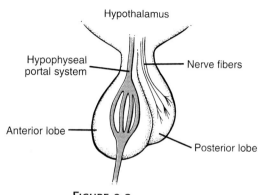

FIGURE 9-2
Lobes of the pituitary gland.

Table 9-1 Pituitary Hormones

Source and Name	Target and Actions
Anterior Lobe	
Thyroid-stimulating hormone (TSH)	Stimulates the thyroid to produce T_3/T_4
Follicle-stimulating (FSH)	Stimulates ovarian follicle growth (female) and spermatogenesis (male).
Luteinizing hormone (LH)	Stimulates ovulation (female) and testosterone production (male)
Growth hormone (somatotropin)	Accelerates body growth and increases milk production
Adrenocorticotropic hormone (ACTH)	Stimulates production of corticosteroids by adrenal cortex
Posterior Lobe	
Oxytocin	Stimulates uterine contraction and milk letdown
Vasopressin (antidiuretic hormone, ADH)	Stimulates water retention

they cause their target organ to produce a second hormone, which in turn influences a second target organ or tissue (Table 9-1). For example, TSH stimulates the thyroid gland to produce triiodothyronine (T_3) and tetraiodothyronine (T_4), which are hormones that in turn influence the metabolic rate of all tissue in the body.

The two hormones of the posterior pituitary are vasopressin (antidiuretic hormone) and oxytocin. These hormones are produced in the hypothalamus and subsequently travel down nerve fibers to the posterior pituitary, where they are stored for release into the circulation. The hormones of the posterior pituitary are called *direct-acting hormones* because they produce the desired activity directly in the target organ (e.g., contraction of the uterus).

Control of the Endocrine System
FEEDBACK MECHANISM
The nervous system is sensitive to levels of hormones through a mechanism called the **feedback** mechanism. By this mechanism, the plasma level of a particular hormone controls the activity of the gland that produces it. The type of feedback may be negative or positive (Figure 9-3).

With negative feedback, high plasma levels of a hormone are sensed by the hypothalamus, which then reduces the amount of the appropriate releasing factor (or hormone). A decreased amount of releasing factor reduces the amount of trophic hormone released from the pituitary, causing less activity in the organ that is producing the hormone

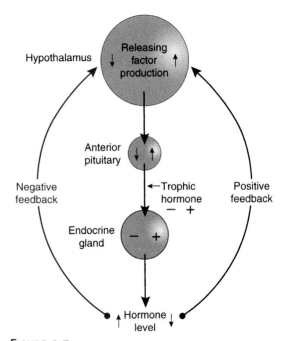

FIGURE 9-3
Feedback control mechanisms. Positive and negative feedback mechanisms control the amount of a particular hormone.

in question. The overall effect is to lower the amount of the hormone in the plasma.

In the positive feedback scheme, low levels of a hormone are sensed by the hypothalamus, and release of the appropriate releasing factor increases. Increased amounts of the corresponding trophic

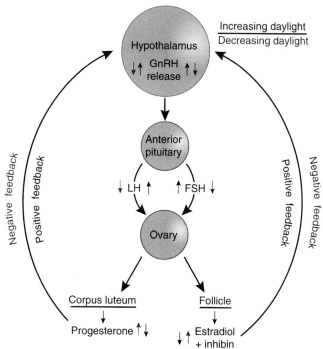

FIGURE 9-4
Control of the reproductive system is primarily through feedback mechanisms and the photoperiod. *GnRH,*
gonadotropin releasing hormone; *LH,* luteinizing hormone; *FSH,* follicle-stimulating hormone.

hormone are then secreted, causing increased activity in the target organ and a corresponding rise in the plasma levels of the hormone.

NEUROHORMONAL REFLEX

The neurohormonal reflex applies to the release of oxytocin by the posterior pituitary. The first step in this reflex can be initiated by (1) stimulation of the udder by a nursing calf or by preparation of the udder for milking, (2) stimulation of the uterus and vagina in parturition, or (3) stimulation of the cerebral cortex by sensory stimuli associated with nursing or milking.

CONTROL OF THE REPRODUCTIVE SYSTEM

The reproductive (estrus) cycle in animals has traditionally been divided into four stages called *proestrus, estrus, diestrus,* and *anestrus.* The cycle may also be divided into a follicular phase and a luteal phase. In the follicular phase, the cycle is under the influence of estrogen produced by a developing follicle, and in the luteal phase it is under the influence of progesterone made by the corpus luteum.

Control of the reproductive system is coordinated in the hypothalamus, where the gonadotropin-releasing hormone (GnRH) is produced in response to various stimuli (Figure 9-4). These stimuli can include the day-night length (photoperiod), pheromones, and positive and negative internal feedback mechanisms. GnRH causes the release of FSH and LH from the anterior pituitary.

FSH causes the growth and maturation of a follicle, which begins to produce increasing amounts of estrogen as it matures. Estrogen causes the changes that occur in proestrus and estrus, including the behavioral characteristics associated with estrus (e.g., standing to be mounted). The follicle also produces inhibin, which—along with estrogen—serves as negative feedback to the hypothalamus to inhibit the release of GnRH.

LH release causes ovulation of the mature follicle and the formation of a corpus luteum in its place. This event signals the beginning of diestrus and the beginning of the luteal phase of the cycle. The corpus luteum produces progesterone, which prepares the uterus for pregnancy. Once pregnancy occurs, the corpus luteum maintains a uterine environment conducive to normal progression of the pregnancy. Progesterone levels in the blood serve as negative feedback to prevent the release of GnRH and the development of new follicles during pregnancy.

When the gestation period nears its end, the fetus begins to produce increasing amounts of ACTH. ACTH causes increased amounts of cortisol to be produced by the adrenal glands. The increased cortisol levels result in increased production of estrogen and prostaglandin by the uterus. These two substances sensitize the uterus to the contraction-producing effects of oxytocin and allow parturition to begin. Prostaglandin also causes the breakdown (lysis) of the corpus luteum at the end of pregnancy and at the end of diestrus if pregnancy does not occur.

HORMONAL DRUGS ASSOCIATED WITH REPRODUCTION

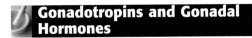
Gonadotropins and Gonadal Hormones

Products in this category are used in veterinary medicine for various reasons. Some of these include synchronization of estrus, suppression of estrus, induction of estrus, treatment of cystic ovaries, and termination of pregnancy.

Gonadotropins

Gonadotropins are drugs that act like GnRH, LH, or FSH. Gonadotropins cause the release of LH and FSH or cause activity like that of LH or FSH. LH may be prepared from the pituitary glands of slaughtered animals or obtained from the urine of pregnant women in the form of human chorionic gonadotropin (hCG). FSH may be obtained from pituitary glands (FSH-P) and from the serum of pregnant mares (PMS) between the 40th and 140th day of pregnancy. GnRH is prepared synthetically.

FSH that is released endogenously by the anterior pituitary causes growth and maturation of the ovarian follicle in females and spermatogenesis in males. LH, also released by the anterior pituitary, causes ovulation in females and production of testosterone in males.

GONADORELIN

Gonadorelin (GnRH) is produced endogenously by the hypothalamus. Gonadorelin causes the release of FSH and LH by the anterior pituitary.

Clinical Uses. Gonadorelin is used to treat cystic (follicular) ovaries in dairy cattle. It has also been used in cats and horses (with limited success) to induce estrus.

Dosage Forms
1. Cystorelin. Gonadorelin for injection
2. Factrel. Gonadorelin for injection
3. Fertagyl. Gonadorelin for injection

Adverse Side Effects. These are minimal with use of this product.

CHORIONIC GONADOTROPIN

Chorionic gonadotropin (hCG) is a hormone secreted by the uterus and obtained from the urine of pregnant women. It mimics the effect of LH, although it has limited FSH activity. In males, it stimulates the production of male hormones by the testicles and may facilitate descent of the testicles.

Clinical Uses. Chorionic gonadotropin is used to treat cystic ovaries (nymphomania) in dairy cattle. In males, it has been used to treat cryptorchidism and infertility caused by low testosterone levels.

Dosage Forms.
1. Follutein. hCG injection
2. P.G. 600. Combination of hCG and PMS; contains both LH and FSH activity

3. Chorulon. hCG injection
4. Chorionic gonadotropin injection (generic)
5. APL. Human label

Adverse Side Effects. These are limited but may include hypersensitivity reactions and abortions in mares if given before the 35th day of pregnancy.

FOLLICLE-STIMULATING HORMONE—PITUITARY
FSHP is obtained from the pituitary glands of slaughtered animals. FSH causes growth and maturation of the ovarian follicle.

Clinical Uses. FSHP is used in veterinary medicine to induce superovulation and for out-of-season breeding.

Dosage Form
FSHP

Adverse Side Effects. These include endometrial hyperplasia, superovulation, and follicular cysts.

Estrogens
Estrogens are a group of hormones synthesized by the ovaries and—to a lesser extent—by the testicles, adrenal cortex, and placenta. The estrogens are classified as sex steroids and are synthesized from a cholesterol precursor. Estrogens are necessary for normal growth and development of the female gonads. They cause secondary female characteristics and are responsible for female sex drive. These hormones inhibit ovulation, increase uterine tone, and cause proliferation of the **endometrium.**

Clinical Uses. In cattle, estrogens are used to treat persistent corpus luteum, to expel purulent material from the uterus, to expel retained placentas and mummified fetuses, and to promote weight gain. In dogs, estrogens are used to induce abortion and to control urinary incontinence. In horses, they may be used for induction of estrus in the nonbreeding season.

Dosage Forms
1. Estradiol cypionate (ECP) injection
2. Estradiol cypionate (generic)

3. Diethylstilbestrol (DES) compounded capsules and tablets
4. Implants to promote weight gain (discussed in a following section)

Adverse Side Effects. These include severe anemia, prolonged estrus, genital irritation, and follicular cysts.

> *Technician's Notes*
> 1. Estrogens should not be given during pregnancy.
> 2. Estrogen administration can cause severe anemia.
> 3. Synthetic DES has been banned from use in food-producing animals because of its possible link with cervical cancer in women.

Androgens
Androgens are male sex hormones produced in the testicles, ovaries, and the adrenal cortex. Like the other gonadal hormones, they have a steroidal parent molecule. These hormones are necessary for growth and development of the male sex organs. They cause secondary male sex characteristics and produce male libido. The androgens promote tissue **anabolism,** weight gain, and red blood cell formation.

TESTOSTERONE CYPIONATE, TESTOSTERONE ENANTHATE, AND TESTOSTERONE PROPIONATE
These injectable testosterone products are available under a human label.

Clinical Uses. These androgens are used to treat urinary incontinence in male dogs and to increase libido and fertility in domestic animals (with generally poor results).

Dosage Forms
1. Danocrine (Danazol—synthetic derivative of ethinyl testosterone) (human label)
2. Testosterone cypionate injection (generic)
3. Testosterone enanthate (generic)
4. Testosterone propionate injection (generic)
5. Depo-Testosterone
6. Combination products with estradiol as growth promoting implants

Adverse Side Effects. These are uncommon when used as directed.

Technician's Notes
Testosterone products are now C-III controlled substances.

MIBOLERONE

Mibolerone is an androgen used for prevention of estrus in dogs. Mibolerone blocks the release of LH by the pituitary and prevents complete development of the follicle. Ovulation does not occur.

Clinical Uses. This product is used for prevention of estrus in adult female dogs and for treatment of pseudocyesis.

Dosage Forms
1. Cheque Drops. Oral liquid preparation
2. Implants to promote weight gain (discussed later)

Adverse Side Effects. Adverse side effects reported in the product insert include premature epiphyseal closure and vaginitis in immature females. In mature females, vulvovaginitis, clitoral hypertrophy, riding behavior, increased body odor, and various other side effects have been reported. It is further reported that the side effects usually resolve with discontinuation of therapy.

Technician's Notes
Mibolerone should not be used in cats because of a very low margin of safety in this species.

Progestins

Progestins are a group of compounds that are similar in effect to progesterone. Endogenous progestins are produced by the corpus luteum. They cause increased secretions by the endometrium, decreased motility in the uterus, and increased secretory development in the mammary glands. They also inhibit the release of gonadotropins by the pituitary to produce an inactive ovary. In some situations, they can cause elevated blood glucose levels (anti-insulin effect) or serious suppression of the adrenal glands. These hormones are used clinically to suppress estrus and to treat false pregnancy, behavioral disorders, and progestin-responsive dermatitis. The root *gest* often allows name recognition of the progestins.

MEGESTROL ACETATE

Megestrol acetate is a synthetic progestin labeled for use in dogs. It is used, however, in cats for some behavioral and dermatologic conditions.

Clinical Uses. Megestrol acetate is labeled for use in dogs to control estrus, treat false pregnancy, prevent vaginal hyperplasia, treat severe galactorrhea, and control unacceptable male behavior. Megestrol acetate has been used in cats for various dermatologic and behavioral problems, and for suppression of estrus.

Dosage Forms
1. Ovaban. Megestrol acetate tablets in bottles or foil strips
2. Megace. Oral tablet preparation of megestrol acetate approved for use in humans

Adverse Side Effects. These can include hyperglycemia, adrenal suppression, endometrial hyperplasia, and increased appetite.

Technician's Notes
Clients should be made aware of the potential dangers associated with the use of this drug and should be asked to report any changes in their pet's health status after initiation of therapy.

MEDROXYPROGESTERONE ACETATE

Medroxyprogesterone acetate (MPA) is a human label progestin that has been used to treat certain behavioral and dermatologic problems and to suppress estrus in dogs and cats.

Clinical Uses. MPA is used for (1) treatment of behavioral problems, such as aggression, roaming, spraying, or mounting in males and (2) treatment of certain dermatologic conditions.

Dosage Forms
1. Depo-Provera. MPA for injection (human label)
2. Provera tablets (human label)
3. Cycrin tablets (human label)

Adverse Side Effects. These are potentially numerous and include pyometra, personality changes, depression, lethargy, mammary changes, and increased appetite.

Technician's Notes
Progestins should be administered with strict adherence to accepted protocol to minimize side effects, such as pyometra.

ALTRENOGEST
Altrenogest is an oral progestin labeled for use in horses. This drug is used to suppress estrus in mares. (Mares stop cycling within 3 days of treatment and begin cycling again 4 to 5 days after treatment is stopped.) It is also used to manage other reproductive conditions that are listed later.

Clinical Uses
1. To suppress estrus for synchronization
2. To suppress estrus for long periods
3. To maintain pregnancy in mares with low levels of progesterone

Dosage Form
Regu-Mate. Altrenogest in oil oral solution

Adverse Side Effects. These have been reported as minimal when used correctly.

Technician's Notes
Altrenogest can be absorbed through the skin and should be used with great caution by pregnant women or anyone with vascular disorders. Read the label carefully before using.

NORGESTOMET
Norgestomet is a synthetic progestin that is used in combination with an estrogen (estradiol valerate) for synchronization of estrus in beef cows and nonlactating dairy cows. A treatment consists of one implant and an injection at the time of implantation.

Clinical Uses. Norgestomet is used for synchronization of estrus in cattle.

Dosage Form
Syncro-Mate-B

Adverse Side Effects. Adverse side effects are not reported in the insert.

MELENGESTROL ACETATE
Melengestrol acetate is a progestin used in implants that promotes weight gain (discussed in a separate section).

Prostaglandins

Prostaglandins are a group of naturally occurring, long-chain fatty acids that mediate various physiologic events in the body. The primary use of prostaglandins in veterinary medicine is for regulation of activity in and treatment of conditions of the female reproductive tract. Of the six classes (A, B, C, D, E, and F), only prostaglandin F_{2alpha} has significant clinical application in the reproductive system.

Prostaglandin F_{2alpha} causes lysis of the corpus luteum, contraction of uterine muscle, and relaxation of the cervix. Lysis of the corpus luteum results in a decline in plasma levels of progesterone and, through the negative feedback mechanism, initiation of a new estrus cycle. Contraction of uterine muscle can facilitate evacuation of uterine contents (pus or a mummified fetus) or produce an abortion.

Bronchoconstriction, increased blood pressure, and smooth muscle contraction have been reported in other species, including humans. For these reasons, pregnant women and asthmatic individuals should handle prostaglandin products with extreme caution because exposure (through injection or skin contact) can cause abortion or an asthma attack.

Name recognition of the prostaglandins is made easier by looking for *prost* in the drug name.

Dinoprost Tromethamine

Dinoprost tromethamine is a salt of the naturally occurring prostaglandin F_{2alpha} and is labeled for use in cattle, horses, and swine. It also has accepted clinical use in dogs, cats, sheep, and goats. It is effective only in animals with a corpus luteum.

Clinical Uses. Labeled clinical uses are as follows:

1. For estrus synchronization, treatment of silent estrus, and pyometra in cattle
2. For abortion of feedlot and other nonlactating cattle
3. For induction of parturition in swine
4. For controlling the timing of estrus in cycling mares and in anestrous mares that have a corpus luteum
5. For treatment of pyometra and endometrial hyperplasia and as an abortion-producing agent in dogs and cats
6. In sheep and goats. Basically has the same uses as in cattle

Dosage Forms
1. Lutalyse. Dinoprost tromethamine for injection
2. Amtech Prostamate
3. In Synch
4. Prostamate

Adverse Side Effects. These can include sweating (horses); abdominal pain (horses, dogs, cats, and swine); urination/defecation (dogs, cats, and swine); dyspnea and panting (dogs and cats); tachycardia (dogs); and increased vocalization (cats and swine). Most of the side effects are self-limiting and disappear within a short time.

Technician's Notes
1. Pregnant women, asthmatic persons, and people with bronchial disease should handle Lutalyse with extreme care.
2. Skin accidentally exposed should be washed off immediately.

Fenprostalene

Fenprostalene is a synthetic **analog** of prostaglandin F_{2alpha}. Fenprostalene produces effects similar to those of dinoprost and the other class F prostaglandins. It is labeled for synchronization of estrus and as an agent to induce abortion (at 150 days or fewer of gestation) in cattle.

Clinical Uses. Fenprostalene is used for induction of abortion in feedlot heifers and for synchronization of estrus in beef and nonlactating dairy cows. It should be administered subcutaneously.

Dosage Form
Bovilene. Fenprostalene for injection

Adverse Side Effects. These can include infections at the injection site and abortion (when not an indication for use).

Technician's Notes
1. Do not administer by intravenous injection.
2. Skin exposure should be washed off immediately.
3. Pregnant women, asthmatics, or people with bronchial disease should handle this product with great caution.

Fluprostenol

Fluprostenol is a synthetic analog of prostaglandin F_{2alpha} for use in mares.

Clinical Uses
1. Estrus synchronization in cycling mares
2. To establish estrus cycles in anestrus mares
3. To induce parturition in mares
4. To treat lactational anestrus

5. For facilitation of postpartum (after foal-heat) breeding

Dosage Form
Equimate. Fluprostenol for injection

Adverse Side Effects. These can include sweating, increased respiration, abdominal discomfort, and defecation.

Technician's Notes
See the sections on dinoprost and fenprostalene.

Cloprostenol Sodium
Cloprostenol sodium is an analog of prostaglandin F_{2alpha} for use in cattle. This product is chemically very similar to dinoprost and fenprostalene and is labeled for uses in cattle that are very similar to those of dinoprost and fenprostalene. The same precautions should be taken when using this drug as with the other prostaglandins.

Clinical Uses. This drug is used for treatment of luteal cysts and mummified fetuses, termination of pregnancy, and estrus synchronization.

Dosage Form
1. Estrumate. Cloprostenol for injection

Adverse Side Effects. At high doses, adverse side effects may include uneasiness, frothing at the mouth, and milk letdown.

Drugs Affecting Uterine Contractility

Several drugs have the ability to increase the contractility of uterine muscle. Some are used during pregnancy to cause abortion, and others are used at term to induce parturition, to aid in delivery of the fetus or the placenta, and to cause **involution** of the uterus after delivery. Great care should be taken to ensure that the cervix is dilated before administering these drugs.

One of these drugs, oxytocin, also causes contraction of the myoepithelial cells in the mammary glands to facilitate milk letdown.

Oxytocin
Oxytocin is a polypeptide made in the hypothalamus and stored in the posterior pituitary for release in response to appropriate stimuli from the reproductive tract or mammary glands. This hormone causes stronger uterine contractions by increasing the contractility of uterine **myofibrils.** The uterus must be primed for a period by progesterone and estrogen before oxytocin is effective in stimulating the uterus.

Oxytocin is used clinically to cause more forceful uterine contractions as an aid in delivery of a fetus. It is also used to assist delivery of the placenta, to cause uterine involution, and to reduce bleeding of the uterus after delivery. It should be used only when the cervix is sufficiently dilated and when it can be determined that the fetus can be delivered through the pelvic canal normally.

This hormone is responsible for milk letdown from the mammary glands through its stimulation of myoepithelial cells in the alveolar wall of the glands. It is released endogenously after stimulation of the udder or in response to environmental stimuli, such as the sound of milking machines or other sights, sounds, or smells associated with nursing/milking.

Clinical Uses
1. To augment the force of uterine contractions during delivery
2. To aid in delivery of the placenta
3. To facilitate involution of the uterus (to reduce bleeding or to facilitate replacement of a prolapse)
4. To induce milk letdown
5. To assist in the treatment of agalactia in sows

Dosage Form. Oxytocin injection is available in generic form from many sources.

Adverse Side Effects. These are minimal when used according to recommendations.

Technician's Notes

1. Oxytocin should be used in **dystocia** only when the reproductive tract has been adequately examined. Inappropriate use can result in uterine torsion or rupture, and can lead to death.
2. A single dose of oxytocin lasts approximately 15 minutes.

Ergot

Ergot is a fungus that grows on rye grass and possibly on some pasture grasses. It causes smooth muscle contraction and can cause intense vasoconstriction. If the vasoconstriction is severe enough, gangrene and sloughing may occur.

Ergonovine maleate has been used in veterinary medicine because it produces uterine contractions much like oxytocin. It results in very little vasoconstrictive action, however. This product is not commonly used.

Prostaglandins

Prostaglandins, as mentioned in a previous section, stimulate uterine smooth muscle and can be used to induce parturition or abortion.

Corticosteroids

Corticosteroids are a group of hormones produced by the adrenal cortex that are used primarily for their antiinflammatory effect but can cause induction of parturition in the last trimester of pregnancy. This effect occurs because exogenous administration of the drug mimics the natural rise in the production of corticosteroids by the fetus as the time for delivery draws near. Induction of parturition or abortion is not a labeled use for the corticosteroids, but they have been applied clinically for this purpose.

Miscellaneous Reproductive Drugs
BROMOCRIPTINE

Bromocriptine is a dopamine agonist and prolactin inhibitor that has been used mainly in dogs for pregnancy termination after mismating or for the treatment of pseudopregnancy.

LEUPROLIDE

Leuprolide is a synthetic analog of gonadotropin releasing hormone that is used for the treatment of adrenal endocrinopathy in ferrets and for treatment of inappropriate egg laying in cockatiels.

MELATONIN

Melatonin is a naturally occurring hormone produced in the pineal gland. In addition to its use in the treatment of alopecia in dogs and sleep disorders in cats and dogs, melatonin has been used to improve early breeding and ovulation in sheep and goats.

NEUTERSOL

Neutersol is an FDA approved product containing the amino acid l-arginine and a zinc salt that is administered directly into the testicles of puppies to cause permanent sterility. It reportedly does not eliminate testosterone production and its associated behavioral characteristics, however.

 Pheromones

Pheromones are odors released by animals that influence the behavior of other animals of the same species. Although pheromones do not fit exactly into the endocrine category, they are considered in this section.

The first pheromone made commercially available was a boar odor aerosol called SOA/Sex. This product is a synthetic version of the natural pheromone that causes the typical boar odor and is used for heat detection in sows and gilts. Label instructions call for spraying the pheromone directly at the nostrils of the sow or gilt for 2 seconds. If the sow or gilt is in heat, she will demonstrate mating reflexes—such as rigid posture, deviations of the tail, and erect ears.

Another pheromone product is Feliway. Feliway is an analog of the feline facial pheromone. It is labeled for use in stopping or preventing urinary marking by the cat and to comfort the cat in an unknown or stressful environment. Cats deposit facial pheromones by rubbing an object with the side of the face. The manufacturer recommends spraying this product directly onto the places soiled by the cat and also on prominent objects that could be attractive to the cat. The product should be applied daily at a height of 8 inches from the floor until the cat is seen rubbing the area with its head. Feliway can also be used to familiarize cats with new environments, such as carriers and cages. It also may be dispensed over a large area using a plug-in diffuser.

The latest pheromone available in the veterinary market is called D.A.P. (dog appeasing hormone). The manufacturer indicates this product mimics the appeasement pheromones, which female dogs secrete to comfort and reassure their nursing puppies. Label indications for use include calming dogs during stressful situations, such as thunderstorms, fireworks, visits by strangers, or moving the dog to a new environment. It is dispensed via a plug-in diffuser.

THYROID HORMONES

The thyroid gland is made up of two lobes (one on each side of the trachea) and is located near the thyroid cartilage of the larynx. Microscopically, the thyroid is composed of follicles that, on stimulation by TSH from the anterior pituitary, produce two metabolically active hormones. The thyroid synthesizes these hormones by first trapping iodide from the blood and then oxidizing the iodide to iodine. The iodine is then combined with the amino acid tyrosine to form (through several intermediary steps) T_3 and T_4. T_3 is considered to be the active form at the cellular level. Although both T_3 and T_4 are released from the thyroid gland, some of the T_4 is converted to T_3 after release. T_4, also called *thyroxine,* is found in higher levels than T_3 in **euthyroid** animals.

Thyroid hormones control many events in the body, including metabolic rate, growth and development, body temperature, heart rate, metabolism of nutrients, skin condition, resistance to infection, and others. Two abnormalities of thyroid function that are encountered in veterinary medicine are hypothyroidism and hyperthyroidism.

Hypothyroidism is noted most often in dogs and is characterized by lethargy, cold intolerance, dry haircoat, and bradycardia. Hyperthyroidism is encountered more often in older cats and is accompanied by weight loss, increased appetite, restlessness, hyperexcitability, and tachycardia. Diagnosis of thyroid conditions is made through the observation of clinical signs and by measuring serum levels of T_3 and T_4 before and after TSH administration.

Goiter is a condition caused by inadequate levels of iodide in the diet. Lack of iodide causes the thyroid to be unable to produce T_3 or T_4. The thyroid attempts to increase its output by enlarging, often to a size that can be palpated and visualized. Goiter is almost nonexistent in animals receiving a commercial diet.

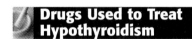

Drugs Used to Treat Hypothyroidism

Treatment of hypothyroidism consists of supplementation of thyroid hormones on a daily basis. Clinical signs usually resolve within a short time of initiating treatment, but lifelong therapy is required.

Thyroid hormones can be extracted from thyroid glands or can be prepared synthetically. Purification of the animal source hormones is difficult and has led to the common use of the synthetic products. Synthetic thyroxine (T_4) is considered to be the compound of choice in the treatment of hypothyroidism. T_3 products are recommended only when a poor response to T_4 occurs.

Levothyroxine Sodium (T_4)
Levothyroxine is a synthetic **levo isomer** of T_4. It is the compound of choice in treating hypothyroidism in all species.

Clinical Uses. Levothyroxine is used for the treatment of hypothyroid conditions.

Dosage Forms
1. Soloxine. Levothyroxine tablets, approved for dogs

2. Thyro-Form. Levothyroxine chewable tablets, approved for dogs
3. Thyro-L. Levothyroxine powder, approved for horses
4. NutriVed T-4 Chewables. Levothyroxine chewable tablets, approved for dogs
5. Thyro-Tab. Levothyroxine tablets for dogs
6. Equine Thyroid Supplement
7. Thyrozine Tablets. Levothyroxine tablets for dogs
8. Synthroid. Levothyroxine tablets approved for humans

Adverse Side Effects. These are rare when used according to recommendations.

Liothyronine Sodium

Liothyronine sodium (T_3) is a synthetic salt of endogenous T_3. T_3 is not the compound of choice when treating hypothyroidism. It may be useful, however, in cases that do not respond well to T_4.

Clinical Uses. T_3 is used for treatment of hypothyroidism in cases that respond poorly to T_4.

Dosage Forms
1. Cytobin Tablets. Liothyronine sodium tablets, approved for dogs
2. Cytomel. Human label

Adverse Side Effects. These are probably minimal with careful use.

Thyroid-Stimulating Hormone

Thyrotropin is a purified form of TSH obtained form the anterior pituitary in cattle. It is used as an aid in the diagnosis of hypothyroidism.

Clinical Uses. In veterinary medicine, thyrotropin is used for diagnosis of **primary hypothyroidism** in the TSH stimulation test.

Dosage Forms
1. Dermathycin. TSH approved for use in dogs
2. Thytropar. TSH approved for use in humans

Adverse Side Effects. Allergic reactions may occur in animals sensitive to bovine protein.

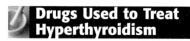

Drugs Used to Treat Hyperthyroidism

Treatment of hyperthyroidism is directed at lowering blood levels of T_3 and T_4. This can be accomplished by destruction or removal of the overproducing thyroid or by blocking production of the hormones. The thyroid can be removed surgically or destroyed with radioactive iodine. Drug therapy to block hormone production can be effective but is continuous and not curative.

The two antithyroid drugs used most often are methimazole and carbimazole. These compounds are used for long-term therapy and for presurgical preparation of patients. Hyperthyroid cats are often high surgical risks, primarily because of tachycardia and other potential cardiac abnormalities.

Methimazole

Methimazole is a compound that interferes with incorporation of iodine into the precursor molecules of T_3 and T_4. It does not alter thyroid hormones already released into the bloodstream.

Clinical Uses. Methimazole is used for the treatment of feline hyperthyroidism.

Dosage Form
Tapazole. Methimazole tablets (human approved)

Adverse Side Effects. These include anorexia, vomiting, and skin eruptions. Kittens should be placed on a milk replacement after receiving colostrum from mothers on methimazole.

Carbimazole

Carbimazole is a product similar to methimazole that is used in Canada and other countries. Most of this drug is converted to methimazole after administration to the cat. It inhibits the synthesis of thyroid hormones.

Clinical Uses. Carbimazole is used for the treatment of feline hyperthyroidism.

Dosage Forms
1. Carbazole. Human label
2. Neo-Carbazole. Human label

Adverse Side Effects. Side effects are similar to methimazole.

Ipodate

Ipodate is an orally administered, radiopaque, organic iodine compound that is thought to inhibit the conversion of T_4 to T_3.

Clinical Uses. Ipodate may be helpful in the treatment of hyperthyroidism in cats that are not tolerant of methimazole or carbimazole.

Dosage Form
Oragrafin. Human label

Propylthiouracil

Propylthiouracil has been used as an antithyroid drug but is considered dangerous to use in cats because of potential hematologic complications.

Radioactive Iodine

Radioactive iodine (I-131) may be given intravenously to destroy overproductive thyroid tissue. I-131 concentrates in the thyroid, where it remains and destroys thyroid tissue. This method has appeal because it is performed only once and is not especially stressful to patients. However, it must be done at facilities that can handle radioactive materials.

Propranolol

Propranolol (Inderal) may be used preoperatively to treat the tachycardia associated with hyperthyroidism in cats.

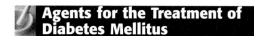
Agents for the Treatment of Diabetes Mellitus

Insulin

The pancreas produces two principal hormones in special cells of the islets of Langerhans: insulin and glucagon. Insulin is produced by beta cells, and glucagon is produced by alpha cells. Insulin causes a decrease in blood glucose levels, while glucagon promotes an increase. Only insulin is used clinically.

Insulin facilitates cellular uptake of glucose and its storage in the form of glycogen and fat. It inhibits the breakdown of fat, protein, and glycogen into forms that may be used as energy sources. Further, it promotes synthesis of protein, fatty acids, and glycogen. In the absence of insulin, the body cannot use glucose and must break down its own fat and protein to use for energy.

Diabetes mellitus is a complex disease that results from inability of the beta cells of the pancreas to produce enough insulin or from altered insulin action in cells. Diabetes mellitus that results from inadequate secretion of insulin is called *type I,* or *insulin-dependent diabetes mellitus.* This is the most common type of diabetes mellitus in dogs and cats. Diabetes mellitus that results from resistance of tissue to the action of insulin is called *type II,* or *non*insulin-dependent diabetes mellitus (NIDDM). NIDDM is rare in dogs but is occasionally encountered in cats.

Both forms of diabetes mellitus eventually cause polydipsia, polyuria, polyphagia, and weight loss. Untreated diabetes mellitus proceeds to the condition called *diabetic ketoacidosis,* in which body fat is metabolized as a substitute energy source. Metabolism of body fat results in accumulation of byproducts of this process called *ketone bodies,* which promote a metabolic acidosis that can lead to death.

Because blood glucose levels can be increased by corticosteroids, epinephrine, and progesterone, these drugs should be given with caution to diabetic animals. Sudden changes in diet and exercise level should also be avoided because they can alter blood glucose levels and cause an imbalance in the ratio of insulin to glucose.

Insulin is not effective when given orally because the digestive tract breaks down the protein molecule before it can be absorbed. Insulin is usually administered by subcutaneous injection. However, some forms may be given intravenously or intramuscularly.

Sources of insulin have traditionally included beef or pork pancreas and preparations comprised of a purified (pure beef source or pure pork source) form or a combination beef/pork form. The beef/pork form is best suited to treat diabetes mellitus in dogs and cats. Pork insulin is very close in structure to dog and human insulins, whereas beef insulin is very similar to cat insulin.

Most human insulin products are now prepared through recombinant DNA or synthetic processes. Only one animal labeled product is currently approved for use in the United States. The availability of insulin products is subject to change and technicians should always consult current information when dealing with diabetic patients.

Insulin concentration is measured in units of insulin per milliliter. It is available in concentrations of 40 (U-40), 100 (U-100), and 500 (U-500) U/ml. All products for human use are U-100 concentrations.

A U-40 concentration makes administering the small amounts of insulin needed for cats and small dogs much easier. When insulin is drawn into the syringes, each mark on the syringe barrel denotes 1 U of insulin. Drawing up 5 U on a scale of 40, for example, is easier than drawing up 5 U on a scale of 100. Small-volume U-100 syringes are available, however, to facilitate administration of small doses of U-100 insulin.

U-40 syringes must be used with U-40 insulin, and U-100 syringes must be used with U-100 insulin. Table 9-2 lists the available insulin syringes.

Table 9-2 Insulin Syringes

Name and Manufacturer	Insulin	Needle Gauge	Needle Size	Packaging
1-ml Syringes				
B-D Microfine IV	U-100	28	½ inch	100 (10 packs of 10)
B-D Microfine	U-100	27	⅝ inch	100 (10 packs of 10)
B-D Microfine IV	U-40	28	½ inch	100 (10 packs of 10)
Can-Am E-Z Ject	U-100	27	½ inch	100 (individually wrapped)
Can-Am E-Z Ject	U-100	28	½ inch	100 (individually wrapped)
Monoject Ultra Comfort 28	U-100	28	½ inch	100 or 30 (individually wrapped)
Pharma-Plast	U-100	28	½ inch	100 (10 packs of 10)
Terumo	U-100	29	½ inch	100 (individually wrapped)
Terumo	U-100	27	½ inch	100 (individually wrapped)
0.25-ml Syringes				
Terumo	U-100	29	½ inch	100 (individually wrapped)
0.5-ml Syringes				
B-D Microfine IV	U-100	28	½ inch	100 (10 packs of 10)
Can-Am E-Z Ject	U-50	28	½ inch	100 (individually wrapped)
Monoject Ultra Comfort 28	U-100	28	½ inch	100 or 30 (individually wrapped)
Pharma-Plast	U-100	28	½ inch	100 (10 packs of 10)
Terumo	U-100	29	½ inch	100 (individually wrapped)
Terumo	U-100	27	½ inch	100 (individually wrapped)
0.3-ml Syringes				
B-D Microfine IV	U-100	28	½ inch	100 (10 packs of 10)

From Peterson ME: Insulin and insulin syringes. In Kirk RW, Bonagura JD, editors: Current veterinary therapy XI: small animal practice, Philadelphia, 1992, WB Saunders Co, p. 358.

INSULIN CLASSIFICATIONS

Insulin is usually classified according to its duration of action as short acting, intermediate acting, or long acting. Short-acting insulins include regular crystalline and Semilente. NPH and Lente are intermediate-acting insulins. PZI and Ultralente are long-acting products. Two different forms are sometimes combined in the same preparation. See Table 9-3 for a partial listing of insulin products in each category.

The onset of effect and route of administration are other important characteristics of insulin preparations to be considered. For an in-depth discussion of insulin forms and characteristics, consult *Small Animal Clinical Pharmacology and Therapeutics* (Boothe, 2001).

Short-Acting Insulin
Regular crystalline insulin/semilente
Regular insulin is a fast-acting insulin that is made from zinc insulin crystals and is a clear solution which may be administered intravenously, intramuscularly, or subcutaneously. It is used mainly to treat diabetic ketoacidosis until blood glucose levels are reduced and the animal is metabolically stable. At that time, the animal is usually switched to a longer-acting form. Semilente insulin is similar in effect to regular insulin but is prepared by a different process.

Clinical Uses. Semilente is primarily used for the treatment of diabetic ketoacidosis.

Dosage Forms. Many products approved for humans are available. The following is a partial listing:

1. Humalog. Very short acting.
2. Novolog. Very short acting.
3. Purified Pork R (purified pork)
4. Humilin R
5. Novolin R

Adverse Side Effects. These are usually related to overdose and may include weakness, ataxia, shaking, and seizures.

> *Technician's Notes*
> 1. Although not required by label in the newer products, refrigeration probably enhances storage life. Do not freeze.
> 2. Do not use regular insulin preparations if discoloration or precipitates are present.

Intermediate-Acting Insulin
NPH (isophane) insulin/lente
NPH insulin is a cloudy suspension of zinc insulin crystals and protamine zinc. It is longer acting than regular insulin and takes effect faster than PZI insulin. It is a commonly used insulin for the control of uncomplicated diabetes in dogs and cats. Lente insulin is similar in activity to NPH insulin but is made without the use of protamine.

A Lente insulin called Caninsulin (U-40) is licensed for dogs and cats in the United Kingdom.

Clinical Uses. NPH insulin is used for treatment of uncomplicated diabetes mellitus.

Dosage Forms. A partial listing follows:
1. Humalin L
2. Novolin L
3. Lente Iletin II (purified pork)
4. NPH Iletin II (pork)
5. Lente Purified Pork
6. Humilin N
7. Novolin N

Adverse Side Effects. These are similar to those of regular insulin.

> *Technician's Notes*
> 1. Resuspension, by gently rolling the bottle, is required before withdrawing the product from the bottle.
> 2. Store like regular insulin. Do not freeze.
> 3. NPH insulin is usually administered once a day.

Table 9-3 Insulins

Product	Manufacturer	Form	Strength
Rapid Acting (onset <15 minutes)			
Humalog	Lilly	Human	U-100
Humalog Cartridges	Lilly	Human	U-100
Novolog	Novo Nordisk	Human	U-100
Short Acting (onset ½-2 hours)			
Humulin R (Regular)	Lilly	Human	U-100, U-500
Iletin I Regular DISCONTINUED/Supply Limited	Lilly	Beef/Pork	U-100
Iletin II Regular	Lilly	Pork	U-100
Humulin R Cartridges (1.5 ml)	Lilly	Human	U-100
Novolin R (Regular)	Novo Nordisk	Human	U-100
Novolin R Penfill (Regular)	Novo Nordisk	Human	U-100
Purified Pork R (Regular)	Novo Nordisk	Pork	U-100
Velosulin Human (Regular) (Buffered)	Novo Nordisk	Human	U-100
Novolin R (Regular) Prefilled	Novo Nordisk	Human	U-100
Intermediate Acting (onset 2-4 hours)			
Humulin L (Lente)	Lilly	Human	U-100
Humulin N (NPH)	Lilly	Human	U-100
Iletin Lente DISCONTINUED/Supply Limited	Lilly	Beef/Pork	U-100
Iletin I NPH DISCONTINUED/Supply Limited	Lilly	Beef/Pork	U-100
Iletin II Lente	Lilly	Pork	U-100
Iletin II NPH	Lilly	Pork	U-100
Humulin N Cartridges (1.5 ml)	Lilly	Human	U-100
Novolin L (Lente)	Novo Nordisk	Human	U-100
Novolin N (NPH)	Novo Nordisk	Human	U-100
Novolin N PenFill (NPH)	Novo Nordisk	Human	U-100
Novolin N Prefilled (NPH)	Novo Nordisk	Human	U-100
Purified Pork Lente	Novo Nordisk	Pork	U-100
Purified Pork N (NPH)	Novo Nordisk	Pork	U-100
Caninsulin	Intervet	Pork	U-40
Long Acting (onset 4-6 hours)			
PZI VET	IDEXX	Pork	U-40
Humulin U (Ultralente)	Lilly	Human	U-100
Lantus	Adventis	Human	U-100
Mixtures			
Humulin 50/50 (50% NPH, 50% Regular)	Lilly	Human	U-100
Humulin 70/30 (70% NPH, 30% Regular)	Lilly	Human	U-100
Humulin 70/30 Cartridges (1.5 ml)	Lilly	Human	U-100
Novolin 70/30 (70% NPH, 30% Regular)	Novo Nordisk	Human	U-100
Novolin 70/30 PenFill (70% NPH, 30% Regular)	Novo Nordisk	Human	U-100
Novolin 70/30 Prefilled (70% NPH, 30% Regular)	Novo Nordisk	Human	U-100

Modified from American Diabetes Association: 1999 buyer's guide to diabetes products, Alexandria, Va, 1999.

Long-Acting Insulin
Protamine zinc insulin (PZI), ultralente, and glargine

PZI is a cloudy suspension of a protamine-insulin-zinc precipitate that has poor solubility and is poorly absorbed from tissue. Because of this relative insolubility, this preparation is slowly absorbed from the injection site and therefore maintains a long-lasting blood level. The manufacturer removed the human label product from the market in 1991 because of declining demand.

Ultralente insulin is similar in effect and duration to PZI insulin. Unlike PZI, ultralente does not contain protamine.

Glargine (Lantus) insulin is a new, long-acting insulin with a human label. It is a clear insulin that is unlike other long- acting insulins that are all cloudy. Care should be taken to avoid confusing Lantus with other clear insulins.

Clinical Uses. PZI is used for the treatment of uncomplicated diabetes mellitus.

Dosage Forms
1. Ultralente (Humulin U)
2. PZI VET. U-40 insulin that carries a veterinary label for cats
3. Lantus. Clear, long-acting insulin

Adverse Side Effects. These are similar to those of regular and NPH insulin.

> ### Technician's Notes
> PZI is considered by some to be the insulin form of choice for use in cats.

USE OF INSULIN PRODUCTS
Technicians who are counseling clients about the use of insulin products should take great care to become thoroughly familiar with the products they are using. The onset of action of various insulin products can vary from a few minutes to a few hours. Peak activity time and duration of activity can also vary greatly between products. Exercise levels and eating patterns may influence insulin activity. An overdose of insulin can lead to various degrees of hypoglycemia, which produce clinical signs ranging from mild weakness to coma. Clients should be shown how to give subcutaneous injections of insulin and they should be given written instructions about monitoring insulin response and making appropriate adjustments. Tips regarding the use of insulin products follow as technician's notes.

> ### Technician's Notes
> 1. It is usually best to feed the animal 30 minutes before giving the insulin injection.
> 2. Roll "cloudy" insulins between your palms; do not shake.
> 3. NPH insulin should not be mixed with any Lente insulin.
> 4. It is the opinion of some people that insulin should be disposed of after 30 days or 100 injections.
> 5. Rotation of injection sites should be practiced.
> 6. Clients should be advised to use insulin syringes only once.
> 7. Mild to moderate hypoglycemia resulting from an overdose can be treated by feeding the animal or administering Karo syrup.

Oral Hypoglycemic Agents
Oral hypoglycemic agents, such as the sulfonylureas, are extensively used in human diabetic patients to control type II diabetes mellitus (NIDDM). They have little apparent effectiveness in diabetic dogs but may be useful in some cats with type II diabetes. Drugs in this category include glipizide (Glucotrol) and metformin (Glucophage XR).

 Hyperglycemc Agents

Several drugs, such as corticosteroids, epinephrine, and progesterone, incidentally elevate blood glucose levels. Two products that are marketed for this purpose, however, are diazoxide (Proglycem)

and octreotide (Sandostatin). They are used to treat the low blood glucose levels associated with hypersecretion of insulin that occurs in tumors of the beta cells of the pancreas (insulinoma) in dogs and ferrets (Plumb, 2002). These products act by inhibiting the release of insulin from the beta cells of the pancreas.

HORMONES THAT ACT AS GROWTH PROMOTERS

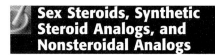

Sex Steroids, Synthetic Steroid Analogs, and Nonsteroidal Analogs

The factors that control growth, **feed efficiency,** and carcass composition in animals involve a complex interrelationship between genetic, metabolic, and hormonal mechanisms that are not always totally understood. It is possible, however, to increase growth (weight gain) in ruminants by administering sex steroid hormones (estrogen, testosterone, or progesterone), synthetic steroid hormone analogs (trenbolone), or certain nonsteroidal hormone analogs (zeranol).

The primary sex steroid used to promote weight gain is estrogen (estradiol). The mechanisms by which estradiol promotes weight gain include (1) increased water retention, (2) increased protein synthesis, (3) increased fat deposition, and (4) possible increased release of growth hormone (bovine somatotropin).

Testosterone is used as an adjunct to estradiol in some growth promotion products because it is an anabolic agent in itself and because a second component in the compound slows down the release of the estradiol and prolongs its effective life span.

Progesterone is also added to growth promoters to slow the release of estradiol. It apparently has little anabolic effect of its own.

Trenbolone is a synthetic anabolic agent that improves feed efficiency and promotes weight gain in steers. It is used as the sole agent in some growth-promoting preparations.

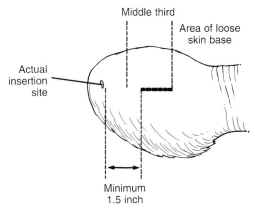

FIGURE 9-5
Implantation site for growth-promoting pellets (posterior view of ear).

Zeranol is an analog of a naturally occurring plant estrogen that increases feed efficiency, protein synthesis, and growth rate.

All of the growth-promoting products for use in cattle and sheep are prepared as compressed pellets that are implanted in the subcutaneous tissue of the dorsal, middle third of the ear (Figure 9-5). These pellets are designed for use with corresponding needle devices and should be implanted with close adherence to product instructions (failure to do so is a violation of federal law in some cases).

The growth promotion products are considered here as a group, and minimal information is provided about each product.

Clinical Uses. These drugs are used to promote feed efficiency and weight gain in calves, steers, heifers, or sheep (depending on the product).

Dosage Forms
1. Synovex C. Estradiol/progesterone implant for use in calves older than 45 days
2. Synovex H. Estradiol/testosterone implant for use in heifers
3. Synovex S. Estradiol/testosterone implant for use in steers
4. Compudose. Estradiol implant for use in steers
5. Implus-H. Estradiol/testosterone implant for use in heifers

6. Implus-S. Estradiol/progesterone for use in steers
7. CALF-oid Implant. Progesterone/estradiol implant for calves older than 45 days
8. Finaplix-H. Trenbolone implant for use in feedlot heifers
9. Finaplix-S. Trenbolone implant for steers
10. Revalor-S. Trenbolone and estradiol implant for use in feedlot steers
11. Ralgro beef cattle implant. Zeranol implant for use in growing cattle, feedlot heifers, feedlot steers, and suckling and weaned calves
12. Ralgro feedlot lamb implant. Zeranol implant for feedlot lambs

Adverse Side Effects. These may include mounting, elevated tailheads, rectal prolapse, and udder development.

Technician's Notes

1. Most growth-promoting implants should not be given to animals intended for breeding purposes or to dairy cattle.
2. Product insert instructions should be read and followed carefully with these products.

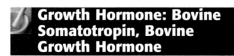

Growth Hormone: Bovine Somatotropin, Bovine Growth Hormone

Growth hormone, also called *somatotropin*, is a hormone produced by the anterior pituitary. Its function before the onset of puberty is to stimulate growth. It is released throughout life to promote anabolic activity (e.g., to increase protein synthesis). It has been shown to increase growth rate and feed efficiency in farm animals. Many of the growth-promoting agents listed in the previous section may work by stimulating the release of somatotropin. Somatotropin is a potent stimulator of milk production as well. Claims have been made of a 20% boost in milk production in dairy cows after administration of somatotropin.

The Food and Drug Administration (FDA) approved a recombinant (genetically engineered) bovine somatotropin (BST) for commercial production in 1993. This product, Posilac, is manufactured by the Monsanto Co. Its market availability has sparked intense debate between certain groups. Some dairy producers have opposed its use because of their fear that increased production would drive milk prices down and reduce their overall income. Other groups have resisted the use of BST because of their concerns about residues of the hormone in milk products, even though the FDA has stated that milk from cows receiving BST is completely safe. Time and the workings of the marketplace should resolve the debates.

ANABOLIC STEROIDS

Anabolic steroids are steroids that cause a tissue building (anabolic) effect. Testosterone is a naturally occurring anabolic steroid that produces masculinization in addition to the anabolic effects. Synthetic anabolic steroids are designed to prevent most of the masculinizing effects.

Anabolic steroid administration causes positive **nitrogen balance** and reverses processes that break down tissue. An increase in appetite, weight gain, improved overall condition, and recovery are promoted. These products are labeled for clinical use in dogs, cats, and horses for anorexia, weight loss, and debilitation. In working animals, they may be used in cases of overwork or overtraining. Anabolic steroids also promote red blood cell formation and are used to treat some forms of anemia. The product insert for a commonly used product states that "anabolic therapy is intended primarily as an adjunct to other specific and supportive therapy, including nutritional therapy."

Because of the potential for abuse by bodybuilders and other athletes, the FDA has now classified anabolic steroids as C-III controlled substances.

Stanozolol

Stanozolol is an anabolic steroid found to have an unusual pattern of biologic activity in that its anabolic effect far outweighs its weak androgenic influence.

Clinical Uses. Stanozolol is used for treatment of anorexia, debilitation, weight loss, overwork, and anemia.

Dosage Forms
1. Winstrol-V. Stanozolol sterile suspension for injection in dogs, cats, and horses
2. Winstrol-V. Stanozolol tablets for use in dogs and cats

Adverse Side Effects. These may include mild androgenic effects after prolonged use or overdose.

Technician's Notes
1. Winstrol-V should not be used in pregnant dogs, mares, or in stallions.
2. Winstrol-V should not be given to horses intended for use in food.

Boldenone Undecylenate

Boldenone undecylenate is a steroid ester that possesses marked anabolic activity and a minimal amount of androgenic activity. It is labeled for use in horses.

Clinical Uses. Boldenone undecylenate acts as an aid in the treatment of debilitated horses.

Dosage Form
Equipose. Boldenone injection for horses

Adverse Side Effects. These include androgenic effects such as overaggressiveness.

Technician's Notes
1. Boldenone should not be used in horses intended as food.
2. Boldenone should not be used in stallions or pregnant mares.

Nandrolone Decanoate

Nandrolone decanoate is an injectable anabolic steroid sold under the human label Deca-Durabolin. It has activity similar to the other anabolic agents.

REFERENCES

Boothe DM: Drug therapy for endocrinopathies. In Boothe DM, editor: small animal clinical pharmacology, Philadelphia, 2001, WB Saunders Co.
Plumb DC: Veterinary drug handbook, Ames, 2002, Iowa State University Press.

REVIEW QUESTIONS

1. Describe the relationship between hormonal releasing factors, trophic hormones, and the hormones produced by specific tissues or glands. _____
2. List the major endocrine glands. _____

3. What are the reasons for using hormonal therapy in veterinary medicine? _____

4. Endogenous hormones are those produced _____, whereas exogenous hormones come from _____ sources.
5. Where is the pituitary gland located, and what is its function? _____
6. Describe the difference between a negative and a positive feedback control mechanism in the endocrine system. _____

7. The release of oxytocin by the posterior pituitary is controlled through the _____ mechanism.
8. GnRH is classified as a/an _____.
9. Hormonal products with *gest* in their name are classified as _____.
10. List three potential uses of the prostaglandins in veterinary medicine. _____

11. Human skin contact or injection with prostaglandins can be a serious health risk to _____ women and _____.
12. Before oxytocin can exert its effects on the uterus, the uterus must first be primed by _____.
13. What precautions should be taken before oxytocin is administered? _____

14. What are the two active hormones produced by the thyroid gland? _____
15. List two drugs used in the treatment of hypothyroidism. _____
16. List the three major classes of insulin. _____
17. Which form of insulin is used in the treatment of diabetic ketoacidosis? _____
18. Which form(s) of insulin must be resuspended before administration? _____
19. What are some signs of insulin overdose? _____
20. Growth promoters generally should not be used in animals intended for _____.
21. Why are anabolic steroids classified as controlled substances? _____
22. _____ are odors released by animals that influence the behavior of other animals of the same species.
23. What precautions should be taken by pregnant women when administering Regu-Mate? _____
24. Why was synthetic DES banned from use in food-producing animals? _____
25. Prostaglandin causes lysis of the _____ at the end of pregnancy or at the end of diestrus if pregnancy does not occur.

OPHTHALMIC AGENTS
Mydriatics and Cycloplegics
    Phenylephrine Hydrochloride
    Atropine Sulfate
    Homatropine Hydrobromide
    Cyclopentolate Hydrochloride
    Tropicamide
    Epinephrine
Miotics
    Pilocarpine
    Carbachol
    Echothiophate Iodide
Other Agents that Reduce Intraocular
  Pressure
    Carbonic Anhydrase Inhibitors
        TIMOLOL MALEATE
    Mannitol
    Glycerol
Topical Anesthetics
    Proparacaine Hydrochloride
    Tetracaine and Tetracaine Hydrochloride
Ophthalmic Stains
Collagen Shields
Topical Ophthalmic Antiinfectives
    Antiviral Agents
Antifungal Agents
Antibacterial Agents
Topical Ophthalmic Antiinflammatory
  Agents
    Nonsteroidal Agents
    Topical Corticosteroid Agents
Agents for the Treatment of
  Keratoconjunctivitis Sicca
    Cyclosporine
    Artificial Tear Products and Ocular
      Lubricants
OTIC DRUGS
Topical Otic Antiinfective Agents
    Gentamicin Sulfate
    Chloramphenicol
    Neomycin Sulfate
    Enrofloxin
Antiparasitics
    Pyrethrins
    Rotenone
    Ivermectin
Drying Agents
Cleaning Agents
Miscellaneous Otic Agents
    Tris-EDTA
    Silver Sulfadiazine

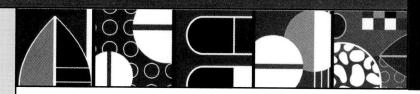

CHAPTER **10**

Drugs Used in Ophthalmic and Otic Disorders

LEARNING OBJECTIVES

After studying this chapter, you should be able to:

1. Understand the clinical indications for common ophthalmic and otic agents
2. Identify the different classes of ophthalmic and otic agents
3. Identify the possible adverse reactions and contraindications of many commonly used agents

KEY TERMS

CLOSED-ANGLE GLAUCOMA A type of primary glaucoma of the eye characterized by a shallow anterior chamber and a narrow angle that compromises filtration because of the iris' blocking the angle and causing an increase in intraocular pressure.

CONJUNCTIVITIS Inflammation of the conjunctiva.

CYCLOPLEGIA Paralysis of the ciliary muscle.

ECTROPION A rolling outward (i.e., away from the eye) or sagging of the eyelid. Many times the conjunctiva is plainly visible.

ENTROPION A rolling inward (i.e., towards the cornea) of the eyelid.

GLAUCOMA A group of eye diseases characterized by increased intraocular pressure resulting in damage to the retina and the optic nerve.

KERATITIS Inflammation of the cornea.

MIOSIS Contraction of the pupil.

MYDRIASIS Dilation of the pupil.

OPEN-ANGLE GLAUCOMA A type of primary glaucoma of the eye in which the angle of the anterior chamber remains open, but filtration of the aqueous humor is gradually reduced—causing an increase in intraocular pressure.

UVEA The vascular layer of the eye comprising the iris, ciliary body, and choroid.

UVEITIS Inflammation of the uvea.

OPHTHALMIC AGENTS

Although the sense of smell is highly developed in many animals, the sense of sight plays an important aspect in an animal's health and well-being. Cats rely on excellent eyesight because they are prey animals. This prey trait provides many cat owners with amusement and laughter, as a string or feather toy is pulled around the house with a cat running behind in rapid pursuit. Horses rely on good eyesight to perform their best for human companions. Police dogs, hunting dogs, seeing-eye dogs, and herd-working dogs rely on their eyesight to interpret their owner's hand signals when working in the field.

A good ocular examination includes an examination of the external ocular features (eyelids, sclera, cornea, third eyelid [nictitating membrane]) and internal ocular features (anterior chamber, iris, lens), all of which can be seen without highly specialized equipment (McCurnin, 2002). Some dog breeds (Sharpei, cocker spaniels, English bulldogs, and others) are genetically predisposed to conditions that may require surgery. Two of these conditions are known as **entropion** and **ectropion.**

Topical administration of eye drops or ointment is the most common method of treatment involving disorders of the eye. It is the veterinary technician's duty to educate the client by demonstrating the proper way to administer eye medication. Products for ocular treatment are usually available as solutions or ointments. Drug penetration is one factor that veterinarians must consider when choosing a topical ophthalmic agent. Topical agents are more readily absorbed into the anterior chamber than the posterior chamber. For this reason, these agents have limited use in posterior eye disorders. Systemic agents may be more effective. Lipid-soluble agents readily penetrate the corneal epithelium and endothelium layers. Water-soluble agents readily penetrate the corneal stroma layer (Figure 10-1). Most topical ophthalmic medications require several applications per day because the eye continuously secretes tears that wash away the medication. Ointments tend to necessitate less frequent applications than do drops. However, ointments may blur an animal's vision for a short period after application. Client education is invaluable when treating an eye disorder.

Clients placing telephone calls to the veterinary hospital to discuss a potential eye problem in a patient should be made to realize that these situations may be considered an emergency. Unfortunately, some clients tend to let an ocular problem progress to severe stages before treatment is sought.

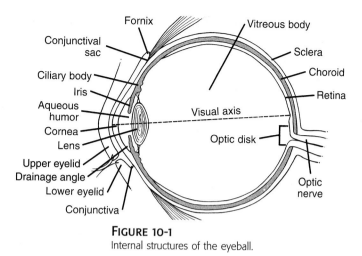

FIGURE 10-1
Internal structures of the eyeball.

Veterinary technicians should remind clients that animals have only two eyes and the importance of vision should not be minimized.

 Mydriatics and Cycloplegics

Mydriatic agents are used to dilate the pupils (Figure 10-2). This action facilitates examination of the posterior segment and the fundus of the eye. Cycloplegic agents paralyze the accommodative muscle of the ciliary body. In some cases, the action can minimize pain associated with ciliary spasms. These agents are often used before and after ophthalmic surgery.

Phenylephrine Hydrochloride
Phenylephrine hydrochloride is used to produce **mydriasis** but does not produce **cycloplegia.**

Clinical Uses. Phenylephrine HCl is used in the evaluation of uveitis, glaucoma, or scleritis. It may also be used before conjunctival surgery to reduce hemorrhage or used in combination with atropine before cataract or intraocular surgery. It can be used to determine the presence of Horner's syndrome.

Dosage Form
Mydfrin (human label)

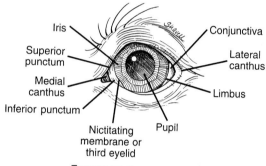

FIGURE 10-2
External structures of the eye.

Adverse Side Effects. These include local discomfort after application. Frequent use may lead to inflammation.

Technician's Notes
Phenylephrine HCl is also used in cough preparations but at a higher concentration.

Atropine Sulfate
Atropine sulfate is one of the ophthalmic agents most commonly used to produce mydriasis and cycloplegia.

Clinical Uses. Atropine sulfate is used for refraction or for the treatment of acute inflammatory conditions of the anterior uveal tract.

Dosage Form
Atrophate

Adverse Side Effects. These include salivation. Atropine is contraindicated in **glaucoma** and keratoconjunctivitis sicca (KCS or dry eye).

Homatropine Hydrobromide
Homatropine hydrobromide produces mydriasis and cycloplegia but is less potent than atropine.

Clinical Uses. Homatropine hydrobromide is used for refraction and the treatment of **uveitis.**

Dosage Forms
1. Homatrocel Ophthalmic (human label)
2. Isopto Homatropine (human label)

Adverse Side Effects. These are the same as for atropine.

Cyclopentolate Hydrochloride
Cyclopentolate hydrochloride produces mydriasis and cycloplegia.

Clinical Uses. Cyclopentolate hydrochloride is used for refraction.

Dosage Form
Cyclogyl (human label)

Adverse Side Effects. These are the same as for atropine.

Tropicamide
Tropicamide is a rapid-acting mydriatic but has less cycloplegic effect than the previously mentioned drugs.

Clinical Uses. Tropicamide is used for ocular fundus examination.

Dosage Form
Mydriacyl (human label)

Adverse Side Effects. These include local discomfort after application and salivation. Contraindications are the same as for atropine.

Epinephrine
Epinephrine is administered topically and is available as epinephrine and dipivalyl epinephrine. Dipivalyl epinephrine more readily penetrates the corneal barrier and is converted to epinephrine in the cornea.

Clinical Uses. Epinephrine is used to reduce intraocular pressure, produce mydriasis, or aid in the diagnosis of Horner's syndrome.

Dosage Form
Epifrin (human label)

Adverse Side Effects. These include local irritation. Epinephrine is contraindicated in **closed-angle glaucoma.**

 ## Miotics

Miotics produce pupillary constriction. These drugs are commonly used in the treatment of chronic **open-angle glaucoma,** acute and chronic closed-angle glaucoma, and some cases of secondary glaucoma. Miotics reduce intraocular pressure by increasing the outflow of aqueous humor.

Pilocarpine
Pilocarpine is a cholinergic drug commonly used to treat chronic open-angle glaucoma.

Clinical Uses. These include stimulation of tear production in some cases of keratoconjunctivitis sicca.

Dosage Form
Piloptic

Adverse Side Effects. These include local irritation and discomfort. Repeated use may cause vomiting, diarrhea, and salivation.

Carbachol

Carbachol is a cholinergic drug and is used less commonly than pilocarpine.

Clinical Uses. Carbachol is used to treat glaucoma.

Dosage Form
Carbacel (human label)

Adverse Side Effects. These are uncommon.

Echothiophate Iodide

Echothiophate iodide is an organophosphate that also produces **miosis** when applied topically to the eyes. This solution has a longer duration of action than pilocarpine.

Clinical Uses. These include the treatment of open-angle glaucoma.

Dosage Forms
1. Echodids (human label)
2. Phospholine Iodide (human label)

Adverse Side Effects. Systemic organophosphate toxicity is possible in smaller patients.

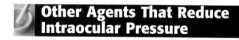
Other Agents That Reduce Intraocular Pressure

Carbonic Anhydrase Inhibitors

Carbonic anhydrase inhibitors reduce intraocular pressure by reducing the production of aqueous humor. These products, like those previously mentioned, are used to control glaucoma. However, some are administered orally and intravenously rather than topically.

Dosage Forms
1. Dichlorphenamide (Daranide—human label)
2. Acetazolamide (Diamox—human label)
3. Methazolamide (Neptazane—human label)
4. Dorzolamide (Trusopt—human label)
5. Diamox

Adverse Side Effects. These include vomiting, diarrhea, panting, and weakness.

TIMOLOL MALEATE

Timolol maleate is an ophthalmic beta blocker with action that results in decreased production of aqueous humor.

Clinical Uses. Timolol maleate is used in the contralateral eye of a dog with primary glaucoma to prevent the development of bilateral disease. It does reduce intraocular pressure some, but it is not as effective in the treatment of glaucoma.

Dosage Form
Timoptic (human label)

Adverse Side Effects. Adverse side effects are uncommon. See the Technician's Notes below.

> *Technician's Notes*
> Timolol may be contraindicated in some patients with cardiovascular disease or bronchoconstrictive disease.

Mannitol

Mannitol is an osmotic diuretic that is administered intravenously to reduce intraocular pressure in emergency situations.

Dosage Form
Mannitol injection

Adverse Side Effects. These include fluid and electrolyte imbalance, nausea, vomiting, pulmonary edema, congestive heart failure, and tachycardia.

Glycerol

Glycerol (glycerin) is an osmotic diuretic that is administered orally to reduce intraocular pressure in emergency situations.

Dosage Form
Osmoglyn (human label)

Adverse Side Effects. Vomiting may occur after administration.

Technician's Notes
Glycerol acts more slowly than mannitol.

 Topical Anesthetics

Topical anesthetics anesthetize the corneal surface and are commonly used to allow removal of a foreign body or sutures, to allow the use of instruments to measure intraocular pressure, or to aid in the application of a hydrophilic contact lens.

Proparacaine Hydrochloride

Proparacaine hydrochloride is a commonly used topical anesthetic. Anesthesia lasts 5 to 10 minutes.

Dosage Form
Ophthaine

Adverse Side Effects. These are very uncommon.

Technician's Notes
Unopened bottles may be stored at room temperature, but opened bottles should be refrigerated. Any discolored solutions should be discarded.

Ophthalmic solutions should be warmed (i.e., those stored in the refrigerator) to room temperature before administration into the patient's eye. This can be facilitated by rolling the bottle between the palms of the hands or placing the bottle under the arm, until the desired temperatured is achieved.

Tetracaine and Tetracaine Hydrochloride

Tetracaine and tetracaine hydrochloride are also used for anesthetizing the cornea.

Dosage Forms
1. Pontocaine (human label)
2. Pontocaine hydrochloride (human label)

Adverse Side Effects. These include irritation, which usually is resolved within a short period after administration.

Technician's Notes
Unlike proparacaine, tetracaine inhibits the growth of microorganisms, and cultures should be obtained before its administration.

 Ophthalmic Stains

Ophthalmic stains are used as diagnostic aids for detecting disease in both the anterior and posterior segments and in the nasolacrimal system. Fluorescein stain (i.e., strips) is the most commonly used dye for the detection of corneal epithelial defects. By wetting the strip with sterile water or saline, the stain is allowed to cover the eye. The strip should not be allowed to touch the cornea. Excess dye is rinsed from the eye with sterile eye wash. Fluorescein stain is a water-soluble agent. The outer (epithelial) layer of the cornea is a fat-soluble layer, and the stroma, just beneath the epithelium, is a water-soluble layer. If the epithelium is intact, the stain does not adhere because of the difference in solubilities. If the epithelium is eroded, as in the case of a corneal ulcer, the stain gains access to the water-soluble stroma where it adheres and remains after the eye is rinsed. Appearance of fluorescein stain at the nostril opening indicates functional patency of the nasolacrimal drainage system.

Technician's Notes
1. Do not allow the fluorescein strip to touch the cornea, because this could potentially produce a paper cut on the cornea.
2. A good idea is to obtain a sterile 6-cc syringe and place the fluorescein strip into the syringe barrel. Fill the syringe with sterile water and replace the plunger. Invert the syringe several times until the water turns yellow. Simply administer this solution into the eye for the staining procedure.
3. Horses have strong palpebral muscles. If stain is to be used in this species, it may be necessary to have another person keep the eyelids spread apart while the stain is introduced into the eye.
4. Fluorescein stains the hair if allowed to drain on the face. Use cotton to wipe away excess fluorescein stain, as it is softer than a paper towel.

Collagen Shields

Collagen shields are biodegradable contact lens–shaped films made from porcine or bovine collagen. They dissolve in 12 to 72 hours because of the naturally occurring enzymes found in tears.

Clinical Uses. A collagen shield may be used in the treatment of superficial corneal ulcers.

Dosage Form
Vet-Shield 72

> ### Technician's Notes
> A topical ophthalmic anesthetic should be used before placing the shield onto the eye. It may be necessary to sedate the animal with a short-acting general anesthetic.

Topical Ophthalmic Antiinfectives

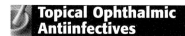

Antiviral Agents
Antiviral agents may be used to treat viral infections of the eye, such as herpes simplex **keratitis** (e.g., feline ocular herpes).

Dosage Forms
1. Idoxuridine (Stoxil—human label)
2. Trifluridine (Viroptic ophthalmic solution—human label)
3. Vidarabine (Vir-A Ophthalmic—human label)

Antifungal Agents

Antifungal agents are used to treat ophthalmic fungal infections, such as mycotic keratitis, mycotic endophthalmitis, and blepharodermatomycosis. Mycotic keratitis occurs most commonly in horses.

Dosage Forms
1. Natamycin (Natacyn—human label)
2. Miconazole injection (Monistat-IV—human label)

> ### Technician's Notes
> Miconazole injection is applied topically to the cornea in the treatment of mycotic keratitis (Plumb, 2002).

Antibacterial Agents

Antibacterial agents are used to treat superficial ocular infections resulting from bacterial organisms. These drugs are often used in combination with each other to provide broad-spectrum activity.

1. Bacitracin is used topically to treat superficial ocular infections resulting primarily from gram-positive bacteria and is often combined with other antibacterial agents, such as neomycin and polymyxin B.
2. Chloramphenicol is available for topical ophthalmic administration and provides broad-spectrum activity. This agent is antagonistic with aminoglycosides.
3. Gentamicin is used topically to treat **conjunctivitis** caused by susceptible bacterial agents.
4. Polymyxin B sulfate is effective against gram-negative organisms and may be combined with other antibacterial agents to provide broad-spectrum activity.
5. Oxytetracycline is used to treat superficial ocular infections and provides broad-spectrum activity. It may be used in combination with other agents, such as polymyxin B.
6. Neomycin provides broad-spectrum activity and is often used in combination with other topical ophthalmic antibacterials.
7. Fluoroquinolone ophthalmic antibiotics are used to treat established gram-negative corneal infections. Ciprofloxacin, Norfloxacin, and ofloxacin are available as human products. They are not recommended for prophylactic use before or after surgery (Plumb, 2002).

> ### Technician's Notes
> Chloramphenicol must not be used in animals raised for food production.

Topical Ophthalmic Antiinflammatory Agents

Nonsteroidal Agents

Nonsteroidal antiinflammatory agents (NSAIDs) are used in the treatment of uveitis. They are commonly used for postsurgical inflammation following cataract surgery.

Dosage Forms
1. Flurbiprofen sodium (Ocufen—human label)
2. Ketorolac tromethamine (Acular—human label)
3. Diclofenac sodium (Voltaren—human label)

Adverse Side Effects. These are uncommon, but flurbiprofen can cause immunosuppression.

Topical Corticosteroid Agents

Corticosteroid agents are used to treat inflammatory conditions of the cornea, iris, conjunctiva, sclera, and anterior uvea. Topical corticosteroids have poor penetration into the eyelid and the posterior segment of the eye (Plumb, 2002). They may be combined with antibacterial agents to manage ocular infections. Some common corticosteroid agents for ophthalmic use include prednisolone, hydrocortisone, dexamethasone, betamethasone, and flumethasone.

Dosage Forms
1. Prednisolone acetate drops—human label
2. Prednisolone sodium phosphate drops—human label
3. Gentocin Durafilm solution
4. Anaprime ophthalmic solution
5. Neo-Predef

Adverse Side Effects. Topical corticosteroids can cause problems similar to those caused by systemic corticosteroids. These include delayed healing, steroid dependency, and corneal complications—such as ulcerative keratitis.

Technician's Notes
Ophthalmic products containing corticosteroids are contraindicated in the treatment of deep corneal ulcers, fungal infections, and viral infections.

Agents for the Treatment of Keratoconjunctivitis Sicca

Keratoconjunctivitis sicca (KCS) is a common ocular disorder in dogs. With this disorder, there is reduced secretion of the lacrimal glands resulting in corneal dryness. If left untreated, corneal ulceration and eventual perforation may occur (Tizard, 2000).

Cyclosporine

Cyclosporine is used for the management of KCS and chronic superficial keratitis (CSK, or German Shepherd pannus). It stimulates increased tear production, although its mechanism of action is not fully understood.

Dosage Forms
1. Optimmune Ophthalmic Ointment
2. Cyclosporin A
3. Neoral
4. Sandimmune

Adverse Side Effects. Adverse side effects are uncommon.

Technician's Notes
It may take several days to a few weeks before the effects of cyclosporine therapy are evident.

Artificial Tear Products and Ocular Lubricants

Before the availability of cyclosporine, artificial tears were used in the treatment of KCS and CSK. These products serve as lubricants for dry eyes and are commonly used in conjunction with cyclosporine therapy. Ocular lubricants are petroleum-based products used to lubricate and protect the eyes. They are commonly used during anesthetic procedures in which the eyes may remain open and may become dry.

Dosage Forms
1. Bion Tears (human label)
2. Liquifilm Tears (human label)

Adverse Side Effects. These are uncommon.

OTIC DRUGS

When a client obtains a new puppy, the veterinary technician should educate the client regarding the proper way to clean the pup's ears. Performing the ear cleaning process at an early age will allow the puppy to submit more readily to the task as an adult dog. Unfortunately, those breeds with pendulous ears may tend to have otic problems. The long ear flaps (i.e., pinnae) tend to keep air from circulating into the ear canal and consequently the ear canal remains moist, creating a perfect environment for yeast formation. Yeast is not the only problem veterinarians encounter in dogs and cats. External parasites, such as *Otodectes cyanotis* and *Otodectes procyonis* (i.e., ear mites), can lead to extreme discomfort in animals parasitized by these creatures. Patients whose ears remain untreated often experience aural hematomas caused by extreme shaking of the head.

Generally, ear problems are treated with topical medications. Sometimes ear infections must be treated with systemic medication as well. Topical preparations used to treat ear infections are often a combination of different types of drugs, such as an antibacterial, antifungal, antipruritic, and antiinflammatory. Still other preparations are cleansers, drying agents, and parasiticides. When a ruptured eardrum is suspected or confirmed, oil-based or irritating external ear preparations (e.g., chlorhexidine) and aminoglycosides should be avoided.

When educating clients about cleaning ears and using otic medications, the veterinary technician should demonstrate how to clean the ear canal. Assure the client that because of the anatomy of

the ear, the eardrum is difficult to reach. Emphasize that preventive care is much easier than having to treat infections continually, especially in those dog breeds predisposed to having ear problems (Figure 10-3).

Topical Otic Antiinfective Agents

Many topical otic preparations with antibacterial or antifungal properties are manufactured and available for placing in inventory. Topical otic preparations often contain antiinflammatory agents to reduce inflammation and decrease pruritus. A good idea consists of clipping the hair on the inside of the pinna and any hair that may block the external ear canal. It is also a good idea to use a cleanser before medicating the ear. By cleansing the ear first, cerumen and debris are removed from the external canal so that the medicine can work effectively. After the ear is cleaned, it should be dried before treatment.

Gentamicin Sulfate
Gentamicin sulfate is an antibacterial agent found in otic preparations. It is commonly combined with a corticosteroid, such as betamethasone valerate. Some products also have antifungal properties because of the addition of clotrimazole.

Clinical Uses. These include the treatment of acute and chronic otitis in dogs. In cats, it may be used to treat superficial infected lesions caused by bacteria susceptible to gentamicin.

Dosage Forms
1. GentaVed Otic Solution
2. Gentocin Otic Solution
3. Otomax
4. Tri-Otic

Adverse Side Effects. These include possible ototoxicity because gentamicin is an aminoglycoside.

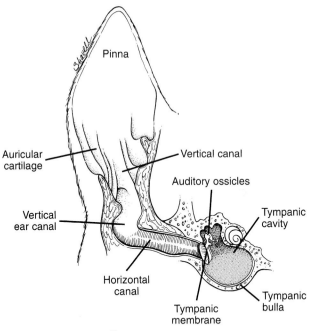

FIGURE 10-3
Structures of the ear.

Technician's Notes
1. Patients should be carefully monitored for signs of ototoxicity. Products that lower the pH or produce an acidic environment in the ear can reduce the efficacy of gentamicin.
2. Do not use these products with other agents that may cause ototoxicity.
3. Do not use in the presence of a ruptured eardrum.

Dosage Forms
1. Liquichlor
2. Chlora-Otic

Technician's Notes
Products containing chloramphenicol cannot be used in animals raised for food production.

Chloramphenicol
Chloramphenicol is an antibacterial agent often combined with a corticosteroid such as prednisolone. Products may also contain an anesthetic (tetracaine) and squalane (cerumene). Squalane enhances the product by speeding up percutaneous penetration of the active ingredients.

Clinical Uses. These include treatment for acute otitis externa and pyodermas in dogs and cats.

Neomycin Sulfate
Neomycin sulfate is an antibacterial agent often combined with drugs such as corticosteroids, antifungals, and/or anesthetics.

Clinical Uses. Clinical uses of this antibacterial, antifungal/antiparasitic, and antiinflammatory combination include the treatment of otitis externa and certain bacterial, fungal, and inflammatory skin disorders.

Dosage Forms
1. Tresaderm
2. Tritop
3. Panalog

Adverse Side Effects. These include sensitivity resulting from the neomycin. If such signs (e.g., erythema) develop after treatment, the medication should be discontinued. Ototoxicity is also a potential side effect.

> ### Technician's Notes
> 1. Do not use in the presence of a ruptured tympanic membrane (i.e., eardrum).
> 2. Observe the patient for signs of ototoxicity.

Enrofloxin

Enrofloxin is available as a combination otic product with silver sulfadiazine.

Dosage Form
Baytril Otic

 Antiparasitics

Ear mites are ubiquitous in the environment. They are the most common parasite affecting the ears of dogs, cats, and rabbits. These mites are macroscopic, white, and freely motile. Although they occur primarily in the external ear canal, ear mites may be found on any area of the body (Hendrix, 1998). Ear mites can be identified using an otoscope and will appear as white, motile creatures within the external ear canal. Ear mites can also be observed microscopically by placing exudate, which can be removed from the ear canal with a cotton-tipped applicator stick, into mineral oil on a microscope slide.

The spinose ear tick (*Otobius megnini*) affects the external ear canal of cattle and horses, and occasionally dogs and cats. The immature ticks pack the ear canal, which causes discomfort, and should be removed. Periodically treating the animal with an insecticide, such as a flea and tick spray, prevents reinfection. Cattle and horses can be treated with topical sprays, such as Catron IV. This product should not be used in lactating dairy animals or on household pets.

> ### Technician's Note
> Ticks should not be removed with bare hands. Technicians should educate clients not to remove ticks without wearing gloves. Donning a pair of exam gloves (or Playtex gloves for clients at home) and then extracting ticks is better. A pair of thumb forceps can also be employed.

Pyrethrins

Some products containing pyrethrins are indicated for the treatment of ticks and mites in the ears of dogs and cats.

Dosage Forms
1. Cerumite
2. Aurimite
3. Mita-Clear
4. Tresaderm
5. Nolvamite

Rotenone

Rotenone is an effective agent for the treatment of ear mites in dogs, cats, and rabbits.

Dosage Forms
1. Ear miticide
2. Mitaplex-R

Ivermectin

Ivermectin has been indicated as an effective treatment for ear mites in dogs and cats. This is an extralabel use of the bovine injectable product Ivomec. The dose is most often given by subcutaneous injection, although some practitioners place it directly into the external ear canal. In recent years, a product that contains .01% Ivomec (Acarexx) has been developed for the treatment of ear mites.

Dosage Form
Acarexx 0.01%

Drying Agents

Drying agents are used to reduce moisture in the ears. Excess moisture provides a warm, moist environment that is ideal for the growth of certain bacterial and yeast agents, which can cause infection or inflammation. These preparations may also contain an antimicrobial or a corticosteroid. Tannic acid, salicylic acid, acetic acid, and boric acid are commonly used in drying solutions.

Dosage Forms
1. Dermal Dry
2. Ace-Otic Cleanser

Technician's Notes

1. It is recommended that the ears be cleaned before applying a drying agent or other medication.
2. Some ear cleansing products also contain drying agents.

Cleaning Agents

Ear cleansers are used to clean the ears and provide odor control. In the presence of otitis externa, they help to remove necrotic tissue, debris, and wax. Many breeds, as mentioned before, are predisposed to ear problems, and routine cleaning can often reduce or prevent these problems. These cleansers may also contain an antimicrobial agent, anesthetic, or drying agent. Many cleansers contain an agent such as squalane (cerumene), which helps to break up and soften wax and debris and facilitate cleaning. If wax and debris are impacted in the horizontal canal, it may be necessary to flush the ear canal to remove the wax and debris before starting routine cleaning. The ears may be too painful for this type of cleaning without general anesthesia. A common solution for flushing the ear canal is a mixture of warm water and chlorhexidine surgical solution diluted 1:100. Flushing may be accomplished using a bulb syringe, a soft rubber feeding tube, or a regular tip syringe. It is very important to use gentle pressure when flushing the ear canal to reduce the possibility of damaging the eardrum. Thorough drying of the canal after flushing provides better visualization of the eardrum.

Dosage Forms
1. Epi-Otic ear cleanser
2. Fresh-Ear
3. Oti-Clens

Miscellaneous Otic Agents

Tris-EDTA
Tris-EDTA (ethylenediaminetetraacetic acid) is a topically applied buffer that contains a chelating agent (EDTA), which removes calcium and magnesium ions from the lipopolysaccharide covering of gram-negative organisms and the cell wall of gram-negative and gram-positive organisms (Boothe, 2001). This action facilitates the penetration of antiinfectives. Treatment with tris-EDTA should be carried out before treatment with antibacterials.

Silver Sulfadiazine
Silver sulfadiazine is a broad-spectrum agent that is effective against gram-positive and gram-negative bacteria and fungi. It has been used extensively in treating people with skin burns. It is available in one veterinary labeled product (Baytril Otic) and is also used off label in formulated products by some clinicians.

Dosage Forms
1. Baytril Otic
2. Silvadene

REFERENCES

Boothe DM: Treatment of bacterial infections. In Boothe DM, editor: Small animal clinical pharmacology and therapeutics, Philadelphia, 2001, WB Saunders Co.

Gelatt KN: Textbook of veterinary ophthalmology, Philadelphia, 1981, Lea & Febiger.

Hendrix CM, et al, editors: Diagnostic veterinary parasitology, ed 2, St. Louis, 1998, Mosby.

McCurnin DM and Bassert JM, editors: Clinical textbook for veterinary technicians, ed 5, Philadelphia, 2002, WB Saunders Co.

Papich MG: Handbook of veterinary drugs, Philadelphia, 2002, WB Saunders Co.

Plumb DC: Veterinary drug handbook, ed 4, Ames, 2002, Iowa State University Press.

Tizard I: Veterinary immunology: an introduction, ed 6, Philadelphia, 2000, WB Saunders Co.

REVIEW QUESTIONS

1. Mydriatic agents are used to _____ the pupils.

2. Atropine is contraindicated in _____ and _____.

3. Miotic agents produce _____ constriction.

4. Why are ophthalmic stains used? _____

5. _____ stain is the most commonly used dye for the detection of corneal epithelial defects.

6. Patients with ear mites, whose ears are left untreated, often experience _____ hematomas caused by excessive shaking of the head.

7. What type of administration is the most common method of treating disorders of the eye? _____

8. Why do most topical ophthalmic medications require several applications per day? _____

9. What is Ophthaine used for? _____

10. True or False: The appearance of fluorescein stain at the nostril opening is an abnormal finding when performing a fluorescein stain test. _____

INTRODUCTION
ANATOMY AND PHYSIOLOGY
Topical Antiseborrheics
    Sulfur
    Salicylic Acid
    Coal Tar
    Benzoyl Peroxide
    Selenium Sulfide
Topical Medications Mixed with Water
    Aluminum Acetate
    Magnesium Sulfate
    Bath Oils
Topical Antipruritics
    Nonsteroidal Antipruritics
    Topical Corticosteroids
Astringents
Antiseptics for the Skin
    Alcohols
    Propylene Glycol
    Chlorhexidine
    Acetic Acid
    Iodine
    Benzalkonium Chloride
WOUND HEALING
Topical Wound Dressings
    Healing Stimulators
    Wound Cleansers
    Protectants
Other Drugs Used In Dermatologic Therapy
    Systemic Corticosteroids
    Topical Antibacterial Agents
    Topical Antifungal Agents
    Fatty Acid Supplements
Counterirritants
Caustics
Miscellaneous Drugs

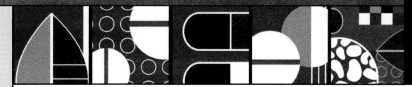

CHAPTER **11**

Drugs Used in Skin Disorders

LEARNING OBJECTIVES

After studying this chapter, you should be able to:

1. Develop a basic understanding of the anatomy and physiology of the skin
2. Be knowledgeable about the common ingredients of topical antiseborrheics
3. Understand the use of topical antipruritics
4. Understand the use of fatty acid supplements
5. Understand the use of astringents
6. Understand the use of skin antiseptics
7. Develop a basic understanding of wound healing
8. Understand the use of topical wound dressings
9. Understand the use of irritants

KEY TERMS

ANGIOGENESIS The development of blood vessels.

ASTRINGENT An agent that causes contraction after application to tissue.

CALLUS Hypertrophy of the horny layer of the epidermis in a localized area resulting from pressure or friction.

COLLAGEN A fibrous substance found in skin, tendon, bone, cartilage, and all other connective tissues.

COMEDO (PL. COMEDONES) A plug of keratin and sebum within a hair follicle of the skin.

DERMATITIS Inflammation of the skin.

ERYTHEMA Redness of the skin caused by congestion of the capillaries.

EXUDATION Leakage of fluid, cells, or cellular debris from blood vessels and their deposition in or on the tissue.

GRANULATION TISSUE New tissue formed in the healing of wounds of the soft tissue, consisting of connective tissue cells and ingrowing young vessels, ultimately forming a scar.

HYPERPIGMENTATION Abnormally increased pigmentation.

INTEGUMENTARY SYSTEM Pertaining to, or composed of skin.

KERATOLYTIC An agent that promotes loosening or separation of the horny layer of the epidermis.

KERATOPLASTIC An agent that promotes normalization of the development of keratin.

PRURITUS Itching.

PYODERMA Any skin disease characterized by the presence or formation of pus.

SEBORRHEA An increase in scaling of the skin; sebum production may or may not be increased.

SEBORRHEA OLEOSA Characterized by scaling and excess lipid production that forms brownish yellow clumps, which adhere to the hair and skin.

SEBORRHEA SICCA Characterized by dry skin and white to gray scales that do not adhere to the hair or skin.

SEBORRHEIC DERMATITIS An inflammatory type of seborrhea characterized by scaling and greasiness.

INTRODUCTION

Dermatologic conditions are frequently seen in veterinary practice. From ectoparasitic problems to allergies, veterinarians are continually combating companion animal skin problems. As a veterinary technician, this is one area where your expertise will be used, because clients will ask many questions about shampoos, dips, conditioners, soaks, lotions, creams, ointments, sprays, and powders. Each of these products may be used to treat a full spectrum of dermatologic problems (e.g., parasites to **pyoderma**). Patients are often presented for examination of a skin disease when in reality they have an underlying systemic illness. Veterinarians use various diagnostic procedures to determine the cause of skin disease (e.g., skin scrapings, allergy testing, and dermatophyte tests). Technicians play a vital role by obtaining a complete history, knowing how to perform the diagnostic procedures used in a dermatologic workup, and providing client education. Client education is essential when treating skin disease, because clients must understand the purpose of medications and how they are properly used.

ANATOMY AND PHYSIOLOGY

The skin is the largest organ in the body. It consists of three layers and is part of the **integumentary system** (Figure 11-1). The epidermis is the outer layer, and it provides protection from injurious external agents. An open and unhealthy epidermis may allow other organisms, bacteria, fungi, or viruses to enter the body. When the epidermis is initially injured, the body begins the healing process. Sometimes this healing may result in a scab. A scab later develops into scar tissue, which may never be as strong as the original tissue. Additionally, increased irritation (e.g., flea allergy dermatitis [FAD]) may result in **hyperpigmentation.** The dermis (corium) lies beneath the epidermis and is made up of connective tissue that contains blood vessels and nerves. Hair follicles, sebaceous glands, apocrine sweat glands, arrector pili muscles, and

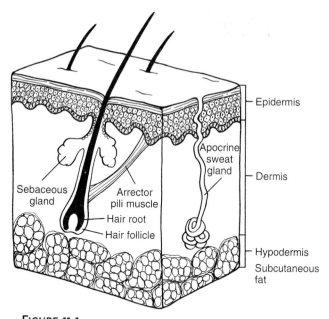

FIGURE 11-1
Schematic representation of the skin layers of normal canine skin.

lymph glands are also located within this layer. Without healthy skin, the haircoat (also a part of the integumentary system) may have no luster or shine. Proper nutrition is essential for healthy skin. The hypodermis (subcutaneous layer) consists of fat cells interwoven with connective tissue. The skin has several functions including protection, temperature regulation, storage, immunoregulation, secretion, vitamin D production, and sensory perception. Various skin diseases that veterinarians may treat include blisters received from a burn, skin parasites (e.g., chiggers, fleas, lice, ticks, flies, cattle grubs) dermatophilosis, dermatophytosis, contact dermatitis, hives, sarcoids, squamous cell carcinoma, melanoma, warts, proud flesh, and photodermatitis (to name a few). The ability of the skin to perform properly is determined not only by its external health, but also by the health of the body's internal systems. Proper nutrition and grooming are precursors to healthy skin.

Drugs used to treat dermatologic disorders can be administered topically or systemically. Topically applied drugs are absorbed by three routes. The first is through the stratum corneum; the second is through the hair follicles; and the third is through the sweat or sebaceous glands (Boothe, 2001). Only a small percentage of topically applied agents are able to penetrate the stratum corneum because of its tough keratinized outer layer. The degree of penetration of a drug depends greatly on the vehicle in which it is delivered.

The therapeutic advantages of shampooing are numerous. Shampooing can provide such extras as enhancing the haircoat, cleansing the skin, improving odor, and treating flea infestations. Sometimes it may be necessary to clip long-haired animals. Shortening the length of the hair may facilitate rapid healing of the skin, as therapeutic shampoos will more readily reach the skin's surface. It is best to use tepid water when bathing animals. There are three broad classes of shampoos: cleansing, antiparasitic, and medicated (Merck, 2000). Cleansing shampoos clean the skin by removing dirt and oils. Additionally, the act of bathing rids the animal of shedding hair. There are many types of shampoos available. Some of the most commonly used include grooming shampoos and flea and tick shampoos. Shampoos do not usually have any residual effect and should be rinsed well. If shampoo is not rinsed well, a hot spot may develop on the skin's surface. Antiparasitic shampoos are those shampoos containing chemicals (e.g., pyrethrins, permethrins) that rid the animal of unwanted fleas or ticks. Most shampoo manufacturers recommend that shampoos be left on the animal for up to 10 minutes (Merck, 2002) before they are rinsed off. In this manner, more parasites will be killed. Medicated shampoos may be either antimicrobial or antiseborrheic products. Some medicated shampoos may contain chlorhexidine or benzoyl peroxide.

If the animal is to be bathed in a medicated shampoo, it should be bathed in a cleansing or antiparasitic shampoo before the medicated shampoo is applied. Usually a medicated shampoo does not remove dirt as well as a cleansing shampoo. All shampoo products should have up to 10 minutes of contact with the skin before they are rinsed off. Care should be taken when rinsing to make sure all shampoo is rinsed off so that no skin irritation occurs. Depending on the manufacturer of the medicated shampoo, it may be used up to 2 to 3 times per week during the first stages of therapy (Merck, 2002).

Topical Antiseborrheics

Keratolytics and **keratoplastics** are known as *antiseborrheic* drugs. These drugs are most often found in medicated shampoos and are available in combinations. Table 11-1 compares products and their uses.

Sulfur

Sulfur is commonly found in shampoos and is also available in ointments. It is nonirritating, nonstaining, and safe for cats. Primarily it is keratolytic and keratoplastic. It is also antipruritic, antibacterial, antifungal, and antiparasitic. It is a mild follicular flusher but is not degreasing.

Client education consists of making sure the client understands the importance of lathering the shampoo well and letting it (the lather) stay on the pet's body for at least 5 to 10 minutes before rinsing. In this manner, the medication in these shampoos will have a greater therapeutic effect. Technicians can bring this to the client's attention most notably by advising the use of a timer set for a 5- to 10-minute time span.

Clinical Uses. Sulfur is used to treat **seborrhea sicca.**

Dosage Forms
1. SebaLyt Shampoo
2. NuSal-T Shampoo
3. Sebolux Shampoo
4. Allerseb-T Shampoo

Adverse Side Effects. These include local irritation, resulting from excessive and prolonged treatment. Sulfur is not recommended for routine bathing.

> ### Technician's Notes
> 1. Products that contain sulfur are not recommended for routine bathing.
> 2. Manufacturers of most products recommend allowing the shampoo to remain on the coat for 5 to 10 minutes before rinsing. Before using this or any other therapeutic shampoo on very dirty pets, it is best to bathe them first in a good cleansing type of shampoo and rinse well. Then, the therapeutic shampoo (sulfur or other) is applied. In this manner, the sulfur will not need to compete with dirt, grease, or parasites to penetrate to the skin to do its job.

Salicylic Acid

Salicylic acid is a common ingredient also found in many antiseborrheic products. It is nonirritating, nonstaining, and safe for cats. It is primarily keratoplastic, but it also has keratolytic, antipruritic, and antibacterial properties.

Clinical Uses. These include its combination with sulfur to treat seborrhea sicca. It may also be used to treat hyperkeratotic skin disorders, such as **calluses,** thickened foot pads, and planum nasale. It is also an ingredient in many otic preparations.

Table 11-1 Common Skin Disorders with Suggested Treatments and Various Products Available

Disease	Sulfur	Salicylic Acid	Coal Tar	Benzoyl Peroxide	Chlorhexidine	Hydrocortisone	Therapeutic Products
Seborrhea sicca	✓	✓					SebaLyt Shampoo Sebolux Shampoo Allerseb-T Shampoo
Seborrhea oleosa	✓	✓	✓	✓			LyTar Shampoo Pyoben Shampoo Sulf/OxyDex Shampoo
Hot spots				✓	✓	✓	ChlorHex Shampoo Pyoben Gel Gentocin Topical Spray
Skinfold dermatitis				✓			OxyDex Gel Pyoben Gel
Deep pyoderma				✓			Pyoben Shampoo Sulf/OxyDex Shampoo Systemic antibiotics
Superficial pustular dermatitis				✓			Pyoben Shampoo OxyDex Shampoo Sulf/OxyDex Shampoo
Superficial folliculitis				✓	✓		ChlorHex Shampoo Pyoben Shampoo Sulf/OxyDex Shampoo
Atopy/allergic contact dermatitis	✓	✓	✓			✓	Micro Pearls Advantage Seba-Moist Moisturizing Shampoo DermaCool-HC Spray
Schnauzer comedo syndrome				✓			Micro Pearls Advantage Benzoyl Plus Shampoo OxyDex Shampoo

Dosage Forms
1. SebaLyt Shampoo
2. Micro Pearls Advantage Seba-Moist Shampoo
3. KeraSolv Gel

Adverse Side Effects. Adverse side effects are uncommon.

Technician's Notes
Products containing salicylic acid as an active ingredient are not recommended for routine bathing.

Coal Tar
Coal tar is potentially irritating and may stain some light-colored haircoats. It is primarily keratolytic and keratoplastic and is mildly degreasing. The refining process used to produce coal tar solutions helps to decrease the staining effect, strong odor, and potential carcinogenic effect.

Clinical Uses. Coal tar is used to treat seborrhea sicca.

Dosage Forms
1. LyTar Shampoo
2. LyTar Therapeutic Spray
3. Mycodex Tar and Sulfur Shampoo

Adverse Side Effects. These include toxicity in cats.

Technician's Notes
1. Products containing coal tar should not be used on cats.
2. Manufacturers of most products recommend allowing the shampoo to remain on the haircoat for 5 to 10 minutes before rinsing.

Benzoyl Peroxide
Benzoyl peroxide is primarily keratolytic, antipruritic, follicular flushing, and degreasing. It is also antibacterial.

Clinical Uses. Benzoyl peroxide is used to treat **seborrhea oleosa,** hot spots, skinfold **dermatitis,** deep pyoderma, superficial pustular dermatitis, superficial folliculitis, schnauzer **comedo** syndrome, tail gland hyperplasia, and stud tail.

Dosage Forms
1. OxyDex Gel and Shampoo
2. Micro Pearls Benzoyl Plus Shampoo
3. Pyoben Gel and Shampoo
4. Sulf/OxyDex Shampoo

Adverse Side Effects. These include hypersensitivity in some humans.

Technician's Notes
1. Manufacturers of most products recommend allowing the shampoo to remain on the haircoat for 5 to 10 minutes before rinsing.
2. Benzoyl peroxide is safe for cats.
3. Benzoyl peroxide may bleach colored fabrics.

Selenium Sulfide
Selenium sulfide is primarily keratolytic, keratoplastic, and degreasing. It is also antifungal.

Clinical Uses. Selenium sulfide is used to treat dry eczema and **seborrhea.**

Dosage Forms
1. Seleen Plus Medicated Shampoo
2. Selsun Blue Shampoo (human label)
3. Selsun Shampoo (human label)

Adverse Side Effects. These include possible rash or irritation after use.

Technician's Notes
1. Selenium sulfide can be irritating and may stain.
2. Do not use selenium sulfide on cats.
3. Manufacturers of most products recommend allowing the shampoo to remain on the haircoat for 5 to 10 minutes before rinsing.
4. Human label products tend to be less irritating and tend to stain less.

Topical Medications Mixed With Water

These products may be used in baths or applied with compresses. They possess a number of uses in veterinary medicines.

Aluminum Acetate

Aluminum acetate (Burow's solution [USP]) is drying, **astringent,** and mildly antiseptic.

Clinical Uses. Aluminum acetate is used in cool water soaks to prevent **exudation** resulting from inflammation and to relieve itching.

Dosage Forms
1. Domeboro powder
2. Domeboro tablets

Adverse Side Effects. Adverse side effects are uncommon.

> **Technician's Notes**
> One pack of powder or one tablet is mixed with ½ to 1 L of water.

Magnesium Sulfate

Magnesium sulfate is mixed with water to produce a mildly hypertonic solution for wet dressings.

Clinical Uses. Wet dressings that contain magnesium sulfate are used to dehydrate or "draw" water from tissues.

Dosage Form
Epsom salt

Adverse Side Effects. Adverse side effects are uncommon.

> **Technician's Notes**
> To produce a 1:65 solution, mix 1 tbsp of magnesium sulfate with 1 L of water.

Bath Oils

Bath oils may be used to manage seborrhea sicca by normalizing keratinization. These may be applied as sprays or diluted and used as a bath rinse. They contain ingredients such as sodium lactate, lanolin, and mineral oil.

Clinical Uses. Bath oils are used in the treatment of dry skin and haircoat.

Dosage Forms
1. HyLyt efa Bath Oil/Coat Conditioner
2. Alpha Keri Therapeutic Bath Oil (human label)
3. Humilac

Adverse Side Effects. Adverse side effects are uncommon.

> **Technician's Notes**
> 1. Excessive use makes the haircoat greasy and causes it to collect dirt.
> 2. Humilac is an oil-free humectant and does not cause the haircoat to become greasy.

Topical Antipruritics

Nonsteroidal Antipruritics

Topical antipruritics provide only temporary relief of itching. They are often used in conjunction with systemic or topical corticosteroids or systemic antihistamines. Colloidal oatmeal provides a soothing effect and may be beneficial for a few hours to days. Pramoxine HCl is also used topically as a palliative treatment for itching. These products provide safe and often effective alternatives to corticosteroids.

Clinical Uses. Topical antipruritics are used to provide relief of itching discomfort.

Dosage Forms
1. Epi-Soothe Shampoo
2. Epi-Soothe Bath Treatment
3. Relief Shampoo

4. Relief Spray
5. Relief Lotion

Adverse Side Effects. Adverse side effects are uncommon.

Topical Corticosteroids

Topical corticosteroids provide relief from itching, burning, and inflammation. They are often combined with other ingredients, such as antimicrobial agents and astringents. Hydrocortisone, triamcinolone, fluocinolone, and betamethasone are corticosteroids commonly used in topical preparations. These steroids differ in their potency and duration of action.

Clinical Uses. They are used in the treatment of inflammation and pruritus associated with conditions such as moist dermatosis (hot spots) and allergic dermatitis.

Dosage Forms
1. Gentocin Topical Spray
2. DermaCool-HC
3. Vetalog Cream

Adverse Side Effects. Adverse side effects are uncommon.

 Astringents

Astringents have very little penetration and act to precipitate proteins. They may be used alone or combined with other ingredients. Tannic acid, iodine, alcohol, and phenol are common astringents used in veterinary medicine.

Clinical Uses. These include the treatment of moist dermatitis in dogs and cats, and weeping skin wounds in large animals. They also are used to toughen the foot pads of dogs.

Dosage Forms
1. Tanisol
2. Tanni-Gel
3. Stanisol

Adverse Side Effects. Astringents may cause irritation.

 Antiseptics For The Skin

Antiseptics inhibit the growth of bacteria and are found in many dermatologic preparations. They are used in the cleansing and treatment of wounds and may be found in products such as surgical scrubs and shampoos.

Alcohols

Alcohols are bactericidal, astringent, cooling, and rubefacient.

Dosage Forms
1. 70% ethyl alcohol
2. 70% to 90% isopropyl alcohol

Adverse Side Effects. Alcohols may cause irritation of denuded skin surfaces.

Propylene Glycol

Propylene glycol is antibacterial and antifungal. Concentrations greater than 50% are keratolytic. Propylene glycol is primarily used as a solvent and a vehicle for other drugs.

Dosage Forms
1. Propylene glycol
2. Topical preparations

Adverse Side Effects. **Erythema** can result when using propylene glycol concentrations greater than 50%.

Chlorhexidine

Chlorhexidine is bactericidal, fungicidal, and effective against many viruses. It is nonirritating, is not affected by organic debris, and is safe for cats. Concentrations of 0.5% to 2% may be found in forms such as shampoos, ointments, surgical scrub, and solution.

Dosage Forms
1. ChlorhexiDerm Maximum Shampoo
2. Nolvasan Antiseptic Ointment

Adverse Side Effects. Adverse side effects are uncommon.

Acetic Acid

Acetic acid may be found in many otic preparations. It is effective against superficial *Pseudomonas spp* infections of the skin and ears.

Dosage Forms
1. Fresh-Ear
2. Clear_x Ear Cleansing Solution and Drying Solution

Adverse Side Effects. Adverse side effects are uncommon.

Iodine

Iodine is bactericidal, fungicidal, virucidal, and sporicidal. It may be found in shampoos, surgical scrubs, surgical preparations, ointments, and sprays.

Dosage Forms
1. Iodine Tincture
2. Lugol's Solution
3. Betadine
4. Xenodine Spray

Adverse Side Effects. Iodine can be irritating and sensitizing, especially in cats. Most products stain.

Technician's Notes
1. Providone-iodine is nonstaining.
2. Xenodine is not as irritating as other iodines.

Benzalkonium Chloride

Benzalkonium chloride is antifungal and antibacterial but is not effective against *Pseudomonas* spp. Soap or other anionic compounds inactivate it.

Dosage Forms
1. Topical wound spray
2. Myosan Cream
3. Dermacide

Adverse Side Effects. Toxicity can occur in cats.

Technician's Notes
This product is not approved for use in food-producing animals or animals intended for food.

WOUND HEALING

A wound is created when an insult—either purposeful, such as surgery, or incidental, such as trauma—disrupts the normal integrity of the tissue (McCurnin, 2002). Normal wound healing can be divided into four stages: inflammatory, debridement, repair, and maturation. However, more than one phase of wound healing is usually occurring at any time (McCurnin, 2002). The inflammatory phase usually begins with hemorrhage and is limited by vessel contraction and constriction. Serum leakage into the wound deposits fibrinogen and other clotting elements. Later, this serum provides enzymes, proteins, antibodies, and complement. The debridement phase begins about 6 hours after injury and is facilitated with the appearance of neutrophils and monocytes migrating to the wound. Neutrophils phagocytize bacteria, then die. Monocytes become macrophages and phagocytize necrotic debris. The repair phase is marked by the formation of a blood clot and is usually active by 3 to 5 days post-injury. During the repair phase, fibroblasts produce **collagen** and other connective tissue proteins. Capillaries infiltrate the wound to provide blood supply and oxygen. This process forms **granulation tissue.** Epithelial cells proliferate beneath the scab, and the wound begins to contract. The maturation phase is the end of wound healing and is a period of remodeling. During this time, the wound consolidates and strengthens. Many factors contribute to proper wound healing. These include patient factors, such as the age of the patient, nutritional status, rest, environment, general health, and wound factors—including wound characteristics (i.e., contaminated wounds vs. noncontaminated wounds), external factors (e.g., temperature regulation [i.e., bandage]), whether or not lavage is performed, and how the wound is closed (e.g., primary or secondary). A veterinarian must consider all these factors when determining how to treat a wound and how well it will heal.

 ## Topical Wound Dressings

The treatment of wounds may include systemic therapy, bandages, topical medications, or a combination of treatments. Topical dressings are commonly used in the treatment of wounds. These wound dressings are available as ointments, solutions, gels, creams, lotions, sprays, powders, and dressing sheets. The type of dressing and length of therapy is dependent on the previously mentioned factors that affect wound healing. For example, a degloving injury will take weeks to months for complete healing to occur, whereas a small abrasion may heal in a few days.

Healing Stimulators

Some dressings stimulate the activities of wound healing. These products may be used on simple wounds or may be most helpful during the later stages of large wound healing, when there is less exudate produced. Some products may be used alone or in combination with other products. Depending on the wound, a bandage may be applied. Many times a bandage is applied to keep a wound warm because warmth advances the healing process. Advances in products that stimulate healing include the addition of products containing acemannan or bovine collagen. Acemannan promotes fibroblast proliferation, collagen deposition, **angiogenesis,** and epithelialization. Products containing bovine collagen also promote fibroblast proliferation and collagen deposition (Swaim and Gillette, 1998).

Dosage Forms
1. Scarlet Oil
2. Zinc oxide
3. Carravet Wound Dressing

4. BioDres
5. Collamend

Adverse Side Effects. Adverse side effects are uncommon.

Technician's Notes
1. It is very important to follow manufacturer recommendations regarding application frequency.
2. Keep bandages dry and clean.
3. Some products may not be suitable for deep or puncture wounds.

Wound Cleansers

Wound cleansers are used during the lavage of wounds in an effort to remove necrotic tissue, debris, and bacteria. Some products also act as healing stimulants. These products may be used in the initial cleansing of a wound before applying a wound dressing. (It should be noted that great benefit is given to the healing process when warm water lavage lasting 15 minutes or more is performed on the wound!) More extensive wounds will require cleansing at every treatment because of the large amounts of exudate, which may be produced during the early stages of healing. It is important that necrotic tissue and purulent debris be removed during cleansing. Some products are applied directly to the wound after cleansing or the removal of necrotic tissue. A nonadherent bandage may be applied and these products will absorb exudate and stimulate the healing process.

Dosage Forms
1. Oti-Clens
2. C-Stat
3. Intracell
4. Dakin's solution—a 0.5% solution of sodium hypochlorite (bleach)
5. Granulex-V

Adverse Side Effects. These are uncommon, but some products may cause temporary stinging after application.

Technician's Notes

1. These products should not be used on fresh arterial clots.
2. Keep bandages dry and clean.
3. Some products may not be suitable for deep or puncture wounds.

Protectants

Protectants provide a protective environment to assist healing of noninfected wounds. Some products protect the skin from irritation caused by urine, feces, and tape. They act as a barrier to prevent irritation and allow healing of previously irritated intact skin.

Dosage Forms

1. Dermal Wound Gel
2. Thuja-Zinc Oxide Ointment
3. Nexaband
4. Tissuemend
5. No Sting Barrier Film

Technician's Notes

1. These products should be applied to clean, dry skin.
2. These products are not suitable for deep or puncture wounds.
3. Products containing zinc oxide may cause zinc toxicity if ingested.

Other Drugs Used in Dermatologic Therapy

Systemic Corticosteroids

Sometimes it may be necessary to use systemic corticosteroids in the treatment of some dermatosis and dermatitis conditions. These drugs affect immunologic and inflammatory activity. Systemic steroids are available for oral and parenteral administration. The effect of systemic steroids may last from a few hours up to several weeks depending on the type of steroid used. Chapter 9 provides an in-depth discussion of systemic corticosteroids and their effects on the body.

Clinical Uses. In the treatment of dermatologic conditions, systemic corticosteroids are indicated for allergic reactions (e.g., flea bite hypersensitivity, atopy) moist dermatosis (hot spot) **seborrheic dermatitis**, and acral lick dermatitis.

Dosage Forms

1. Dexamethasone injection
2. Depo-Medrol injection
3. Prednisone generic tablets
4. Medrol tablets
5. Vetalog

Adverse Side Effects. Adverse side effects are numerous. Many occur with misuse and long-term use. Side effects most commonly seen with doses used in the treatment of skin inflammation and **pruritus** include polyuria, polydipsia, and polyphagia, which may result in weight gain.

Technician's Notes

The technician should alert clients to the side effects seen with systemic corticosteroids. Polyuria and polydipsia may be problematic for some household pets. Technicians should always consult the veterinarian when refilling each prescription of systemic corticosteroids and should note the doctor's approval of the refill on the medical record.

Topical Antibacterial Agents

Topical antibacterial agents are used in the treatment and prevention of superficial bacterial infections of wounds. These products may also contain corticosteroids and antifungal agents. They may require frequent application (i.e., 2 to 3 times daily) and can be used under bandages.

Dosage Forms

1. Bactoderm
2. Nitrofurazone dressing

3. Forte-Topical
4. Prodine solution

Topical Antifungal Agents

Topical antifungal agents are used in the treatment of superficial fungal infections. They are effective in the treatment of ringworm and for thrush in equines. They are often found in combination with antibacterial agents and corticosteroids. They may necessitate frequent application (i.e., 2 to 3 times daily) and can be used under bandages. Local treatment of fungal infections is not always effective, and the use of systemic antifungal agents may be necessary.

Dosage Forms
1. Conofite
2. Kopertox
3. Miconazole
3. Panalog
4. Iodine Shampoo

Fatty Acid Supplements

Fatty acids consist of long chains of carbon atoms with a methyl group ($-CH_3$) at one end. Polyunsaturated fatty acids have varying numbers of double bonds connecting the carbon atoms. Formulas used to identify fatty acids give the number of carbon atoms, followed by the number of double bonds, and finally the distance of the first double bond from the methyl group. The formula for arachidonic acid is (20:4N-6) and indicates that this fatty acid has 20 carbon atoms and four double bonds and that the first double bond is six carbon atoms from the methyl group.

Fatty acids that have the first double bond six carbon atoms away from the methyl group are called *omega-6 (N-6) fatty acids*. Those that have the first double bond three carbon atoms away are called the *omega-3 (N-3) fatty acids*. (Scott, Miller, and Griffin, 1995). Linoleic acid (18:2N-6) and linolenic acid (18:3N-3) cannot be synthesized by the dog and must be supplied in the diet. For this reason, linoleic and linolenic acids are called *essential fatty acids*. Arachidonic acid is an essential fatty acid in the cat.

Fatty acids are responsible for the shine of the haircoat and the smooth texture of the skin. It has also been well documented that fatty acid supplementation can play an important role in managing the itching dog or cat. The exact mechanism by which the fatty acids help to control itching is not known, but it has been proposed that the fatty acids may tie up cyclooxygenase and/or phospholipase (see Chapter 14) and therefore inhibit prostaglandin formation in the skin. A synergistic effect may be achieved by combining fatty acid therapy with the administration of antihistamines or glucocorticosteroids.

Fatty acid supplements are usually derived from fish oil or vegetable oil and may be combined with antioxidant vitamins, such as A and E.

Clinical Uses. Fatty acid supplements are used to control itching (pruritus) associated with certain dermatologic conditions of dogs and cats. They may also be used to improve the luster of the skin.

Dosage Forms
1. Dermcaps
2. Dermcaps ES
3. Dermcaps ES liquid
4. EFA-Caps
5. Pet Tabs FA liquid

Adverse Side Effects. Side effects may include vomiting, diarrhea, or increased bleeding times.

Counterirritants

Counterirritants are substances that are applied to the skin of horses to produce local irritation and inflammation. These compounds are sometimes used to treat chronic inflammatory conditions of bone, joints, ligaments, tendons, or other tissue below the surface. The rationale for their use is that creating an acute inflammatory condition increases blood supply to the inflamed area and adjacent tissue. This increased blood supply brings with it more oxygen, white blood cells, antibodies, complement, and other factors to promote healing. The proper use of counterirritants is complicated because underuse may have little effect and overuse may cause severe tissue damage. The beneficial effects of using counterirritants is controversial, and many clinicians claim the period of enforced rest (1 to 3 months) for treated animals is actually responsible for the healing effect.

When counterirritants are applied to the skin, three stages of irritation result, depending on the agent applied, the quantity applied, or the way in which it is applied. The three stages are listed below.

1. Rubefaction
2. Vesication
3. Blistering

Rubefaction (reddening) indicates mild irritation accompanied by an increase in blood congestion in the skin. Liniments and "braces" are alcohol-based products that produce a rubefacient effect when massaged into the skin. Liniments and braces usually have alcohol as the primary ingredient and may include oil of wintergreen, camphor, turpentine, thymol, menthol, or ammonia. The major benefits of these products may be a result of the massage used in their application rather than the medicinal effect. A *tightener* is a rubefacient compound, similar to a liniment or a brace, that is applied under a cotton leg wrap in an effort to reduce edema around tendons or joints. A *sweat* usually contains alcohol and glycerin and is applied under a moisture-proof bandage to reduce edema.

Clinical Uses. Counterirritants are used for reducing "filling" (edema) around joints or tendons and the associated soreness.

Dosage Forms
1. White Liniment
2. Isopropyl alcohol
3. Lin-O-Gel
4. Shin-O-Gel
5. Absorbine Veterinary Liniment
6. Equ-Lin
7. BIGEOIL
8. SU-PER Sweat
9. Antiphlogistine Poultice
10. SU-PER Poultice

Adverse Side Effects. Tissue irritation may be caused by counterirritants.

Vesication is the second stage of counterirritation, and it is achieved by applying irritating substances under a bandage. Severe irritation accompanied by capillary damage results in vesication or blister formation. Mercuric oxide and cantharide ointments are commonly used as blistering agents. Since the application of vesicants is a painful process that can lead to self-mutilation, they should be applied only under the supervision of a veterinarian.

Clinical Uses. Vesication is used in the treatment of chronic inflammatory musculoskeletal conditions in horses.

Dosage Forms
1. Mercuric oxide
2. Cantharide

Adverse Side Effects. These may include severe tissue damage, worsening of the original condition, and self-mutilation.

Technician's Notes
Petroleum jelly should not be applied around the site where a vesicant is applied. To do so may damage adjacent tissue.

Caustics

Caustics are substances that destroy tissue at the application site. They are used to destroy excessive granulation tissue (proud flesh), superficial tumors (warts), or horn buds. They should be applied by knowledgeable persons because they can cause damage to adjacent tissue.

Clinical Uses. Caustics are used for the control of proud flesh, the removal of warts, and the removal of horn buds in calves.

Dosage Forms
1. Copper sulfate
2. Silver nitrate
3. Proudsoff
4. Wartsoff
5. Caustic Powder
6. Acidified Copper Sulfate
7. Caustic Dressing Powder
8. Equi-Phar Proud Blue Liquid
9. Dehorning Paste

Adverse Side Effects. These may include damage to adjacent tissue, especially the eye when used on the horn buds.

Miscellaneous Drugs

Some drugs used for behavior modification in cats and dogs can be used in dermatologic conditions, such as feline psychogenic alopecia and canine acral lick dermatitis (Merck, 2002). These conditions occur because of excessive self-licking. Tricyclic antidepressants are potent H_1 blockers and they also inhibit the uptake of serotonin and norepinephrine.

Clinical Uses. These drugs are used to modify behavior in such a way that excessive self-licking may decrease. They may be used in the treatment of feline psychogenic alopecia and canine acral lick dermatitis.

Dosage Forms
1. Phenobarbital
2. Diazepam (Valium)
3. Amitriptyline
4. Fluoxetine
5. Naloxone
6. Naltrexone

Adverse Side Effects. Side effects include sedation, idiosyncratic fatal hepatic necrosis in cats, dry mouth, hypersalivation, vomiting, constipation, urinary retention, ataxia, disorientation, depression, and anorexia.

REFERENCES

Boothe DM: Dermatologic therapy. In Boothe DM: Small animal clinical pharmacology and therapeutics, Philadelphia, 2001, WB Saunders Co.

McCurnin DM and Bassert JM, editors: Clinical textbook for veterinary technicians, ed 5, Philadelphia, 2002, WB Saunders Co.

Merck veterinary manual, CD-ROM, ed 8, Whitehouse Station, NJ, 2000, Merck & Co.

Pasquini C, Spurgeon T, and Pasquini S, editors: Anatomy of domestic animals, ed 7, Pilot Point, Tex, 1995, Sudz Publishing.

Scott DW, Miller WH, and Griffin CE: Dermatologic therapy. In Small animal dermatology, ed 5, Philadelphia, 1995, WB Saunders Co.

Scott DW, Miller WT, and Griffin CE: Small animal dermatology, ed 6, Philadelphia, 2001, WB Saunders Co.

Swaim SF, Gillette RL: An update on wound medications and dressings, Compend Cont Educ Pract Vet 20(10): 1133-1145, 1998.

REVIEW QUESTIONS

1. The skin consists of
   _____ layers and is part
   of the _____ system.
2. _____ is essential for
   healthy skin.
3. Name seven functions of the skin.
   _____
4. Shampoos are more effective if left on the
   skin about _____ minutes
   before rinsing.
5. Keratolytics and keratoplastics are known as
   _____ agents.

6. Name the four stages of wound healing.
   _____
7. What does an astringent do to the skin?
   _____
8. True or False: Tissue irritation may be cased by
   counterirritants. _____
9. Patients are commonly presented for skin
   problems when in reality they may have a
   _____ illness.
10. Why are behavioral-type drugs used in
    treating skin illness?
    _____

INTRODUCTION
MECHANISM OF ACTION
Penicillins
    Pharmacokinetics
    Pharmacodynamics
        AMOXICILLIN + CLAVULANATE
        POTASSIUM
Cephalosporins
    Pharmacokinetics
    Pharmacodynamics
Tetracyclines
    Pharmacokinetics
    Pharmacodynamics
Aminoglycosides
    Pharmacokinetics
    Pharmacodynamics
Fluoroquinolones
    Pharmacokinetics
    Pharmacodynamics
Other Antiinfectives
    Chloramphenicol
    Florfenicol
    Macrolides and Lincosamides
        MACROLIDES
        LINCOSAMIDES
    Vancomycin
    Spectinomycin
    Polymyxin B and Bacitracin
    Sulfonamides
    Nitrofurans
Antifungal Drugs
    Polyene Antifungal Agents
        AMPHOTERICIN B
        NYSTATIN
    Imidazole Antifungal Agents
        KETOCONAZOLE AND MICONAZOLE
        ITRACONAZOLE
    Antimetabolic Antifungal Agents
        FLUCYTOSINE
    Superficial Antifungal Agents
        GRISEOFULVIN
    Other Antifungal Agents
Antiviral Drugs
    Acyclovir
    Interferon Alfa-2A, Human Recombinant
Disinfectants/Antiseptics
    Alcohols
    Ethylene Oxide
    Formaldehyde
    Chlorines and Iodines
    Phenolics: Saponated Cresol,
      Semisynthetic Phenols
    Quaternary Ammonium Compounds:
      Cationic Detergents
    Biguanide Compounds
    Other Disinfectants
        SOAPS
        ORGANIC MERCURY COMPOUNDS
        ALKALIS
        HYDROGEN PEROXIDE
        GLUTARALDEHYDE

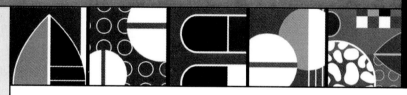

CHAPTER **12**

Antiinfective Drugs

LEARNING OBJECTIVES

After studying this chapter, you should be able to:

1. Identify the classes of the antiinfective drugs
2. Understand the adverse side effects of the antiinfective drugs
3. Understand the clinical uses of the antiinfective drugs
4. Be familiar with the antiviral drugs
5. Be familiar with how disinfectants and antiseptics are used

KEY TERMS

ANTIBACTERIAL An agent that inhibits bacterial growth, impedes replication of bacteria, or kills bacteria.

ANTIBIOTIC An agent produced by a microorganism or semisynthetically that has the ability to inhibit the growth of or kill microorganisms.

ANTIMICROBIAL An agent that kills microorganisms or suppresses their multiplication or growth.

BACTERIA Single-celled microorganisms that usually have a rigid cell wall and a round, rodlike, or spiral shape.

BACTERICIDAL An agent with the capability to kill bacteria.

BACTERIOSTATIC An agent that inhibits the growth or reproduction of bacteria.

BETA-LACTAMASE Enzymes that reduce the effectiveness of certain antibiotics; beta-lactamase I is penicillinase; beta-lactamase II is cephalosporinase.

DERMATOPHYTOSIS A fungal skin infection.

DETERGENT An agent that cleanses.

DISINFECT To make free of pathogens or make them inactive.

FUNGICIDAL An agent that kills fungi.

FUNGISTATIC An agent that inhibits the growth of fungi.

IN VITRO Within an artificial environment.

IN VIVO Within the living body.

IODOPHOR An iodine compound with a longer activity period resulting from the combination of iodine and a carrier molecule that releases iodine over a period of time.

MICROORGANISM An organism that is microscopic (e.g., bacterium, protozoan, *Rickettsia*, virus, and fungus).

SPORICIDAL An agent capable of killing spores.

INTRODUCTION

Microorganisms are ubiquitous in the environment. Some microorganisms have pathogenic potential, while others do not. Animals usually make initial contact with an infectious agent beginning somewhere on the body's surface (e.g., mucous membranes, skin, respiratory tract, or digestive tract). In the fight against infection, several hundred **antimicrobial** drugs have been developed since the early 1900s. These drugs have helped to overcome disease in both humans and animals.

Not all antimicrobials have the same degree of effectiveness against **microorganisms.** A determination can be made to distinguish different types of bacteria, by employing a Gram stain. The Gram stain is a laboratory procedure using dyes to stain **bacteria** (Figure 12-1).* Gram-positive bacteria will stain a dark-blue to purple color. Gram-negative bacteria will stain a pink to red color. However, some bacteria cannot be identified with the Gram stain technique. To differentiate acid-fast bacilli, carbolfuchsin stain can be used and then decolorized with ethyl alcohol and hydrochloric acid. Other bacteria must be identified using special techniques, such as dark-field examination or Gimenez stain. Giemsa's and Wright's stain may be used to identify parasites and intracellular microorganisms. Bacteria with similar staining properties tend to respond to the same antimicrobial therapy. Still other bacteria are classified by the ability to survive with or without oxygen. Aerobes are bacteria that must have oxygen to live and replicate. Other bacteria are able to live and multiply without oxygen, and are known as anaerobes. Anaerobes may be quite hardy and difficult to eradicate.

MECHANISM OF ACTION

By basing the effects a drug's action poses on bacteria, we can divide antimicrobial drugs into two categories: **bactericidal** or **bacteriostatic.** However, some strains of mutant bacteria have higher resistance to some antimicrobials. Resistant strains of bacteria can make antimicrobial therapy difficult. Therefore to prevent mutant strains from developing, it is important not to use antimicrobial drugs indiscriminately. Sometimes it may be necessary to use two different types of antimicrobial drugs to

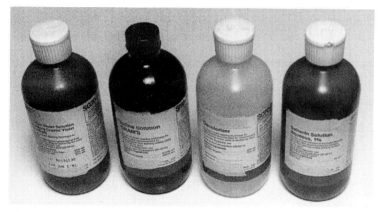

FIGURE 12-1
The Gram stain is a common laboratory test for distinguishing different types of bacteria. This procedure is as follows: (1) After preparing the slide and heat fixing, flood smear with crystal violet solution and let stand 1 minute. (2) Rinse gently with tap water. (3) Flood smear with Gram's iodine and let stand 1 minute. (4) Rinse gently with tap water and flood with Gram's decolorizer for 5 to 10 seconds. (5) Wash gently with tap water. (6) Flood smear with safranin counterstain for 30 to 60 seconds. (7) Wash gently with tap water, blot dry, and examine under oil immersion (i.e., using the microscope's 100× objective). The staining solutions are shown above in the order in which they are used.

treat infections caused by two or more different organisms.

After a laboratory determines the type of organism causing an infection, a sensitivity test may be performed. Several tests are available for susceptibility testing of an organism to a specific antimicrobial drug. Most commonly, the disc susceptibility test is used in small laboratories (Figure 12-2). This test employs an agar plate with a standard amount of cultured organism. Using a dispenser, paper discs impregnated with various antimicrobial drugs are placed within the agar plate. Incubation is carried out along with measurement of the zones of inhibition. These zones show which antimicrobial agents are susceptible or resistant to each particular antimicrobial, and how effectively they may perform **in vitro.** The Kirby-Bauer procedure is commonly used in many laboratories.

The broth dilution susceptibility test is used in many laboratories (Figure 12-3). An organism is inoculated into a series of tubes or wells in a microculture plate. These tubes or wells contain different concentrations of antimicrobials. The lowest concentration that macroscopically inhibits growth of an organism is the minimal inhibitory concentra-

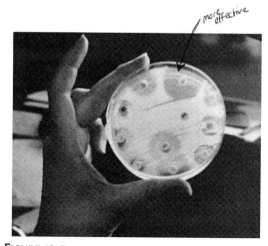

more effective

FIGURE 12-2
The agar diffusion test measures the in vitro susceptibility of a microorganism to specific antibiotics. Note the zones of inhibition surrounding the antibiotic disks.

tion (MIC). The MIC represents the degree of susceptibility of the organism to a specific concentration of a particular antimicrobial drug. The antimicrobials that are effective in vitro may not always be the best choice to use **in vivo.** A clinician chooses which agent to use by considering the

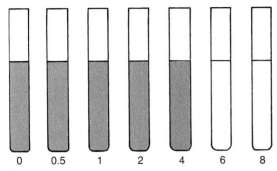

FIGURE 12-3
The broth dilution susceptibility test. Note that the organism grew in broth containing 0, 0.5, 1, 2, and 4 mg/ml of antibiotic. The organism was inhibited in the tube containing 6 mg/ml. The minimal inhibitory concentration is 6 mg/ml.

diagnosis and knowing each agent's pharmacodynamics and pharmacokinetics. This information allows a clinician to choose the most efficient and efficacious drug to treat a specific condition.

Technician's Notes
Special Considerations When Using Antimicrobial Drugs

1. Do not use antimicrobial drugs for mild infections.
2. Antimicrobials should be used only for individuals at risk of severe infection.
3. Do not dismiss the principles of asepsis just because there are many antibiotics to choose from.
4. The use of antimicrobials should be based upon a definitive diagnosis.
5. Do not use a broad-spectrum antibiotic if the infecting organism is sensitive to a specific antibiotic.
6. Antimicrobial drugs should be administered in full therapeutic doses.
7. If an antimicrobial can be used topically or locally, do so. This reserves the use of systemic drugs for serious disease.
8. Be careful regarding antibiotic withdrawal times in animals to be slaughtered for human consumption and antibiotic withdrawal times in dairy cows.
   a. Penicillin G benzathine is long-acting (48 hours) and is not approved for use in dairy animals.

 Penicillins

Penicillin was developed during the 1940s and remains very important as an antimicrobial drug, even though the advent of many other antimicrobials are available in today's arsenal of drugs. Today, researchers have developed natural and semisynthetic compounds that display varied antimicrobial spectrums (Table 12-1).

Many penicillin formulations may "settle out" (i.e., precipitate) during nonuse and must be shaken well before use. Additionally, when reconstituting oral preparations, it is important to add accurate amounts of water so that dilution does not occur (e.g., when mixing amoxicillin oral preparations). Many oral preparations are stable for only 7 to 14 days. Most penicillin formulations must be stored in the refrigerator, and the veterinary technician must tell clients that oral prescriptions for pets should be administered until the entire therapeutic time frame is finished.

Pharmacokinetics

The absorption of most penicillins administered orally takes place in the stomach and small intestine (i.e., the duodenum). Most injected penicillins are rapidly absorbed at the injection site and are distributed through most tissue quite rapidly. The kidneys are the primary organs for excretion of penicillins, although the liver metabolizes other penicillins. Withdrawal times for dairy cows must be adhered to since penicillins are excreted through the milk. Veterinary technicians should be aware of the withdrawal rates of penicillin and should ensure that proper directions are included on the prescription label, especially for clients who are beef and dairy producers.

Pharmacodynamics

Research has shown that penicillins bind reversibly with enzymes, called *penicillin-binding proteins (PBPs)*, outside the bacterial cytoplasmic membrane. These enzymes are involved in cell-wall synthesis and cell division, and when this binding occurs, it increases the internal osmotic pressure

Table 12-1 Penicillin Preparations, Indications, and Antagonistic Drugs

Drug	Indications	Antagonist	Comments
Narrow-Spectrum Penicillins			
Penicillin G sodium	Infections caused by penicillin-sensitive organisms: bacterial pneumonia, upper respiratory tract infections, equine strangles, blackleg, infected wounds, urinary tract infections (at high doses)	Tetracyclines, chloramphenicol, and paromomycin	May add to sodium load
Penicillin G potassium	Same as for penicillin G sodium	Same as for penicillin G sodium	May produce hyperkalemia (IV); delayed absorption in horses (IM); unreliable absorption
Penicillin G procaine	Same as for penicillin G sodium	Same as for penicillin G sodium	Never give IV; contraindicated in some exotics and horses that race; preslaughter withdrawal and milk withholding periods
Penicillin G benzathine	Same as for penicillin G sodium	Same as for penicillin G sodium	Never give IV; preslaughter withdrawal required, and may persist in dairy cattle milk for 2 weeks
Narrow-Spectrum, Acid-Resistant Penicillins			
Penicillin V	Mild infections already controlled by parenteral therapy	Same as for penicillin G sodium	Should not be administered with food; less active against gram-negative bacteria than penicillin G
Beta-Lactamase-Resistant Penicillins			
Methicillin	Pyodermatitis, otitis externa, and other conditions caused by *Staphylococcus aureus*	Same as for penicillin G sodium	Not stable in solution; many incompatibilities in vitro
Cloxacillin	Same as for methicillin	Same as for penicillin G sodium	Frequently used in dry-cow intramammary preparations
Dicloxacillin and floxacillin	Same as for methicillin	Same as for penicillin G sodium	Absorbed from GI tract better than cloxacillin
Oxacillin	Same as for methicillin	Sulfonamides	Not absorbed as well as cloxacillin
Broad-Spectrum Penicillins			
Ampicillin and hetacillin	Infection of organs and tissues caused by ampicillin-sensitive bacteria	Chloramphenicol, erythromycin, tetracyclines, cephaloridine	Incompatible with many drugs and solutions; food impairs absorption; milk withholding and preslaughter withdrawal times
Amoxicillin	Same as for ampicillin	Same as for ampicillin	Absorbed from GI tract better than ampicillin

Continued on next page

Table 12-1 Penicillin Preparations, Indications, and Antagonistic Drugs—cont'd

Drug	Indications	Antagonist	Comments
Piperacillin	Same as for ampicillin	Aminoglycosides	
Carbenicillin sodium	Same as for ampicillin, but especially *Pseudomonas* infections	Same as for ampicillin	Freshly mixed solutions should be used
Broad-Spectrum Penicillins			
Carbenicillin indanyl sodium	Same as for carbenicillin sodium	Same as for ampicillin	Absorbed rapidly from the GI tract
Ticarcillin	Same as for carbenicillin sodium	Same as for ampicillin	Used as an intrauterine infusion in mares
Potentiated Penicillins			
Amoxicillin-potassium clavulanate (4:1)	Wide range of infections when used in combination	Same for ampicillin	Capsules/tablets that are not kept in air-tight containers lose activity; do not give to patients allergic to penicillins or cephalosporins
Inhibitor of Tubular Secretion of Penicillins			
Probenecid	Prolongs blood levels of penicillins that have very short plasma half-lives or that are extremely costly	Same as for ampicillin	

and ruptures the cell. Some bacteria produce **beta-lactamase** (penicillinase), which increases the bacteria's resistance by converting penicillin to inactive penicillic acid. Some penicillins are more resistant to beta-lactamase hydrolysis and are referred to as *beta-lactamase–resistant* or *penicillinase-resistant penicillins*. Penicillins are usually very effective against gram-positive bacteria, but gram-negative bacteria have an outer membrane around the cell wall that limits the PBPs' permeability. Some penicillins that have been developed have an increased ability to penetrate this outer membrane and be more effective against the gram-negative bacteria.

Clinical Uses. Penicillins are used to treat bacterial infections resulting from penicillin-susceptible microorganisms.

Dosage Forms
1. Amoxicillin (tablets and oral liquids for dogs and cats)
   a. Amoxicillin
   b. Amoxi-Tabs
   c. Amoxi-Drops
   d. Amoxi-Inject
   e. Robamox
   f. Biomox
   g. Amoxicillin trihydrate
      i. Many brands are available
   h. Withdrawal times (cattle only)
      i. Meat = 25 days
      ii. Milk = 96 hours
2. Ampicillin (Veterinary)
   a. Amp-Equine
   b. Ampicillin trihydrate (Polyflex)
   c. Withdrawal times (at 6 mg/kg)

i. Meat = 6 days
ii. Milk = 48 hours

3. Carbenicillin
   a. Geopen
   b. Pyopen
4. Cloxacillin
   a. Cloxapen
   b. Orbenin
   c. Tegopen
5. Dicloxacillin
   a. Dynapen
6. Penicillin G
   a. Many brands available
   b. Penicillin G, potassium or sodium
   c. Penicillin G, benzathine: Benza-Pen, Benzylpenicillin; (many brands available)
   d. Penicillin G, procaine
      i. Many brands available
   e. Penicillin V: Pen-Vee
   f. Amoxicillin trihydrate
      i. Many brands available
   g. Withdrawal time (cattle)
      i. Meat = 4 days
      ii. Milk = 48 hours
      iii. Calves = 7 days
   h. Withdrawal time (sheep)
      i. 8 days
   i. Withdrawal time (swine)
      i. 6 days
   j. Withdrawal time at higher doses (i.e., off-label doses)
      i. Meat = 21 days
7. Ticarcillin
   a. Ticar
   b. Ticillin

Adverse Side Effects. Allergic reactions, vomiting and diarrhea, or enteritis may occur in cattle and horses when administered orally. Hives or respiratory distress may also occur because of possible sensitivity reactions to penicillin. Epinephrine should be administered STAT if respiratory distress is severe.

> **Technician's Notes**
> 1. The SC administration of penicillin-G or benzathine penicillin should be avoided because of potential tissue injury or residue potential in food animals.
> 2. Penicillin should not be used in horses intended for food.
> 3. Carefully read labels concerning milk withholding times and treating animals to be slaughtered for food.
> 4. Penicillin G benzathine is long-acting (48 hours) and is not approved for use in dairy cattle.

AMOXICILLIN + CLAVULANATE POTASSIUM

Known as Augmentin in human medicine, Clavamox (veterinary) is a beta-lactam antibiotic + beta-lactamase inhibitor. Clavamox is a broad-spectrum antibiotic used to treat skin infections, urinary tract infections, wound infections, and respiratory infections. Clavamox is supplied in tablets and liquid for oral administration.

Dosage Form
1. Amoxicillin + clavulanate potassium
   a. Clavamox tablets
   b. Clavamox liquid

Adverse Side Effects. Although allergic reactions may occur, this drug is usually well tolerated. Vomiting and diarrhea may occur in some animals when this drug is administered orally.

> **Technician's Notes**
> Use with caution in animals with allergies to penicillin.

 Cephalosporins

Cephalosporins are primarily used in small-animal medicine. However, a few have been developed for use in large animal medicine. This group of drugs is classified into generations according to the drug's spectrum of activity (Table 12-2).

Pharmacokinetics

Most cephalosporins are administered parenterally because they lack the ability to be well absorbed by the gastrointestinal (GI) tract. Once absorbed, cephalosporins are distributed to tissues and fluids, with the exception of the central nervous system (CNS). Some cephalosporins are absorbed into the cerebrospinal fluid, but this absorption is limited. Metabolism occurs in the liver, with elimination occurring in the kidneys by glomerular filtration and tubular secretion into the urine. Therefore doses must be modified for patients in renal failure. In a few exceptions, cephalosporins are excreted through the feces from the biliary system.

Pharmacodynamics

Like penicillins, the cephalosporins interfere with cell-wall synthesis by binding to the bacterial enzymes (PBPs). A cephalosporin's spectrum of activity is determined by the drug's ability to penetrate the bacterial cell wall and bind with proteins

Table 12-2 Cephalosporin Preparations, Indications, and Antagonistic Drugs

Drug	Indications	Antagonist	Comments
Cefadroxil	Infections caused by sensitive organisms in the respiratory tract, skin, urinary tract, soft tissue, bones, joints, etc.	All cephalosporins: gentamicin	Ingestion of food does not impair absorption
Cephalexin	Urinary tract infections		Ingestion of food may delay absorption
Cephalothin	Infections caused by sensitive organisms in the respiratory tract, skin, urinary tract, soft tissue, bones, joints, etc.		IM injection painful; inactivated in liver
Cefazolin	Same as for cephalothin		Highly protein bound; very rarely nephrotoxic
Cephapirin	Same as for cephalothin		Intramammary infusion for mastitis
Cefamandole	Life-threatening, gram-negative infections		Dose should be reduced in patients with renal failure
Cefoxitin (a cephamycin)	Treatment of susceptible infections		Local reaction may occur at injection site
Ceftiofur HCl	Treatment of respiratory disease in cattle and swine; broad spectrum against gram-positive and gram-negative bacteria including beta-lactamase-producing strains		May be used in lactating dairy animals
Ceftiofur sodium	Treatment of respiratory disease in cattle, sheep, horses, and swine; urinary tract infections in dogs; and for control of early mortality associated with E. coli organisms in day-old chicks and day-old turkey poults; broad spectrum against gram-positive and gram-negative bacteria including beta-lactamase-producing strains		May be used in lactating dairy animals

in the cytoplasmic membrane. Another similarity between cephalosporins and penicillins is the cephalosporin's susceptibility to beta-lactamases (cephalosporinases), which can be produced by certain bacteria. Some cephalosporins are more effective in treating infections caused by bacteria that produce beta-lactamase II.

Technician's Notes

1. Naxcel is approved for use in lactating dairy animals.
2. Remember to read package inserts regarding milk withholding time and withholding time in animals to be slaughtered.

Clinical Uses. Cephalosporins are used to treat cystitis, skin and soft tissue infections in dogs and cats, bovine mastitis, shipping fever, and other respiratory infections in cattle, horses, sheep, and swine. Ceftiofur sodium (Naxcel) is also approved for use in day-old chicks and day-old turkey poults for control of early mortality associated with *Escherichia coli* organisms.

Dosage Forms

1. Cefaclor (second-generation cephalosporin antibiotic)
   a. Ceclor
2. Cefadroxil (first-generation cephalosporin antibiotic)
   a. Cefa-Tabs
   b. Cefa-Drops
3. Cefazolin (first-generation cephalosporin antibiotic)
   a. Ancef
   b. Kefzol
   c. Many other brands available
4. Cefepime (fourth-generation cephalosporin antibiotic)
   a. Maxipime
5. Cefotaxime (third-generation cephalosporin antibiotic)
   a. Claforan
6. Cefotetan (second-generation cephalosporin antibiotic)
   a. Cefotan
7. Cefoxitin (second-generation cephalosporin antibiotic)
   a. Mefoxin
8. Ceftazidime (third-generation cephalosporin antibiotic)
   a. Fortaz
   b. Ceptaz
   c. Tazicef
   d. Tazidime
9. Ceftiofur (third-generation cephalosporin antibiotic)
   a. Naxcel
   b. Excenel
10. Cephalexin (first-generation cephalosporin antibiotic)
    a. Keflex and generic forms
11. Cephalothin (first-generation cephalosporin antibiotic)
    a. Keflin
12. Cephradine (first-generation cephalosporin antibiotic)
    a. Velosef

Adverse Side Effects. Cephalosporins are usually safe to use in animals. However, allergic reactions can occur. Rare bleeding disorders have been reported with some cephalosporins. Some cephalosporins have caused seizures, although these are rare. Vomiting and diarrhea may occur in some individuals.

Technician's Notes

1. Carefully read labels regarding milk-withholding time after mastitis treatment and use in animals to be slaughtered.
2. Naxcel is approved for use in lactating dairy animals.

Tetracyclines

Tetracyclines can be administered either parenterally or orally. The most common tetracyclines used in clinical practice are tetracycline, oxytetracycline, doxycycline, and minocycline (Table 12-3).

Pharmacokinetics

When tetracyclines are administered, they are quickly distributed throughout the tissue and sometimes may penetrate into the CNS. Decreased metabolism occurs with most tetracyclines, and thus they are eliminated from the body in the active form. Elimination occurs mostly by glomerular filtration but sometimes may include biliary excretion routes as well.

Pharmacodynamics

Tetracyclines work by inhibiting protein synthesis, thereby impeding bacterial cell division. They offer a broad spectrum of activity against gram-positive and gram-negative bacteria. They are bacteriostatic, although at high dose concentrations they may become bactericidal.

Clinical Uses. Tetracyclines are used to treat respiratory tract infections, bacterial enteritis, and urinary tract infections caused by tetracycline-susceptible microorganisms. Tetracyclines are also used to treat rickettsial diseases (e.g., borreliosis [i.e., Lyme disease] and Rocky Mountain spotted-tick fever).

Dosage Forms
1. Chlortetracycline
   a. Anaplasmosis block
   b. Aureomycin soluble powder
   c. Aureomycin tablets
   d. Aureomycin soluble calf oblets
   e. Calf scour bolus
   f. Fermycin
2. Doxycycline
   a. Vibramycin
   b. Monodox
   c. Doxy caps
   d. Many other brands available
3. Minocycline
   a. Minocin
4. Oxytetracycline

Table 12-3 Tetracycline Preparations, Indications, and Antagonistic Drugs

Drug	Indications	Antagonist	Comments
Oxytetracycline	Infections of organs or tissues caused by tetracycline-sensitive strains; anaplasmosis; often ineffective for endocarditis, empyema, meningitis, septic arthritis, and osteomyelitis	Antacids, milk, diuretics, methoxyflurane, penicillins, ferrous sulfate	Long withdrawal times in cattle; shock reaction may occur when given intravenously in horses; diarrhea also common in horses
Chlortetracycline	Same as for oxytetracycline	Antacids, milk, diuretics, methoxyflurane, penicillins	
Tetracycline	Same as for oxytetracycline	Same as for oxytetracycline	
Doxycycline, minocycline	Same as for oxytetracycline, but much better tissue penetration; doxycycline is especially useful for canine ehrlichiosis	Minocycline—same as for chlortetracycline; doxycycline—same as for oxytetracycline, barbiturates, and carbamazepine	These drugs are potent broad-spectrum tetracyclines

a. Biomycin
b. Oxybiotic
c. Oxy-Tet
d. Terramycin
e. Terramycin scours tablets
f. Terramycin soluble powder
g. Long-acting formulations include:
   i. Liquamycin-LA 200
   ii. Biomycin 200
5. Tetracycline
  a. Panmycin
  b. Duramycin powder

Adverse Side Effects. Tetracyclines may cause renal problems when administered at high doses, can affect bone and teeth formation (causes staining of teeth) in young animals, should never be given to horses intravenously, may cause drug fever in cats, and some hepatotoxicity may occur at increased doses, especially in susceptible individuals.

Technician's Notes

1. Never give tetracycline intravenously to a horse
2. Absorption of tetracyclines by the GI tract is dramatically decreased by the presence of food, milk products, and antacids.
3. Carefully read labels about use in animals to be slaughtered.
4. Not approved for use in lactating dairy animals or poultry that produce eggs for human consumption.

Aminoglycosides

Aminoglycosides provide broad-spectrum activity, and those commonly used include amikacin, gentamicin, kanamycin, and neomycin. They are used for treatment of large, small, and exotic animals. When aminoglycosides are used in reptiles and birds, it is important that intravenous fluid therapy be administered along with the **antibiotic** therapy to reduce the nephrotoxic effects. Although aminoglycosides are effective against most gram-negative and many gram-positive bacteria, their use should be restricted to treating primarily gram-negative infections. Aminoglycosides have the potential to cause serious side effects, such as nephrotoxicity, ototoxicity, and neuromuscular synaptic dysfunction (Table 12-4).

Pharmacokinetics

Since aminoglycosides are not readily absorbed through the GI tract, aminoglycosides are administered parenterally—except for neomycin, which is administered orally. When aminoglycosides are administered, they are absorbed into the bloodstream and then distributed into extracellular fluid. After parenteral administration, aminoglycosides do not reach therapeutic levels in bile, cerebrospinal fluid, respiratory secretions, prostatic or ocular fluids, or fetal tissue (Beech et al, 1987). Elimination occurs by glomerular filtration into the urine. Since aminoglycosides have a tendency to accumulate at high concentrations in the renal cortical tissue, adequate renal function is necessary for their use. Ettinger (2001) recommends monitoring nephrotoxicity by obtaining a pretreatment serum creatinine level and comparing that with samples taken during treatment. Any significant change in the serum creatinine level could indicate the need to terminate treatment. Another area of concentration is in the inner ear, in which concentration levels do not diminish until the conclusion of treatment. The ototoxicity that occurs may be vestibular or auditory.

Pharmacodynamics

Aminoglycosides work like tetracyclines by inhibiting protein synthesis and impeding bacterial cell division. Aminoglycosides have a broad spectrum but should be used only in specific cases of gram-negative infections. Streptococcal bacteria species do not show much sensitivity to aminoglycosides (Ettinger, 2001). They are mostly effective against anaerobic bacteria.

Clinical Uses. Aminoglycosides are used to treat pneumonia, endometritis, urinary tract infections, bacterial enteritis, conjunctivitis, and skin and

Table 12-4 Aminoglycoside Preparations, Indications, and Antagonistic Drugs

Drug	Indications	Antagonist	Comments
All aminoglycosides	Infections caused by susceptible pathogens, pneumonias, urinary tract infections, endometritis, and septicemias that are resistant to other antibiotics	Dimenhydrinate and ethacrynic acid affect hearing loss; methoxyflurane	Monitor patient for hearing loss; do not administer with methoxyflurane
Kanamycin, tobramycin, gentamicin, neomycin, streptomycin		Neuromuscular blocking agents	Administer calcium and anticholinergic agents as prescribed
Gentamicin		Amphotericin B and cephalosporins produce nephrotoxicity	Monitor renal function test results frequently when combining these agents
Neomycin		Digitalis glycosides, penicillin V	Doses may need to be adjusted when combining these agents
Gentamicin, tobramycin		Carbenicillin, ticarcillin, axlocillin, mezlocillin, piperacillin	Never mix these two types of antibiotics; if a patient is receiving combined therapy, administer the doses at least 1 hour apart

soft tissue infections caused by aminoglycoside-susceptible microorganisms.

Dosage Forms
1. Amikacin
   a. Amiglyde-V
2. Gentamicin
   a. Gentocin
3. Kanamycin
   a. Kantrim
4. Neomycin
   a. Biosol

Adverse Side Effects. Since intestinal bacterial flora may be disrupted during therapy with this drug, diarrhea may occur. Other side effects include neuromuscular blockage (when used with anesthetic agents), nephrotoxicity, and ototoxicity.

Technician's Notes
1. Since aminoglycosides enhance the effects of neuromuscular blocking drugs, it is best to not use these drugs at the same time. Aminoglycoside blood levels can be determined before use of neuromuscular blocking drugs to prevent the development of muscular collapse.
2. Aminoglycosides are contraindicated in animals with renal insufficiency.
3. Aminoglycosides are not approved for use in food-producing animals.
4. Do not mix vials or syringes with other antibiotics.
5. May cause problems, such as ototoxicity or nephrotoxicity in animals, especially if the patient is currently on furosemide therapy.

Fluoroquinolones

Fluoroquinolones are relatively new to veterinary medicine and have been approved for use in dogs, cats, turkeys, chickens, and cattle. Their use in horses continues to be controversial and is not approved (Plumb, 2002). The fluoroquinolones approved for use in veterinary medicine include enrofloxacin, difloxacin hydrochloride, orbifloxacin, sarafloxacin, and marbofloxacin. Fluoroquinolones exhibit broad-spectrum activity against gram-positive and gram-negative bacteria.

Pharmacokinetics

Fluoroquinolones are available for oral and parenteral administration. After administration, they are readily absorbed into tissue and body fluids. Metabolism occurs in the liver, and elimination occurs by the kidneys into the urine or the bile into the intestines.

Pharmacodynamics

The broad spectrum of activity offered by fluoroquinolones is bactericidal against many different pathogens. The effect of fluoroquinolones is achieved through inhibition or interference of the bacterial enzyme DNA-gyrase.

Clinical Uses. Clinical uses in dogs and cats include the treatment of bacterial skin and soft tissue infections, respiratory infections, and cystitis (dogs). Fluoroquinolones are used in cattle for the treatment of bovine respiratory disease, in chickens to control mortality associated with *E. coli*, and in turkeys to control mortality associated with *E. coli* and *Pasteurella multocida*.

Dosage Forms

1. Ciprofloxacin
   a. Cipro
2. Difloxacin
   a. Dicural
3. Enrofloxacin
   a. Baytril
4. Marbofloxacin
   a. Zeniquin
   b. Marbocyl (European name)
5. Norfloxacin
   a. Noroxin
6. Orbifloxacin
   a. Orbax

Adverse Side Effects. Adverse side effects of fluoroquinolones include the formation of lesions in the joint articular cartilage during rapid growth phases of dogs. Fluoroquinolones have been associated with CNS stimulation and should be used with caution in animals with known or suspected CNS disorders.

Technician's Notes
1. The safety of fluoroquinolones in breeding or pregnant dogs and cats has not been determined.
2. Fluoroquinolones cannot be used in cattle intended for dairy production or in veal calves.
3. Fluoroquinolones cannot be used in laying hens that produce eggs for human consumption.
4. Carefully read labels regarding withdrawal periods for animals intended for slaughter.

Other Antiinfectives

Chloramphenicol

Chloramphenicol is available in tablet, capsule, and ophthalmic formulations. It is a broad-spectrum antibiotic that acts against gram-negative and gram-positive bacteria. It is readily absorbed into tissue and body fluids after administration. Chloramphenicol is metabolized by the liver and excreted through the kidneys into the urine.

Clinical Uses. Chloramphenicol is used to treat bacterial respiratory tract infections, urinary tract infections, enteritis, and bacterial conjunctivitis caused by chloramphenicol-susceptible organisms.

Dosage Forms
1. Chloramphenicol 1% Ophthalmic Ointment
2. Duricol Chloramphenicol Capsules
3. Chloromycetin (many brands available)

Adverse Side Effects. These include blood dyscrasias in cats after prolonged treatment.

Technician's Notes
1. Chloramphenicol is very stable and should not be used in food-producing animals because residual amounts of the drug can be left in meat, milk, or eggs.
2. Chloramphenicol is not recommended for dogs maintained for breeding purposes.
3. Chloramphenicol should not be administered simultaneously with penicillin, streptomycin, or cephalosporins.

Florfenicol

Florfenicol is available as an injectable solution. It has broad-spectrum activity against many gram-positive and gram-negative bacteria. It is primarily bacteriostatic and acts by inhibiting bacterial protein synthesis. Florfenicol is well distributed in the body and can achieve therapeutic levels in the cerebrospinal fluid (Plumb, 2002).

Clinical Uses. Florfenicol is approved for the treatment of bovine respiratory disease associated with *Pasteurella haemolytica*, *Pasteurella multocida*, and *Haemophilus somnus*.

Dosage Form
Nuflor Injectable Solution

Adverse Side Effects. Adverse side effects include transient inappetence, decreased water consumption, or diarrhea.

Technician's Notes
1. Florfenicol is not approved for use in female dairy cattle 20 months of age or older and should not be used in veal calves, calves less than 1 month old, or calves receiving an all-milk diet.
2. Florfenicol is for intramuscular injection only. Injection should be administered in the neck with no more than 10 ml/site.

Macrolides and Lincosamides

Macrolides and lincosamides are primarily effective against gram-positive organisms. The most common macrolides used in veterinary medicine are tilmicosin phosphate, erythromycin, and tylosin. The lincosamides include lincomycin, clindamycin, and pirlimycin. Clindamycin is also effective in treating anaerobic infections and is used to treat deep pyodermas, wounds, abscesses, and osteomyelitis.

MACROLIDES

Clinical Uses. Macrolides are used to treat upper respiratory tract infections, mastitis, metritis, and foot rot caused by microorganisms susceptible to macrolides.

Dosage Forms
1. Erythro
2. Gallimycin
3. Illotycin (many brands available)
4. Micotil
5. Tylan
6. Tylocine
7. Tylosin

Adverse Side Effects. These include diarrhea, vomiting, and anorexia in small animals after oral administration of erythromycin and tylosin. Severe diarrhea may result after oral administration of erythromycin and tylosin in ruminants and horses. Intramuscular injection of erythromycin and tylosin is very painful. Adverse side effects are uncommon after subcutaneous injection of tilmicosin phosphate (Micotil) in cattle.

LINCOSAMIDES

Clinical Uses. Lincosamides are used to treat upper respiratory tract infections and skin infections in dogs, cats, and swine, and mastitis in cattle. Lincomycin may also be found in combination with other agents for use in chickens. Clindamycin is approved for use in dogs and cats to treat deep pyoderma, wound infections, abscesses, dental infections, and osteomyelitis.

Dosage Forms
1. Clindamycin
   a. Antirobe (capsules, oral liquid)
2. Lincomycin
   a. Lincocin (capsules, oral liquid)
   b. Lincocin sterile solution (swine)
   c. Lincomix
   d. Pirsue aqueous gel

Adverse Side Effects. These include occasional vomiting and diarrhea.

Vancomycin

Vancomycin is not commonly used in veterinary medicine. It is very effective against gram-positive pathogens, particularly coccus organisms. It is administered intravenously or orally. Oral administration (not absorbed) is only to control *Clostridium difficile*.

Clinical Uses. Vancomycin is used to treat resistant staphylococcal and streptococcal infections.

Dosage Forms
1. Vancocin Powder
2. Vancocin Injection

Adverse Side Effects. These include possible thrombophlebitis and febrile reactions (Beech et al, 1987). Ototoxicity, nephrotoxicity, and hypersensitivity are other possible side effects.

Spectinomycin

Spectinomycin is an aminocyclitol antibiotic that is primarily effective against gram-negative bacteria, some mycoplasma, and some gram-positive bacteria. Its action inhibits protein synthesis in susceptible bacteria. It is not generally effective against anaerobic bacteria.

Clinical Uses. These include control of air sacculitis and chronic respiratory disease in turkey poults and chicks caused by organisms sensitive to spectinomycin. In baby pigs, it is used to control and treat infectious diarrhea caused by *Escherichia coli*. In cattle, it is indicated for the treatment of bovine respiratory disease associated with *Pasteurella haemolytica*, *Pasteurella multocida*, and *Haemophilus somnus*.

Dosage Forms
1. Spectam Injectable (turkey poults and chicks)
2. Spectam Scour-Halt (swine)
3. Adspec Sterile Solution (cattle)

Adverse Side Effects. These are uncommon. Mild swelling at the injection site may occur in cattle.

Polymyxin B and Bacitracin

Polymyxin B and bacitracin are restricted to topical skin and ophthalmic applications. These drugs are often combined with other drugs (e.g., neomycin) in topical skin and ophthalmic ointments.

Clinical Uses. These include treatment of superficial bacterial infections of the eye, conjunctiva, and skin.

Dosage Forms

1. Mycitracin Sterile Ointment
2. Forte Topical
3. Neobacimyx Ophthalmic Solution

Adverse Side Effects. Adverse side effects of polymyxin B include nephrotoxicity and neurotoxicity if administered parenterally (Beech et al, 1987). Bacitracin is limited to topical application because it causes nephrotoxicity.

Technician's Notes
Care should be taken to avoid contaminating the applicator tip when administering ophthalmic preparations.

Sulfonamides

Sulfonamides, or sulfa drugs, are **antibacterials** that offer a relatively broad spectrum of activity against gram-positive and gram-negative bacteria. The most common sulfonamides used in veterinary medicine are sulfadiazine, sulfisoxazole, and sulfadimethoxine. Trimethoprim, pyrimethamine, and ormetoprim are commonly combined with sulfonamides to enhance their effect.

Clinical Uses. Sulfonamides are used to treat acute urinary tract infections, respiratory tract infections, wound infections, coccidiosis, and foot rot.

Dosage Forms

1. Tribrissen 48% Injection
2. Primor Tablets
3. Albon Boluses

4. Albon Oral Suspension 5%
5. Sustain III Cattle Bolus

Adverse Side Effects. These include urticaria (hives), vomiting, diarrhea, anorexia, fever, and crystal formation within the kidneys, which can result in hematuria, proteinuria, and renal tubular damage. Keratoconjunctivitis sicca has been reported in dogs. The use of these drugs has been limited in food-producing animals because of residues of the drug in meat, milk, and eggs.

Technician's Notes
Maintaining normal hydration can decrease the risk of crystal formation in the kidneys.

Nitrofurans

Nitrofurans are a group of antibacterials with broad-spectrum activity. The most common nitrofurans used in clinical practice are nitrofurazone, nitrofurantoin, and furazolidone.

Clinical Uses. These include treatment of superficial bacterial infections of wounds, necrotic enteritis in swine, coccidiosis in chickens, and bacterial enteritis in pigs less than 4 weeks old. Nitrofurazone may also be used to treat pink eye in cattle, sheep, and goats, and eye and ear infections in dogs and cats.

Dosage Forms

1. NFZ Puffer
2. Nitrofurazone Soluble Dressing
3. Nitrofurazone 0.2% Solution

Adverse Side Effects. Adverse side effects are uncommon.

Technician's Notes
1. The use of nitrofurans has been prohibited in food-producing animals except for approved topical use.
2. Nitrofurans should not be used in veal calves.

Antifungal Drugs

Fungal infections (mycoses) are classified into two types: topical (superficial), affecting the skin and mucous membranes, and systemic, affecting such areas as the blood, lungs, or CNS. The diagnosis of a topical fungal infection may be determined by direct microscopic examination for the presence of delicate hyphae in skin cells or the presence of spores on the surface of an infected hair. Dermatophyte test medium is available for topical fungal identification at in-hospital laboratories (Figure 12-4). Systemic mycosis is usually diagnosed in large laboratories by serologic testing. Fungal infections are treated by oral, topical, or parenteral administration of drugs that are suitable for these infections. The antifungal, or antimycotic, drugs are divided into four classes: (1) polyene, (2) imidazole, (3) antimetabolic, and (4) superficial agents.

Polyene Antifungal Agents
AMPHOTERICIN B
Amphotericin B is an antifungal drug, which may be **fungistatic** or **fungicidal.**

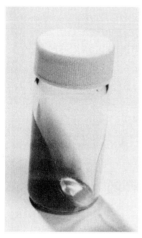

FIGURE 12-4
Dermatophyte test medium may be used to culture topical fungal infections. This medium contains a phenol red indicator that turns red as a dermatophyte grows and produces alkaline metabolic products.

Clinical Uses. These drugs are used to treat systemic mycotic infections in dogs and cats.

Dosage Form
Fungizone (human label)

Adverse Side Effects. Numerous toxicities, such as anorexia, vomiting, seizures, anemia, and cardiac arrest, have been reported with the use of amphotericin B. Nephrotoxicity also occurs in most patients that receive this drug (Beech et al, 1987).

Technician's Notes

1. Amphotericin B is administered intravenously by diluting in 5% dextrose.
2. Renal function should be monitored closely during treatment.

NYSTATIN
Nystatin may be fungistatic or fungicidal. It is often combined with other drugs, such as neomycin, thiostrepton, and triamcinolone acetonide.

Clinical Uses. Nystatin is used to treat candidiasis infections of the skin, mucous membranes, and the intestinal tract in dogs and cats.

Dosage Forms
1. Animax Ointment
2. Dermalone Ointment
3. Panolog Cream

Adverse Side Effects. Adverse side effects are uncommon.

Imidazole Antifungal Agents
KETOCONAZOLE AND MICONAZOLE
Ketoconazole and miconazole are two of the most commonly used drugs in this class. Ketoconazole is available in oral and topical preparations, and miconazole is available in parenteral and topical preparations.

Clinical Uses. These include the treatment of some systemic mycotic infections and some dermatophytoses and *Candida* infections in dogs and cats.

Dosage Forms
1. Nizoral Tablets (human label)—ketoconazole
2. Nizoral Cream (human label)—ketoconazole
3. Monistat (human label)—miconazole
4. Conofite Lotion or Spray—miconazole

Adverse Side Effects. Adverse side effects are not as severe as those of amphotericin B and are uncommon. Ketoconazole may produce hepatotoxicity. Miconazole may produce tachycardia, arrhythmias, fever, nausea, and thrombophlebitis after intravenous administration.

Technician's Notes
Ketoconazole may cause infertility in male dogs.

ITRACONAZOLE
Itraconazole is the most recent imidazole available for use in veterinary medicine.

Clinical Uses. Itraconazole is used to treat systemic mycotic infections in dogs and cats.

Dosage Form
Sporanox Capsules (human label)

Adverse Side Effects. These include anorexia associated with hepatotoxicity, ulcerative dermatitis resulting from vasculitis, and possible cardiotoxicity. Severe adverse reactions are uncommon.

Antimetabolic Antifungal Agents
FLUCYTOSINE
Flucytosine is a fungistatic oral antifungal agent. This drug may be used in combination with other antifungal agents for the treatment of some yeast infections.

Clinical Uses. Flucytosine is used to treat cryptococcal infections, but it inhibits the growth of other fungi as well.

Dosage Form
Ancobon (human label)

Adverse Side Effects. These include bone marrow depression, anemia, leukopenia, and thrombocytopenia. Severe reactions may occur in patients with renal insufficiency.

Superficial Antifungal Agents

GRISEOFULVIN
Griseofulvin is primarily used in dogs, cats, and horses as an antifungal. It is administered orally in the form of a tablet or powder.

Clinical Uses. Griseofulvin is used to treat **dermatophytosis.**

Dosage Forms
1. Fulvicin-U/F Tablets
2. Fulvicin-U/F Powder

Adverse Side Effects. Adverse side effects are uncommon.

Technician's Notes
1. Griseofulvin should not be administered to pregnant or breeding animals.
2. Absorption of griseofulvin is enhanced by administering it with a fatty meal.

Other Antifungal Agents
Several agents that have other uses are also effective as topical antifungal drugs. A topical preparation is often used in conjunction with systemic antifungal drugs. Commonly used topical preparations include chlorhexidine, iodine, tolnaftate, benzoic acid, salicylic acid, and thiabendazole.

Antiviral Drugs

Antiviral drugs are used to treat viral infections. Their use in veterinary medicine is still limited, but research is increasing the use of these drugs for treatment of viral infections in animals. Since there are not any veterinary-approved antiviral agents, human-approved antiviral agents are used. Antivirals may be used for treating optic viral infections and nonneoplastic feline leukemia virus (FeLV)–associated disease. Antiviral drugs are available for topical and systematic use. Other antiviral drugs that also may be beneficial to veterinary medicine include amantadine, ganciclovir, idoxuridine, and azidothymidine.

Acyclovir

Clinical Uses. In veterinary medicine, acyclovir may be used in birds for the treatment of Pacheco's disease and in cats for confirmed feline herpes virus infection of the conjunctiva or cornea in which other treatments have failed (Plumb, 2002).

Dosage Forms
1. Zovirax tablets and capsules (human label)
2. Zovirax suspension (human label)
3. Zovirax injectable (human label)
4. Valacyclovir (human label)

Adverse Side Effects. Adverse side effects include leukopenia and anemias in treated cats. In birds, tissue necrosis can occur at the injection site if used parenterally for more than 72 hours (Oglesbee and Bishop, 2000).

Interferon Alfa-2A, Human Recombinant

Clinical Uses. In veterinary medicine, interferon alfa-2A is administered orally to treat nonneoplastic FeLV disease in cats.

Dosage Form
Roferon-A

Adverse Side Effects. No adverse side effects have been noted (Plumb, 2002).

Disinfectants/Antiseptics

The use of disinfectants in a veterinary hospital ranges from table sprays to premise cleaners (Figure 12-5). A disinfectant destroys disease-producing microorganisms or inactivates viruses. Its application is primarily for use on inanimate objects. Disinfection time is the time required for a particular agent to produce its maximum effect. This time varies with different agents but can be affected by a range of factors, such as the type of material being disinfected, the amount of soil and microbial contamination, and the concentration of the disinfectant and its germicidal potency. Antiseptics are used on live tissue to destroy microorganisms. The terms *disinfectant* and *antiseptic* are commonly used interchangeably, although disinfectants should be used on inanimate surfaces (e.g., counter tops, feed bowls, etc.), whereas antiseptics are used on living tissue (e.g., skin). Table 12-5 illustrates common products and their uses.

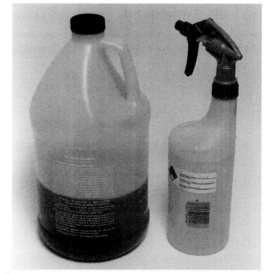

FIGURE 12-5
The concentrations of disinfectants vary from dilutions for disinfecting kennels, floors, and so forth to dilutions for use as table sprays.

Table 12-5 Disinfectant Preparations and Their Activity

Disinfectant Group	Proprietary Products	Recommendations	Bactericidal	General Virucide	Fungicidal	Sporicidal at Room Temperature
Quaternary ammonium compounds	Q-Cide Roccal-D Plus D-128	Instruments, dairy equipment, rubber goods	M	M	M	N
Phenolics	Panteck Cleanser Lysol I.C. Disinfectant Spray Beaucoup	Laundry rinse, floors, walls, equipment	M	M	H	N
Halogens	*Chlorines:* Clorox Purex	Floors, spot disinfection	M	H	H	S
	Iodophors: Betadine Povidine Iosan	Presurgical skin preparation, thermometers, dairy operation	H	H	M	S
Glutaraldehyde	Cidex	Instruments	H	H	H	M
Chlorhexidine	Nolvasan Virosan	Instruments, surgical scrub, dairy operation	M	M	M	N
Alcohols	Isopropyl alcohol 70%	Instruments, thermometers, skin preparation	H	N	S	N

M, Moderate activity; N, no activity; H, high activity; S, slight activity.

Alcohols

Alcohols, such as ethyl and isopropyl, work by protein coagulation and dissociation of membrane lipids. They are bactericidal, tuberculocidal, and active against some viruses, but they are not **sporicidal** or active against fungi. Alcohols do not penetrate organic material.

Clinical Uses. These include disinfection of thermometers and instruments for skin preparations and for spot disinfections.

Adverse Side Effects. Alcohols can corrode metal and can be drying to skin.

Technician's Notes

1. Iodine (1% to 2%) can be added to alcohol for thermometer disinfection to increase its activity against spores and viruses.
2. Alcohols should not be applied to open wounds.
3. Never use alcohol as a part (i.e., a step) of the surgical scrubbing procedure if electrocautery will be employed during the surgical procedure.

Ethylene Oxide

Ethylene oxide works by substitution of the cell alkyl groups for labile hydrogen atoms. It sterilizes against bacteria, fungi, and viruses. This is a gas that should be handled carefully when used by veterinary personnel. The gas may irritate the lungs and cause chemical burns if skin contact occurs. The gas is flammable and is considered to be a human carcinogen. When using this gas to sterilize inanimate objects, it must be used under proper ventilation and according to proper Occupational Health and Safety Administration (OSHA) standards.

Clinical Uses. Ethylene oxide is used to sterilize inanimate objects, such as blankets, pillows, mattresses, lensed instruments, rubber goods, thermolabile plastics, books, and papers.

Adverse Side Effects. Adverse side effects are uncommon if used according to proper OSHA standards and with good ventilation.

Technician's Notes

Special equipment is required to use ethylene oxide as a sterilization gas.

1. After sterilizing rubber boots with this gas, it is best to let them "air" for several hours before donning them, to prevent chemical burns to the skin of the feet.
2. Proper ventilation (refer to OSHA standards) must be employed when using this gas.

Formaldehyde

The mode of action for formaldehyde is the same as for ethylene oxide. It is noncorrosive and is effective against bacteria, fungi, spores, and viruses. It is considered to be carcinogenic to humans and must be used only in diluted amounts.

Clinical Uses. Formaldehyde is used as a disinfecting gas or solution. The gas can be used to **disinfect** large areas, such as a cabinet or incubator. The solution is appropriate for instrument disinfection. Delicate instruments may be vapor disinfected.

Technician's Notes

1. For adequate disinfection, formaldehyde requires long contact time.
2. Organic material inactivates its effectiveness.

Adverse Side Effects. These include toxicity to skin and mucous membranes because of its strong odor.

Chlorines and Iodines

Chlorines and iodines are halogens that inactivate pathogens by oxidizing free sulfhydryl groups on bacterial enzymes. Chlorines are bactericidal, have high activity against viruses, and are fungicidal and tuberculocidal unless highly diluted. Iodines and **iodophors** are bactericidal, have high activity against viruses, are fungicidal and tuberculocidal, and are effective against bacterial spores.

Clinical Uses. Chlorines are recommended for floors, plumbing fixtures, spot disinfection, and fabrics not harmed by bleaching. Iodine tincture is used for skin preparations and thermometers. Iodophors are used to disinfect thermometers, utensils, rubber goods, and dishes, and for presurgical skin preparation.

Dosage Forms
1. Sodium hypochlorite
   a. Clorox bleach
2. Iodine tincture (7%)
3. Betadine surgical scrub
4. Povidone solution

Adverse Side Effects. The strong vapor of chlorines may irritate the eyes and mucous membranes. Skin irritation may result by failing to rinse a chlorine-disinfected surface. Chlorine bleaches colored fabrics and is corrosive to most metals. Tinctures of iodine contain alcohol and are drying to the skin. They stain and may corrode metal. Iodophors may corrode metal; iodine solutions stain and may corrode metal, and high concentrations (3.5%) may irritate living tissue.

Phenolics: Saponated Cresol, Semisynthetic Phenols

The mode of action of phenolics is protein coagulation. They destroy selective permeability of cell membranes and leakage of cell constituents results. They are effective against bacteria, fungi, and some viruses, but they are not sporicidal and are only weakly effective against nonenveloped viruses (e.g., parvovirus). Cresol must be used in soft water and is slow acting. Organic matter, soap, or hard water (except cresol) does not inactivate phenolics. They have high detergency and a residual effect if allowed to dry on surfaces.

Clinical Uses. These include use as a general disinfectant for laundry, floors, walls, and equipment.

Dosage Forms
1. Panteck Cleanser
2. Beaucoup
3. Lysol I.C. Disinfectant Spray

Adverse Side Effects. Adverse side effects are uncommon, but repeated and prolonged skin exposure may cause accumulation in tissue and eventual toxic effects, such as neurotoxicity or teratogenic effects.

Quaternary Ammonium Compounds: Cationic Detergents

Cationic **detergents** concentrate at the cell membrane and are thought to act by dissolving lipids in cell walls and membranes. They are more active against gram-positive than against gram-negative organisms. They are bacteriostatic at high dilutions, but spores, viruses, mycobacteria, and *Pseudomonas aeruginosa* are relatively resistant. Organic debris, hard water, and anionic soaps and detergents inactivate quaternary ammonium compounds.

Clinical Uses. These include cleaning instruments, utensils, inanimate objects, and rubber goods. They may be used for instrument soaks except for instruments with cemented lenses.

Dosage Forms
1. Roccal-D Plus
2. Q-Cide
3. D-128

Adverse Side Effects. Adverse side effects are uncommon.

Biguanide Compounds

Chlorhexidine is the most common disinfectant in this group. In high dilutions, it is bactericidal, fungicidal, and active against enveloped viruses (e.g., the feline infectious peritonitis virus and feline leukemia virus). Other viruses, spores, and mycobacteria are relatively resistant.

Clinical Uses. These include disinfecting surgical instruments, anesthetic equipment, and kennels. It is also available as a surgical scrub and teat dip.

Dosage Forms
1. Nolvasan cap tabs
2. Nolvadent oral solution
3. Nolvalube (lubricating jelly)
4. Nolvasan solution

5. Nolvasan surgical scrub
6. Virosan solution

Adverse Side Effects. Adverse side effects are uncommon.

Other Disinfectants
SOAPS
Soaps, or anionic detergents, have only slight bactericidal activity but are effective in the mechanical removal of organisms. They are not sporicidal or tuberculocidal and have limited virucidal activity. They often contain germicides, such as triclosan, to decrease the number of resident flora after washing. Their mode of action is the same as for cationic detergents.

ORGANIC MERCURY COMPOUNDS
These compounds, such as merbromin (Mercurochrome) and thimerosal (Merthiolate), may be used as antiseptics. These compounds have only slight bactericidal activity.

ALKALIS
Alkalis, such as lye and quicklime, may be used for disinfecting stables and premises.

HYDROGEN PEROXIDE
Hydrogen peroxide is an oxidizing agent available as a 3% aqueous solution and may be used for cleaning and disinfecting wounds and as a mouthwash for septic stomatitis.

GLUTARALDEHYDE
Glutaraldehyde is a dialdehyde and is bactericidal, virucidal, fungicidal, and sporicidal. It is not inactivated by organic debris. Its uses include disinfecting surgical instruments, anesthetic equipment, floors, walls, and nonfood contact surfaces.

REFERENCES
Beech J, Bistner S, Boothe DM et al: The Bristol veterinary handbook of antimicrobial therapy, ed 2, Trenton, NJ, 1987, Veterinary Learning Systems Co.

Carter GR et al, editors: Essentials of veterinary microbiology, Baltimore, 1995, Williams and Wilkins.

Ettinger SJ: Pocket companion to textbook of veterinary internal medicine, ed 3, Philadelphia, 2001, WB Saunders Co.

Olglesbee B, Bishop C: Avian infectious diseases. In Birchard S, Sherding R, editors: Saunders manual of small animal practice, ed 2, Philadelphia, 2000, WB Saunders Co.

Papich MG: Handbook of veterinary drugs, Philadelphia, 2002, WB Saunders Co.

Plumb DV: Veterinary drug handbook, ed 4, Ames, Iowa, 2002, Iowa State University Press.

Quinn PJ et al, editors: Microbial and parasitic diseases of the dog and cat, London, 1997, Saunders.

Williams BR, Baer CL: Essential of clinical pharmacology in nursing, Springhouse, Pa, 1990, Springhouse.

REVIEW QUESTIONS

1. A determination can be made to distinguish different types of bacteria by employing a _____ stain.
2. Gram-positive bacteria will stain what color?
3. Gram-negative bacteria will stain what color?
4. _____ is approved for use in lactating dairy animals.
5. _____ can cause staining of teeth in young animals.
6. _____ should never be given intravenously to horses.
7. Some aminoglycosides may be _____-toxic and/or _____-toxic.
8. Griseofulvin is used to treat _____.
9. A drug's _____ of activity is the range of bacteria affected by its action.
10. True or False: Aerobes are bacteria that require oxygen to live.

INTRODUCTION
ENDOPARASITES
Antinematodal
  Benzimidazoles
  Organophosphates
  Tetrahydropyrimidines
  Imidazothiazoles
  Avermectins
    IVERMECTIN
    MOXIDECTIN
    DORAMECTIN
  Other Agents
    PIPERAZINE (PIPA-TABS, PIP-POP 320)
    PRAZIQUANTEL/PYRANTEL
    PAMOATE/FEBANTEL (DRONTAL PLUS)
Anticestodal
  Bunamidine(Scolaban)
  Epsiprantel (Cestex)
Antitrematodal
  Clorsulon (Curatrem)
  Albendazole (Valbazen)
  Praziquantel (Droncit)
Antiprotozoal
  Drugs for Treating *Coccidia* and Other
    Protozoans
  Drugs for Treating *Giardia*
  Drugs for Preventing *Giardia*
  Drugs for Treating *Babesia*
HEARTWORM DISEASE
Adulticides
  Melarsomine Dihydrochloride
    (Immiticide)
Microfilaricides
Preventatives
  Ivermectin (Heartgard, Heartgard Plus,
    Heartgard for Cats)
  Milbemycin Oxime (Interceptor,
    Sentinel)
  Moxidectin (ProHeart)
  Selamectin (Revolution)
  Diethylcarbamazine Citrate (Carbam,
    Filaribits, Filaribits Plus)
ECTOPARASITES
Application Systems
  Prediluted Sprays
  Emulsifiable Concentrates
    DIPS
    YARD AND KENNEL SPRAYS
  Shampoos
  Dusts
  Foggers
  Monthly Flea and Tick Products
    FIPRONIL (FRONTLINE TOP SPOT FOR
      DOGS, FRONTLINE TOP SPOT FOR
      CATS)
    IMIDACLOPRID (ADVANTAGE)
    IMIDACLOPRID AND PERMETHRIN (K9
      ADVANTIX)
    LUFENURON (PROGRAM TABLETS,
      PROGRAM 6 MONTH INJECTABLE FOR
      CATS, PROGRAM SUSPENSION,
      SENTINEL)
    PERMETHRIN (DEFEND EXSPOT
      INSECTICIDE FOR DOGS)
    SELAMECTIN (REVOLUTION)
Insecticides
  Pyrethrins
  Synthetic Pyrethroids
  Chlorinated Hydrocarbons
  Carbamates
  Organophosphates
  Formamidines
  Synergists
  Repellents
  Insect Growth Regulators ([IGRs], Insect
    Growth Hormones)
  Other Insecticides

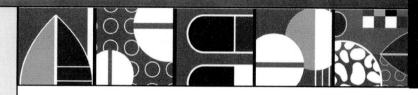

CHAPTER **13**

Antiparasitic Drugs

LEARNING OBJECTIVES

After studying this chapter, you should be able to:

1. Know the ingredients found in common anthelmintics and insecticides
2. Understand the delivery systems of insecticides
3. Educate clients about products covered in this chapter
4. Know the importance of reading and understanding product labels
5. Know the different classes of parasiticides and any contraindications for each particular class

KEY TERMS

ANTHELMINTIC Drug used to eliminate helminth parasites (e.g., roundworms) from a host.

BOTS Larvae of several fly species (e.g., *Gastrophilus,* horse bot).

CESTODE A tapeworm.

ECTOPARASITE A parasite that lives on the outside body surface of its host.

ENDOPARASITE A parasite that lives inside the body of its host.

HELMINTHS Parasite worms, including nematodes, cestodes, and trematodes.

MICROFILARIA A prelarval stage of a filarial worm transmitted to the biting insect from the principal host (e.g., filarial stage of *Dirofilaria immitis*).

NEMATODES Parasitic worms, including the intestinal roundworms, filarial worms, lungworms, kidney worms, heartworms, and others.

ORGANOPHOSPHATE A substance that can interfere with the function of the nervous system by inhibiting the enzyme cholinesterase.

SYMBIOSIS Two living organisms of different species living together.

TREMATODE Any parasitic organism belonging to the class Trematoda, including flukes.

INTRODUCTION

Controlling parasites in companion animals is a high priority for most clients. Owners want to make sure their pets do not have parasites of any kind. Most people get squeamish talking about "worms," but somehow once the subject is broached, most clients listen intently to what is being said. Veterinary technicians play an important role in educating clients about parasites' life cycles and the anthelmintics used to eradicate them. Veterinary technicians can also educate children by allowing them to view parasite eggs under the microscope during their pet's physical examination. Not only does this interaction get the point across, it also provides good public relations for the veterinary hospital. A formaldehyde-preserved heart filled with *Dirofilaria immitis* adults adds a great visual aid when discussing the subject of heartworm prevention. Serum bottles with *Toxocara canis* adults or *Dipylidium caninum* proglottids (or the whole worm for that matter) also make good visual aids when performing client education.

Parasites live on this earth in many diverse forms and relationships. Some parasites lead a symbiotic (**symbiosis**) life. There are five types of symbiotic relationships: (1) predator-prey, (2) phoresis, (3) mutualism, (4) commensalism, and (5) parasitism (Hendrix, 1998). An example of a predator-prey

relationship is that of a hawk finding, capturing, and eating a mouse running in a field. The word form *phore,* from which phoresis is derived, means "to carry." An example of phoresis is the bacterium *Moraxella bovis,* the etiologic agent of infectious bovine keratoconjunctivitis, or "pinkeye," being mechanically carried from the eyes of one cow to those of another on the sticky foot pads of the face fly, *Musca autumnalis* (Hendrix, 1998). Mutualism is what occurs when both members of a symbiotic relationship gain from each other. An example of mutualism is the ciliated protozoans living in the rumen of a cow. The cow benefits by having bulk and fiber digested more readily, and the ciliates benefit because the rumen provides a warm, liquid environment in which to live. Commensalism is a type of symbiotic relationship in which one symbiont benefits, but the other symbiont is not harmed. An example of commensalism is mistletoe growing in the top of a tree. Lastly, parasitism is when one species lives at the expense of another. An example of parasitism is *Trichuris vulpis* living in the cecum of the canine.

Sometimes an animal may harbor a parasite on or within its body that is potentially pathogenic, but does not exhibit any outward signs (i.e., clinical disease) of parasitism. This is known as parasitiasis. If, however, the animal harbors a parasite on or within its body, and injury occurs to the animal because of the parasite, this is known as parasitosis. Parasites living on the outside of an animal's body are known as **ectoparasites** (e.g., fleas and ticks). Parasites living on the inside of an animal's body are known as **endoparasites** (e.g., canine heartworms). An animal with ectoparasites is said to be infested, while an animal with endoparasites is said to be infected. Sometimes a parasite may wander from its normal location in the body to another location where it does not normally live. These parasites are said to be aberrant (erratic). While most veterinary personnel use the lay term given to parasites when speaking with a client, it is important for them to know the genus and species name as well. The Linnaean classification scheme is fundamental in keeping parasites organized (i.e., kingdom, phylum, class, order, family, genus, and species).

Each parasite has its own individual life cycle, which may consist of several stages. Every parasite has at least a definitive host and, depending on the species, may have one or more intermediate hosts. The host that contains the adult (sexually mature) stage of the parasite is known as the definitive host, while the host that contains the immature (not sexually mature) stage of the parasite is known as the intermediate host. Knowing the life cycle of parasites helps veterinarians determine which anthelmintics to use and how many doses will be needed to eradicate the parasite from the host animal's body.

Some parasites have zoonotic potential. This means they may be transmissible from animals to humans. Veterinary technicians should be familiar with which parasites have this ability in order to properly educate clients. Examples of parasites with zoonotic potential include *T. gondii*, *Trichinella spiralis*, *Ancylostoma caninum*, and *Toxocara canis* (Hendrix, 1998).

Ectoparasites have been, and will probably continue to be, an ongoing problem that companion animal owners face. There are numerous products manufactured for the removal of fleas and ticks from an animal's body. Since there are so many products available, veterinary technicians play an important role in educating clients about the effectiveness of each product. Client education is important in the area of ectoparasites, because misusing a flea or tick dip bought over-the-counter can be fatal. Clients should be taught to ask veterinary personnel about the correct use of shampoos, dips, sprays and powders, and the proper use of topical parasiticides (e.g., fipronil, imidacloprid, etc.).

Parasitology is a very fascinating subject. However, for most clients there is no fascination at all because they just want their pet free from "worms and bugs." It is up to veterinary personnel to have knowledge about the products available, and to remember that—as technology evolves—lifelong learning must be a goal to remain current with how each drug or parasiticide works. Reading package inserts also helps veterinary personnel understand how a particular drug works. Tables 13-1 to 13-9 will help identify products and their uses for various species.

ENDOPARASITES

Endoparasites found in the gastrointestinal tracts of animals benefit not only from the foodstuffs the animal ingests, but from body fluids (e.g., blood) as well. Horses with increased numbers of endoparasites in the GI tract may develop colic. Puppies and kittens with increased numbers of intestinal parasites may have anemia to such an extent that fatalities may occur. Heartworms in the heart of a dog can cause disruption to the normal movement of blood in the heart from chamber to chamber, resulting in clinical signs similar to congestive heart failure. Without treatment, a dog with heartworms may be facing a shortened life span.

The following section discusses some of the most common **anthelmintics** used in veterinary practice today. As a veterinary technician, you may come into contact with products not mentioned in this section. The charts in this section list various products, their trade names, and their effectiveness. Since the numbers of anthelmintics are so numerous, many veterinarians keep only a few products to meet their needs and to limit inventory. Some products are available under many different names. Experience will provide familiarity with the different brands available.

Text continued on p. 253

Table 13-1 Parasiticides Used for Treatment and Control of Internal Parasites in Dogs and Cats*

	PARASITE									
Drug	**Toxocara, Toxascaris**	**Ancylostoma, Uncinaria**	**Strongyloides**	**Trichuris**	**Dirofilaria Adults**	**Dirofilaria Microfilariae**	**Taenia**	**Dipylidium**	**Giardia**	**Coccidia**
Albendazole	+	+	−	+	−	−	+	−	+	−
Amprolium	−	−	−	−	−	−	−	−	−	+
Butamisole hydrochloride	−	+	−	+	−	−	−	−	−	−
Dichlorophen	−	−	−	−	−	−	+	+	−	−
Dichlorophen/toluene	+	+	−	−	−	−	+	+	−	−
Dichlorvos	+	+	−	+	−	−	−	−	−	−
Diethylcarbamazine	+	−	−	−	−	+	−	−	−	−
Epsiprantel	−	−	−	−	−	−	+	+	−	−
Febantel	+	+	−	+	−	−	+	−	−	−
Febantel/praziquantel	+	+	−	+	−	−	+	+	−	−
Fenbendazole	+	+	−	+	−	−	+	−	+	−
Furazolidone	−	−	−	−	−	−	−	−	−	−
Ivermectin	+	+	−	+	−	+	−	−	−	−
Mebendazole	+	+	−	+	−	−	+	−	−	−
Melarsomine dihydrochloride	−	−	−	−	+	−	−	−	−	−
Metronidazole	−	−	−	−	−	−	−	−	+	−
Milbemycin oxime	+	+	−	+	−	+	−	−	−	−
N-Butyl chloride	+	+	−	−	−	−	−	−	−	−
Nitroscanate	+	+	−	+	−	−	+	+	−	−
Oxibendazole/diethylcarbamazine	+	+	−	+	−	+	−	−	−	−
Piperazine salts	+	−	−	−	−	−	−	−	−	−
Praziquantel	−	−	−	−	−	−	+	+	−	−
Praziquantel/pyrantel pamoate	+	+	−	−	−	−	+	+	−	−
Praziquantel/pyrantel pamoate/febantel	+	+	−	+	−	−	+	+	−	−
Pyrantel pamoate	+	+	−	−	−	−	−	−	−	−
Quinacrine hydrochloride	−	−	−	−	−	−	−	−	+	−
Selamectin	+	+	−	−	−	+	−	−	−	−
Sulfadiazine/trimethoprim	−	−	−	−	−	−	−	−	−	+
Sulfadimethoxine	−	−	−	−	−	−	−	−	−	+
Thiabendazole	−	−	+	−	−	−	−	−	−	−

+, Indicated for use; −, not indicated for use.
*Paromomycin, an antibiotic, is being used to manage *Cryptosporidium* infections and resistant *Giardia* infections in dogs and cats.
From McCurnin DM, Bassert JM: Clinical textbook for veterinary technicians, ed 5, Philadelphia, 2002, WB Saunders.

Table 13-2 Parasiticides Used to Treat Internal Parasites in Horses

Drug	Gasterophilus	Ascarids	Strongylus vulgaris	Strongylus edentalus	Small Strongyles	Pinworms	Strongyloides
Cambendazole	−	+	+	+	+	+	+
Dichlorvos	+	+	+	+	+	+	−
Febantel	−	+	+	+	+	+	+
Fenbendazole	−	+	+	+	+	+	+
Ivermectin	+	+	+	+	+	+	−
Moxidectin	+	+	+	+	+	+	+
Oxibendazole	−	+	+	+	+	+	+
Oxifendazole	−	+	+	+	+	+	+
Phenothiazine	−	−	+	+	+	−	−
Piperazine salts	−	+	−	−	+	+	−
Pyrantel salts	−	+	+	−	+	−	+
Thiabendazole	−	−	+	+	+	+	+
Thiabendazole/piperazine	−	+	+	+	+	+	+
Thiabendazole/trichlorfon	+	+	+	+	+	+	+
Trichlorfon	+	+	−	−	−	+	−
Trichlorfon/phenothiazine/piperazine	+	+	+	−	+	+	−

+, Indicated for use; −, not indicated for use.
From McCurnin DM, Bassert JM: Clinical textbook for veterinary technicians, ed 5, Philadelphia, 2002, WB Saunders.

Table 13-3 Parasiticides Used to Treat Internal Parasites in Cattle, Sheep, and Goats

	PARASITE													
Drug	Haemon-chus	Oster-tagia	Tricho-strongylus	Cooperia	Nema-todirus	Strongy-loides	Bunos-tomum	Trich-uris	Oesopha-gostomum	Cha-bertia	Dicty-ocaulus	Monezia	Fas-ciola	Coc-cidia
Albendazole	+	+	+	+	+	−	+	−	+	+	+	+	+	−
Amprolium	−	−	−	−	−	−	−	−	−	−	−	−	−	+
Chlorsulon	−	−	−	−	−	−	−	−	−	−	−	−	+	−
Decoquinate	−	−	−	−	−	−	−	−	−	−	−	−	−	+
Fenbendazole	+	+	+	+	+	+	+	+	+	+	+	+	−	−
Haloxon	+	+	+	+	−	−	−	−	−	+	−	−	−	−
Ivermectin	+	+	+	+	+	+	+	−	+	+	+	−	−	−
Lasolacid	−	−	−	−	−	−	−	−	−	−	−	−	−	+
Levamisole	+	+	+	+	+	+	+	+	+	+	+	−	−	−
Moxidectin	+	+	+	+	+	−	+	−	+	−	+	−	−	−
Monensin	−	−	−	−	−	−	−	−	−	−	−	−	−	+
Morantel tartrate	+	+	+	+	+	+	+	−	+	+	+	−	−	−
Phenothiazine	+	+	+	−	−	−	−	−	+	−	−	−	−	−
Sulfonamides	−	−	−	−	−	−	−	−	−	−	−	−	−	+
Thiabendazole	+	+	+	+	+	+	+	−	+	+	−	−	−	−

+, Indicated for use; −, not indicated for use.
From McCurnin DM, Bassert JM: Clinical textbook for veterinary technicians, ed 5, Philadelphia, 2002, WB Saunders.

Table 13-4 Parasiticides Used to Treat Internal Parasites in Swine

| | PARASITE | | | | | | | |
Drug	Ascaris	Strongyloides	Oesophagostomum	Trichuris	Hyostrongylus	Metastrongylus	Stephanurus	Coccidia
Dichlorvos	+	−	+	+	+	−	−	−
Fenbendazole	+	−	+	+	+	+	−	−
Hygromycin B	+	−	+	+	−	−	−	−
Ivermectin	+	+	+	−	+	+	+	−
Levamisole	+	+	+	−	+	+	+	−
Piperazine salts	+	−	−	−	−	−	−	−
Pyrantel tartrate	+	−	+	−	−	−	−	−
Sulfonamides	−	−	−	−	−	−	−	+
Thiabendazole	−	+	+	−	+	−	−	−

+, Indicated for use; −, not indicated for use.
From McCurnin DM, Bassert JM: Clinical textbook for veterinary technicians, ed 5, Philadelphia, 2002, WB Saunders.

Table 13-5 Drugs Used to Treat Internal Parasites in Reptiles

Drug	PARASITE						
	Ectoparasites	Nematodes	Trematodes	Cestodes	Cryptosporidia	Coccidia	Amoebae and Trichomonads
Metronidazole (Flagyl)	–	–	–	–	–	–	+
Humatin 400 (Paromomycin)	–	–	–	–	–	–	+
Praziquantel (Droncit)	–	–	+	–	–	–	–
Febantel plus Praziquantel (Vercom)	–	+	+	+	–	–	–
Dichlorvos (Task)	–	+	–	–	–	–	–
Levamisole (Tramisol, Ripercol)	–	+	–	–	–	–	–
Thiabendazole (Thibenzole)	–	+	–	–	–	–	–
Fenbendazole (Panacur)	–	+	–	–	–	–	–
Mebendazole (Telmin)	–	+	–	–	–	–	–
Ivermectin* (Ivomec)	+	+	–	–	–	–	–
Dithiazanine iodide (Dizan)	–	+	–	–	–	–	–
Vapona Strip	+	–	–	–	–	–	–
Sulfadiazine (many trade names)	–	–	–	–	–	+	–
Sulfamerazine (many trade names)	–	–	–	–	–	+	–
Sulfamethazine (many trade names)	–	–	–	–	–	+	–
Sulfadimethoxine (Albon)	–	–	–	–	–	+	–
Trimethoprim plus Sulfadiazine (Di-Trim, Tribrissen)	–	–	–	–	+	+	–

+ Effective.

– Not effective.

*Do not use in chelonians. Contraindicated in animals that have been given diazepam or will receive diazepam within 10 days of administration of ivermectin.

Data from Frye FL. Reptile care, Neptune City, NJ, 1991, T.F.H. Publications.

Table 13-6 Parasiticides Used for Control of External Parasites on Dogs and Cats

Drug	Fleas	Lice	Miles	Ticks	Drug	Fleas	Lice	Miles	Ticks
Allethrin	+	−	−	−	Linalool	+	−	−	−
Amaitraz	−	−	+	−	Lufenuron	+	−	−	−
Carbaril	+	+	+	+	Malathion	+	+	−	+
Chlorpyrifos	+	+	+	+	Methylcarbamate	+	+	−	+
Cythioate	+	−	−	−	Permethrin	+	+	−	+
d-Limonene	+	+	−	−	Phosmet	+	+	+	+
Diazinon	+	+	−	+	Pyrethrins	+	+	−	+
Fenthion	+	−	−	−	Resmethrin	+	+	−	−
Fipronil	+	+	−	+	Rotenone	+	+	−	+
Imidacloprid	+	+	−	−	Selamectin	+	−	+	+
Lime-sulfur	−	−	+	−					
Lindane (not legal in United States)	+	+	+	+					

+, Indicated for use; −, not indicated for use.
From McCurnin DM, Bassert JM: Clinical textbook for veterinary technicians, ed 5, Philadelphia, 2002, WB Saunders.

Table 13-7 Parasiticides Used for Control of External Parasites on Horses

Drug	Lice	Flies	Mites	Ticks	Maggots
Coumaphos	+	+	−	+	+
Malathion	+	+	+	+	−
Permethrin	+	+	−	+	−
Pyrethrins	+	+	−	−	−

+, Indicated for use; −, not indicated for use.
From McCurnin DM, Bassert JM: Clinical textbook for veterinary technicians, ed 5, Philadelphia, 2002, WB Saunders.

Table 13-8 Parasiticides Used for Control of External Parasites on Cattle, Sheep, and Goats

	PARASITE											
Drug	Cattle Grub	Horn Fly	Face Fly	Other Flies	Maggots	Chewing Lice	Sucking Lice	Psoroptic Mite	Other Mites	Ear Ticks	Other Ticks	Sheep Ked
Carbaril	−	+	+	+	−	+	+	−	−	+	+	+
Coumaphos	+	+	+	+	+	+	+	+	−	+	+	+
Chlorpyrifos	−	+	−	−	−	+	+	−	−	−	−	−
Dichlorvos	−	+	+	+	−	−	−	−	−	−	+	−
Famphur	+	−	−	−	−	+	+	−	−	+	+	−
Doramectin	−	−	−	−	−	+	+	−	−	−	−	−
Fenthion	+	−	−	−	−	+	+	−	−	+	+	−
Fenvalerate	−	+	+	−	−	−	−	−	−	+	−	−
Ivermectin	+	−	−	−	−	+	+	+	+	+	+	−
Methoxychlor	−	+	+	+	−	+	+	+	+	+	+	−
Moxidectin	+	+	−	−	−	+	+	+	+	+	−	−
Permethrin	−	+	+	−	−	+	−	−	−	+	−	−
Phosmet	+	+	−	−	−	+	+	+	+	+	+	−
Pyrethrins	−	+	+	+	−	−	−	−	−	−	−	−
Rotenone	−	−	−	−	−	+	+	−	−	−	−	+
Trichlorfon	+	+	−	−	+	+	+	−	−	+	+	−

+, Indicated for use; −, not indicated for use.
From McCurnin DM, Bassert JM: Clinical textbook for veterinary technicians, ed 5, Philadelphia, 2002, WB Saunders.

Table 13-9 Parasiticides Used for Control of External Parasites on Swine

	PARASITE			
Drug	**Lice**	**Flies**	**Mites**	**Maggots**
Coumaphos	+	+	−	+
Fenthion	+	−	−	−
Ivermectin	+	−	+	−
Malathion	+	−	+	−
Methoxychlor	+	−	−	−
Permethrin	+	+	+	−
Pyrethrins	−	+	−	−

+, Indicated for use; −, not indicated for use.
From McCurnin DM, Bassert JM: Clinical textbook for veterinary technicians, ed 5, Philadelphia, 2002, WB Saunders.

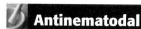

Antinematodal

Benzimidazoles

Dosage Forms. This class includes the following products:

1. Thiabendazole (Equizole, TBZ, Omnizole)
2. Oxibendazole (Anthelcide EQ)
3. Mebendazole (Telmin, Telmintic)
4. Fenbendazole (Panacur)
5. Cambendazole (Camvet)
6. Oxfendazole (Benzelmin, Synanthic)
7. Albendazole (Valbazen)

Clinical Uses. Benzimidazoles are used in the following species:

1. Horses. Effective against strongyli, pinworms, and ascarids.
2. Cattle. Ascarids, several species of strongyli and other stomach worms; albendazole is also effective against adult liver flukes and tapeworms; fenbendazole is also effective against lungworms.
3. Sheep and goats. Ascarids, several species of strongyli and other stomach worms; Panacur is also effective against lungworms.

4. Dogs. Hookworms, roundworms, whipworms; some are effective against *Taenia pisiformis* but not *Dipylidium caninum*.
5. Swine. *Strongyloides* and lungworms.
6. Many of the benzimidazoles are used as anthelmintics for exotics, such as snakes and birds.

Adverse Side Effects. These are uncommon but include vomiting and diarrhea. Mebendazole has clinically produced hepatotoxicity in dogs.

Technician's Notes
1. Read labels carefully regarding use in lactating dairy animals and animals to be slaughtered.
2. None of these products are approved for use in cats.

Organophosphates

Dosage Forms. This class includes the following products:

1. Trichlorfon (Combot, Dyrex T.F., Equibot TC)
2. Coumaphos (Baymix, Dairy Dewormer BX Crumbles)
3. Haloxon (Loxon)
4. Dichlorvos (Task, Atgard)

Clinical Uses. Organophosphates are used in the following species:

1. Horses. Effective against **bots,** roundworms, strongyli, and pinworms but less effective against *Strongyloides*.
2. Cattle, sheep, and goats. Strongyli.
3. Dogs and cats. Hookworms, roundworms, whipworms.
4. Swine. Ascarids, whipworms, nodule worms, strongyli.

Adverse Side Effects. Adverse side effects include those expected with any organophosphate poisoning: excessive salivation, vomiting, diarrhea, muscle tremors, and miosis.

Technician's Notes

1. It is very important that these anthelmintics not be administered concurrently or within a few days of the use of other cholinesterase inhibitors, other organophosphates, succinylcholine, or phenothiazine derivative agents.
2. Atropine and pralidoxime (2-PAM) are antidotal.
3. Read labels carefully regarding use in lactating dairy animals and animals to be slaughtered.

Tetrahydropyrimidines

Dosage Forms. This class includes the following products:

1. Pyrantel pamoate (Nemex, Strongid-T, Anthelban)
2. Pyrantel tartrate (Banminth 48)
3. Morantel tartrate (Nematel, Rumatel)

Clinical Uses. Tetrahydropyrimidines are used in the following species:

1. Horses. Ascarids, strongyli, pinworms.
2. Cattle, sheep, and goats. Strongyli.
3. Dogs and cats. Hookworms, roundworms.
4. Swine. Roundworms, strongyli.

Adverse Side Effects. These are uncommon but may include increased respiration, profuse sweating, or incoordination.

Technician's Notes
Read labels carefully regarding use in lactating dairy animals and animals to be slaughtered.

Imidazothiazoles

Dosage Forms. This class includes the following products:

1. Febantel (Rintal)
2. Levamisole (Tramisol, Levasole)

Clinical Uses. Imidazothiazoles are used in the following species:

1. Horses. Ascarids, strongyli.
2. Cattle, sheep, and goats. Strongyli, lungworms.
3. Dogs and cats. Febantel—hookworms, roundworms, whipworms; levamisole has been used in dogs as a microfilaricide.
4. Swine. Strongyli, *Strongyloides*, lungworms, nodule worms.
5. These products may also be used effectively in some exotic species.

Adverse Side Effects. These include transient foaming at the mouth.

Technician's Notes
Read labels carefully regarding use in lactating dairy animals and animals to be slaughtered.

Avermectins

Dosage Forms. This class includes the following products:

1. Ivermectin (Heartgard, Heartgard Plus, Heartgard for Cats, Eqvalan, Ivomec)
2. Moxidectin (ProHeart, Quest 2% Equine Oral Gel, Cydectin Pour-On)
3. Doramectin (Dectomax Injectable Solution, Dectomax Pour-On)

Clinical Uses
IVERMECTIN

1. Horses. Large and small strongyles, pinworms, ascarids, hairworms, large-mouth stomach worms, neck threadworms, bots, lungworms, intestinal threadworms, and summer sores secondary to *Habronema* or *Draschia* spp.
2. Cattle. Gastrointestinal roundworms, lungworms, cattle grubs, sucking lice, and mites.
3. Swine. Gastrointestinal roundworms, lungworms, lice, and mange mites.
4. Dogs. Effective preventative for *Dirofilaria immitis*; Heartgard Plus contains pyrantel

pamoate and is effective against hookworms and roundworms.

5. Cats. Effective preventative for *D. immitis* and for the removal of hookworms.

6. Birds and snakes. Effective against some endoparasites and ectoparasites.

MOXIDECTIN

1. Horses. Large and small strongyles, encysted cyathostomes, ascarids, pinworms, hairworms, large-mouth stomach worms, and bots.
2. Cattle. Gastrointestinal roundworms, lungworms, cattle grubs, mites, lice, and horn flies.
3. Dogs. Effective preventative for *D. immitis*.

DORAMECTIN

1. Cattle. Gastrointestinal roundworms, lungworms, eyeworms, grubs, biting and sucking lice, horn flies, and mange mites.
2. Swine. Gastrointestinal roundworms, lungworms, kidney worms, sucking lice, and mange mites.

Adverse Side Effects. These are uncommon. Toxic signs include mydriasis, ataxia, tremors, and depression.

Technician's Notes
1. Although not approved, Ivomec is sometimes used for the treatment of ear mites in cats and scabies in dogs.
2. Because of the small amount of medication in the heartworm preventatives, crumbling or breaking the tablets or a chewable version is not recommended.
3. Read labels carefully regarding use in lactating dairy animals and animals for slaughter. Moxidectin is approved for use in dairy cattle of all ages and stages of lactation, except for veal calves.

Other Agents
PIPERAZINE (PIPA-TABS, PIP-POP 320)
1. Dogs and cats. Roundworms.
2. Used effectively in exotics, such as birds and snakes.

3. Commonly combined in large-animal dewormers to broaden its spectrum and increase its efficacy.

PRAZIQUANTEL/PYRANTEL PAMOATE/FEBANTEL (DRONTAL PLUS)
Dogs. It is effective for the removal of tapeworms, hookworms, roundworms, and whipworms.

Adverse Side Effects. These are uncommon.

Technician's Notes
1. Do not use in dogs weighing less than 2 lb or puppies younger than 3 weeks old.
2. Do not use in pregnant animals.

 Anticestodal

Drugs used for treating tapeworms have greatly improved over the years. These newer agents are more effective and do not necessitate fasting before their administration.

Bunamidine (Scolaban)
1. Dogs. *Taenia pisiformis, Dipylidium caninum, Echinococcus granulosus,* and *Echinococcus multilocularis.*
2. Cats. *D. caninum, T. taeniaeformis.*

Adverse Side Effects. These are uncommon but include vomiting, anorexia, diarrhea, and lethargy.

Technician's Notes
1. No adverse reactions have been reported in pregnant or breeding animals.
2. Not for use in puppies younger than 4 weeks or kittens younger than 6 weeks old.

Epsiprantel (Cestex)
1. Dogs. *T. pisiformis* and *D. caninum*.
2. Cats. *T. taeniaeformis* and *D. caninum*.

Adverse Side Effects. These are uncommon.

> ## Technician's Notes
> 1. Safety in pregnant or breeding animals has not been established.
> 2. Not for use in puppies or kittens younger than 7 weeks old.

 ## Antitrematodal

Clorsulon (Curatrem)
1. Cattle. Liver flukes.
2. Effective against immature and adult flukes.

Adverse Side Effects. These are uncommon.

> ## Technician's Notes
> 1. Not approved for use in female dairy cattle of breeding age.
> 2. Read label regarding use in animals to be slaughtered.

Albendazole (Valbazen)
1. Cattle. Liver flukes.
2. Effective against adult flukes and many intestinal worms.

Praziquantel (Droncit)
Praziquantel may be used for lung flukes in dogs and cats.

 ## Antiprotozoal

Protozoa are single-celled organisms found at various body sites that have the ability to replicate rapidly. *Coccidia* and *Giardia* are the most common protozoans associated with diarrhea in many species of animals. Protozoans are most commonly transmitted via contaminated feed and/or water. Prevention of these parasites includes providing uncontaminated food and water, clean housing, and avoiding overcrowding. A vaccine is also available for the prevention of giardiasis in dogs. *Babesia* is a hematozoan protozoa that is transmitted by ticks and also affects many species of animals. An injectable treatment for babesiosis is available for dogs.

Drugs for Treating Coccidia and Other Protozoans
1. Monensin (Coban 60). Turkeys and chickens
2. Amprolium (Corid). Calves
3. Clopidol (Coyden 25). Chickens
4. Diclazuril (Clincox) Horses
5. Maduramicin ammonium (Cygro Type A Medicated Article). Chickens
6. Decoquinate (Deccox). Cattle, calves, and goats
7. Narasin/nicarbazine (Maxiban 72). Chickens
8. Ponazuril (Marquis) Horses
9. Robenidine hydrochloride (Robenz Type A Medicated Article). Chickens
10. Sulfadimethoxine (Albon). Chickens, turkeys, dogs, and cats

Adverse Side Effects. These are uncommon.

> ## Technician's Notes
> Read labels carefully regarding use in food-producing animals and animals to be slaughtered.

Drugs for Treating Giardia
1. Metronidazole (Flagyl). Dogs and cats
2. Albendazole (Valbazen). Dogs and cats

Adverse Side Effects. These are uncommon, but vomiting and diarrhea may occur in some animals treated with metronidazole.

Drugs for Preventing Giardia

A vaccine for dogs is available as an aid in the prevention of *Giardia lamblia* infection and reduction in the duration of cyst shedding. The vaccine is administered subcutaneously with a booster given 2 to 4 weeks after the first vaccination. Annual revaccination is recommended.

Dosage Form
GiardiaVax

Adverse Side Effects. These are uncommon.

Drugs for Treating Babesia

Imidocarb dipropionate is available for the treatment of clinical signs of babesiosis and/or evidence of *Babesia* organisms in the blood. The product is indicated for use in dogs, and treatment consists of two injections given in a 2-week interval.

Dosage Form
Imizol

Adverse Side Effects. These may include injection pain and mild cholinergic signs, such as salivation, nasal drip, or vomiting. Other less common side effects are panting, restlessness, diarrhea, and mild injection site inflammation.

HEARTWORM DISEASE

Heartworm disease is commonly found throughout the United States. This disease primarily affects dogs and wild Canidae, although cats and ferrets may become infected also. *D. immitis* is the filarial **nematode** that causes heartworm disease. *Dipetalonema reconditum* is a subcutaneous filarial nematode but does not require any therapeutic treatment because it is nonpathogenic. Prevention is the key word for controlling heartworm disease. Dogs not on an approved heartworm disease prevention program should be tested for the presence of adult heartworms before beginning preventative treatment. Clients should be educated about the importance of treating an existing infection if one exists, preventing infection or reinfection, and periodic testing that may be necessary. (Many veterinarians will not prescribe heartworm prevention without an annual heartworm antigen test.) In the past several years, the number of cats diagnosed with heartworm disease has increased. The treatment and justification of prevention of heartworms in cats continues to be controversial (Smith, 1999). Products for the prevention of *D. immitis* infection in cats are available. There are no adulticide products approved for use in cats. Table 13-10 provides a comparison of several heartworm preventatives on the market at this time.

 Adulticides

Melarsomine Dihydrochloride (Immiticide)
1. An arsenic compound administered by deep intramuscular injection in the lumbar region.
2. Administration schedule is based on the classification of the severity of heartworm disease.
3. Melarsomine appears to be more efficacious than thiacetarsamide (Caparsolate) and less irritating to tissue and does not cause hepatic necrosis (Plumb, 2002).

Adverse Side Effects. Some dogs experience reactions, such as pain, swelling, and tenderness, at the injection site. Firm nodules may form at the

Table 13-10 Comparision of Products Indicated for Heartworm Prevention

	What is the mode of administration?	What are the age parameters?	Is the product safe for use in pregnant animals?	What is the effectiveness after swimming?	What action should be taken if a dose is late?	What is the safety of the drug if given mistakenly to HW+ dogs?	Are other parasites affected?	What stage of the HW life cycle is acted upon?
Heartgard Plus	Chewable tablet given PO on the same day every month	*Puppies:* 6 weeks *Kittens:* 6 weeks	Yes	N/A	15-day grace period (one dose protects against infection up to 45 days)	Not approved for such use; probably won't cause problems	*Dogs* Roundworms Hookworms *Cats* Hookworms	3rd and 4th stage microfilaria larvae
Interceptor	Flavored tablet given PO on the same day every month	*Puppies:* 8 weeks *Cats:* Not approved for use in cats	Yes	N/A	Can pick up next dose when mistake is noted but shouldn't wait longer than 2-3 weeks	Probably safe if microfilaria counts aren't too high; may be dangerous if microfilaria counts are high	Hookworms Roundworms Whipworms	Microfilaria larvae stages, 3rd, 4th and some 5th larvae stages
Revolution	Topical application on the same day every month	*Puppies:* 6 weeks *Kittens:* 6 weeks	Yes	No effect, but pet must be dry when product is applied	Up to 2 months is grace period	Is safe because product is FDA-approved for use in heartworm-positive dogs	Sarcoptic mange mites, ear mites, fleas, roundworms in cats, and hookworms in dogs	Microfilaria 4th stage larvae
Sentinel	Flavored tablet given PO on the same day every month	*Puppies:* 8 weeks *Cats:* Not approved for use in cats	Yes	N/A	Can pick up next dose when mistake is noted but shouldn't wait longer than 2-3 weeks	Probably safe if microfilaria counts aren't too high; may be dangerous if microfilaria counts are high	Hookworms Roundworms Whipworms *Sentinel has lufenuron in it, which breaks down the chitin within the flea's shell rendering it harmless	Microfilaria 4th stage larvae
ProHeart	Tablet given PO on the same day every month; injection given by DVM which lasts 6 months	*Puppies:* 8 weeks *Cats:* Not approved for use in cats	Yes	N/A	Up to 84-days grace period	Safe because product is approved by FDA for use in HW$^+$ dogs	*Tablets:* Heartworms only *Injectable:* Heartworms and hookworms	Microfilaria 3rd stage larvae

injection site. Coughing, gagging, depression, lethargy, anorexia, fever, lung congestion, and vomiting are also common reactions.

> ### Technician's Notes
> 1. The manufacturer recommends using a 23-gauge, 1-inch needle for dogs equal to or less than 22 lb and a 22-gauge, 1½-inch needle for dogs greater than 22 lb.
> 2. The safety in breeding, lactating, or pregnant bitches has not been determined.
> 3. Melarsomine is contraindicated in dogs with very severe heartworm disease (Class 4, according to manufacturer disease classification).
> 4. Clients must be informed of the potential of morbidity and mortality associated with heartworm treatment.
> 5. Dogs should have exercise restricted after treatment.

Microfilaricides

1. Given 6 weeks after administration of the adulticide.
2. Kill circulating **microfilaria.**
3. Although not approved as a microfilaricide, ivermectin and milbemycin oxime have been used.
4. Levamisole has also been used as a microfilaricide.

Preventatives

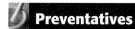

Ivermectin (Heartgard, Heartgard Plus, Heartgard for Cats)
1. Dogs. Monthly preventative; the Plus formula contains pyrantel pamoate and is effective against hookworms and roundworms.
2. Cats. Monthly preventative for *D. immitis* and for the removal of hookworms.
3. Eliminates the tissue stage of heartworm larvae.

Adverse Side Effects. These are uncommon. Toxic signs include mydriasis, depression, and ataxia.

> ### Technician's Notes
> 1. If replacing diethylcarbamazine citrate (DEC), the first dose should be given within a month after stopping DEC treatment.
> 2. This product is safe to use in pregnant and breeding animals.
> 3. Do not use in puppies or kittens younger than 6 weeks old.

Milbemycin Oxime (Interceptor, Sentinel)
1. Dogs. Monthly preventative; also controls hookworms, roundworms, and whipworms.
2. Eliminates the tissue stage of heartworm larvae.
3. Sentinel product contains lufenuron for flea control.

Adverse Side Effects. These are uncommon.

> ### Technician's Notes
> 1. If replacing DEC, the first dose should be given within 1 month after stopping DEC treatment.
> 2. This product is safe to use in pregnant and breeding animals.
> 3. Do not use in puppies younger than 4 weeks old.

Moxidectin (ProHeart)
1. Dogs. Monthly preventative used for *D. immitis*.
2. Eliminates the tissue stage of heartworm larvae.

Adverse Side Effects. Adverse side effects may include lethargy, vomiting, ataxia, anorexia, diarrhea, nervousness, weakness, polydipsia, and itching.

> ### Technician's Notes
> 1. If replacing DEC, the first dose should be given within 1 month after stopping DEC treatment.
> 2. This product is safe to use in pregnant and breeding animals.
> 3. Do not use in puppies younger than 8 weeks old.

Selamectin (Revolution)
1. Dogs and cats. Used as a monthly preventative.
2. Available as a solution for topical administration.
3. Indications include the prevention of heartworm disease caused by *D. immitis*, prevention and control of flea infestations, treatment and control of ear mites (*Otodectes cynotis*) infestation, treatment and control of sarcoptic (*Sarcoptes scabiei*) mange in dogs, and hookworm and roundworm treatment in cats.

Adverse Side Effects. These are uncommon but include transient, localized alopecia at the application site of some treated cats.

Technician's Notes
1. If replacing diethycarbamazine citrate (DEC), the first dose should be given within 1 month after stopping DEC treatment.
2. This product is safe to use in pregnant and breeding animals and in avermectin-sensitive collies.
3. Do not use in puppies or kittens younger than 6 weeks old.
4. This product should not be applied if the haircoat is wet. Bathing the animal 2 or more hours after treatment will not reduce the effectiveness.

Diethylcarbamazine Citrate (Carbam, Filaribits, Filaribits Plus)
1. Daily preventative; also controls roundworms.
2. Filaribits Plus also contains oxibendazole for the control of hookworms, whipworms, and roundworms.
3. Eliminates the tissue stage of heartworm larvae.

Adverse Side Effects. These include occasional vomiting. Filaribits Plus has been linked with hepatic dysfunction.

Technician's Notes
1. Administering with food or directly after a meal reduces the possibility of vomiting.
2. This product is safe to use in pregnant and breeding animals.
3. Missing just 2 to 3 days can affect the efficacy of this product.
4. Do not use in puppies younger than 8 weeks old.

ECTOPARASITES

Most ectoparasites are ubiquitous in the environment and therefore control is often difficult. Environmental factors, such as housing (indoor or outdoor) and geographic location, affect the incidence of many ectoparasites, such as fleas and ticks. When trying to control ectoparasites, the veterinary technician must be familiar with the products used to eradicate these parasites to educate clients about how to properly combat their pet's problem. Not only do ectoparasites cause misery to their host, but many dermatologic problems arise from their infestation. Additionally, increased infestation of fleas may affect owners since fleas are not particular about where their next blood meal comes from (i.e., they are not host specific). Table 13-11 provides a comparison of various topical products on the market at this time.

 Application Systems

Prediluted Sprays
1. Consumers like the convenience of sprays.
2. Sprays are available for animal and environmental use.
3. These formulations are only for the use specified on the label and should be used accordingly.
4. Sprays are available as water based or alcohol based.
   a. Water-based sprays do not penetrate oily coats or fabrics as well and do not dry as quickly as alcohol-based sprays.

Table 13-11 Comparision of Products Indicated for Flea and Tick Control

	Revolution	Advantage	Frontline and Frontline Plus	K9 Advantix
Active ingredient	Selamectin	Imidacloprid	*Frontline:* Fipronil *Frontline Plus:* Fipronil Methoprene	Imidacloprid Permethrin
Age animal must be for safe application	*Puppies:* 6 weeks *Kittens:* 6 weeks	*Puppies:* 7 weeks *Kittens:* 8 weeks	*Puppies:* 10 weeks *Kittens:* 12 weeks	*Puppies:* 7 weeks *Cats* Do not use on cats
Safety in pregnant or lactating animals	Safe	Not safe *Safety has been approved in other countries, but the U.S. EPA does not recognize this testing. No studies have been done in U.S.	Not safe	Not safe
Time needed to kill all fleas after first application	42 hours	24 hours	42 hours	12 hours
Does product wash off easily?	No	Yes Can be washed of completely with a degreasing shampoo	No	No
How soon after a bath can the product be applied?	As soon as pet is dry	As soon as pet is dry	Wait 2 days	As soon as pet is dry
Effectiveness on ticks	Yes *Dermacentor variabilis*	No	Yes *Amblyomma americanum* Deer tick *Dermacentor variabilis Rhipicephalus sanguineus* Fleas and ticks only	Yes Deer ticks *Dermacentor variabilis Amblyomma americanum Rhipicephalus sanguineus* Fleas and ticks Repels mosquitoes
Other parasites affected	Ear mites Sarcoptic mange mites Roundworms in cats Hookworms in cats	Fleas only		
Duration of strength in one application	1 month	1 month	1 month for ticks 1 month for fleas on cats 1-3 months for fleas on dogs	1 month
Is a prescription needed?	Prescription drug	No Product is an insecticide, not a drug	No Product is an insecticide, not a drug	Can be obtained from a licensed veterinarian only
Manufacturer's website	*www.revolutionpet.com*	*www.nofleas.com*	*www.frontline.com*	*www.bayerus.com*

b. Alcohol-based sprays may be irritating and drying to the skin. They usually kill ectoparasites quickly.

5. Environmental sprays are usually residual. Most pet sprays require application daily or every 2 to 3 days for adequate parasite control.

Adverse Side Effects. These vary among products. Carefully read warning labels.

Technician's Notes

1. Spray the pet from head to tail, including the legs and abdomen. Avoid only the eyes, mouth, and nose. For best results, spray against the natural lay of the hair.
2. Educate clients about environmental control and treating the pet.
3. Read labels before applying to young, sick, or pregnant animals. Some products are not safe for certain species (e.g., cats).
4. Water-based flea sprays are best used on young animals because the alcohol-based sprays tend to evaporate quickly and may cause the loss of body heat.

Emulsifiable Concentrates
DIPS

1. Concentrates need to be diluted with water.
2. Dips are usually used after a shampoo.
3. Dips are generally considered residual.

Adverse Side Effects. These vary among products. Read labels carefully for animal and user safety and precautions.

Technician's Notes

1. Removing excess water or drying the coat before dipping is recommended to prevent further dilution of the product.
2. For best results, do not rinse after applying the dip.
3. Organophosphate dips should *never* be applied on cats.

YARD AND KENNEL SPRAYS

1. These are designed for environmental use and should not be used on animals.
2. These products are residual.

Adverse Side Effects. These vary among products. Directions for application should be followed carefully for the safety of the user and animals.

Shampoos

1. These products may contain insecticides or medications, or may be effective only for cleaning the coat.
2. Some shampoos are available as concentrates and require dilution before use.
3. Shampoos are not considered to be residual.
4. Rinse shampoos well; water hardness/softness affects how quickly some shampoos rinse away.

Adverse Side Effects. These vary among products. Shampoos containing carbamates or organophosphates should not be used with other products of the same origin.

Technician's Notes

1. Read labels carefully. Shampoos may seem harmless, but they can be harmful if used improperly.
2. It is recommended that most shampoos be left on the haircoat for 5 to 10 minutes before rinsing.
3. If shampoo is not rinsed well, a "hot spot" may develop on the dog's skin.

Dusts

1. Popularity has decreased with the availability of effective sprays.
2. Dusts do not provide a quick kill.

Adverse Side Effects. These include irritation to mucous membranes and drying of the skin and haircoat.

Technician's Notes
Read labels carefully.

Foggers

1. Foggers work best in large, open rooms.
2. Remind clients that foggers do not go around corners, under couches, or into closets.
3. Combination use of foggers with a premises spray enhances results.
4. Read labels carefully.

Monthly Flea and Tick Products

FIPRONIL (FRONTLINE TOP SPOT FOR DOGS, FRONTLINE TOP SPOT FOR CATS)

1. Topical solution that provides flea and tick control; according to the manufacturer, the product collects in the oils of the skin and hair follicles.
2. Controls less severe flea infestations for up to 3 months.
3. Controls ticks for 1 month.
4. Kills newly emerged adult fleas and all stages of ticks.

Adverse Side Effects. Adverse side effects are uncommon.

> ### Technician's Notes
> 1. Remains effective after bathing, water immersion, or exposure to sunlight.
> 2. Do not use on kittens younger than 12 weeks old or on puppies younger than 10 weeks old.
> 3. This product may be harmful to debilitated, aged, pregnant, or nursing animals.
> 4. Do not use more often than once every 30 days.
> 5. It is recommended that gloves be worn when applying the product.

IMIDACLOPRID (ADVANTAGE)

1. Topical solution that provides flea control, and according to the manufacturer, is not absorbed into the bloodstream or other internal organs.
2. Controls less severe flea infestations for up to 4 weeks.
3. Kills newly emerged adult fleas.

Adverse Side Effects. Adverse side effects are uncommon.

> ### Technician's Notes
> 1. Remains effective after bathing, water immersion, or exposure to sunlight.
> 2. Do not use on kittens younger than 8 weeks old or on puppies younger than 7 weeks old.
> 3. This product should not be used in pregnant animals.
> 4. May be used weekly for severe infestations.
> 5. It is not necessary to wear gloves when applying the product.

IMIDACLOPRID AND PERMETHRIN (K9 ADVANTIX)

1. A once-a-month topical product for dogs used to treat ticks, fleas, and repel mosquitoes.
2. Can be used on puppies 7 weeks of age or older.
3. K9 Advantix is effective after swimming.

LUFENURON (PROGRAM TABLETS, PROGRAM 6 MONTH INJECTABLE FOR CATS, PROGRAM SUSPENSION, SENTINEL)

1. Monthly flea control administered orally; it is absorbed into fatty tissue and slowly released into the bloodstream.
2. Sentinel contains milbemycin for the prevention of heartworms and control of some intestinal parasites in dogs.
3. Controls fleas by preventing the development of flea eggs. Does not kill adult fleas.
4. Fleas must take a blood meal to ingest the product.

Adverse Side Effects. Adverse side effects are uncommon. Cats may develop a small lump at the injection site.

> ### Technician's Notes
> 1. Do not use in puppies or kittens younger than 6 weeks old. Sentinel is approved for use in puppies 4 weeks old.
> 2. The oral products are considered to be safe for use in pregnant, breeding, or lactating animals.
> 3. The safety of the injectable product in reproducing animals has not been established.

PERMETHRIN (DEFEND EXSPOT INSECTICIDE FOR DOGS)

1. Topical solution that provides flea and tick control, and according to the manufacturer, migration of permethrin occurs on the skin surface.
2. Controls fleas, deer ticks, and brown dog ticks for up to 4 weeks.
3. Controls American dog ticks for 2 to 3 weeks.
4. Dogs should be tested for heartworm disease before initial treatment with Sentinel.

Adverse Side Effects. Adverse side effects include skin sensitivity and lethargy.

Technician's Notes
1. Efficacy is reduced with bathing.
2. Do not use more often than once every 7 days.
3. Do not use on cats.

SELAMECTIN (REVOLUTION)

1. Topical solution applied monthly that provides prevention and control of flea infestations in dogs and cats.
2. Kills adult fleas and prevents flea eggs from hatching.
3. Also indicated for prevention of heartworm disease in dogs and cats, treatment and control of ear mite infestations in dogs and cats, and the treatment of hookworm and roundworm infections in cats.

Adverse Side Effects. These are uncommon but include transient, localized alopecia at the application site of some treated cats.

Technician's Notes
1. This product is safe to use in pregnant and breeding animals and in avermectin-sensitive collies.
2. Do not use in puppies or kittens younger than 6 weeks old.
3. Should not be applied if the haircoat is wet. Bathing the animal 2 or more hours after treatment will not reduce the effectiveness.
4. Dogs should be tested for heartworm disease before initial treatment.

 Insecticides

Pyrethrins
1. Extracted from pyrethrum or chrysanthemum flowers.
2. Generally considered safe for most mammals.
3. Have a quick-kill effect; low residual (stabilized or microencapsulated pyrethrins have increased residual).
4. Commonly found in pet sprays, dips, shampoos, dusts, foggers, premises sprays, and yard and kennel sprays.
5. Often used in conjunction with other insecticides.
6. Always used with synergists to maximize effects.

Synthetic Pyrethroids
1. Kirk (1986) identifies pyrethroids as "synthesized chemicals modeled on the chrysanthemate molecule of natural pyrethrins, with various substitutions and modifications."
2. Commonly used in pet sprays, dips, foggers, premises sprays, and yard and kennel sprays.
3. The following are common pyrethroids:
   a. D-trans allethrin (Duocide spray; Mycodex Pet Shampoo)
   b. Resmethrin (Durakyl pet spray and shampoo)
   c. Tetramethrin (Ectokyl IGR Pressurized Spray)
   d. D-Phenothrin (Duocide spray; Mycodex minifog)
   e. Permethrin (Defend EXspot; Permectrin spray; Ectokyl IGR Total Release Fogger)
4. Most have a quick-kill effect, and some have limited residual.
5. Safety is comparable to that of natural pyrethrins.
6. Synergists are not always needed with pyrethroids.

Technician's Notes
Read labels carefully; concentrations affect the use of certain products in some species (e.g., cats).

Chlorinated Hydrocarbons

1. Once common, most have been banned because of their instability (e.g., dichlorodiphenyl trichlorethane [DDT]).
2. They now have limited uses, and efforts are still being made to ban them completely.
3. The following are common chlorinated hydrocarbons:
   a. Lindane (Happy Jack Kennel Dip)
   b. Methoxychlor (Purina Cattle Dust, 2.5x Flea and Tick Powder)

Adverse Side Effects. These vary among products, but these products are considered very hazardous to humans and domestic animals. Read labels carefully before using.

Technician's Notes

Educate clients on the availability of safer products.

Carbamates

1. Act as cholinesterase inhibitors and should not be used with other cholinesterase inhibitors, phenothiazine derivatives, and succinylcholine.
2. Found in dusts, sprays, shampoos, flea and tick collars.
3. The following are common carbamates:
   a. Carbaryl. Mycodex Pet Shampoo with Carbaryl, Sevin Dust, Adams Flea and Tick Dust II (used on birds)
   b. Bendiocarb. Mainly large-animal products
   c. Propoxur. Mainly small-animal products

Adverse Side Effects. These include excessive salivation, vomiting, diarrhea, muscle tremors, and miosis.

Technician's Notes

1. Read labels carefully.
2. Atropine and 2-PAM are antidotal.

Organophosphates

1. Act as cholinesterase inhibitors and should not be used with other organophosphates, carbamates, phenothiazine derivatives, or succinylcholine.
2. Found in dips, pet sprays, dusts, yard and kennel sprays, premises sprays, and systemics.
3. The following are common organophosphates:
   a. Chlorpyrifos (Adams Flea and Tick Dip, Yard & Kennel Spray)
   b. Dichlorvos (Vapona)
   c. Cythioate (Proban tablets and liquid—oral systemic flea control for dogs)
   d. Diazinon (Escort, Escort Plus, Terminator; used on snakes—Diazinon 25-E)
   e. Fenthion (Spotton)
   f. Phosmet (Paramite Dip for Dogs)

Adverse Side Effects. These include excessive salivation, vomiting, diarrhea, muscle tremors, and miosis.

Technician's Notes

1. These products should not be used in dogs prone to seizure.
2. Read labels carefully for user and animal safety.
3. Atropine and 2-PAM are antidotal.

Formamidines

1. Amitraz is the most commonly used formamidine in veterinary medicine.
2. The following are products containing amitraz:
   a. Mitaban. Treatment for canine demodicosis
   b. Preventic Tick Collar for dogs
   c. Taktic. Large-animal insecticide
3. Amitraz is not an organophosphate.

Adverse Side Effects. These include transient sedation, lowered rectal temperature, increased blood glucose level, and seizures.

Technician's Notes

Read labels carefully.

Synergists

1. Increase efficacy of pyrethrins and some pyrethroids
2. The following are common synergists:
   a. Piperonyl butoxide
   b. N-octyl bicycloheptene dicarboximide

Adverse Side Effects. Piperonyl butoxide has shown evidence of toxicity to cats and a low incidence of chronic neurologic side effects (tremors, incoordination, lethargy) with sprays having levels equal to or greater than 1.5% (Kirk, 1986).

Repellents

1. Commonly used in human, equine, and companion animal products.
2. Most repel gnats, mosquitoes, and flies; when combined with pyrethrins and pyrethroids, they repel new fleas and ticks longer than the active ingredient alone.
3. The following are common repellents:
   a. 2,3,4,5-bis(2-butenylene)tetrahydro-2-furaldehyde (MGK 11)
   b. Di-n-propyl isocinchomeronate (MGK 326)
   c. Butoxypolypropylene glycol

Insect Growth Regulators ([IGRs], Insect Growth Hormones)

1. Maturation and pupation of flea larvae normally require a low level of natural IGRs.
2. Products containing IGRs mimic natural IGRs. They cause a high level of IGRs and interrupt the natural development of flea larvae.
3. The following are common IGRs:
   a. Methoprene
   b. Fenoxycarb
   c. Nylar

4. Found in pet sprays, flea collars, premises sprays.

Other Insecticides

1. Rotenone (Rotenone Shampoo, Ear Mite Lotion)
   a. Very toxic to fish and swine
   b. Commonly used in combination with other insecticides
2. Ivermectin (Ivomec 1% Injection for Cattle, Ivomec 1% Sterile Solution for Swine)
   a. Systemic injectable for the control of ectoparasites and some **helminths**
   b. Studies show efficacy against *Sarcoptes scabiei* and *Otodectes cynotis*; not approved for these uses in dogs or cats
3. D-Limonene (VIP Flea Dip, VIP Flea Control Shampoo)
   a. Extract of citrus peel
   b. Found in sprays, shampoos, and dips
   c. Provides a quick kill but is not residual
4. Benzyl benzoate. Effective against many ectoparasites and may be combined with other agents
5. Petroleum distillate. Usually added to products as the solvent for pyrethrin and pyrethroid products

REFERENCES

Kirk RW: Current veterinary IX: small animal practice, Philadelphia, 1986, WB Saunders Co.

Hendrix CM, editor: Diagnostic veterinary parasitology, ed 2, St. Louis, 1998, Mosby.

McCurnin DM, Bassert JM: Clinical textbook for veterinary technicians, ed 5, Philadelphia, 2002, WB Saunders Co.

Plumb DC: Veterinary drug handbook, ed 3, Ames, Iowa, 1999, Iowa State University Press.

Smith P: New studies, products fuel heartworm debate, Veterinary Product News 11(4):34-36, 1999.

REVIEW QUESTIONS

1. Name five types of symbiotic relationships.
   _____

2. What is parasitiasis?
   _____

3. What is parasitosis?
   _____

4. What are ectoparasites?
   _____

5. What are endoparasites?
   _____

6. An animal with endoparasites is said to be
   _____, while an animal
   with ectoparasites is said to be
   _____.

7. What is an anthelmintic?
   _____

8. _____ dips should never
   be used on cats.

9. IGR is an acronym for
   _____.

10. Praziquantel is a drug used to rid the body of
    _____.

INTRODUCTION
ANATOMY AND PHYSIOLOGY
Nonsteroidal Antiinflammatory Agents
  Salicylates
  Pyrazolone Derivatives
    PHENYLBUTAZONE
  Flunixin Meglumine (Banamine)
  Dimethyl Sulfoxide
  Acetaminophen
  Propionic Acid Derivatives
    CARPROFEN
    KETOPROFEN
    NAPROXEN
    IBUPROFEN
Other Nonsteroidal Antiinflammatory
Drugs
  Etodolac
  Deracoxib
  Tepoxalin
Opioid Analgesics
  Opioid Agonists
    TRANSDERMAL FENTANYL USE
  Opioid Agonists-Antagonists
  Opioid Partial Agonists
Antihistamines
  H$_1$ Blockers
  H$_2$ Blockers
Muscle Relaxants
  Methocarbamol (Robaxin-V)
  Other Muscle Relaxants
Corticosteroids
  Injectables
  Oral
  Topical
**LOCAL, REGIONAL, AND TOPICAL
ANESTHETIC AGENTS**
  Injectable
  Topical

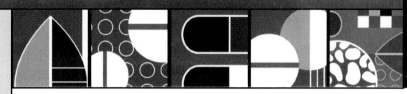

CHAPTER **14**

Drugs Used to Relieve Pain and Inflammation

LEARNING OBJECTIVES

After studying this chapter, you should be able to:

1. Define terms related to the pharmacology of drugs used to relieve pain and inflammation
2. Develop an understanding of the anatomy and physiology associated with pain production and relief
3. Describe the mechanism of action of the category of drugs known as nonsteroidal antiinflammatory drugs (NSAIDs)
4. List indications for the use of NSAIDs
5. List potential adverse side effects of the NSAIDs
6. Describe the mechanism of action of the antihistamines
7. Differentiate between the action of H$_1$ and H$_2$ histamine receptors
8. List indications for muscle relaxants
9. List the two major categories of corticosteroids and the effects of each
10. Describe the hypothalamic-pituitary-adrenal axis, which controls the release of corticosteroids in the body
11. List indications for the use of corticosteroids
12. Describe potential adverse side effects of short-term and long-term corticosteroid use
13. Describe the mechanism of action of local anesthetic agents
14. List some indications for local anesthetic agents

KEY TERMS

ANALGESIA The absence of the sensation of pain.

ADDISON'S DISEASE A disease or syndrome characterized by inadequate amounts of corticosteroid hormones.

CUSHING'S DISEASE A disease or syndrome characterized by an overabundance of corticosteroid hormones.

DEEP PAIN Pain arising from deep receptors in the periosteum, tendons, and joint structures.

HISTAMINE A chemical mediator of the inflammatory response released from mast cells. Histamine may cause dilation and increased permeability of small blood vessels, constriction of small airways, increased secretion of mucus in airways, and pain.

IATROGENIC Caused by the physician (veterinarian).

NERVE BLOCK A loss of feeling or sensation produced by injecting an anesthetic agent around a nerve to interfere with its ability to conduct impulses.

MODULATION The modification of nociceptive transmission.

PROSTAGLANDIN A substance synthesized by cells from arachidonic acid that serves as a mediator of inflammation and has other physiologic functions.

REGIONAL ANESTHESIA Loss of feeling or sensation in a large area (region) of the body after injection of an anesthetic agent into the spinal canal or around peripheral nerves.

TRANSDERMAL ADMINISTRATION The use of a patch applied to the skin to deliver a drug through an intact cutaneous surface to the systemic circulation.

TRANSDUCTION The process that involves translation of noxious stimuli into electrical activity at sensory nerve endings.

INTRODUCTION

Pain has been defined by the International Association for the Study of Pain as "an unpleasant sensory and emotional experience associated with actual or potential tissue damage." It may occur alone or in combination with inflammation. Pain sensation arises in free nerve endings called *nociceptors,* which are located in the skin, joints, blood vessel walls, periosteum, hollow organs (e.g., stomach, intestines, and bladder), and parietal surfaces of the thorax and abdomen. These free nerve endings may be activated through mechanical, thermal, and chemical stimulation. Chemical stimulation may be from an exogenous source or from those endogenous chemicals like eicosanoids (prostaglandins), bradykinin, serotonin, and others released in response to tissue damage. Pain can have varying degrees of severity and can be acute or chronic.

Pain is sensed in terms of its intensity, duration, location, and quality. Pain arising in subcutaneous tissue is called superficial pain. Deep pain is associated with skeletal muscles, tendons, and bones and joints. Visceral pain arises from hollow abdominal organs, peritoneum, heart, liver, and lungs. Pain can be beneficial in that it can allow the animal to avoid damaging stimuli. It has an emotional content and activates sympathetic stimulation. It can be harmful, because it can lead to stress and its related problems like gastrointestinal lesions, immunosuppression, delayed healing, hypertension, and potential dysrhythmias. Pain also has a motivational content and can be used to force behavior and compliance (Kamerling, 2001).

Assessment of pain in animals can be very difficult because of the dependence on nonverbal communication in veterinary medicine. Furthermore, animals differ from people in their pain response. It is important in wild animals to control the expression of pain to avoid predation or abandonment. Response to pain varies among individuals and may include increased heart rate, increased respiratory rate, mydriasis, salivation, vocalization, changes in facial expression, guarding the painful site, restlessness, unresponsiveness, failure to groom, abnormal gait, abnormal stance, and rolling. A patient that is pain-free will be quiet and calm (Paddleford, 1999).

Drugs used to control pain (analgesics) include the NSAIDs and the narcotics (see Chapter 4). The body is able to produce its own opiate-like analgesic agents called *endorphins* and *enkephalins*. Efforts to synthesize these substances for commercial production have been unsuccessful.

Even though some people believe that masking pain with analgesics can interfere with the diagnosis or treatment course of a disease, pain should be treated for humane reasons and to reduce the harmful side effects that accompany it. The treatment regimen may vary according to the assessment of the severity and the etiology of the pain. For best results, pain management intervention should be preemptive when possible.

Inflammation is a basic process that occurs in the body in response to tissue injury from physical, chemical, or biologic trauma. The objectives of this process are to counteract the injury by removing or walling off the cause of the injury and to repair or replace the damaged tissue. The clinical manifestations (cardinal signs) of inflammation include *redness*, *heat*, *swelling*, and *pain*. Although the process is designed to be protective, it can continue to become a source of further injury or damage (e.g., allergy, shock, and "proud flesh").

Damage to cells from any source results in the release of several chemical mediators that may initiate or prolong the inflammatory response. These chemicals include **prostaglandins,** leukotrienes, **histamine,** cytokines, and other mediators. These substances cause helpful responses, such as dilation and increased permeability of blood vessels, that result in increased blood flow to the injured tissue. The increased blood flow brings plasma to dilute the offending agent, fibrin to immobilize it, and phagocytic cells to remove it. The redness, heat, swelling, and to some extent the pain of inflammation are a result of the increased amount of blood in the damaged tissue. The chemical mediators serve other beneficial functions, such as attracting phagocytic cells to the area of concern (chemotaxis), but also several potentially harmful ones—such as initiation of bronchoconstriction (histamine), anaphylactic shock, pain (histamine), cell death, platelet aggregation, and intestinal spasm. The inflammatory process can be acute (anaphylaxis) or chronic (flea allergy and arthritis).

Drugs that are used to decrease the inflammatory process include the NSAIDs, the glucocorticosteroids, and several miscellaneous agents including dimethyl sulfoxide (DMSO). Another process mediated by a chemical (or chemicals) released from damaged cells is fever. Fever is an increase in body temperature above normal; it is an important clinical indicator of disease. The purpose of fever may include destruction of invading microorganisms by heat inactivation and facilitation of biochemical reactions in the body. (Most chemical reactions are speeded up by increased heat.)

Heat is generated by the metabolic activity of muscle and glands and is lost through radiation or conduction loss from the skin, sweat evaporation, and evaporation during panting. A "thermostat" in the hypothalamus regulates these mechanisms, which control body temperature.

A substance that can initiate a fever is called a *pyrogen*. An exogenous pyrogen is a foreign substance (e.g., bacteria and viruses) that when introduced into the body causes the release of an endogenous pyrogen (a chemical mediator, such as prostaglandin) from white blood cells, and this endogenous pyrogen causes a resetting of the hypothalamic thermostat. The hypothalamus then activates processes to generate or conserve body heat: shivering to generate more heat, constriction of blood vessels in the skin to prevent radiation and conduction loss, and decreased sweating or panting to reduce evaporation loss. Damaged cells in some instances may release endogenous pyrogens in the absence of exogenous pyrogens. The drugs used to control fever are primarily the NSAIDs.

ANATOMY AND PHYSIOLOGY

Pain sensation arises in nociceptors—"naked" nerve endings found in almost every tissue of the body. Pain impulses are carried to the central nervous system by two fiber systems: type C unmyelinated fibers are responsible for dull, poorly localized pain (in humans), and type A delta fibers are responsible for sharp, localized pain (Ganong, 2003). Both type A and C fibers carry impulses to the dorsal horn of the spinal cord (Figure 14-1), and

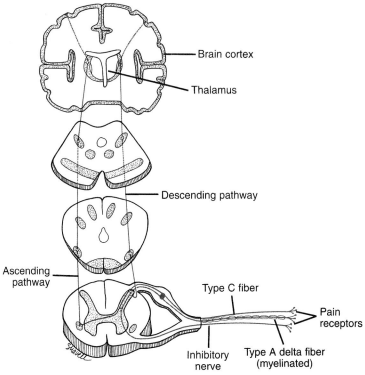

FIGURE 14-1

Pain Pathways and relevant receptors. (From Boothe DM: Control of pain in small animals. In Small animal clinical pharmacology and therapeutics, Philadelphia, 2001, WB Saunders Co.)

the information is then relayed up the cord via the spinothalamic tract through the thalamus to the cerebral cortex, where it is interpreted as pain. If any part of this neuronal chain or the cortical interpretive area is nonfunctional, pain sensation does not occur. Since an active cortex is required, the perception of pain can occur only in a conscious animal. It should be remembered that reflexive activity without pain recognition can occur as a result of nociceptor stimulation (Chapter 4).

The perception of pain can be enhanced by phenomena called hyperalgesia and central sensitization (Boothe, 2001). Hyperalgesia occurs when the area of tissue injury becomes more sensitive and the threshold for subsequent stimuli decreases. This sensitivity can also spread to surrounding uninjured tissue (secondary hyperalgesia). When the neurons of the spinothalamic tract of the spinal cord are stimulated repeatedly they apparently become sensitized and discharge at a much lower threshold. This activity is called central sensitization or "wind-up" and is the rationale for the idea that pain control is enhanced if the analgesic is given before the generation of pain.

When spinal cord lesions occur, superficial pain is inhibited before **deep pain** as lesion severity worsens. The absence of deep pain is often a poor prognostic sign.

Nonsteroidal Antiinflammatory Agents

The NSAIDs are thought to work by inhibiting an enzyme called *cyclooxygenase (cox)*. Two forms (cox-1 and cox-2) of cyclooxygenase exist. Cyclooxygenase 1 maintains physiologic functions like modulation of renal blood flow and the synthesis of gastric mucosa (Paddleford, 1999). Cyclooxygenase 2 promotes the formation of prostaglandin from cell membrane arachidonic acid (Figure 14-2). NSAIDs that selectively inhibit cox-2 are thought to produce fewer gastrointestinal side effects. The glucocorticoids exert their effect by blocking phospholipase, an enzyme necessary for the production of both the prostaglandins and the leukotrienes (intervention comes earlier in the sequence of the formation of the inflammatory mediators). Because the inflammatory reaction is blocked earlier by the glucocorticoids, they are more effective antiinflammatory agents than the NSAIDs (Langston and Mercer, 1988). NSAIDs are often preferred, however, because they have fewer side effects and they promote **analgesia** and fever reduction. At this time, it is not known why the glucocorticoids do not induce the analgesic and antipyretic effects of the NSAIDs. It is also unknown why some NSAIDs provide relief of only mild pain (aspirin) and others provide relief of moderate to severe pain (flunixin). Some clinicians speculate that NSAIDs may act to varying degrees centrally to modulate spinal transmission of pain impulses (Paddleford, 1999).

The most common side effect of the NSAIDs is gastrointestinal ulceration and bleeding, which are probably a result of interference with the normal mucous coating of the stomach. Other side effects may include nephrotoxicity, inhibition of cartilage metabolism, bone marrow suppression,

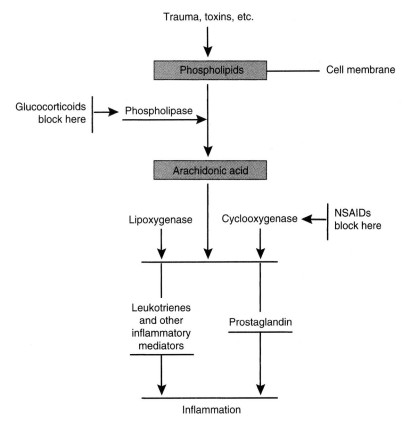

FIGURE 14-2
Action of nonsteroidal antiinflammatory drugs and the glucocorticoids to interrupt the inflammatory response.

and bleeding tendencies (from reduced platelet aggregation).

Technician's Notes

1. NSAIDs should be used with caution in geriatric animals.
2. Combining NSAIDs or combining NSAIDs with corticosteroids should be used with great caution or avoided.

Salicylates

Aspirin, a salicylate, is also known as acetylsalicylic acid. Its actions include the following:

1. Relief of pain (analgesia)
2. Reduction of fever (antipyrexia)
3. Inhibition of inflammation (antiinflammatory)
4. Reduction of platelet aggregation

These effects are thought to occur as a result of aspirin's ability to inhibit an enzyme (cyclooxygenase), which is responsible for the synthesis of prostaglandin. Prostaglandin is a chemical mediator of the processes that lead to pain, fever, inflammation, and platelet aggregation. Its inhibition results in a diminishing of each process.

Clinical Uses. Clinical uses of aspirin exist for most animal species and may include the following:

1. Relief of mild to moderate pain resulting from musculoskeletal conditions, such as arthritis or hip dysplasia
2. Postadulticide treatment for heartworm disease
3. Analgesia/antipyrexia
4. Treatment of cardiomyopathy in cats
5. Treatment of endotoxic shock

Dosage Forms. These include plain uncoated tablets, buffered uncoated tablets, enteric coated forms, and boluses (large-animal applications). Many generic or brand names in many different strengths are available, including the following:

1. Aspirin bolus
2. Aspirin tablets
3. Cortaba (a combination of aspirin and methylprednisolone)

Adverse Side Effects. Adverse side effects of aspirin include gastric irritation, which can lead to ulceration and bleeding. *Cats are very susceptible to aspirin overdose because of their inability to metabolize it rapidly, and they should receive this drug only under the supervision of a veterinarian.*

Technician's Notes

1. Enteric coated aspirin, such as Ecotrin, may be used to prevent gastric irritation.
2. A 1-grain "baby" aspirin contains 65 mg; a 1.25-grain baby aspirin contains 81 mg.
3. There is no withdrawal time for aspirin in food animals.

Pyrazolone Derivatives
PHENYLBUTAZONE

Phenylbutazone, a pyrazolone derivative, is a commonly used NSAID in veterinary medicine. Its actions include the following:

1. Analgesia for mild to moderate pain
2. Antiinflammatory action
3. Antipyrexia

Clinical Uses. These include relief of inflammatory conditions of the musculoskeletal system of horses and dogs. Phenylbutazone is used extensively in horses for the treatment of lameness and for the relief of pain associated with colic. It is sometimes used in dogs and cattle for its antiinflammatory, analgesic, and antipyretic effects.

Dosage Forms. Dosage forms of phenylbutazone include a parenteral injection, tablets, boluses, an oral paste, an oral gel, and powder.

1. Butazolidin Tablets, Boluses, Paste, Injection
2. Phenylzone Paste

3. Equipalazone Powder
4. Equi-Phar Phenylbutazone Gel, Tablets
5. Phenylbutazone Tablets
6. Pro-Bute
7. Phenylbutazone Injection

Adverse Side Effects. These include gastrointestinal bleeding and bone marrow suppression.

Technician's Notes

1. Phenylbutazone injection should be administered by the intravenous route only. Subcutaneous and intramuscular injection may lead to sloughing of tissue.
2. Prolonged use or overdose can lead to bone marrow suppression in humans.
3. Prolonged use may also lead to ulcer formation.
4. Because of the possible bone marrow suppression and potential ulcer formation, animals that are receiving long-term treatment with phenylbutazone should be monitored carefully.

Flunixin Meglumine (Banamine)

Flunixin is an NSAID labeled for use in horses and cattle. It has extralabel uses in other species. Its actions are related to its ability to inhibit cyclooxygenase and include the following:

1. Analgesia
2. Antipyrexia
3. Antiinflammatory

Clinical Uses. Clinical uses of flunixin in horses include alleviation of pain associated with musculoskeletal disorders and colic. (Flunixin apparently has great ability to inhibit visceral pain.) Other uses in horses and other species include treatment of the following:

1. Disk disease
2. Endotoxic shock
3. Calf diarrhea
4. Parvovirus disease
5. Heatstroke

6. Ophthalmic conditions
7. Postsurgical pain

Dosage Forms. Dosage forms of flunixin include injectable, oral paste, and oral granule formulations.

1. Banamine Injection
2. Banamine Oral Paste
3. Banamine Oral Granules
4. Finadyne

Adverse Side Effects. These are limited in horses but may include swelling at the injection site and sweating. In dogs, vomiting, diarrhea, nephrotoxicity, and gastric ulceration may occur with long-term use.

Technician's Notes

1. Flunixin is labeled for intravenous and intramuscular use in horses.
2. Some equine clinicians believe that flunixin relieves abdominal pain so well in horses that it may cause a sense of false security about the condition of an animal with colic.
3. Small-animal patients receiving flunixin should be well hydrated and should be receiving intravenous fluids and ulcer prophylaxis (Paddleford, 1999).

Dimethyl Sulfoxide

DMSO is a clear liquid that was originally developed as a commercial solvent. It is noted for its antiinflammatory action and its ability to act as a carrier of other agents through the skin. Its antiinflammatory actions may be related to its ability to trap products associated with the inflammatory response. DMSO causes vasodilation when applied topically.

Clinical Uses. Clinical uses of DMSO are varied; however, the only labeled use for DMSO is for topical application to reduce acute swelling resulting from trauma in dogs and horses. DMSO has reportedly been used as the following:

1. An adjunct to intestinal surgery (intravenously)
2. A treatment for cerebral edema or spinal cord injury (intravenously)
3. A treatment for perivascular injection of sodium caparsolate or other irritating substances (topical)
4. A carrier of drugs across the skin

Dosage Forms. Dosage forms of DMSO include a solution (90%) and a gel (90%).

1. DMSO Gel and Solution (90%)
2. Synotic (DMSO and a steroid)

Adverse Side Effects. Adverse side effects of DMSO are probably minimal with limited use or exposure but may include the following:

1. Garlic taste, which occurs very shortly after the agent is applied to the skin
2. Skin irritation accompanied by a burning sensation
3. Induction of birth defects (teratogenic) in some species

Technician's Notes
1. Rubber gloves should be worn while applying DMSO.
2. Bandaging over an application of DMSO may cause skin irritation.
3. DMSO should be used carefully when cholinesterase inhibitors have been used.

Acetaminophen
Acetaminophen is an analgesic with limited antipyretic and antiinflammatory activity.

Clinical Uses. Clinical uses of acetaminophen are limited in veterinary medicine, and acetaminophen use should be discouraged because of the risk of potential toxicity and the availability of acceptable substitutes.

Dosage Forms. Dosage forms of acetaminophen include tablets, caplets, and liquid formulations.

The following is a list of some of the human label brand names:

1. Tylenol
2. Datril
3. Tempra

Technician's Notes
1. Acetaminophen should never be given to cats.
2. Over-the-counter products should be checked carefully for the presence of acetaminophen before use in cats.

Adverse Side Effects. Adverse side effects of acetaminophen use in cats include the formation of methemoglobinemia, cyanosis, anemia, and liver damage. *Cats have a limited ability to biotransform acetaminophen and may succumb to a single dose.*

Propionic Acid Derivatives
CARPROFEN
Carprofen is a propionic acid derivative NSAID approved for oral use in dogs. Carprofen has been approved for oral and injectable use in dogs and cats in Europe. It has a half-life of 8 hours and is thought to work by inhibiting cyclooxygenase. An injectable form is now available for use in the United States as well.

Clinical Uses. Uses include the relief of pain associated with degenerative joint disease or postoperative pain resulting from soft tissue or orthopedic pain.

Dosage Form
Carprofen (Rimadyl). Available in tablets, caplets, injection, and chewable tablets.

Adverse Side Effects. Side effects, such as gastrointestinal ulceration or bleeding, are apparently rare with this agent.

KETOPROFEN
Ketoprofen is a propionic acid derivative with analgesic, antipyretic, and antiinflammatory activity. It

is labeled for use in horses in the United States but has been used a great deal in dogs and cats in Europe and Canada.

Clinical Uses. In horses ketoprofen is used for treatment of pain and inflammation associated with musculoskeletal disorders. It has been used for postoperative and chronic pain in dogs and cats.

Dosage Forms
1. Ketofen (horses)
2. Orudis (human label)

Adverse Side Effects. Side effects may include gastrointestinal bleeding or ulceration, renal dysfunction, and generalized bleeding.

NAPROXEN

Naproxen is a propionic acid derivative similar to ketoprofen and ibuprofen. It is labeled for use in horses, although it has been used in dogs.

Clinical Uses. Naproxen is labeled for the "relief of pain, inflammation, and lameness associated with myositis and other soft tissue diseases of the musculoskeletal system of horses."

Dosage Forms
1. Equiproxen (horses)
2. Naprosyn (human)

Adverse Side Effects. Few side effects are reported in horses. GI ulceration has been reported in dogs.

IBUPROFEN

Ibuprofen is reported to have potential for serious side effects in dogs and cats and is not recommended for use in these species.

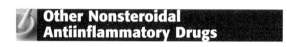

Other Nonsteroidal Antiinflammatory Drugs

Etodolac

Etodolac is an indole acetic acid derivative NSAID labeled for use in dogs.

Clinical Use. This drug is labeled for the management of pain and inflammation associated with osteoarthritis in dogs.

Dosage Form
EtoGesic

Adverse Side Effects. Side effects include anorexia, vomiting, diarrhea, and lethargy.

Deracoxib

Deracoxib is an analgesic and a nonsteroidal anti-inflammatory agent of the coxib class.

Clinical Use. Deracoxib is labeled for the control of pain and inflammation associated with orthopedic surgery in dogs with 4 lb body weight or greater, and for the control of pain and inflammation associated with osteoarthritis in dogs weighting 14 lb or greater.

Dosage Form
Deramaxx

Tepoxalin

Tepoxalin is a nonsteroidal anti-inflammatory drug for oral use in dogs only. The manufacturer claims that this product is the only NSAID to block both arms of the arachidonic acid cascade (cyclooxygenase and lipoxygenase). It is manufactured as a "rapidly disintegrating" tablet that breaks down quickly upon contact with the moisture of the animal's mouth and cannot be spit out. This dosage form is designed to improve owner/animal dosage compliance.

Clinical Use. Tepoxalin is labeled for the control of pain and inflammation associated with osteoarthritis in dogs.

Dosage Form
Zubrin

Other agents that are classified as NSAIDs or that have similar activity include the following:

Polysulfated Glycosaminoglycan (Adequan). Adequan is a semisynthetic mixture of glycosaminoglycans derived from bovine cartilage. This drug reduces degenerative changes induced by noninfectious or traumatic joint diseases and promotes activity of the synovial membrane. It is available in intraarticular and intramuscular forms and is labeled for use in horses and dogs.

Hyaluronate Sodium (Hyalovet). Hyalovet is a glycosaminoglycan that is labeled for intraarticular injection. It has activities similar to that of Adequan.

Legend. A solution of hyaluronate that may be given by intravenous or intraarticular injection for synovitis associated with osteoarthritis.

Meclofenamic Acid (Arquel Granules). This NSAID is labeled for oral treatment of acute or chronic inflammatory disease in horses.

Selenium and Vitamin E (Seletoc). Seletoc is labeled for relief of acute symptoms of arthritic conditions in dogs.

Ketorolac. Ketorolac is an NSAID with efficacy similar to that of morphine. It carries a human label and may cause serious side effects.

Orgotein (Palosein). Palosein is labeled for acute and chronic inflammatory conditions in horses and dogs.

Cosequin. Cosequin contains glucosamine, chondroitin sulfate, and manganese sulfate. It is a neutraceutical and has similar benefits on osteoarthritis, as do the polysulfated glycosaminoglycans.

Opioid Analgesics

The opioids and opioid receptors are discussed in a general fashion in Chapter 4. This section deals only with opioid use to control pain.

Opioids relieve pain by binding with specific receptor sites in the brain, spinal cord, and in peripheral tissue. By altering neurotransmitter release, they alter nerve impulse formation and transmission at many levels within the CNS. The ultimate effect is that the opioids block or inhibit pain impulses to the higher CNS centers responsible for the perception of pain.

Opioid Agonists

Opioid agonists remain one of the most effective drug classes in relieving moderate to severe pain (Paddleford, 1999). Opioid agonists are drugs that bind with all opioid receptor sites and produce opioid effects and respiratory depression, sedation, and addiction. The opioid agonists include alfentanil, carfentanil, codeine, etorphine, fentanyl, hydromorphone, meperidine, methadone, morphine, oxymorphone, and sufentanil. Even though some of these drugs are considered more potent than morphine, morphine is still considered to be one of the most effective of the opioids. All of the agonists are C-II controlled substances.

Clinical Uses. Opioid agonists are used to control moderate to severe pain in animals.

Selected Dosage Forms
1. Morphine sulfate (Infumorph, Astramorph PF) (human labels)
2. Oxymorphone (Numorphan)
3. Meperidine (Demerol)
4. Codeine (codeine phosphate, codeine sulfate, Tylenol with codeine)
5. Fentanyl transdermal (Duragesic)

Adverse Side Effects. Side effects can include respiratory depression, sedation, excitement, and addiction. Cats are more sensitive to the excitatory effects of the opioid agonists than other species but do tolerate low doses well.

TRANSDERMAL FENTANYL USE
Transdermal application of fentanyl has been successfully used in humans for control of chronic pain for some time. This use has recently been adapted for the control of postoperative and chronic pain in dogs and cats (extralabel).

Care must be taken when using the transdermal patches to ensure that the animal does not eat or lick the patch (causing possible overdosage) or that accidental exposure to humans (especially children) does not occur. To apply the patch, gloves should be worn; the skin over the dorsum of the neck should be clipped, cleansed, and allowed to dry well; good skin contact with the patch should be achieved; and a snug bandage should be applied to hold the patch in place. The patch should never be cut because this interferes with the rate of release of the fentanyl. The patch should be carefully disposed of after use.

Opioid Agonists-Antagonists

The opioid agonist-antagonist drugs bind with opioid kappa receptors but antagonize opioid mu receptors. Opioid agonists-antagonists include butorphanol (C-IV), pentazocine (C-IV), and nalbuphine. These drugs are considered effective for mild to moderate pain and have few side effects.

Clinical Uses. The primary use is the relief of mild to moderate pain.

Dosage Forms
1. Butorphanol (Torbugesic, Torbutrol, Stadol)
2. Pentazocine (Talwin-V)
3. Nalbuphine (Nubain)

Adverse Side Effects. Side effects include sedation, ataxia, and salivation (pentazocine).

Opioid Partial Agonists

The opioid partial agonists bind with the mu receptors but only partially activate them. Buprenorphine is the primary drug in this category. Recent studies have shown that buprenorphine may be effectively administered by the sublingual/buccal route in cats (Robertson, 2001).

Clinical Uses. Uses include relief of mild to moderate pain in dogs and horses.

Dosage Form
Buprenex (human label)

Adverse Side Effects. Side effects include sedation and respiratory depression.

Antihistamines

Antihistamines are drugs that are used to inhibit the effects or the spread of the inflammatory process. These drugs do not inhibit the formation of prostaglandins or other inflammatory mediators. They work by preventing histamine from combining with tissue receptors or by displacing histamine from receptor sites.

Because histamine is a major chemical mediator of the allergic response, antihistamines may be useful in controlling allergic responses.

Histamine is a chemical that is released from mast cells when they are adequately stimulated by immunoglobulin E (IgE) antibodies to allergens (Figure 14-3). Histamine then combines with tissue receptors and causes dilation of small blood vessels,

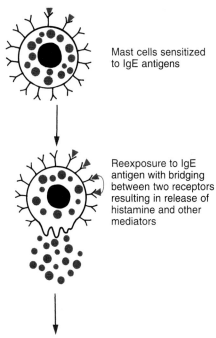

Mast cells sensitized to IgE antigens

Reexposure to IgE antigen with bridging between two receptors resulting in release of histamine and other mediators

Activation of H_1 receptors with dilation of blood vessels, increased capillary permeability, pain, and other inflammatory responses

FIGURE 14-3
The release of histamine from mast cells when stimulated by IgE antibodies.

increased permeability of capillaries, smooth muscle spasm, and increased secretion of glands. Two types of antihistamine receptors have been identified: H_1 and H_2.

Antihistamines competitively block the binding of histamine to H_1 receptors, which may block the progression of the allergic response. Some antihistamines also block H_1 receptors that may contribute to motion sickness or nausea. Some antihistamines have a high affinity for H_1 receptors in the brain and cause a sedative effect.

Stimulation of H_2 receptors causes an increase in flow of hydrochloric acid by the gastric mucosa. H_2 blockers reduce secretion of hydrochloric acid and may be used to treat gastrointestinal irritation and ulceration.

Clinical Uses. Antihistamines are used to treat the following:

1. Pruritus
2. Urticaria and angioedema associated with acute allergic reactions
3. Laminitis in horses and cattle
4. "Downer" cow syndrome
5. Motion sickness
6. "Reverse sneeze" syndrome
7. Anaphylactic shock
8. Upper respiratory tract conditions

Dosage Forms. These include injectables, oral preparations, and topical agents. Many brand names are available under veterinary and human labels. A partial list of the formulations follows:

H_1 Blockers
1. Pyrilamine maleate (antihistamine injection)
2. Pyrilamine maleate injection
3. Pyrilamine maleate injection (Histavet-P)
4. Tripelennamine hydrochloride (Re-Covr Injection)
5. Pyrilamine maleate, phenylephrine hydrochloride with a decongestant and an expectorant (cough syrup)
6. Probahist Syrup (same ingredients as in No. 5)
7. Diphenhydramine HCl (Histacalm Shampoo, Spray)

8. Diphenhydramine (Benadryl)
9. Dimenhydrinate (Dramamine)
10. Meclizine (Bonine)
11. Promethazine (Phenergan)
12. Terfenadine (Seldane)
13. Hydroxyzine HCl (Atarax)
14. Chlorpheniramine maleate (Chlor-Trimeton)

H_2 Blockers
1. Cimetidine (Tagamet)
2. Ranitidine (Zantac)

Adverse Side Effects. Adverse side effects of the antihistamines include drowsiness, weakness, dry mucous membranes, urinary retention, and CNS stimulation on overdose.

Technician's Notes
Antihistamines are not as effective in controlling pruritus in animals as they are in humans.

 Muscle Relaxants

Skeletal muscle relaxants may be used as an aid in the treatment of acute inflammatory and traumatic conditions of muscle and the resulting spasms that may occur in these situations. They are thought to work by decreasing muscle hyperactivity without interfering with normal muscle tone. This action may be brought about by selective action on the internuncial neurons of the spinal cord.

Methocarbamol (Robaxin-V)
Robaxin-V is labeled for use in dogs, cats, and horses.

Clinical Uses. This product is used to treat the following:

1. Intervertebral disk syndrome
2. Strains and sprains
3. Myositis and bursitis
4. Muscle spasm
5. Tying up in horses

Table 14-1 Mineralocorticoid Versus Glucocorticoid Classification of Corticosteroids

Drug	Glucocorticoid Potency (Antiinflammatory Effect)	Mineralocorticoid Potency
Hydrocortisone	1.0	1.00
Cortisone	0.8	0.80
Prednisone	4.0	0.25
Prednisolone	4.0	0.25
Methylprednisolone	5.0	0.00
Triamcinolone	5.0	0.00
Paramethasone	10.0	0.00
Flumethasone	15.0	0.00
Dexamethasone	30.0	0.00
Betamethasone	35.0	0.00

Dosage Forms. Dosage forms of Robaxin-V include tablets and an injectable.

Other Muscle Relaxants
1. Myotrol
2. Spasgesic

Adverse Side Effects. These include excessive salivation, emesis, muscle weakness, and ataxia when overdosed. The package insert states that adverse side effects are seldom encountered.

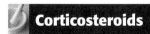

Corticosteroids

Corticosteroid drugs are used in veterinary medicine to treat inflammatory, pruritic, and immune-mediated diseases. These drugs are also used to treat shock, laminitis, anorexia, adrenal insufficiency, and various other conditions. The technician should remember that corticosteroid therapy involves the treatment of the signs of disease; it is seldom, if ever, curative.

Natural corticosteroids are hormones that are produced by the adrenal cortex, whereas corticosteroids used clinically are synthetic reproductions (analogs) of the naturally occurring hormones. Corticosteroids are classified according to their activity as either mineralocorticoids or glucocorticoids

Table 14-2 Duration of Action of Corticosteroids

Short Acting (<12 Hours)	Intermediate Acting (12-36 Hours)	Long Acting (>48 Hours)
Hydrocortisone	Prednisone	Betamethasone
Cortisone	Prednisolone	Dexamethasone
	Methylprednisolone	Flumethasone
	Tramcinolone	Paramethasone

(Table 14-1) and, according to their duration of action (Table 14-2), as short, intermediate, or long acting. Mineralocorticoids, such as aldosterone, regulate electrolyte and water balance in the body. Glucocorticoids, such as cortisone, exert antiinflammatory and immunosuppressive effects and influence the metabolism of carbohydrate, fat, and protein. No corticosteroid has complete glucocorticoid or mineralocorticoid activity, but each has a predominant activity that determines its classification. Because mineralocorticoids are seldom used clinically, this discussion focuses on the glucocorticoids.

Control of the release of the naturally occurring corticosteroids (cortisol, corticosterone, and deoxycortisol) is complex and occurs through the hypothalamic-pituitary-adrenal axis (Figure 14-4). Control is exerted through this axis by two basic mechanisms. The first is a feedback mechanism related to the level of cortisol in the bloodstream. When the level of cortisol in the blood is lowered, the hypothalamus sends a chemical messenger called *corticotropin-releasing factor (CRF)* to the anterior pituitary gland. This causes the pituitary to release a substance called *adrenocorticotropic hormone (ACTH)* into the bloodstream. The blood then carries ACTH to the adrenal cortex, where it stimulates this structure to release cortisol to raise the amount in the blood to appropriate levels. On the other hand, a high level of blood cortisol inhibits release of CRF by the hypothalamus, and the blood level is thus prevented from reaching excessive levels. It should be noted that the hypothalamus cannot distinguish between naturally occurring cortisol and the synthetic analogs administered by veterinarians.

The second mechanism for the control of the release of cortisol by the adrenal gland is through the stress response. External and internal stressors, such as crowding, weaning, transporting, disease, surgery, trauma, pain, fear, anxiety, and many others, can stimulate the hypothalamus—through impulses from the higher brain centers—to release CRF. The control mechanism then proceeds in a similar fashion as illustrated in Figure 14-4.

One of the major indications for the clinical use of corticosteroids is for their antiinflammatory effects. These effects are brought about by their ability to block the enzyme phospholipase, which promotes the reaction that results in the formation of prostaglandin—a primary mediator of the immune response. Corticosteroids also protect cells from inflammatory trauma by various mechanisms that include but are not limited to the following:

1. Stabilizing cell membranes to help prevent their breakdown
2. Stabilizing lysosomal membranes so that they do not release their harmful enzymes
3. Disrupting histamine synthesis
4. Inhibiting interleukin synthesis
5. Reducing exudative processes

Corticosteroids are also used clinically for their immunosuppressive effects. They are used to suppress the immune system in allergic conditions, such as flea allergy dermatitis, atopy, autoimmune hemolytic anemia, rheumatoid arthritis, and uveitis. The immunosuppressive effect comes from the ability of corticosteroids to do the following:

1. Inhibit antibody formation
2. Decrease the concentration of lymphocytes and eosinophils
3. Suppress the migration of neutrophils
4. Inhibit phagocytosis

Although the immunosuppressive qualities are very useful clinically, they can also mask the signs of serious infections that are simultaneously present.

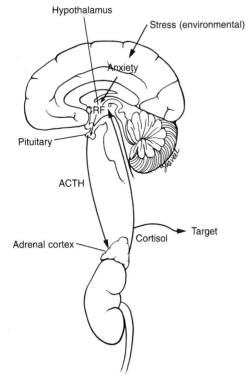

FIGURE 14-4
The release of corticosteroids is under the control of the hypothalamic-pituitary-adrenal (HPA) axis.

Corticosteroids are useful in the treatment of lymphoid tumors by causing a direct lymphotoxic effect. (Barton, 2001).

All steroid compounds are synthesized from a basic parent compound, which has been described as resembling three rooms and a bath (Figure 14-5). Steroids are formed in three regions in the adrenal gland. Those regions and their respective products include the following:

1. Zona glomerulosa—mineralocorticoids
2. Zona fasciculata—glucocorticoids
3. Zona reticularis—sex hormones (androgen and estrogen)

An increased number of double bonds in the parent compound, the addition of certain side chains, or the addition of fluorine atoms to the parent molecule usually increases the antiinflammatory effects of corticosteroids.

Clinical Uses. Corticosteroids are used for the treatment of the following conditions:

1. Allergic reactions/conditions
2. Inflammatory conditions of the musculoskeletal system
3. Shock/toxemia
4. Laminitis
5. Inflammatory ocular conditions, such as conjunctivitis and uveitis
6. Addison's disease

7. Autoimmune disease, such as autoimmune hemolytic anemia, lupus, and rheumatoid arthritis
8. Lymphocytic neoplasms

Dosage Forms. Corticosteroids are available in injectable, oral, and topical forms and in preparations containing antibiotic, antifungal, and corticosteroid products. These products may be applied to the skin or mucous membranes, injected into lesions, given orally, or administered parenterally. When emergency conditions call for administration of corticosteroids, the intravenous route is normally used with a water-soluble product in a water-soluble vehicle. Water-soluble products can be injected via the intramuscular or subcutaneous route when life-threatening conditions do not exist. The long-acting depot (repositol) products are prepared in a poorly soluble vehicle to prolong their effects. The justification for these long-acting products has been questioned by some clinicians.

A list of some of the many corticosteroid products available follows.

Injectables
1. Azium
2. Azium Sodium Phosphate
3. Betasone
4. Cortisate-20
5. Depo-Medrol
6. Dexamethasone Injection
7. Dexamethasone Sodium Phosphate
8. Dex-A-Vet Injection
9. Dexasone
10. Flucort Solution
11. Meticorten
12. Percorten-V
13. Predef
14. Solu-Delta-Cortef
15. Vetalog Parenteral

Oral
1. Azium Powder
2. Medrol
3. Methylprednisolone Tablets
4. Pet-Derm III
5. Temaril-P Tablets

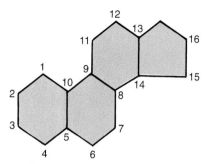

FIGURE 14-5
The configuration of the parent molecule of all steroid molecules including corticosteroids.

6. Triamcinolone Tablets
7. Vetalog Oral Powder/Tablets
8. Prednisone generic tablets
9. Prednisolone generic tablets

Topical
1. Cort/Astrin Solution
2. CortiSpray
3. Hydro-Plus
4. Synalar Cream
5. Synalar Otic Solution
6. Vetalog Cream

Adverse Side Effects. Adverse side effects of the corticosteroids are numerous:

1. Polyuria and polydipsia
2. Thinning of the skin and muscle wasting resulting from the ability of corticosteroids to convert protein into glucose (seen with long-term administration)
3. Depressed healing
4. Polyphagia and resulting weight gain
5. Iatrogenic (caused by the veterinarian) hyperadrenocorticism, iatrogenic **Cushing's disease**
6. Hypoadrenocorticism (iatrogenic) resulting from suppression of the hypothalamic-pituitary-adrenal axis by long-term administration of exogenous corticosteroids and then sudden cessation of the treatment (**Addison's disease**)
7. Gastric ulcers with or without bleeding
8. Osteoporosis (long-term)
9. Abnormal behavior

Because administration of corticosteroids is fraught with many potential side effects, clinicians must give careful consideration to their use. Much information has been written about the appropriate use of corticosteroids in veterinary medicine, and a selection of the principles of use follows:

1. Alternate-day dosing may help prevent iatrogenic hypoadrenocorticism.
2. Administration should never be stopped abruptly but tapered off gradually.
3. Very large doses may be used in emergency situations.

4. Corticosteroids are generally not used for the treatment of corneal ulcers.
5. When corticosteroids are injected into joint spaces, extreme care should be given to aseptic technique.

LOCAL, REGIONAL, AND TOPICAL ANESTHETIC AGENTS

Many clinical situations call for the use of local or topical anesthesia to prevent or relieve pain. We have chosen to discuss these agents in this chapter on pain relief rather than in the traditional context of anesthesia.

In some situations, general anesthesia is not available or is too dangerous to a client. In others, repair of a small laceration may not justify general anesthesia. In equine medicine, lameness may be diagnosed by administering a **nerve block** to an area and then observing abatement of the lameness. In bovine medicine, it may be useful to administer a regional nerve block to prevent straining in order to replace a prolapsed uterus. In cats, it may be useful to apply a local anesthetic to the larynx to facilitate placement of an endotracheal tube.

Local anesthetics work by preventing the generation and conduction of nerve impulses in peripheral nerves. These anesthetics are administered by the following routes:

1. Topically to the skin or mucous membranes of the ear, eye, larynx, or other appropriate areas
2. By infiltration in a localized area, such as the margin of a wound, to anesthetize nerve endings (Figure 14-6)
3. Dripping or "splashing" into a surgical site
4. By injection into joint spaces
5. For intravenous regional nerve block; may be used for foot surgery in cattle by applying a tourniquet to the proximal area of a limb and then infusing a local anesthetic into the limb
6. Around nerve bodies
   a. Epidural anesthesia—injection of a local anesthetic into the epidural space (see Figure 14-6) of the spinal canal to provide anesthesia to the area around the anus and perineum for

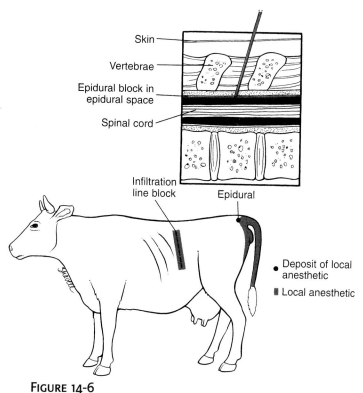

FIGURE 14-6
The use of local anesthetics to provide local and regional anesthesia.

obstetric manipulations and to stop straining for the replacement of a prolapsed uterus

b. Nerve block—local anesthetic deposited around a specific nerve (Figure 14-7) to facilitate minor procedures (e.g., lameness diagnosis, dehorning, lid or lip suturing)

c. Paravertebral block—placement of a local anesthetic around a spinal nerve near where it leaves the intervertebral space; this procedure blocks a larger area and may be used for procedures such as cesarean sections and rumenotomies

The onset and duration of action of the various agents vary. Lidocaine has a rapid onset of action (5 to 10 minutes) and a somewhat short duration (1 to 2 hours). Lidocaine may also cause a stinging sensation when injected. The onset of bupivacaine takes 20 minutes but it lasts 4 to 6 hours. The effects

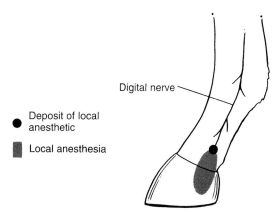

FIGURE 14-7
Local anesthesia to diagnose lameness in horses.

of local anesthetics can be prolonged by adding epinephrine, which causes vasoconstriction and therefore prolongs the absorption time owing to a reduced blood supply in the area. Using ethyl alcohol as a local anesthetic agent may considerably prolong the duration of the anesthesia. Some clinicians prefer to use xylazine or a narcotic agent for administering epidural anesthesia.

Clinical Uses. Local anesthetics are used for the following purposes:

1. Infiltration of local areas
2. Epidural anesthesia
3. Topical application in the eye, ear, larynx, and so forth
4. Nerve blocks
5. Their antiarrhythmic effects

Dosage Forms. Local anesthetic agents are available in injectable and topical forms. A partial list of these agents follows:

Injectable
1. Anthocaine Injection (lidocaine)
2. Marcaine (bupivacaine)
3. Epidural Injection (procaine HCl)
4. Lidocaine hydrochloride injection
5. Other generic local anesthetics, including tetracaine and dibucaine

Topical
1. Ophthaine Solution Veterinary
2. Ophthetic

Adverse Side Effects. Local anesthetics can have adverse side effects if the total maximum dose for the species being treated is exceeded. The side effects may include restlessness, excitement, hypotension, and seizures.

Technician's Notes

1. Lidocaine with epinephrine should never be used if an antiarrhythmic is indicated.
2. Exceeding the total recommended dose of local analgesics may cause toxicity.

REFERENCES

Barton CL: Chemotherapy. In Boothe DM, editor: Small animal clinical pharmacology and therapeutics, Philadelphia, 2001, WB Saunders Co.

Boothe DM: Control of pain in small animals. In Small animal clinical pharmacology and therapeutics, Philadelphia, 2001, WB Saunders Co.

Ganong WF: Cutaneous, deep, and visceral sensation. In Ganong WF, editor: Review of medical physiology, ed 21, New York, 2003, McGraw-Hill.

Kamerling SG: Pain recognition and relief. In Proceedings of the annual meeting of the American Veterinary Medical Association, Boston, 2001.

Langston VC, Mercer HD: Non-steroidal anti-inflammatory drugs. In Proceedings of the 17th seminar for veterinary technicians, The Western Veterinary Conference, Las Vegas, 1988.

Paddleford RR: Analgesia and pain management. In Manual of small animal anesthesia, Philadelphia, 1999, WB Saunders Co.

Robertson SA: Systemic uptake of buprenorphine after buccal administration in cats. In Proceedings of the annual meeting of the College of Veterinary Anesthesiologists, New Orleans, 2001.

REVIEW QUESTIONS

1. Pain sensation arises in free nerve endings called _____.
2. List some signs associated with pain in animals. _____
3. NSAIDs that selectively inhibit _____ are thought to produce fewer gastrointestinal side effects.
4. What is the most common side effect of the NSAIDs? _____
5. Why are cats so susceptible to aspirin overdose? _____
6. True or False: Phenylbutazone should be administered parenterally by the SQ route only. _____
7. What C-II opioid is administered in a transdermal patch? _____
8. True or False: Corticosteroid therapy involves the treatment of the signs of disease and often times cures the disease as well. _____
9. What function do mineralocorticoids serve in the body? _____
10. List some principles that should be followed concerning corticosteroid therapy. _____
11. What does the term iatrogenic mean? _____
12. Describe the side effects of short-term and long-term corticosteroid use. _____
13. What is the mechanism of action of the local anesthetic agents? _____
14. What are some indications for the use of local anesthetics? _____

INTRODUCTION
ANATOMY, PHYSIOLOGY, AND CHEMISTRY
    Distribution of Body Water and Electrolytes
    Composition of Body and Therapeutic Fluids
    Osmotic Pressure and Tonicity of Fluids
PRINCIPLES OF FLUID THERAPY
    Indications for Fluid Therapy
    Fluid Balance
    History, Physical Examination, and Laboratory Findings
    Determining the Amount of Fluid to Administer
    Routes of Fluid Administration
    Rate of Administration
    Monitoring Fluid Administration
    Preparing Fluid Administration Equipment
TYPES OF SOLUTIONS USED IN FLUID THERAPY
Crystalloid Solutions
    Physiologic Saline
    Lactated Ringer's Solution
    Dextrose 5% in Water
    Ringer's Solution
    2.5% Dextrose in Half-Strength (0.45%) Saline/Potassium Added
    Multisol-R/Normosol-R
    Normosol-M in 5% Dextrose
    Plasma-Lyte/Plasma-Lyte M in 5% Dextrose
Colloid Solutions
Hypertonic Solutions
Fluid Additives
    Sodium Bicarbonate
    Potassium Chloride
    Calcium Supplements
    50% Dextrose
    Vitamin Supplements
ORAL ELECTROLYTE PREPARATIONS
PARENTERAL NUTRITION
PARENTERAL VITAMIN/MINERAL PRODUCTS
Water-Soluble Vitamins
    Vitamin B Complex
    Thiamine Hydrochloride (Vitamin B_1)
    Vitamin B_{12} (Cyanocobalamin)
Fat-Soluble Vitamins
    Vitamin A
    Vitamin D
    Vitamin E
    Vitamin K

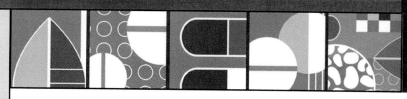

CHAPTER **15**

Therapeutic Nutritional, Fluid, and Electrolyte Replacements

LEARNING OBJECTIVES

After studying this chapter, you should be able to:

1. Define terms related to fluid, electrolyte, and selected therapeutic nutritional preparations
2. Describe the distribution of water in the body
3. Describe the composition of body and therapeutic fluids
4. Define osmotic pressure and tonicity as they apply to fluids
5. Discuss the basic principles of fluid therapy
6. Describe fluid equipment and its use
7. Categorize and provide examples of the fluids used in fluid therapy
8. List and describe selected fluid additives
9. List and describe selected oral electrolyte preparations
10. List and describe selected parenteral vitamin/mineral products

KEY TERMS

BUFFER A substance that decreases the change in pH when an acid or base is added.

COLLOID A chemical system composed of a continuous medium throughout which small particles are distributed and do not settle out under the influence of gravity.

DISSOCIATION The act of separating into ionic components (NaCl → Na and Cl).

ELECTROLYTE A substance that dissociates into ions when placed in solution, becoming capable of conducting electricity.

EMPIRICAL Based on observation and personal experience.

HYPERKALEMIA An excess of potassium in the blood.

HYPERNATREMIA An excess of sodium in the blood.

HYPOKALEMIA A deficiency of potassium in the blood.

HYPONATREMIA A deficiency of sodium in the blood.

HYPOVOLEMIA Decreased volume of circulating blood.

METABOLIC ACIDOSIS Decreased body pH caused by excess hydrogen ions in the extracellular fluid.

METABOLIC ALKALOSIS Increased body pH caused by excess bicarbonate in the extracellular fluid (ECF).

ONCOTIC PRESSURE The osmotic pressure generated by plasma proteins in the blood.

SOLUTE A substance dissolved in a solvent to form a solution.

TOTAL NUTRIENT ADMIXTURE A solution used for parenteral administration containing amino acids, lipids, dextrose, vitamins, and minerals.

TRANSCELLULAR FLUID Cerebrospinal fluid, aqueous humor of the eye, synovial fluid, gastrointestinal fluid, lymph, bile, and glandular and respiratory secretions.

TURGOR Degree of fullness or congestion; describes the degree of elasticity of the skin.

INTRODUCTION

Veterinary technicians often have an important role in fluid, electrolyte, and therapeutic nutritional therapy. They administer parenteral or oral fluid or nutritional products and monitor patients' responses under the direction of a veterinarian. Because the use of the products can be critically important to the outcome of a case, technicians should have a thorough knowledge of these products and their use.

ANATOMY, PHYSIOLOGY, AND CHEMISTRY

Distribution of Body Water and Electrolytes

Measurements of total body water (TBW) have shown that water represents 50% to 70% of the total body weight in adult animals; 60% is often used as the average figure. As much as 80% of a neonatal animal's body weight may be water, a factor that makes fluid loss in young animals potentially very serious. An increase in body fat decreases the amount of TBW, and makes it important to estimate fluid needs based on lean body mass to avoid overhydration.

TBW is distributed in several compartments within the body (Figure 15-1). Sixty percent of the TBW is found within cells and is called *intracellular fluid* (ICF). ICF makes up 40% of the total body weight. The other 40% of the TBW is found outside the cells and is called *extracellular fluid* (ECF). The ECF accounts for 20% of the total body weight.

The ECF (discounting the relatively small **transcellular** component) distributes itself between the interstitial fluid (15% of body weight) and the intravascular fluid or plasma (5% of body weight).

Body fluid compartments should be thought of as volumes of fluid and electrolytes in dynamic equilibrium, with fluids and electrolytes moving back and forth across semipermeable cell membranes. Changes in the quantity of fluid or electrolytes in one compartment usually result in changes in the quantities in other compartments.

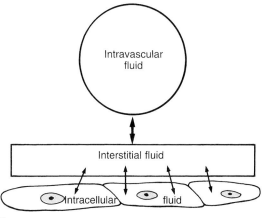

FIGURE 15-1
Body fluid compartments. TBW, total body water.

FIGURE 15-2
Schematic showing movement of fluid between compartments.

Table 15-1 Composition of Plasma and Interstitial Fluid

Ion	Plasma (mEq/L)	Interstitial Fluid (mEq/L)
Cations		
Na$^+$	142	145.1
K$^+$	4.3	4.4
Ca^{2+}	2.5	2.4
Mg^{2+}	1.1	1.1
Total	**149.9**	**153.0**
Anions		
Cl$^-$	104	117.4
HCO$_3^-$	24	27.1
H$_2$PO$_4$	2	2.3
Protein	14	(none)
Other	5.9	6.2
Total	**149.9**	**153.0**

Fluids administered intravenously to an animal first enter the intravascular space of the ECF, move into the interstitial space, and then enter the ICF (Figure 15-2). In most cases, the loss of fluid occurs first from the ECF and then from the other compartments.

Composition of Body and Therapeutic Fluids

Body water contains an array of **solutes** varying in quantity from compartment to compartment. A solute is a substance that dissolves in a solvent; this solvent is usually water in biologic systems. The molecules of substances called **electrolytes** break down (dissociate) into charged particles called *ions*. Electrolytes are either positively charged (cations) or negatively charged (anions). The number of cations always equals the number of anions in normal animals (Table 15-1). In the ECF, the most abundant cation is sodium and the most abundant anions are chloride and bicarbonate. In the ICF, the major cations are potassium and magnesium and the major anions are phosphates and proteins. Therapeutic fluids are described as balanced if they resemble ECF in composition and unbalanced if they do not. Lactated Ringer's solution is an example of a balanced solution, and saline is an example of an unbalanced solution. Table 15-2 lists the composition of solutions used in fluid therapy.

It is important for readers to have a basic understanding of the way in which solute particles, such as electrolytes, are quantified in fluids. One of the oldest ways of measuring solute concentration is by describing the weight of the solute per 100 ml of solution (g%). A 0.9% sodium chloride (NaCl) solution (saline) would contain 0.9 g/100 ml or 900 mg/100 ml. Other clinically significant ways of describing the quantity of solute particles include use of the concepts of (1) the milliequivalent, (2) osmolality, (3) osmolarity, and (4) tonicity.

The milliequivalent is the unit of measurement used to express the concentration of electrolytes, such as sodium, potassium, and calcium, in solutions. The concentration of these substances is usually expressed as milliequivalents per liter (mEq/L) in fluids and milliequivalents per milliliter in supplements. The milliequivalent describes the tendency of a particle to combine with another particle and is defined as 1:1000 of an equivalent. An *equivalent* is defined as the weight in grams of an element that will combine with 1 g of hydrogen ion. For all practical purposes, the equivalent weight of a compound is equal to the gram molecular weight of the substance divided by the total positive valence of the material in question (Blankenship and Campbell, 1976). For example, the equivalent weight of NaCl is 58.5/1 = 58.5, and 1 L of fluid containing 58.5 g of NaCl contains 1 equivalent weight or 1000 mEq of NaCl. The equivalent weight of sulfuric acid (H_2SO_4) is 98.1/2 = 49; therefore, 49 g of H_2SO_4 in 1 L of fluid contains 1 equivalent or 1000 mEq. The following formulas allow determination of milliequivalents of solute in a solution when the concentration in grams or milligrams is known:

$$mEq/L = \frac{\text{milligrams per liter}}{\text{molecular weight}} \times \text{valence}$$

or

$$mEq/L = \frac{\text{milligrams per deciliter} \times 10}{\text{molecular weight}} \times \text{valence}$$

Osmotic Pressure and Tonicity of Fluids

Body fluid compartments are usually separated by a semipermeable (cell) membrane, which permits the passage of water and some solutes. Solutes that can cross the membrane tend to move from an area of higher to an area of lower concentration by the process called *diffusion*. Solutes that cannot cross the cell membrane tend to attract water toward them. This movement of water across a cell membrane is called *osmosis*, and the ability of particles to attract water is called *osmotic pressure*.

Osmolality is a determination of the osmotic pressure of a solution based on the relative number of solute particles in 1 kg of the solution. The greater the number of particles, the greater the pressure generated. The unit of measurement of osmolality is the osmol (osm), and 1 osm of any substance is equal to 1 g molecular weight divided by the number of particles formed by the **dissociation** of that substance. A substance that dissociates into two particles in solutions creates twice as much osmotic pressure as one that does not dissociate. Because the quantities being measured are very small in biologic systems, the milliosmole (mOsm) is used when describing fluids. One kilogram of a solution containing 29.25 g (58.5/2 particles) of NaCl would generate 1 osm/kg or 1000 mOsm/kg of osmotic pressure.

Osmolarity is also a measure of the osmotic pressure of a solution based on the number of solute particles in that solution. However, osmolarity refers to the number of particles per liter of solvent rather than per kilogram of solvent, as with osmolality. There is very little difference, however, between osmolality and osmolarity of animal fluids, and the terms are frequently used interchangeably. A 1 L solution containing a full gram molecular weight (58.5 g) of NaCl would generate 2 osm or 2000 mOsm/L of osmotic pressure.

Not all solutes contribute to osmotic activity (exert a "pull" on water molecules). Those particles

Table 15-2 Composition of Solutions Used in Fluid Therapy

	Glucose* (g/L)	Na⁺ (mEq/L)	Cl⁻ (mEq/L)	K⁺ (mEq/L)	Ca²⁺ (mEq/L)	Mg²⁺ (mEq/L)	Buffer† (mEq/L)	Osmolarity (mOsm/L)	kcal/L	pH
DEXTROSE ELECTROLYTE SOLUTION COMPOSITION										
5% dextrose	50	0	0	0	0	0	0	252	170	4.0
10% dextrose	100	0	0	0	0	0	0	505	340	4.0
2.5% dextrose in 0.45% NaCl	25	77	77	0	0	0	0	280	85	4.5
5% dextrose in 0.45% NaCl	50	77	77	0	0	0	0	406	170	4.0
5% dextrose and 0.9% NaCl	50	154	154	0	0	0	0	560	170	4.0
0.45% NaCl	0	77	77	0	0	0	0	154	0	5.0
0.85% NaCl (normal saline)	0	145	145	0	0	0	0	290	0	5.0
0.9% NaCl	0	154	154	0	0	0	0	308	0	5.0
3% NaCl	0	513	513	0	0	0	0	1026	0	5.0
Ringer's solution	0	147.5	156	4	4.5	0	0	3.10	0	5.5
Lactated Ringer's solution	0	130	109	4	3	0	23(L)	272	9	6.5
2.5% dextrose in lactated Ringer's solution	25	130	109	4	3	0	28(L)	398	94	5.0
5% dextrose in lactated Ringer's solution	50	130	109	4	3	0	28(L)	524	179	5.0

Continued on next page

Table 15-2 Composition of Solutions Used in Fluid Therapy—cont'd

	Glucose* (g/L)	Na$^+$ (mEq/L)	Cl$^-$ (mEq/L)	K$^+$ (mEq/L)	Ca^{2+} (mEq/L)	Mg^{2+} (mEq/L)	Buffer† (mEq/L)	Osmolarity (mOsm/L)	kcal/L	pH
2.5% dextrose in half-strength lactated Ringer's solution	25	65.5	55	2	1.5	0	14(L)	263	89	5.0
Normosol-M in 5% dextrose‡	50	40	40	13	0	3	16(A)	364	175	5.5
Normosol-R‡	0	140	98	5	0	3	27(A) 23(G)	296	18	6.4
Plasma-Lyte§	0	140	103	10	5	3	47(A) 8(L)	312	17	5.5
Plasma-Lyte M in 5% dextrose‡	50	40	40	16	5	3	12(A) 12(L)	376	178	5.5
Plasma	1	145	105	5	5	3	24(B)	300	—	7.4
ADDITIVES AND SOLUTIONS										
20% mannitol	200(M)	0	0	0	0	0	0	1099	—	
7.5% NaHCO$_3$	0	893(B)	0	0	0	0	893(B)	1786	0	
8.4% NaHCO$_3$	0	1000(B)	0	0	0	0	1000(B)	2000	0	
10% CaCl$_2$	0	0	2720	0	1360	0	0	4080	0	
14.9% KCl	0	0	2000	2000	0	0	0	4000	0	
50% dextrose	500	0	0	0	0	0	0	2780	1700	4.2

*All glucose, with one exception: M, mannitol.
†Buffers used: A, acetate; B, bicarbonate; G, gluconate; L, lactate.
‡CEVA Laboratories.
§Baxter Healthcare.
From Chew DJ, DiBartola SP: Saunders manual of small animal nephrology and urology, Philadelphia, 1986, WB Saunders Co.

that are capable of generating pressure are called *effective osmoles*, and those that are not are called *ineffective osmoles*. Sodium and glucose provide most of the effective osmoles in commercial fluid preparations (Chew, 2000). The total effective osmolarity/osmolality of a solution is called *tonicity*. The osmolarity of dog and cat serum is approximately 300 mOsm/L. Commercial fluids with an osmolarity of 300 mOsm/L are isotonic (e.g., Ringer's solution). Those with an osmolarity greater than 300 mOsm/L are hypertonic (e.g., 10% dextrose); and those with an osmolarity less than 300 mOsm/L are hypotonic (e.g., 0.45% saline). Tonicity can be an important consideration when choosing a fluid or its route of administration, because a hypotonic solution can shift fluid out of the intravascular space and a hypertonic solution can shift fluid into the intravascular space (Figure 15-3).

PRINCIPLES OF FLUID THERAPY

Fluid therapy is a critical but somewhat inexact component of veterinary medical care. It is critical because it is often lifesaving, but it is inexact because its application revolves around estimating the amount of fluid loss and, consequently, the amount of fluid that must be replaced. Fortunately, if the heart and kidneys and the processes that sense and control fluid balance are functioning normally, many errors of estimation are compensated for automatically.

Indications for Fluid Therapy

A basic factor in the decision to administer fluids is the animal's hydration status. The hydration status is determined by evaluating the patient's history,

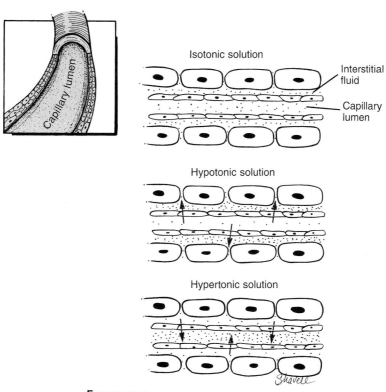

Isotonic solution

Interstitial fluid

Capillary lumen

Hypotonic solution

Hypertonic solution

FIGURE 15-3
Schematic showing the osmotic effects of fluids.

physical examination status, and the results of basic laboratory tests. If it is determined that the animal has lost more water than it has taken in, it is said to be in a state of *dehydration,* and fluids must be administered to compensate. In addition, fluids are often administered to maintain normal hydration status in animals that are losing excessive fluid quantities in order to replace electrolytes and nutrients and to maintain an open intravenous line for administering medications.

Fluid Balance

In normal animals, the intake of fluid and electrolytes is adjusted to offset losses that occur. The sources of water intake include (1) water that is drunk, (2) water ingested in food, and (3) water that results from the metabolism of food (metabolic water). Normal routes of water loss include (1) urine, (2) fecal water, (3) sweat (horses), and (4) respiration. Respiratory loss can potentially be important in dogs because of panting, and sweating can be important in horses. Fluid losses are frequently characterized as sensible, or those that can be easily measured (e.g., urine), and insensible, or those that cannot be easily measured (e.g., fecal and respiratory losses).

Decreased fluid intake often accompanies anorexia, and increased fluid loss occurs in disease states that cause polyuria, vomiting, and diarrhea. Third-space shifts of body water may occasionally cause quantities to be taken out of circulation as they are trapped in body cavities or lost through skin lesions (e.g., intestinal obstruction, body cavity effusions, or hemorrhage). Extensive burns, uncommon in veterinary medicine, can also cause extensive fluid loss.

History, Physical Examination, and Laboratory Findings

A patient's history provides important information about the route and extent of water intake and loss. Knowing the route of loss can aid a clinician in determining the type of fluid to use to correct dehydration and electrolyte imbalances. Table 15-3 lists various causes of dehydration and the fluid indicated for treating the condition. For example, acute vomiting leads to loss of potassium and chloride ions, whereas acute diarrhea causes primarily a potassium loss.

The physical examination provides important information about the extent of fluid loss. The skin **turgor** test, along with other physical findings, is used to determine the percentage of body weight that has been lost via fluid (Table 15-4). This skin turgor test is performed by pinching up a fold of skin over the thoracic or lumbar area and then determining how long it takes to return to a normal position. If the neck area is used in small animals, the extra skin may cause misleading results. The point of the shoulder should be used in horses, because the skin of the neck area can again be misleading. The longer the skin takes to return to normal, the greater the degree of dehydration. Animals with little body fat may appear to be more dehydrated than they really are (slow return to normal skin position) because of low body fat levels, whereas obese animals may appear to be well hydrated when they are not because the increased fat increases skin elasticity. The presence of dry mucous membranes; an increased heart rate; weak, thready pulses; reduced jugular distention (especially in horses); and a reduced capillary refill time all may be indicators of dehydration. Because most of the evaluations mentioned earlier are subjective, simple laboratory tests may be performed to aid in assessing hydration status.

Simple laboratory tests that can aid in evaluating hydration status are the packed cell volume (PCV), total plasma protein (TPP) determination, and urine specific gravity. Dehydration generally results in an increase in the PCV, TPP, and urine specific gravity. Because anemia can make a dehydrated patient appear to be normally hydrated, the PCV should always be evaluated with the TPP. Readers should consult more advanced references for interpretation of laboratory findings related to hydration status.

Determining the Amount of Fluid to Administer

The three values that are calculated to determine the volume of fluid to administer are (1) the hydration deficit, (2) the maintenance requirement, and (3) the contemporary (ongoing) losses.

Table 15-3 Fluid and Electrolyte Disorders and Fluids Used in Their Correction

Abnormality	Type of Dehydration	Electrolyte Balance	Acid-Base Status	Fluid Therapy
Simple dehydration, stress, exercise	Hypertonic			Half-strength or balanced electrolyte solution; 5% dextrose solution
Heatstroke	Hypertonic	K+ variable Na+ variable	Metabolic acidosis	Half-strength electrolyte solution followed by balanced electrolyte solution
Anorexia	Isotonic	K+ loss	Mild metabolic acidosis	Balanced electrolyte solutions; KCl
Starvation	Isotonic	K+ loss	Mild metabolic acidosis	Half-strength or balanced electrolyte solutions; KCl; calories
Vomiting	Isotonic or hypertonic	Na+, K+, and Cl− loss	Metabolic alkalosis; metabolic acidosis chronically	Ringer's solution; 0.9% saline with KCl supplementation
Diarrhea	Isotonic or hypertonic	Na+ loss K+ loss chronically	Metabolic acidosis	Balanced electrolyte solution; HCO₃−; KCl (if chronic)
Diabetes mellitus	Hypertonic	K+ loss	Metabolic acidosis	Balanced electrolyte solution; KCl
Hyperadreno-corticism	Isotonic	K+ loss	Occasionally mild metabolic alkalosis	Balanced electrolyte solutions; KCl
Hypoadreno-corticism	Isotonic or hypertonic	Na+ loss K+ retention	Metabolic acidosis	0.9% saline followed by balanced electrolyte solutions
Urethral obstruction	Isotonic or hypertonic	K+ retention Na+, Cl− variable	Metabolic acidosis	0.9% saline followed by balanced electrolyte solution; KCl post-obstruction
Acute renal failure	Isotonic or hypertonic (with vomiting)	K+ retention Na+, Cl− variable	Metabolic acidosis	Balanced electrolyte solutions
Chronic renal failure	Isotonic or hypertonic (with vomiting)	Na−, K+, Cl− variable	Metabolic acidosis	Balanced electrolyte solutions
Congestive heart failure	Plethoric (Na+, H₂O retention early); hypotonic chronically	Na+ retention (but dilutional hyponatremia)	Metabolic acidosis (chronically)	5% dextrose solution
Hemorrhagic shock	Isotonic		Metabolic acidosis	Balanced electrolyte solutions; blood
Endotoxic shock	Isotonic		Metabolic acidosis	Balanced electrolyte solutions; 0.9% saline

From Muir WW, DiBartola SP: Fluid therapy. In Kirk RW, ed.: Current veterinary therapy VIII: small animal practice, Philadelphia, 1983, WB Saunders Co.

Table 15-4 Clinical Signs of Dehydration

Clinical Signs	Percent Dehydration
Not detectable	<5
Slight loss of skin elasticity	5-6
Noticeable delay in return of skin to normal position. Slight increase in capillary refill time. Dry mucous membranes.	6-8
Skin remains "tented." Continued increase in capillary refill time. Eyes sunken in orbits. Tachycardia and weak pulses.	10-12
Prominent signs of shock and/or death.	12-15

The hydration deficit is the amount of fluid that must be replaced to bring the animal back to a normal hydration status and is calculated by multiplying the percentage of dehydration by the patient's normal body weight. The percentage of dehydration is estimated from the history, physical examination, and laboratory findings. The saying "a pint is a pound the world around" can then be applied, because a pint is roughly equivalent to 500 ml. For example, if a 22 lb beagle is determined to be 5% dehydrated, the hydration deficit is calculated as follows:

$$22\,lb \times 0.05\,(5\%) = 1.1\,lb\ of\ fluid\ loss$$
$$1.1\,lb \times 500\,ml/lb$$
$$= 550\,ml\ replacement\ fluid\ needed$$

If an animal's weight is measured in kilograms, the calculations are made in a similar manner except that the weight of fluid loss (in kilograms) is multiplied times 1000 because 1 kg is roughly equivalent to 1 L (1000 ml). Using the same 22 lb (10 kg) beagle, the calculations are as follows:

$$10\,kg \times 0.05\,(5\%) = 0.5\,kg\ of\ fluid\ loss$$
$$0.5\,kg \times 1000\,ml/kg$$
$$= 500\,ml\ of\ replacement\ fluid$$

The second value needed to calculate the volume of fluids to administer is the maintenance value. Daily maintenance volumes are related to daily energy requirement and can be read from Figure 15-4. Many veterinarians calculate main-tenance values by using thumb rules (20 to 30 ml/lb/day) established by Chew (2000), Muir and DiBartola (1983), DiBartola (2000), and others. Readers should consult these references if more precise calculations are required. Using the thumb rule, our 20 lb beagle would need:

$$22\,lb \times 25\,ml/lb/day$$
$$= 500\,ml/day\ for\ maintenance$$

The final calculation to be made is that for ongoing losses. If we estimate that our beagle is losing 100 ml of fluid per day through vomiting, then we would need to add an additional 100 ml of fluid to our total calculated volume.

The total volume that our beagle would need to be given in 24 hours is:

$$
\begin{aligned}
&550\,ml\ to\ correct\ the\ hydration\ deficit\\
+\ &550\,ml\ for\ normal\ maintenance\\
+\ &100\,ml\ for\ ongoing\ vomiting\ losses\\
\hline
&1200\,ml\ total
\end{aligned}
$$

Routes of Fluid Administration

The route by which fluids are administered depends on several factors, such as the nature of the condition being treated, its duration, and its severity. The routes that may be used are (1) intravenous, (2) subcutaneous, (3) oral, (4) intraperitoneal, and (5) intraosseous.

The intravenous route is preferred when the loss has been great or the disorder is severe. The intravenous route allows quicker, more precise delivery

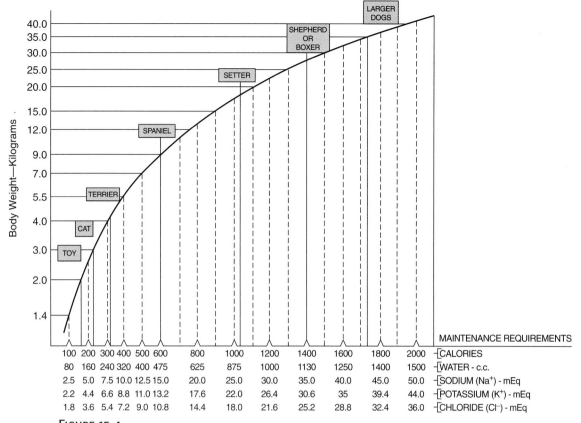

FIGURE 15-4

Daily fluid requirements. (From Harrison JB: Fluid and electrolyte therapy in small animals, JAVMA 137:637-645, 1960.)

of fluids than the other routes. This route does require placement of an intravenous catheter and closer monitoring because of potential complications, such as obstruction or kinking of the catheter, septicemia, embolism, and phlebitis. Catheters should be flushed with heparinized saline (5 U/ml of 0.9% saline) every 6 to 12 hours and should be removed and replaced every 72 hours to minimize complications.

The subcutaneous route is useful when a patient's needs are not severe. The amount of fluid that can be administered subcutaneously depends on the size of the animal and the amount of loose skin that it has. Between 50 and 200 ml can generally be infused at a subcutaneous site. Great care should be taken not to administer enough fluid to

dissect the skin loose from its blood supply, because this can cause sloughing of the skin over the site. Hypertonic or irritating fluids should not be given by the subcutaneous route.

The oral route is a practical means of administering fluids as long as an animal has no severe disorders of the gastrointestinal system. This route allows normal physiologic processes to control the amount of fluid, and the amount and type of electrolytes absorbed. This route is not satisfactory when large volumes of fluid need to be given rapidly.

The intraperitoneal route allows for administration of large volumes of fluid, but the absorption is slow. Peritonitis is a potential complication, and this route is not commonly used.

The intraosseous (femur, ilium, or humerus) route is sometimes used in very small animals or in those with poor access to veins. This route allows rapid delivery of fluids and blood but does require more technical expertise for placing the delivery needle. Careful attention should be paid to sterile technique when this route is used to avoid causing osteomyelitis.

Rate of Administration

Once the volume of fluid needed and the route of administration have been decided, the time frame must be established for delivering the fluids. Rapid losses of fluid usually call for rapid replacement. In veterinary practice, fluid flow rates are often determined **empirically.** However, some generalizations are helpful.

For treating shock, fluids should be administered rapidly (40 ml/lb/hour in dogs and 20 to 30 ml/lb/hour in cats). The use of a pressure administration cuff may allow more rapid infusion in these cases (Figure 15-5).

Fluids should ideally be infused continuously during a 24-hour period. One method of determining fluid flow rate is to calculate the hydration deficit, add maintenance and ongoing losses, and set the drip rate to administer the total during a 24-hour period. Some clinicians prefer to administer the hydration deficit during the first few hours and then give the remainder over a longer period. Some divide the total calculated volume into three equal

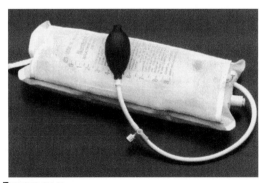

FIGURE 15-5
Pressure administration cuff. (Infusable Pressure Infuser is a registered trademark of Biomedical Dynamics. Sold by Sanofi Animal Health, Inc., Overland Park, Kan.)

parts and administer each in an 8-hour period. In many practices, fluid administration can be monitored for a part of the day only. In this case, the total 24-hour fluid volume can be administered during the period that the patient can be monitored. (Common sense and medical judgment, however, must be exercised.) Portions of the total volume may be administered subcutaneously when appropriate.

Fluids are administered from plastic bags or bottles or from glass bottles through intravenous administration sets (Figures 15-6 and 15-7). Two sizes of administration sets that are commonly used in veterinary medicine are the standard macrodrip set (15 drops/ml) and the minidrip/microdrip set (60 drops/ml). Other sizes (10 drops/ml and 20 drops/ml) are also available. The microdrip sets are suited for use in administering fluids to cats and small dogs. The size of the administration set must be known to calculate the drip or flow rate.

To calculate the drip rate, first divide the total number of milliliters to be administered by the total number of minutes for administration to determine the number of milliliters per minute to deliver. Then multiply the milliliters per minute by the drops per milliliter of the administration set you have chosen to use to arrive at the number of drops (gtt) per minute (gtt/min). For example, if we wish to give our beagle 1200 ml of fluid during a 24-hour period using a standard (15 gtt/ml) administration set:

$$\frac{\text{Volume of infusion (ml)}}{\text{Time of infusion (min)}} \times \text{drop factor (gtt/ml)}$$
$$= \text{gtt/min}$$
$$\frac{1200\,\text{ml}}{24\,\text{hours} \times 60\,\text{min/hour}} = \frac{1200\,\text{ml}}{1440\,\text{min}}$$
$$= 0.83\,\text{ml/min} \times 15\,\text{gtt/ml} = 12.5\,\text{gtt/min}$$

A rate of 12.5 gtt/min can be thought of as 1 drop approximately every 5 seconds $\left(\frac{60}{12} = 5\right)$.

When standard gravity flow bags or bottles are used, drip rates are controlled by devices that are placed on the administration sets to adjust the diameter of the line (e.g., roller clamps, slide clamps, or screw clamps) (Figure 15-8). The flow

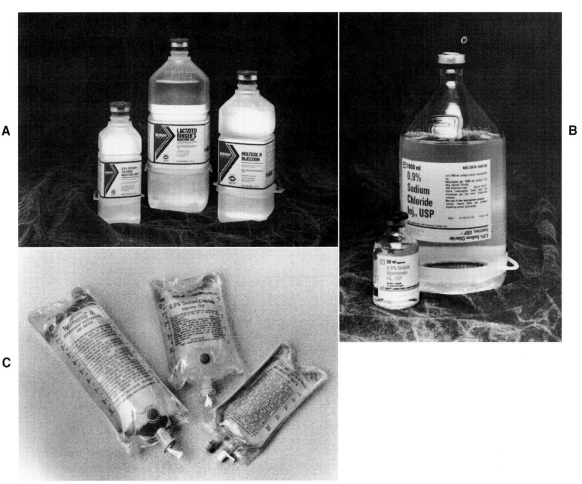

FIGURE 15-6

Types of fluid containers. **A,** RigiCare rigid plastic bottles. **B,** Glass bottles. **C,** LIFECARE flexible plastic bags. (Photo courtesy Sanofi Animal Health, Inc., Overland Park, Kan; RigiCare is a registered trademark of Sanofi Animal Health, Inc., Overland Park, Kan; LIFECARE is a registered trademark of Abbott Laboratories.)

rate is simply dialed in on the machine when fluid infusion pumps (ml/hour) or controllers (ml/min) are used.

Monitoring Fluid Administration

Fluids administered too rapidly or in too great a volume can be life threatening. Careful monitoring of the physical status of the animal is essential. Lung sounds, skin turgor, and the overall status of the animal should be monitored regularly along with the PCV and TPP. When a large volume of fluids is administered rapidly, it is prudent to insert

a urinary catheter to monitor urine output and establish that the kidneys are functioning normally. Some clinicians also choose to insert a jugular catheter to monitor central venous pressure as a way of preventing fluid volume overload.

Signs of overhydration may include restlessness, serous nasal discharge, increased lung sounds (crackles), tachycardia, dyspnea, pitting subcutaneous edema, and an increased "Jello-like" feel to the subcutaneous tissue (Haskins, 2000). Fluid infusion should be slowed or stopped and the veterinarian contacted at the first appearance of these signs.

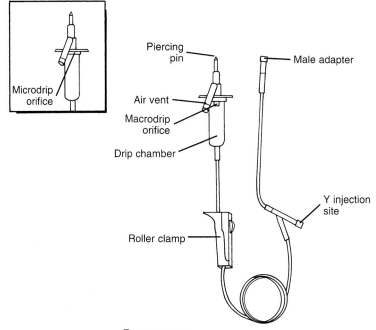

FIGURE 15-7
Intravenous administration set.

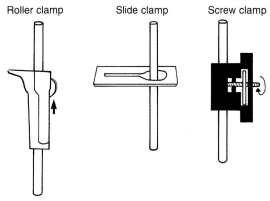

FIGURE 15-8
Clamps for controlling fluid flow.

Labeled adhesive tape should be placed vertically on fluid bottles or bags to allow monitoring of the volume delivered (Figure 15-9). Bottles or bags should also be labeled with all pertinent information, including the presence of any additives. It may be helpful to place a horizontal piece of tape across the fluid container to indicate when fluid delivery is to be stopped.

A volume control system or Buretrol device may be used for administering small volumes of fluid (Figure 15-10). A clamp allows the volume control chamber to be filled with a predetermined amount of fluid from the bag or bottle. The line is then clamped off to prevent entry of additional fluid from the bag. The chamber can be refilled if desired.

Preparing Fluid Administration Equipment

When preparing to administer intravenous fluids, you should follow a standard protocol. After gathering your supplies and preparing the injection site, check to see that you have the correct fluid type and that it is not out of date. Then determine that the container is not cracked or chipped and that the solution is clear. Fluids should never contain precipitates or appear cloudy. After inspecting the container's cap to make sure that it is intact, remove the metal cap (bottle) or insertion port

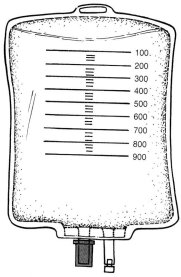

FIGURE 15-9
Labeling (vertical) of fluid bag.

cover (bag), being careful not to contaminate the port. Close the flow clamp on the administration set and remove the cover from the administration set spike. Wipe the port with an alcohol swab and insert the administration set spike into the rubber stopper (bottle) or insertion port (bag). Hang the bottle or bag, and fill the administration set line by opening the flow clamp and allowing fluid to run through the line until all bubbles are cleared. Close the flow clamp and attach the adapter to the intravenous catheter using sterile technique. After the flow clamp is opened to determine that the catheter and the line are patent, the drip rate may be adjusted as required.

If at any time the flow rate slows or stops, check the following: (1) the catheter for correct placement and patency, (2) the position of the patient to determine whether limb position or flexion has occluded the flow, (3) the flow clamp to see whether it is in the open position, (4) the tubing to determine whether it is kinked or crimped, and (5) the fluid level in the bottle.

Two fluid solutions may be administered simultaneously by using a piggyback setup of the containers (Figure 15-11). The secondary bag is hung

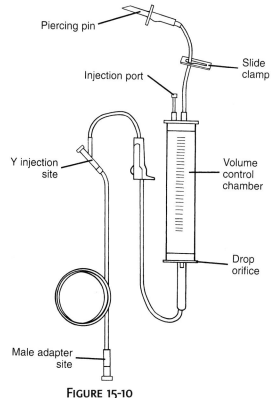

FIGURE 15-10
Volume control administration set.

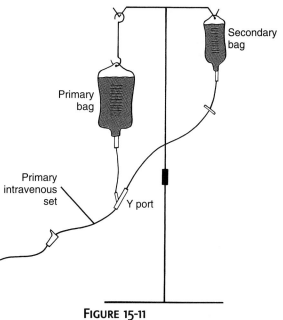

FIGURE 15-11
Piggyback setup of fluids.

higher than the primary bag, and the secondary administration set line is connected to the Y port of the primary administration set.

It is useful for a technician to understand the use of a three-way valve. The three-way valve permits three-way connections to be made. Flow of fluid through the valve depends on the position at which the control handle is placed. The handle points toward the line that is closed. Figure 15-12 illustrates the operation of a three-way valve.

TYPES OF SOLUTIONS USED IN FLUID THERAPY

Crystalloid Solutions

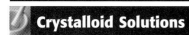

Crystalloids are solutions containing electrolyte and nonelectrolyte substances that are capable of passing through cell membranes and can therefore enter all body fluid compartments. Administration of crystalloid solutions therefore results in rapid equilibration of fluid between the intravascular and the interstitial spaces. Crystalloid solutions are routinely used in veterinary medicine because of their versatility and relatively low cost. Crystalloid solutions can further be classified as replacement or maintenance solutions. Replacement solutions resemble ECF in content, whereas maintenance solutions contain less sodium and more potassium than replacement fluids.

Clinical Uses. Fluids are administered for correction of dehydration, treatment of shock, maintenance of normal hydration, replacement of electrolytes and nutrients, and as a vehicle for administration of intravenous drugs.

Dosage Forms. Dosage forms are numerous. Fluids are available in glass bottles, plastic bottles, and plastic bags that hold 250, 500, and 1000 ml. Containers that hold 3000 and 6000 ml are available for some solutions (see manufacturer product guides). The following section briefly describes the commonly used crystalloid solutions. See Table 15-3 for a listing of the composition and other characteristics of each.

Adverse Side Effects. Adverse side effects of fluid administration are primarily associated with overhydration. Signs of overhydration may include restlessness, shivering, serous nasal discharge, coughing, and pulmonary edema.

Physiologic Saline
Physiologic saline is a 0.9% solution of NaCl and is also called normal saline. It may also be called *isotonic saline*, because it has an osmolarity of 308 mOsm/L. Saline is used to increase plasma volume or to correct a sodium deficiency (**hyponatremia**). It may also be used to bathe tissues during surgery to prevent them from drying out. Because of its high sodium content, saline should not be used in animals with known heart disease.

Lactated Ringer's Solution
Lactated Ringer's solution is one of the most versatile and commonly used fluids in veterinary medicine. It is a balanced electrolyte replacement solution and can be administered by any route that is available. It contains 28 mEq/L of lactate, which is converted by the liver to bicarbonate to act as a **buffer** against acidosis. Theoretically, lactated Ringer's solution should not be administered with blood, because the calcium contents could cause clotting to occur.

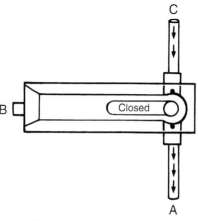

FIGURE 15-12
Operation of a three-way valve.

Dextrose 5% in Water

Dextrose 5% in water (D5W) is a nonbalanced solution that contains only dextrose (50g/L) and water. Administering dextrose 5% is equivalent to administering pure water because the dextrose is metabolized to carbon dioxide and water. Dextrose 5% provides approximately 170kcal/L (a quantity that cannot be relied on to meet the daily caloric needs of most small animals), although it may supplement other caloric sources. Dextrose 5% should not generally be given by the subcutaneous route because it may osmotically "draw" fluid from the vascular space. Dextrose in water should not be used as a maintenance solution because it may dilute out all electrolytes.

Ringer's Solution

Ringer's solution is a balanced replacement solution that contains more sodium, calcium, and chloride than lactated Ringer's solution. It contains no lactate, however, and can be used in cases of **metabolic alkalosis.**

2.5% Dextrose in Half-Strength (0.45%) Saline/Potassium Added

Half-strength (0.45%) saline in 2.5% dextrose with 5mEq/L of potassium chloride is a maintenance solution that is appropriate for use in patients that have sodium restrictions.

Multisol-R/Normosol-R

Multisol-R is the veterinary trademark for Normosol-R. Both are balanced, multiple electrolyte solutions with a dual buffering system (acetate and gluconate). Acetate and gluconate are metabolized outside the liver, a factor that may have advantages in conditions such as liver disorders. Both Multisol-R and Normosol-R are calcium free and thus may help to prevent potential incompatibilities with transfused blood or added sodium bicarbonate.

Normosol-M in 5% Dextrose

Normosol-M in 5% dextrose is a balanced maintenance solution that has acetate as a buffer and contains 175kcal/L.

Plasma-Lyte/Plasma-Lyte M in 5% Dextrose

Plasma-Lyte is a balanced replacement solution with 47mEq/L of acetate and 8mEq/L of lactate as buffers. Plasma-Lyte M in 5% dextrose is a maintenance solution with equal amounts of acetate and lactate (12mEq/L) as buffers and 178kcal/L.

Technician's Notes

1. Fluids containing preservatives such as benzyl alcohol should never be given to cats because of the likelihood of toxic reactions.
2. Some clinicians warn against administering fluids with preservatives to puppies and adult dogs.

 Colloid Solutions

Colloid solutions contain large-molecular-weight particles, which are unable to cross cell membranes and are therefore confined to the vascular space. These confined particles are effective osmoles, and are able to hold fluid in the vascular space and to draw fluid from the interstitial space into the vascular space (expand the plasma volume). They are especially useful when cerebral or pulmonary edema is a potential complication of fluid administration or when crystalloid therapy has not been successful.

Colloids include albumin, plasma, and the synthetic colloids (dextrans and hydroxyethyl starch). Only the commercially available synthetic products are discussed here.

Clinical Uses. Colloid solutions are used for expansion of the plasma volume in the treatment of **hypovolemic** or septic shock.

Dosage Forms

1. The dextrans. Dextran 70 is a large-molecular-weight polysaccharide solution used in the treatment of shock. Dextran 70 (Gentran 70) is supplied as a 6% solution in 0.9% saline and is the most commonly used form of the dextrans in

veterinary medicine. The dextrans may cause allergic reactions or clotting deficits in some animals.

2. Hetastarch (Hespan). Hydroxyethyl starch (hetastarch) is a large-molecular-weight starch that is used in the treatment of hypovolemia and hypoproteinemia. Hetastarch expands the plasma volume longer and has fewer side effects than the dextrans. It is prepared as a 6% solution in 0.9% saline. The primary disadvantage of hetastarch is its expense.

3. Oxypolygelatin (Vetaplasma). Gelatins are modified animal collagens. These molecules are denser than the dextrans and therefore produce greater osmotic action. Coagulopathy is a potential side effect.

Adverse Side Effects. Adverse side effects of colloid administration are usually related to clotting deficiencies or allergic reactions.

> ### Technician's Notes
> 1. Colloids are not intended for maintenance or long-term use.
> 2. References should be checked for determining the appropriate flow rate for colloid solutions.

Hypertonic Solutions

This discussion is confined to the use of hypertonic saline solutions. These solutions have been advocated by some clinicians in the treatment of hemorrhagic and endotoxic shock, and for patients undergoing major surgical procedures (e.g., gastric dilation or volvulus). Like the colloids, the hypertonic saline solutions also may be useful when brain or pulmonary edema is present or is a potential complication.

Clinical Uses. Hypertonic saline solutions are used for the treatment of shock associated with trauma, endotoxemia, burns, pancreatitis, and major surgical procedures.

Dosage Forms. Hypertonic saline solutions are available from commercial sources in 3%, 4%, 5%, 7%, and 23.4% preparations.

Adverse Side Effects. These may include phlebitis, tissue irritation, rehemorrhage in traumatic shock, electrolyte imbalances, and—when the administration rate is too fast—hypotension, bronchoconstriction, and bradycardia.

> ### Technician's Notes
> 1. The rate of administration of the hypertonic saline solutions is a very important consideration because exceeding this rate may cause serious side effects.
> 2. These solutions should be infused through a well-secured intravenous catheter to prevent extravasation of the irritating fluids.

Fluid Additives

In some instances, special substances may be added to intravenous fluid solutions to enhance the solutions' therapeutic effects. These substances may be added to correct acid-base abnormalities and electrolyte imbalances, to supplement calories, and to provide supplemental vitamins to replace those washed out by fluid therapy.

Sodium Bicarbonate

Sodium bicarbonate (baking soda) is an alkalizing agent that may be added to correct **metabolic acidosis** and certain other conditions. Because lactate or acetate in fluid preparations often cannot correct severe metabolic acidosis, supplementation becomes necessary. Normal serum bicarbonate is 24 mEq/L. Required amounts for supplementation are calculated by measuring a patient's bicarbonate (or carbon dioxide) level and subtracting that value from 24 (normal). The difference is called the *bicarbonate deficit*. The bicarbonate deficit is multiplied by 0.6 and then by the animal's weight in kilograms to determine the number of milliequivalents of sodium bicarbonate to administer.

Bicarbonate supplementation (mEq) = bicarbonate deficit $\times$ 0.6 $\times$ weight (kg)

When access to laboratory measurement of bicarbonate or carbon dioxide is not available, **empirical** estimations of supplementation levels are made based on clinical judgment.

Bicarbonate concentration in commercial products is measured in milliequivalents per milliliter.

Clinical Uses. These include the treatment of metabolic acidosis and as an adjunctive therapy for the treatment of hypercalcemia or **hyperkalemia.**

Dosage Forms. Veterinary-approved forms include the following:

1. An 8% (1 mEq/ml) solution for injection, which is available in 50-, 100-, and 500-ml vials
2. A 5% (0.6 mEq/ml) solution for injection

Adverse Side Effects. These may include metabolic alkalosis, hypokalemia, hypocalcemia, and **hypernatremia.**

Technician's Notes

1. Sodium bicarbonate is incompatible with several solutions and should be mixed only after consulting product inserts or appropriate references.
2. Some references indicate that sodium bicarbonate should not be added to solutions containing calcium because of potential for precipitates to form.
3. Replacement of the total number of milliequivalents should be made over several hours.

Potassium Chloride

Potassium chloride is a solution used to supplement potassium deficits **(hypokalemia).** Anorexia, diuresis, and diarrhea are some of the common causes of hypokalemia. Normal serum potassium levels are between 3.5 and 5.5 mEq/L. Table 15-5 provides a guide for potassium supplementation based on the measured serum level of potassium.

Clinical Uses. Potassium chloride is used for the treatment or prevention of potassium deficits.

Dosage Forms. Dosage forms for intravenous use include the following:

1. Potassium chloride for injection (2 mEq/ml) in 10- and 20-ml vials (veterinary approved)
2. Potassium chloride for injection (2 mEq/ml) in 5-, 10-, 20-, 30-, 100-, 200-, and 500-ml vials (human approved)

Adverse Side Effects. These may include hyperkalemia, which is manifested by muscle weakness, and cardiac conduction disturbances, which can be life threatening.

Technician's Notes

1. Potassium chloride solutions must be diluted before administration.
2. The rate of infusion of potassium is critical. Consult product inserts or other references for appropriate rates.

Table 15-5 Potassium Supplementation Guide*

Serum K$^+$ (mEq/L)	mEq K$^+$ (To Add to 250 ml Fluid)	mEq K$^+$ (To Add to 1 L Fluid)	Maximum Infusion Rate of Intravenous Fluids (0.5 mEq/kg/hour)
<2.0	20	80	6
2.1-2.5	15	60	8
2.6-3.0	10	40	12
3.1-3.5	7	28	18
>3.5, <5.0	5	20	25

*For dogs or cats with hypokalemia or for those with potassium depletion and normal serum potassium levels. This regimen is designed to be infused in maintenance volume of fluids.

Calcium Supplements

Calcium gluconate and calcium chloride may be diluted (1:1 with saline) and given as an infusion to correct hypocalcemia. This is not a common procedure in practice, however. It is more common to inject the supplement, without diluting, for the treatment of emergency conditions, such as eclampsia or milk fever.

Clinical Uses. Calcium supplements are used for the treatment of hypocalcemia that may result from various conditions, which may include parathyroid gland disorders, milk fever, eclampsia, and excessive sweating in horses. Calcium in combination with phosphorus, magnesium, potassium, and dextrose is used to treat conditions in cattle, such as grass tetany, milk fever, and downer cow syndrome.

Dosage Forms

1. Calcium gluconate injection (generic and proprietary) 10%, in ampules, syringes, vials, and bottles (veterinary label)
2. Calcium gluconate (various proprietary names), 23%, in 100- and 500-ml bottles (veterinary label)
3. Calcium chloride injection (generic and proprietary), 10%, in ampules, vials, and syringes (human label)
4. Numerous combination products (CalDextro, Norcalciphos) containing calcium, phosphorus, magnesium, potassium, and dextrose

Adverse Side Effects. Adverse side effects that result from hypercalcemia may include hypotension, cardiac arrhythmias, and cardiac arrest. These effects are usually a result of too rapid an infusion of the calcium.

Technician's Notes

1. Any product containing calcium should be given by slow intravenous administration to prevent cardiac complications.
2. Products containing 23% calcium are labeled for large-animal use.

50% Dextrose

When caloric supplementation is indicated, 50% dextrose is often used as a stock solution to add to other fluids to provide a desired percent solution of dextrose. It is not usually possible to meet the total caloric needs of a small-animal patient through dextrose supplementation of intravenous fluids. Supplementation is often indicated, however, in patients that are hypoglycemic because of fever, sepsis, insulin overdose, insulinoma, liver disease, and others. Varying amounts of dextrose may be added in an attempt to keep the blood glucose level near the normal range (80 to 100 mg/dl).

Intravenous administration of 50% dextrose is used in ruminants as a treatment of uncomplicated ketosis.

To prepare a 2.5% solution of dextrose, add 50 ml (25 g) of 50% dextrose to 1 L of fluids. Fifty milliliters of the original fluid solution should be removed before adding the 50% dextrose to keep the dilution correct. To prepare a 5% solution, add 100 ml of 50% dextrose to 1 L of fluids. A formula that may be used to determine the quantity of a stock solution to use in preparing percent solutions follows:

$$\frac{\text{Desired strength}}{\text{Available strength}} = \frac{\text{How much you are going to use}}{\text{How much you are going to make}}$$

or

$$V_1 \times C_1 = V_2 \times C_2$$

For example, if you wish to make 250 ml of a 5% solution of dextrose using your stock supply of 50% dextrose, you would set up your formula in the following way:

$$\frac{5\%}{50\%} = \frac{X}{250}$$

Cross multiplying 50X = 1250

$$X = 25\,ml$$

Therefore, to prepare the 250 ml of 5% solution, draw up 25 ml of 50% dextrose and add 225 ml of a diluting fluid.

Clinical Uses. These include caloric supplementation in small-animal patients and treatment of ketosis in ruminants.

Dosage Forms. Various manufacturers supply 50% dextrose. The most common package is a 500-ml plastic bottle.

Adverse Side Effects. These are few if used according to directions.

Technician's Notes
A 50% solution of dextrose contains 500 mg/ml.

Vitamin Supplements

Patients that have been given large amounts of fluids undergo a diuresis, which may cause a corresponding loss of the water-soluble vitamins (B complex and C), making fluid supplementation desirable. Animals with polyuria resulting from renal failure also lose water-soluble vitamins and benefit from supplementation of their parenteral fluids. Recommendations for supplementation vary from 0.5 to 2 ml/L of fluids.

Clinical Uses. Vitamin supplements are used for restoration of normal levels of the water-soluble vitamins.

Dosage Forms. Several manufacturers produce vitamin B complex. Care should be taken to ensure that the form selected may be given intravenously. Many are labeled for intramuscular or subcutaneous use only.

Adverse Side Effects. These include hypersensitivity reactions to the thiamine in the complex.

ORAL ELECTROLYTE PREPARATIONS

In severely dehydrated animals, fluids must be given by the intravenous route to be effective. In mild to moderate cases of dehydration, however, the oral route is a practical alternative to replenish water and electrolytes.

Oral electrolytes are packaged as powders that are mixed with water to form a solution that can be given free choice or by stomach tube. In some instances, oral pastes or fluids packaged for intravenous use may be given orally. The oral route of administration is especially useful for cases in which the veterinarian wishes to direct the pet or livestock owner in the home or farm treatment of the animal.

Diarrhea in young dairy calves, commonly called *calf scours,* is caused by bacteria, viruses, or nutritional factors and is a condition often treated with oral electrolyte solutions. The diarrhea is commonly a result of the type or amount of milk replacer that the calf is being fed. A calf is treated by eliminating the milk replacer from its diet and by giving it an oral electrolyte solution with glucose or glycine for 24 to 48 hours. Glucose and glycine provide a source of calories and may enhance absorption of the electrolytes. The solution may be administered via an esophageal feeder—a device that has a plastic bag (for mixing the electrolyte solution) attached to a rigid delivery tube (Figure 15-13). The tube has a ball of sufficient diameter on the distal end to prevent introduction of the tube into the trachea.

Oral electrolyte solutions or pastes are often given to performance horses to replace the electrolytes lost through sweating. Horses participating in endurance races, 3-day events, and other athletically demanding events benefit from electrolyte replenishment.

Administration of oral electrolyte solutions may also be helpful as a follow-up to intravenous fluid therapy for dogs recovering from viral enteritis or other diseases causing prolonged vomiting or diarrhea. Hypokalemia in dogs and cats may be treated with oral potassium products.

Clinical Uses. These include electrolyte and water replenishment.

Dosage Forms. Dosage forms are numerous, and the following is only a partial listing:

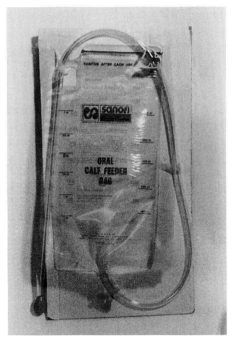

FIGURE 15-13
Esophageal feeder.

1. Avian Bluelite (powder)
2. Biolyte (powder)
3. Elpak-G Electrolyte Gel
4. Equine Bluelite (powder)
5. Entrolyte (powder)
6. Formula 911 (powder)
7. Ora-Lyte (powder)
8. Re-Sorb (powder)
9. Tumil-K (powder, gel, and tablets for dogs and cats)
10. Vedalyte 8X (powder)
11. Ritrol

Adverse Side Effects. These are rare if care is taken not to cause inadvertent administration into the respiratory system.

Technician's Notes
Some of the oral electrolyte products for farm animals also contain antibiotics.

PARENTERAL NUTRITION

The term parenteral indicates the administration of nutrients by a route other than the gastrointestinal tract. Parenteral nutrition (PN) is described in human medicine as total or partial in reference to whether all nutrient requirements are supplied. Diseased and debilitated patients require a daily intake of adequate calories and protein to maintain good immune function, tissue synthesis, and normal metabolic activities. Those patients that are unable or have no desire to eat normally may need parenteral nutrition.

The term total parenteral nutrition (TPN) does not apply to veterinary patients since there is not a need to meet the needs for all essential fatty and amino acids, fat and water soluble vitamins, and macro and trace minerals as there is in people (Remillard, Armstrong, and Davenport, 2000). In veterinary medicine an attempt is made to meet the animal patient's resting energy requirement and most of the requirements for amino and fatty acids, and to provide some of the required vitamins and minerals.

PN solutions must be compounded for the individual patient. A mixture of all the required nutrients, called a **total nutrient admixture** (TNA), can be prepared for the veterinary patient in one fluid bag for convenience. The preparation of these solutions is beyond the scope of most veterinary clinics but may be available through human hospitals, veterinary schools, or specialty practices. For a list of products used in the formulation of the TNA, consult an article entitled "Parenteral Nutrition Products" by Miller and Bartges in Kirk's *Current Veterinary Therapy, XIII*.

PARENTERAL VITAMIN/MINERAL PRODUCTS

Parenteral vitamin/mineral products are used to prevent or treat various conditions in veterinary medicine. They are used as therapeutic agents in large-animal medicine more than in small-animal medicine. White muscle disease, "tying up," polyneuritis, pink eye, reproductive problems, bracken fern poisoning, and polioencephalomalacia are only a few of the conditions prevented or treated with vitamin products in large-animal practice. In small-animal practice, routine vitamin and mineral supplementation is not considered necessary if the animal receives a balanced diet. Many small-animal clinicians consider overuse of vitamin/mineral products a bigger problem than vitamin/mineral deficiencies. Warfarin poisoning (vitamin K) and certain dermatologic conditions (zinc) are exceptions.

Oral multiple vitamin/mineral products are numerous and are not listed here.

Water-Soluble Vitamins

Vitamin B Complex

B complex vitamins are a group of water-soluble vitamins that include thiamine, riboflavin, niacinamide (niacin), d-panthenol (pantothenic acid), pyridoxine, cyanocobalamin (B_{12}), biotin, choline, and folic acid. B vitamins serve as co-enzymes for many metabolic reactions in the body. B complex is often added to intravenous fluids (discussed earlier) and may be given parenterally in an attempt to enhance the biochemical response of stressed or debilitated animals.

Clinical Uses. These vitamins are administered to replace or supplement a deficiency of B complex vitamins.

Dosage Forms
1. Compound 150
2. Vitamin B Complex
3. Vitamin B Complex Fortified
4. Vitamin B Complex Injectable

Adverse Side Effects. These can include allergic reactions and pain at the injection site.

Technician's Notes
1. Check the label before giving B complex intravenously.
2. Observe the animal for allergic reactions.
3. B complex injections may cause pain at the injection site.

Thiamine Hydrochloride (Vitamin B₁)

Thiamine is a water-soluble B complex vitamin that acts as a co-enzyme for biochemical reactions involved in carbohydrate metabolism. Deficiency of thiamine may occur as a consequence of decreased intake or synthesis, or from increased destruction, which may result from bracken fern poisoning, thiamine-destroying factors in the rumen, or thiaminase in raw fish. Polioencephalomalacia of ruminants has also been associated with thiamine deficiency.

Clinical Uses. Thiamine is administered for the treatment of thiamine deficiency in all domestic species and as an aid in the treatment of lead poisoning in cattle.

Dosage Forms
1. Vita-Jec Thiamine HCl
2. Thiamine hydrochloride (generic)
3. Vitamin B₁ Powder

Adverse Side Effects. These may include hypersensitivity reactions and muscle soreness at intramuscular injection sites.

Vitamin B₁₂ (Cyanocobalamin)

Vitamin B_{12} is a B complex vitamin that contains cobalt and is thought to act as a co-enzyme in protein synthesis. Pernicious anemia is a condition that occurs in humans as a result of a failure to absorb B_{12} adequately. A deficiency in any case results in anemia because red blood cells fail to mature properly in the absence of B_{12}. B_{12} deficiencies are rare in veterinary medicine.

Clinical Uses. Vitamin B_{12} is administered for the management of B_{12} deficiencies.

Dosage Forms
1. Vita-Jec Vitamin B_{12}
2. Vitamin B_{12} injection

Adverse Side Effects. These may include allergic reactions to administration.

Fat-Soluble Vitamins

Vitamin A

Vitamin A is an organic alcohol that is converted from plant substances called *carotenoids* (e.g., beta carotene) in the intestine and liver and stored primarily in the liver. It is needed for proper growth and maintenance of surface epithelium, for proper bone growth, and for maintenance of visual pigments in the retina. A deficiency of vitamin A may be associated with many clinical signs, including poor growth and reproductive performance, susceptibility to infectious disease, and poor vision in dim light. Many of the commercial vitamin A products are combined with vitamin D or E.

Clinical Uses. Vitamin A is administered for the prevention or treatment of vitamin A deficiencies.

Dosage Forms
1. Vitamin A-D Injectable
2. Vitamin AD Injection
3. Vita-Ject A-D 500
4. Vitamin AD

Adverse Side Effects. These are uncommon if label directions are followed.

Vitamin D

Vitamin D exists in two forms—D_2 and D_3. Vitamin D_2 is formed when a plant substance (ergosterol) is exposed to sunlight, and D_3 is formed when a provitamin precalciferol in the skin is converted by sunlight. A deficiency of vitamin D is characterized by the development of rickets in young animals or osteomalacia in adults. Vitamin D is often combined commercially with vitamin A or E.

Clinical Uses. Vitamin D is administered for the treatment or prevention of vitamin D deficiencies.

Dosage Forms. Refer to the dosage forms for vitamin A.

Adverse Side Effects. These are uncommon if label directions are followed.

Vitamin E

Vitamin E (alpha-tocopherol) is involved (with selenium) in the metabolism of sulfur and acts as an antioxidant. Vitamin E is used in the prevention or treatment of selenium/vitamin E deficiency syndromes, such as white muscle disease (ewes, lambs, and calves), mulberry heart disease (sows and pigs), and myositis (horses).

Clinical Uses. Vitamin E is administered for the prevention and treatment of vitamin E deficiencies.

Dosage Forms
1. Bo-Se (selenium, vitamin E injection [approved for use in calves, swine, and sheep])
2. E-SE (selenium, vitamin E injection [approved for use in horses])
3. Mu-Se (selenium, vitamin E injection [approved for use in nonlactating dairy cattle and beef cattle])
4. L-Se (selenium, vitamin E injection [approved for use in lambs and baby pigs])
5. Seletoc (selenium, vitamin E injection [approved for use in dogs])

Adverse Side Effects. These include allergic reactions and soreness at injection sites.

Vitamin K

Vitamin K is a fat-soluble vitamin required for the formation of prothrombin and for this reason is very important to the clotting process. Vitamin K is discussed in Chapter 16.

REFERENCES

Blankenship J, Campbell JB: Solutions. In Blankenship J, Campbell JB, editors: Laboratory mathematics: medical and biological applications, St. Louis, 1976, Mosby.

Chew DJ: Fluid therapy for dogs and cats. In Birchard S, Sherding R, editors: Saunders manual of small animal practice, ed 2, Philadelphia, 2000, WB Saunders Co.

DiBartola SP: Introduction to fluid therapy. In DiBartola SP, editor: Fluid therapy in small animal practice, ed 2, Philadelphia, 2000, WB Saunders Co.

Haskins SC: Fluid overload: how to identify and manage. Proceedings of the International Veterinary Emergency and Critical Care symposium, Orlando, Fla, 2000.

Muir WW, DiBartola SP: Fluid therapy. In Kirk RW, editor: Current veterinary therapy VIII: small animal practice, Philadelphia, 1983, WB Saunders Co.

Remillard RL, Armstrong PJ, and Davenport DJ: Assisted feeding in hospitalized patients: enteral and parenteral nutrition. In Hand et al, editors: Small animal clinical nutrition, Marceline, Mo, 2000, Walsworth Publishing Co.

REVIEW QUESTIONS

1. Define hyperkalemia.
   _____

2. Intravascular fluid makes up approximately
   _____ body weight.
   a.   2%
   b.   5%
   c.   15%
   d.   40%

3. Explain the concept of a balanced solution for
   fluid therapy. _____

4. What are three units of measurement for
   quantifying electrolytes in fluids?
   _____

5. Therapeutic fluids with an osmolarity of
   approximately _____
   mOsm/L are isotonic.
   a. 100
   b. 200
   c. 300
   d. 500

6. Give examples of sensible and insensible fluid
   losses. _____

7. Underestimation of the degree of dehydration
   is sometimes a problem in
   _____ animals.

8. One pound of fluid is equivalent to
   _____ milliliters, and 1 kg
   is equivalent to _____
   milliliters.

9. The three volumes that are calculated to
   arrive at the total fluid volume are
   _____.

10. Calculate the fluid needed for a 44 lb dog that
    is 6% dehydrated and losing 100 ml of fluid
    daily through vomiting.
    _____

11. What drip rate should be used to deliver (over
    a 24-hour period) the fluid for the dog in
    question 10 (using a standard administration
    set)? _____

12. Describe how you would set up the first bag of
    fluids for the dog in question 10.
    _____

13. Tell how you would prepare 500 ml of 5%
    dextrose from a 50% stock solution.
    _____

14. What is the purpose of the lactate in lactated
    Ringer's solution? _____

15. Describe the use of an esophageal feeder.
    _____

16. What type of fluid (tonicity) should not be
    given subcutaneously?
    _____

17. Give an example of a balanced solution and
    an example of an unbalanced solution.
    _____

18. _____ is a determination
    of the osmotic pressure of a solution based on
    the relative number of solute particles in 1 kg
    of the solution.

19. The osmolarity of dog and cat serum is
    approximately _____
    mOsm/L.

20. Commercial fluids with an osmolarity of
    300 mOsm/L are _____.

21. How often should intravenous catheters be
    flushed? _____

22. What is the longest time an IV catheter
    should remain in place before it is replaced?
    _____

23. What precaution should be observed when
    administering fluids subcutaneously?
    _____

24. What fluid can be used to bathe tissues in
    during surgery to prevent them from drying
    out? _____

25. Any product containing the electrolyte
    _____ should be given by
    slow IV administration to prevent cardiac
    complications.

INTRODUCTION
BLOOD-MODIFYING
DRUGS/AGENTS
Hematinics
  Iron Compounds
  Erythropoietin
  Androgens
  Blood Substitutes
Anticoagulants
  Heparin
  Ethylenediamine Tetraacetic Acid
    (EDTA)
  Coumarin Derivatives
  Acid Citrate Dextrose (ACD) Solution
    and Citrate Phosphate Dextrose Ad-
    enine (CPDA-1)
  Antiplatelet Drugs
Hemostatics/Anticoagulant Antagonists
  Topical Agents
  Parenteral Agents
    PROTAMINE SULFATE
    VITAMIN K₁ (PHYTONADIONE)
Fibrinolytic (Thrombolytic) Drugs
ANTINEOPLASTIC DRUGS
Alkylating Agents
Antimetabolites
Plant Alkaloids (Mitotic Inhibitors)
Antibiotic Antineoplastic Agents
Platinum Drugs
Miscellaneous Antineoplastic Agents
  Asparaginase
  Glucocorticoids
Biologic Response Modifiers
  Monoclonal Antibodies
  Interferon
  Other Biologic Response Modifiers
Immunosuppressive Drugs
  Azathioprine
  Cyclosporine
  Metronidazole
  Cyclophosphamide
  Corticosteroids
  Other Immunosuppressive Agents

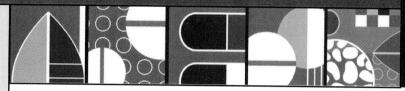

CHAPTER **16**

Blood-Modifying, Antineoplastic, and Immunosuppressant Drugs

LEARNING OBJECTIVES

After studying this chapter, you should be able to:

1. Understand the role of erythropoietin in red blood cell formation
2. Understand the significance of iron in the hemoglobin molecule
3. List an example of iron deficiency anemia that occurs in veterinary medicine
4. Understand the potential indications for and limitations of hematinics and oxygen-carrying solutions
5. Describe the clotting mechanism in general terms
6. List four anticoagulants and their method of action
7. List examples of topical hemostatics
8. Name the antagonist for heparin overdose
9. List the indications for the use of vitamin K₁ and possible adverse side effects of its use
10. Define fibrinolysis and name a fibrinolytic agent
11. Describe the phases of the cell cycle
12. List six categories of antineoplastic drugs and give an example of each
13. Define biologic response modifier (BRM) and list two examples of BRMs
14. List indications for the use of immunosuppressive drugs and provide five examples
15. Discuss the safety precautions involved in the use of antineoplastic drugs

315

KEY TERMS

ALKYLATION Formation of a linkage between a substance and DNA that causes irreversible inhibition of the DNA molecule. Alkylating drugs are used in chemotherapy treatment of cancer.

CELL CYCLE NONSPECIFIC Capable of acting in several or all cell cycle phases.

CELL CYCLE SPECIFIC Capable of acting during a particular cell phase only.

CYTOTOXIC Capable of destroying cells.

DISSEMINATED INTRAVASCULAR COAGULATION (DIC) Widespread formation of clots (thrombi) in the microscopic blood vessels of the circulatory system. DIC occurs as a complication of a wide variety of disorders and consumes clotting factors, with resultant bleeding.

ENDOTHELIAL LAYER The smooth layer of epithelial cells that line blood vessels.

ERYTHROPOIETIN A substance produced in the kidneys that stimulates the bone marrow to make red blood cells.

FIBRINOLYSIS Fibrin (clot) breakdown through the action of the enzyme plasmin.

HYBRIDOMA A cell culture consisting of a clone of a hybrid cell formed by fusing cells of different kinds, such as stimulated mouse plasma cells and myeloma cells.

METASTASIS Generally refers to the transfer of cancer cells from one site to another.

MYELOMA A malignant neoplasm of plasma cells (B-lymphocytes).

MYELOSUPPRESSION Inhibiting bone marrow activity, resulting in a decreased production of blood cells and platelets.

THROMBOCYTOPENIA A decreased number of platelets.

THROMBOEMBOLISM The condition that occurs when thrombus material becomes dislodged and transported by the bloodstream to another site.

THROMBUS A clot in the circulatory system.

VESICANT A substance that causes blister formation.

INTRODUCTION

The first section of this chapter deals with drugs or agents that influence blood formation or its processes (e.g., clotting and **fibrinolysis**). Hematinics, anticoagulants, anticoagulant antagonists/hemostatics, and fibrinolytic agents are discussed. Because the anticoagulants are used routinely in veterinary practice, veterinary technicians should have a complete working knowledge of their applications and their potential misuse.

The second section covers antineoplastic and immunosuppressant drugs. Antineoplastic drug categories include alkylating agents, antimetabolites, mitotic inhibitors (vinca alkaloids), antibiotics, hormones, and miscellaneous agents. Safe handling techniques for these potentially dangerous agents are listed. Selected immunosuppressant drugs and their clinical applications are discussed at the conclusion of this section.

Separate anatomy/physiology descriptions are used for each section listed earlier to provide continuity of the information.

BLOOD-MODIFYING DRUGS/AGENTS

Hematinics

Red blood cells are formed in the bone marrow in response to stimulation by **erythropoietin**, a chemical released by the kidneys when hypoxia is present in this organ (Ganong, 2003) (Figure 16-1). Their primary function is to carry oxygen to the tissues. This activity is greatly enhanced by the hemoglobin component of the red blood cells. Only a small portion of oxygen is carried in solution in the plasma.

Hemoglobin is made up of a protein and an iron-containing pigment (Figure 16-2). The iron in hemoglobin must be in the ferrous (Fe^{2+}) state to combine with oxygen in the most efficient way. If the iron in the hemoglobin is in the ferric (Fe^{3+}) state, hemoglobin cannot combine with oxygen and is called *methemoglobin*. Adequate amounts of iron, cobalt, copper, B vitamins, trace minerals, and protein are needed for normal hemoglobin and red blood cell formation.

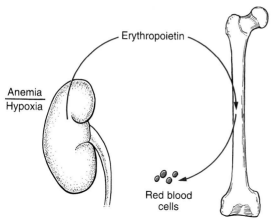

FIGURE 16-1
Erythropoietin stimulates the bone marrow to produce red blood cells.

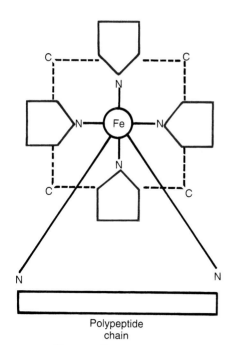

FIGURE 16-2
The structure of hemoglobin.

Anemia can result from excessive loss of red blood cells, formation of inadequate numbers of red blood cells, or inadequate amounts of hemoglobin in the red blood cells. Iron deficiency anemia, a relatively common form in humans, is rare in animals that consume balanced diets. One exception, however, is baby pig anemia, a condition that results because of inadequate assimilation of iron from the placenta of the sow for future hemoglobin formation by the piglet. The piglet is born without adequate stores of iron for its rapid growth phase, and sow's milk is relatively low in this element. Baby pig anemia is a problem of pigs raised in confined environments (concrete or slatted floors), because those raised outdoors usually obtain adequate iron from the soil.

Hematinics are substances that tend to promote an increase in the oxygen-carrying capacity of the blood. Hematinics are used to prevent or treat anemia, and the primary ingredient in most of these products is iron, a vital component of hemoglobin. Some also contain copper and B vitamins to enhance red blood cell formation. The response to hematinic administration is relatively slow, and this factor makes use of hematinics ancillary to whole blood transfusion in acute anemia.

Iron Compounds
Many injectable and oral iron preparations are available for veterinary use under generic and proprietary labels. The form of iron in these products may be iron dextran, ferrous sulfate, peptonized iron, gleptoferron, ferric hydroxide, and others, and the form apparently has little effect on use. Copper, B vitamins, liver fraction (an iron source), and palatability enhancers are often added to the oral products as well. The injectable forms are labeled for intramuscular injection and contain only iron. They may cause discoloration of muscle tissue at the site of injection.

Clinical Uses. Iron compounds are used for prevention or treatment of baby pig anemia or as a nutritional aid, depending on the form.

Dosage Forms
1. Injectable Iron 10%
2. Injectable Iron Dextran
3. Ferrodex 100
4. Iron Dextran Complex
5. Lixotinic
6. Pet Tinic

7. Gleptosil
8. Iron Hydrogenated Dextran Injection

Adverse Side Effects. These are rare but may include muscle weakness, prostration, or muscle discoloration.

> ## Technician's Notes
> Pork quality assurance programs often recommend that iron injections be given in neck muscle rather than in the ham (a higher-quality cut) because of potential meat staining and subsequent condemnation.

Erythropoietin

Erythropoietin, a protein produced in the kidneys, stimulates the division and differentiation of committed erythroid precursors in the bone marrow. A synthetic product, Epogen, has the same properties of erythropoietin and is available commercially. It is approved for human use and is produced by recombinant DNA technology. It is labeled for the treatment of anemia related to chronic renal failure or for that associated with azidothymidine treatment in patients with human immunodeficiency virus infection. No veterinary approved product is available.

Clinical Uses. Erythropoietin is used in dogs and cats for the treatment of anemia associated with chronic renal failure or other causes.

Dosage Forms
1. Epogen (Amagen)
2. Procrit (Ortho Biotech)
3. Epoetin Alfa for Injection

Adverse Side Effects. In humans, adverse side effects may include hypertension, iron deficiency, polycythemia, and seizures. The use of human-coded proteins in dogs or cats could potentially cause allergic reactions.

Androgens

The treatment for anemia associated with chronic renal failure has traditionally been androgen therapy. The results of the use of androgens for chronic anemia have been inconsistent.

Clinical Uses. Androgens are used for the treatment of chronic (nonregenerative) anemia.

Dosage Forms
1. Winstrol-V
2. Equipoise
3. Deca-Durabolin (human approved)

Adverse Side Effects. These have included enlargement of the prostate, hepatic toxicity, and sodium and water retention.

Blood Substitutes

Researchers have looked for an oxygen-carrying substitute for red blood cells practically since it was learned that the hemoglobin in those cells was the transporting vehicle. Only recently has an acceptable substitute been developed.

The Biopure Corp. has prepared a polymerized bovine product with a hemoglobin concentration of 13 g/dl in a modified lactated Ringer's solution. This solution has obvious benefits over blood products, which include availability, a long shelf life, universal compatibility, and freedom from disease-producing agents.

This hemoglobin solution picks up and distributes oxygen in a similar manner to red blood cells, but the oxygen-carrying function is shifted to the plasma. Since the oxygen is carried in the plasma, diffusion of this gas across cell membranes occurs more efficiently than when carried by red blood cells because one fewer membrane must be crossed.

This product is stable for 3 years when unwrapped at room temperature or in the refrigerator (but it should not be frozen). Once the wrapper is removed, the product must be used within 24 hours. It is compatible with any other IV fluid, but other solutions should not be mixed in the same bag. A separate line should be used for these other solutions. No consideration needs to be made for blood typing or crossmatching when using this product.

Clinical Uses. This product is labeled for the treatment of anemia in dogs regardless of the cause. It has been used in cats but is not labeled for such use.

Dosage Form

Oxyglobin (hemoglobin glutamer-200)

Adverse Side Effects. Potential side effects include pulmonary edema, discolored urine, discolored membranes, ventricular arrhythmias, fever, and coagulopathy.

Technician's Notes

1. The recommended administration rate should not be exceeded.
2. Do not administer with other fluids or drugs through the same intravenous set.
3. Do not combine with other fluids in the same bag.

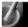 **Anticoagulants**

Blood coagulation is an obviously essential process designed to inhibit the loss of vital blood constituents from the circulatory system. Two separate systems or pathways may initiate the clotting mechanism, the intrinsic (intravascular) and extrinsic (extravascular) systems.

The intrinsic pathway is activated by injury to the **endothelial layer** of a blood vessel, which disrupts blood flow and causes a chain of chemical reactions leading to a **thrombus,** or clot. This process helps to repair damage to blood vessel walls that occurs from routine wear and from pathologic processes.

The extrinsic pathway is activated by injury to tissue and vessels, releasing tissue thromboplastin. Thromboplastin stimulates the clotting mechanism. Vasoconstriction occurs in damaged blood vessels, causing a slowing of blood flow and facilitating clot formation. Platelet aggregation and adherence are also important steps in the clotting process.

The intrinsic and the extrinsic pathways converge into a common pathway in the final steps of clot formation (Figure 16-3). At least 13 clotting factors participate in this series of reactions (called a *cascade*) in which the product of the preceding reaction promotes the next reaction (Table 16-1). The final step in the process is the conversion of fibrinogen to fibrin by thrombin. If any of the clotting factors in the cascade are deficient or missing, clotting does not occur.

A balance must be maintained in the body between clot formation and clot breakdown. Destruction of clots—fibrinolysis—occurs through the action of an enzyme called *plasmin.* Plasmin digests fibrin threads and other clotting products to cause clot lysis and the release of fibrin degradation products into the circulation.

Anticoagulants inhibit clot formation by tying up or inactivating one of the clotting factors to interrupt the cascade reaction. They are used clinically to prevent coagulation of blood (or other body fluid) samples that are collected for testing, to preserve blood for transfusions, to inhibit clotting in intravenous catheters, and to prevent or treat thromboembolic disorders (e.g., thromboembolic cardiomyopathy in cats).

Heparin is used paradoxically to treat the bleeding disorder **disseminated intravascular coagulation (DIC).**

Heparin

Heparin is an anticoagulant that is found in many tissues of the body and is thought to be stored in mast cells. It is obtained from pig intestinal mucosa, and its strength is expressed in terms of heparin units. Heparin acts as an anticoagulant by preventing the conversion of prothrombin (factor II) to thrombin. Without thrombin, fibrinogen is not converted to fibrin and a clot does not form. Heparin does not break down clots but can prevent clots from increasing in size. It is administered therapeutically by intravenous or subcutaneous injection.

Heparin has various uses in veterinary medicine. It is used in vitro as an anticoagulant to preserve blood samples for testing by heparinizing (drawing heparin into the syringe and then forcing all visible quantities out) a syringe before drawing the blood

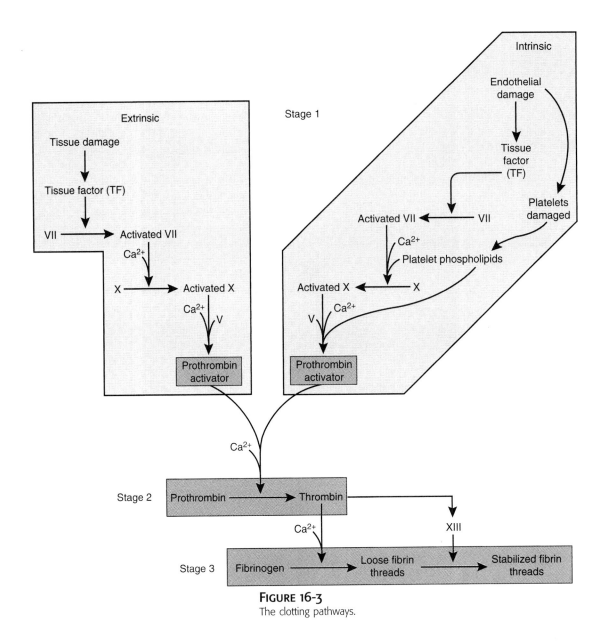

FIGURE 16-3
The clotting pathways.

sample. It is also diluted in saline or sterile water for injection to form a flush solution for preventing clots in intravenous catheters. Heparin is sometimes used to preserve donated blood for transfusions when small quantities are needed (e.g., for cats, small dogs). It is used in vivo to aid in the treatment of DIC and **thromboembolism** and has been advocated for the treatment of laminitis in horses.

Clinical Uses. Clinical uses are listed in the previous paragraph.

Dosage Forms. Forms approved for use in humans are used in veterinary medicine:

1. Heparin sodium injection, 1000 U/ml
2. HepLock flush solution (10 or 100 U/ml)

Adverse Side Effects. These are usually bleeding or **thrombocytopenia**.

Table 16-1 The Clotting Factors

Coagulation Factor	Synonym
I	Fibrinogen
II	Prothrombin
III	Tissue Factor (thromboplastin)
IV	Calcium ions
V	Proaccelerin, labile factor, or accelerator globulin
VI	Activated factor V
VII	Serum prothrombin conversion-accelerator (SPCA), stable factor, or proconvertin
VIII	Antihemophilic factor (AHF), antihemophilic factor A, or antithemophilic globulin factor B
IX	Christmas factor, plasma thromboplastin component (PTC), or antithemophilic factor B
X	Stuart-Prower factor, thrombokinase
XI	Plasma thromboplastin antecedent (PTA) or antihemophilic factor C
XII	Hageman factor, glass factor, or contact factor
XIII	Fibrin-stabilizing factor (FSF) or fibrinase

Technician's Notes

1. Heparin should not be used as an anticoagulant when collecting blood for performing a differential count because white blood cell morphology may be adversely affected.
2. A heparin flush solution may be prepared by diluting heparin in saline at a concentration of 5 U/ml (Crow and Walshaw, 1987).
3. Approximately 750 U of heparin should be drawn into a 60-ml syringe to act as an anticoagulant when collecting blood for transfusion (Norsworthy, 1992).
4. Heparin blood collection tubes have a green top.
5. Protamine sulfate is the antidote for heparin overdose.

Ethylenediamine Tetraacetic Acid (EDTA)

EDTA is an anticoagulant that prevents clotting by chelation of calcium (factor IV). With calcium ions tied up by the EDTA, clotting cannot occur. It is used in vitro to preserve blood samples and is the anticoagulant of choice when a differential count is needed (it preserves white cell morphology well). EDTA is prepared in lavender-topped collection tubes.

The calcium salt of EDTA (calcium disodium versenate) is also used in vivo as a chelating agent to treat lead poisoning. This function does not involve the clotting mechanism (see Chapter 18).

Coumarin Derivatives

Coumarin derivatives such as dicumarol and warfarin are oral anticoagulants that bind vitamin K and therefore inhibit the synthesis of prothrombin (factor II) and factors VII, IX, and X. These compounds are indicated for long-term treatment of thromboembolic conditions. They are used clinically to a greater extent in human medicine than in veterinary medicine.

Dicumarol may be found in moldy sweet clover and has been associated with fatal hemorrhagic disease in cattle. Warfarin and related compounds are used in many rat poisoning products.

Clinical Uses. Coumarin derivatives are used for long-term management of thromboembolic conditions.

Dosage Form
Coumadin tablets or injection

Adverse Side Effects. Adverse side effects are related to hemorrhage.

Technician's Notes
Vitamin K_1 is the antidote for warfarin or dicumarol toxicity.

Acid Citrate Dextrose (ACD) Solution and Citrate Phosphate Dextrose Adenine (CPDA-1)

ACD solution contains dextrose, sodium citrate, and citric acid and prevents clotting by chelating calcium. It is prepared in bottles or plastic bags for blood collection under both veterinary and human labels. Bottles for collecting 250 and 500 ml of blood are available. ACD solution preserves blood for 3 to 4 weeks.

CPDA-1 solution is available in plastic bags for collection of 450 ml of blood. CPDA-1 also prevents clotting by chelating calcium and preserves blood for as long as 6 weeks.

Eight milliliters of ACD or CPDA-1 can be drawn into a syringe to collect 50 ml of blood when small quantities are needed (Norsworthy, 1992).

Antiplatelet Drugs

Antiplatelet drugs, such as aspirin, appear to impair clotting through inhibition of platelet stickiness and clumping. This activity is thought to be mediated through inhibition of the proaggregatory prostaglandin called thromboxane (Pugh, 1991).

Aspirin has been used to prevent thromboembolism associated with heartworm treatment in dogs and to treat cardiomyopathy in cats.

Hemostatics/Anticoagulant Antagonists

Substances that promote blood clotting—hemostatics—may be divided into two categories: (1) those applied topically and (2) those given parenterally.

Topical Agents

Topical agents act by providing a framework in which a clot may form or by coagulating blood protein to initiate clot formation. Framework substances used in topical hemostatics include gelatins and collagens, whereas styptics, hemostatic powders, and solutions are substances that initiate clotting through coagulation. The framework substances are absorbed after clot formation. Topical hemostatics are used to control capillary bleeding or bleeding from other small vessels.

Clinical Uses. These include the control of capillary bleeding in surgical sites or superficial wounds.

Dosage Forms
1. Gelfoam absorbable gelatin sponge
2. Hemopad Absorbable Collagen Hemostat
3. Surgical Absorbable Hemostat
4. Hemostat Powder (ferrous sulfate powder)
5. Clotisol (ferric sulfate)
6. Silver nitrate sticks
7. Thrombogen topical thrombin solution

Adverse Side Effects. These are usually minimal but may include delayed wound healing.

Parenteral Agents

Parenterally administered hemostatic agents act as anticoagulant antagonists because they do not directly activate clotting. These substances either promote the synthesis of clotting factors that have been depleted through poisoning or disease or tie up (inactivate) anticoagulants that have been overdosed. These drugs are not used to control surgical or traumatic bleeding.

PROTAMINE SULFATE

Protamine sulfate is a protein produced from the sperm or testes of salmon or related species (Plumb, 2002). Protamine has a strongly basic pH, and heparin has a strongly acidic pH. Protamine combines with heparin to form inactive complexes (salt).

Clinical Uses. Protamine sulfate is used for the treatment of heparin overdose. Slow intravenous administration is recommended.

Dosage Form
Protamine sulfate injection, USP

Adverse Side Effects. Hypotension and bradycardia can occur if given too rapidly.

VITAMIN K₁ (PHYTONADIONE)

Phytonadione is a synthetic substance that is identical to naturally occurring vitamin K_1. Vitamin K is necessary for the production (in the liver) of active prothrombin (factor II), proconvertin factor (factor VII), plasma thromboplastin component (factor IX), and Stuart factor (factor X). It is used clinically for treating cases in which vitamin K has been tied up or destroyed and in bleeding disorders associated with poor formation of vitamin K-dependent clotting factors. Immediate coagulant effect should not be expected after administration of vitamin K because several hours may pass before synthesis of new clotting factors.

Clinical Uses. In veterinary medicine, vitamin K_1 is used for the treatment of rodenticide toxicity, for bleeding disorders related to faulty synthesis of vitamin K-dependent clotting factors, and for unknown anticoagulant toxicity.

Dosage Forms. Human forms of vitamin K_1 are used:

1. AquaMEPHYTON, phytonadione injection
2. Konakion, phytonadione injection
3. Mephyton, phytonadione tablets

Adverse Side Effects. These include anaphylactoid reactions (intravenous use) and bleeding at the injection site.

Technician's Notes

Because of the possibility of anaphylactoid reactions, many consider intravenous administration of phytonadione to be contraindicated.

 Fibrinolytic (Thrombolytic) Drugs

Thrombolytic drugs are used to break down or dissolve thrombi. Occlusion of an artery by a thromboembolus can cause necrosis of tissue distal to the blockage if the obstruction is not removed quickly. In humans, damage to heart muscle that occurs when a coronary artery is occluded in a heart attack is a classic example of this process. Pulmonary thromboemboli sometimes occur in dogs after

heartworm treatment and may accompany cardiomyopathy in cats.

Thrombolytic agents may help to remove or reduce the size of the occluding thromboembolus and minimize tissue damage. This action is brought about by stimulating conversion of plasminogen to the enzyme plasmin, which lyses the clots. The sooner the therapy is initiated after thromboembolism has occurred, the better the chances of success. Thrombolytic activity of one of the products (alteplase) is activated by the presence of fibrin so that recent clots are targeted.

The expense of these drugs often precludes their use in veterinary medicine.

Clinical Uses
1. Treatment of pulmonary embolism
2. Treatment of arterial thrombosis and emboli
3. Treatment of coronary thrombosis
4. Intravenous catheter clearance

Dosage Forms
1. Streptase, streptokinase
2. Abbokinase, urokinase
3. Activase, alteplase

Adverse Side Effects. These are related to bleeding episodes, especially if anticoagulants have also been used.

ANTINEOPLASTIC DRUGS

Antineoplastic drugs are administered to animal patients to cure or lessen the effects of neoplasms. Anticancer chemotherapy may be used alone or in combination with other treatment methods, such as surgery, radiation, or immune modulation. Chemotherapy can reduce tumor size, relieve pain, destroy microscopic **metastases,** and in some instances prolong periods of remission and survival time (MacEwen and Rosenthal, 2000). The goal of cancer therapy is to kill all of the neoplastic cells, but this is seldom a reality.

Carcinogenesis has been associated with many factors, including (1) aging (improved health care has led to an increasing population of older animals), (2) oncogenes, (3) stress, (4) viruses, (5) chemicals, (6) nutritional factors, and (7) irritation. No matter what the cause, all cancers are characterized by populations of cells with defective growth control: they multiply rapidly, form large growths, and may spread to other sites.

The cytotoxic drugs used in chemotherapy have been developed to interfere with activities such as DNA/RNA synthesis, mitotic spindle formation, or other processes involved with cell division. These effects are not limited to cancer cells. All rapidly dividing cells, such as those of the bone marrow, gastrointestinal tract, reproductive organs, and hair follicles, are affected by antineoplastic drugs.

All cells go through a series of cell cycle phases to replicate themselves (Figure 16-4). These phases are described as G_0, the resting or nonproliferative phase; G_1, presynthesis preparation; S, DNA synthesis; G_2, RNA production; and M, mitosis (Jenkins, 1991). The cytotoxic activity of antineoplastic drugs often targets activity of one or more of these phases to interfere with synthesis of products or with division processes. In general, antineoplastic drugs are divided into two groups: (1) the **cell cycle–nonspecific** drugs, which act at all stages of the cycle except the resting phase (G_0), and (2) the **cell cycle–specific** drugs, which act selectively at a certain phase of the cycle (usually S or M). Cell cycle–specific drugs are most effective against rapidly growing neoplasms. Malignant cells in the resting phase may be difficult to destroy, because they are not very susceptible to chemotherapeutic drugs. This is one reason why prolonged use of antineoplastic drugs may be needed.

Many potential adverse side effects are associated with the use of antineoplastic drugs. These may include anaphylactic reactions, immunosuppression, **myelosuppression**, cardiomyopathy, vomiting, diarrhea, hair loss (poodles and Old English Sheepdogs), cystitis, pain associated with administration, and tissue damage resulting from drug extravasation. Several of the drugs that are administered intravenously (e.g., doxorubicin, vinblastine, and vincristine) are severe **vesicants,** and great care should be taken to avoid extravasation.

Great care also should be taken to prevent accidental exposure to these drugs by technicians, veterinarians, and other employees because of their ability to be teratogenic, mutagenic, and carcinogenic at therapeutic dosages (Dickinson and Ogilvie, 1995). Box 16-1 provides a list of recommendations for safe handling of antineoplastic agents.

Dosage of most antineoplastic agents is based on body surface area as measured in square meters (Barton, 2001). Body surface area can be converted

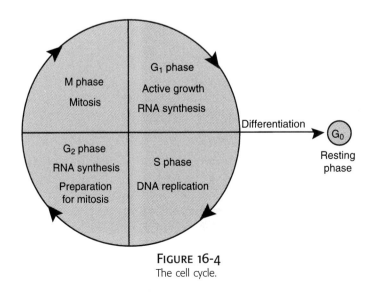

FIGURE 16-4
The cell cycle.

Box 16-1 Recommendations for Safe Handling of Antineoplastic Agents

1. Designate a specific hospital location for drug handling (reconstitution, preparation, disposal, etc.).
2. Use an absorbent, disposable, plastic-backed sheet to cover the work surface; change regularly.
3. Wear latex nonpermeable gloves when handling all cytotoxic agents.
4. Reduce exposed skin surfaces by wearing laboratory coats, gowns, etc. Wear particulate respiratory filtration masks to prevent inhalation of aerosolized drug particles.
5. Reconstitute all materials carefully and safely, avoiding potential contamination of materials or aerosolization.
6. Clean reconstituted material of any contamination and properly mark and date it.
7. Dispose of contaminated materials in leak-proof, puncture-resistant containers. Proper disposal by health regulatory officials is necessary.
8. Wash hands thoroughly after removing gloves.

Table 16-2 Conversion of Body Weight in Kilograms to Body Surface Area in Meters for Dogs

kg	m²	kg	m²
0.5	0.06	26.0	0.88
1.0	0.10	27.0	0.90
2.0	0.15	28.0	0.92
3.0	0.20	29.0	0.94
4.0	0.25	30.0	0.96
5.0	0.29	31.0	0.99
6.0	0.33	32.0	1.01
7.0	0.36	33.0	1.03
8.0	0.40	34.0	1.05
9.0	0.43	35.0	1.07
10.0	0.46	36.0	1.09
11.0	0.49	37.0	1.11
12.0	0.52	38.0	1.13
13.0	0.55	39.0	1.15
14.0	0.58	40.0	1.17
15.0	0.60	41.0	1.19
16.0	0.63	42.0	1.21
17.0	0.66	43.0	1.23
18.0	0.69	44.0	1.25
19.0	0.71	45.0	1.26
20.0	0.74	46.0	1.28
21.0	0.76	47.0	1.30
22.0	0.78	48.0	1.32
23.0	0.81	49.0	1.34
24.0	0.83	50.0	1.36
25.0	0.85		

The conversion table is based on the following formula:

$$\frac{kg^{0.67}}{10} = m^2$$

From Ettinger SJ: Textbook of veterinary internal medicine, Philadelphia, 1975, WB Saunders Co.

from body weight measured in kilograms (Table 16-2). Their narrow therapeutic index and potentially life-threatening side effects make careful dosage calculations a must. The clinician must also carefully take into consideration the dose intensity, schedule of administration, interaction with other drugs, and potential drug resistance. Two or more antineoplastic drugs may be combined and administered according to a carefully designed protocol.

The antineoplastic drugs have been divided into the following major categories: alkylating agents, antimetabolites, plant alkaloids, antibiotics, platinum drugs, and miscellaneous agents. Table 16-3 lists some of the commonly used antineoplastic agents and the indications for their use in veterinary medicine.

its replication. This brings protein synthesis and cell division to a halt; cell death often follows.

Clinical Uses

1. Treatment of various neoplastic disorders, including lymphoproliferative neoplasms, osteosarcoma, hemangiosarcoma, and squamous cell carcinoma

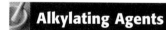

Alkylating Agents

Alkylating agents are cell cycle–nonspecific drugs that are able to cross-link strands of DNA to inhibit

Table 16-3 Common Antineoplastic Drugs and Indications for Their Use

Drugs	Indication	Recommended Dosages	Toxicity
Alkylating Agents			
Cyclophosphamide (Cytoxan; Mead-Johnson)	Lymphoproliferative disorders, mast cell tumors, hemangio-sarcoma, miscellaneous carcinomas	50 mg/m^2/PO every 48 hours 50 mg/m^2 PO every 24 hours for 4 days weekly 100-300 mg/m^2 IV every 3 weeks	BM, GI, hemorrhagic cystitis
Chlorambucil (Leukeran; Burroughs-Wellcome)	Lymphoproliferative disease, macroglo-bulinemia	2-4 mg/m^2 every 24-48 hours	BM
Melphalan (Alkeran; Burroughs-Wellcome)	Multiple myeloma	2-4 mg/m^2 PO every 24-48 hours	BM
Cisplatin (Platinol; Bristol)	Osteosarcoma, transitional cell carcinoma, squamous cell carcinoma	50-70 mg/m^2 IV every 3 weeks (vigorous hydration)	BM, GI, renal; do not use in cats
Carboplatin (Paraplatin; Bristol)	Similar to cisplatin	250-300 mg/m^2 IV every 3 weeks	BM, GI
Antimetabolites			
Methotrexate (Lederle)	Lymphoproliferative disorders	2.5 mg/m^2 PO every 24 hours 15-20 mg/m^2 IV every 3 weeks	BM, GI, renal
5-Fluorouracil (Roche)	GI and hepatic carcinoma	150-200 mg/m^2 IV every 7 days	BM, GI, CNS; do not use in cats
Cytosine arabinoside (Cytosar-U; Upjohn)	Lymphoproliferative disorders, myeloproliferative disorders	100 mg/m^2 IV or SC for 4 days every 3-4 weeks	BM, GI
Plant Alkaloids			
Vincristine (Oncovin; Eli Lilly)	Lymphoproliferative disorders, mast cell tumors, sarcomas, carcinomas	0.5-0.7 mg/m^2 IV every 7 days	GI, peripheral neuropathy; vesicant
Antibiotics			
Doxorubicin (Adriamycin; Adria Labs)	Lymphoproliferative disorders, soft tissue sarcoma, carcinomas	30 mg/m^2 IV every 3 weeks (maximum cumulative dose =180-240 mg/m^2)	BM, GI, cardiac, severe vesicant, urticaria, alopecia
Mitoxantrone (Novantrone; Lederle)	Lymphoproliferative disorders	5-6 mg/m^2 every 3 weeks	BM
Hormones			
Prednisone	Lymphoproliferative disorders, mast cell tumors, brain tumors	20-50 mg/m^2 every 24-48 hours as needed	Iatrogenic Cushing's syndrome, GI
Miscellaneous			
L-Asparaginase (Elspar; Merck, Sharp & Dohme)	Lymphoproliferative disorders	10,000-30,000 IU/m^2 IM, SC, or IP as needed (pretreat with antihistamines, steroids)	Anaphylaxis, pancreatitis, coagulopathy

m^2, body surface area in square meters; *PO*, per os; *IV*, intravenously; *IM*, intramuscularly; *SC*, subcutaneously; *IP*, intraperitoneal; *BM*, bone marrow; *GI*, gastrointestinal; *CNS*, central nervous system.
From Birchard S, Sherding R, editors: Saunders manual of small animal practice, Philadelphia, 1994, WB Saunders Co.

2. Treatment of certain immune-mediated diseases (immunosuppression)

Dosage Forms
1. Cytoxan, cyclophosphamide injection
2. Leukeran, chlorambucil tablets
3. Alkeran, melphalan tablets
4. Nitrosoureas, lomustine and carmustine
5. Dacarbazine

Adverse Side Effects. Adverse side effects of the alkylating agents may include neutropenia, nephrotoxicity, thrombocytopenia, vomiting, and hemorrhagic cystitis.

> *Technician's Notes*
>
> Cyclophosphamide is also used as an immunosuppressant.

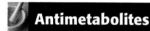

Antimetabolites

The antimetabolites are cell cycle–specific drugs that affect the S phase (DNA synthesis) of the cycle. These drugs are analogs of purines and pyrimidines—naturally occurring bases in DNA—and may be incorporated into the DNA molecule to inhibit protein and enzyme synthesis. Cellular functions needed for normal activity are thus blocked.

Clinical Uses
1. Treatment of lymphoproliferative neoplasms
2. Treatment of gastrointestinal and hepatic neoplasms
3. Treatment of central nervous system lymphoma

Dosage Forms
1. Methotrexate, oral tablet or injection
2. Cytosar-U, cytosine arabinoside injection
3. Fluorouracil injection
4. Hydroxyurea

Adverse Side Effects. These may include anorexia, nausea, vomiting, diarrhea, bone marrow suppression, hepatotoxicity, and neurotoxicity.

> *Technician's Notes*
>
> Fluorouracil is contraindicated in cats because of adverse side effects.

Plant Alkaloids (Mitotic Inhibitors)

The plant alkaloids are cell cycle–specific for the M phase, inhibiting mitosis and causing cell death. They are thought to bind microtubular proteins and inhibit formation of the mitotic spindle, thus suspending mitosis in metaphase.

The two drugs in this category—vincristine and vinblastine—are natural alkaloids derived from the periwinkle plant (*Vinca rosea*, Linn). Protective clothing should be worn when administering these drugs to prevent possible skin contact irritation.

Clinical Uses
1. Treatment of lymphoproliferative neoplasms
2. Treatment of carcinomas
3. Treatment of mast cell tumors
4. Treatment of splenic tumors

Dosage Forms
1. Oncovin, vincristine sulfate injection
2. Alkaban-AQ, vinblastine sulfate for injection

Adverse Side Effects. These may include gastroenteritis, bone marrow suppression, stomatitis, alopecia, and peripheral neuropathy.

> *Technician's Notes*
>
> 1. Extravasation of plant alkaloids may cause tissue necrosis.
> 2. Skin contact causes irritation.

Antibiotic Antineoplastic Agents

The antibiotic antineoplastic agents are derived from soil fungi of the *Streptomyces* genus. They are cell cycle–nonspecific and exert their effects by binding with DNA, thus inhibiting mitotic activity. Doxorubicin is the most commonly used drug in this class in veterinary medicine. It is widely used for various neoplastic conditions.

Clinical Uses. These agents are used for the treatment of lymphoproliferative neoplasms and various carcinomas and sarcomas.

Dosage Forms
1. Adriamycin, doxorubicin hydrochloride for injection
2. Bleomycin
3. Dactinomycin
4. Mitoxantrone

Adverse Side Effects. These include bone marrow suppression, cardiotoxicity (cardiomyopathy), gastroenteritis, and anaphylaxis.

Technician's Notes

1. Some clinicians use antihistamines to premedicate animals to be treated with doxorubicin to suppress allergic reactions.
2. Doxorubicin is a strong vesicant. Tissue sloughing can follow extravasation, and skin irritation can result from contact with the drug.
3. Doxorubicin is commonly used in combination with other antineoplastic agents.

 Platinum Drugs

The platinum drugs are thought to act in a manner similar to the alkylating agents, which interrupt the replication of DNA in tumor cells (Papich, 2002).

Clinical Uses. These products are used for a variety of solid tumors, including osteosarcomas and carcinomas.

1. Treatment of osteosarcoma
2. Treatment of various other tumors, including carcinomas

Dosage Forms
1. Cisplatin (Platinol)
2. Carboplatin (Paraplatin)

Adverse Side Effects
1. Renal toxicity, nausea, anorexia, and vomiting (cisplatin).
2. Dyspnea, pulmonary edema, and death in cats
3. Carboplatin—less nephrotoxicity, nausea, and vomiting than cisplatin

---

Technician's Notes
Cisplatin is contraindicated in cats.

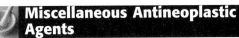 **Miscellaneous Antineoplastic Agents**

Asparaginase
Asparaginase is the most commonly used miscellaneous agent. It is a cell cycle–specific (G_1) enzyme extracted from *Escherichia coli* bacteria. Asparaginase acts as a catalyst in the breakdown of asparagine, an amino acid required by cancer cells. Deprived of a needed amino acid, the cancer cells die. Asparaginase has no effect on normal cells, and it is usually used in combination protocols.

Clinical Uses. Asparaginase is used for the treatment of lymphoproliferative neoplasms.

Dosage Form
Elspar, asparaginase for injection

Adverse Side Effects. The adverse side effects of this drug include immediate hypersensitivity and gastrointestinal disturbances.

Glucocorticoids
The glucocorticoids prednisone and prednisolone are sometimes used for the treatment of neoplastic disorders. They are cell cycle–nonspecific. Corticosteroids have a lympholytic action, which makes them useful for treating lymphoid neoplasms. They are also helpful in the management of secondary complications of neoplastic diseases, such as hypercalcemia and immune-mediated (thrombocytopenia) problems. In addition, they can increase appetite and the overall feeling of well-being in

patients being treated for neoplasm. They are usually used in combination protocols with other antineoplastic drugs.

Biologic Response Modifiers

Biologic response modifiers (BRMs) are agents that alter the relationship between the tumor and the host animal in a way that improves the host's ability to mount an antitumor response (Grant and Shelton, 1989). BRMs are used as an adjunct to conventional chemotherapy protocols, not as the sole agent of treatment.

Cancer develops in many animals because of an immunosuppressed state, and chemotherapy exacerbates the immunosuppression. The BRMs may be used to stimulate or restore the compromised immune response of the host.

Examples of BRMs include bacterial agents, chemical agents, interferons, thymosins, cytokines/lymphokines, and monoclonal antibodies.

Monoclonal Antibodies

Monoclonal antibodies are identical immunoglobulin molecules formed by a single clone of plasma cells. They are produced by a **hybridoma,** a fusion of a specific antibody-producing B cell with **myeloma** cells (Figure 16-5). Hybridomas secrete large quantities of a very specific (for the tumor) antibody. Monoclonal antibodies may have direct cytotoxic effects on tumor cells, or they may be attached (conjugated) to chemotherapeutic agents, such as radioisotopes, BRMs, or other agents, to deliver them directly to the tumor cells. In this way, they become a "magic bullet" directed at the cancer cells (Figure 16-6).

Clinical Uses. Clinical use of monoclonal antibodies in practice is confined primarily to the treatment of canine lymphoma.

Dosage Form

Canine Lymphoma Monoclonal Antibody 231 (CL/MAb 231)

Adverse Side Effects. Adverse side effects of the sequential intravenous infusions may include pruri-

tus, facial edema, vomiting, diarrhea, or anxious behavior. Reactions are usually a result of infusing the agent too rapidly.

Interferon

Interferons are chemicals produced by leukocytes, fibroblasts, and epithelial cells. Interferons can exert antitumor, antiviral, and immunoregulatory effects. Several categories of interferons have been identified. The products that are available are approved for use in humans and have been used in humans to treat hairy cell leukemia, Kaposi's sarcoma, genital warts, and certain granulomatous diseases. In veterinary medicine, they have been used to attempt to prevent the development of fatal disease in feline leukemia virus (FeLV)-infected cats and to attempt to extend the survival time of cats infected with feline infectious peritonitis (FIP).

Clinical Uses. These may include the amelioration of FeLV- and FIP-related conditions.

Dosage Forms
1. Roferon-A injection, recombinant interferon alfa-2a
2. Intron A, recombinant interferon alfa-2b for injection
3. Alferon N injection, human leukocyte–derived interferon alfa-N3
4. Actimmune injection, recombinant interferon gamma-1b

Adverse Side Effects. Adverse side effects in humans have included fever and flulike symptoms.

Other Biologic Response Modifiers
1. Acemannan. This product is licensed for the treatment of fibrosarcoma in dogs and cats.
2. Interleukins. There are 17 identified interleukins. Their functions include various activities in the immune system, such as cell enhancement or suppression, hematopoietic growth, or regulation of leukocyte function.
   a. Interleukin 2. This substance's primary function is the promotion of the clonal expansion of antigen-specific T cells and may be useful

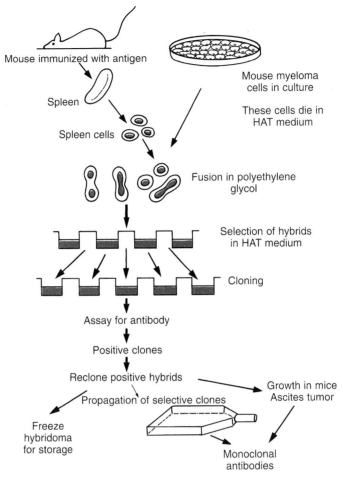

Mouse immunized with antigen

Mouse myeloma cells in culture

These cells die in HAT medium

Spleen

Spleen cells

Fusion in polyethylene glycol

Selection of hybrids in HAT medium

Cloning

Assay for antibody

Positive clones

Reclone positive hybrids

Growth in mice Ascites tumor

Propagation of selective clones

Freeze hybridoma for storage

Monoclonal antibodies

FIGURE 16-5
Production of monoclonal antibodies. *HAT,* hypoxanthine-aminopterin-thymidine. (From Tizard I: Veterinary immunology: an introduction, ed 3, Philadelphia, 1987, WB Saunders Co.)

in treating certain canine and feline neoplasias (Kruth, 1998).

3. Granulocyte Colony Stimulating Factor (G-CSF)—Filgrastrim. These growth factors affect specific myeloid cell lines and may have some use in the treatment of neutropenia associated with the chemotherapy of canine or feline neoplasia or in the management of feline panleukopenia.

4. *Bacillus Calmette-Guerin (BCG)*—BCG is a live, attenuated strain of *Mycobacterium bovis* that activates B and T cells.

5 Levamisole—Use of levamisole as an immunostimulant is controversial.

6. *Propionibacterium acnes* — Immunoregulin is a killed suspension of *Propionibacterium acnes* approved for use in veterinary medicine. It causes nonspecific immunostimulation.

7. Staphylococcal Protein A—This product initiates T and B lymphocyte proliferation.

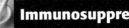

Immunosuppressive Drugs

The immunosuppressive drugs are used in veterinary medicine to treat various immune-mediated disorders. Some of the diseases related to an overactive or improperly responding immune system

Direct destruction

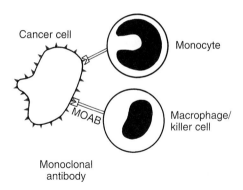

Delivery of cytotoxic drugs to cancer cells

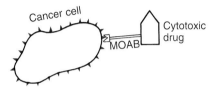

FIGURE 16-6
Antitumor mechanisms of monoclonal antibodies. *MOAB,* monoclonal antibody.

include lupus erythematosus, lymphocytic-plasmacytic enteritis, rheumatoid arthritis, immune-mediated skin disease, and hemolytic anemia. Many of the immunosuppressive drugs work by interfering with one of the stages of the cell cycle or by affecting cellular messengers.

Azathioprine
Azathioprine is an antimetabolite that affects cells in the S phase of the cell cycle. It inhibits both T- and B-lymphocytes to bring about immunosuppression. It has fewer side effects than cyclophosphamide and some of the other immunosuppressants. It is often used in combination with prednisone or prednisolone. Because cats are more likely to be affected by the side effects of this drug, it should not be used in this species.

Clinical Uses. Azathioprine is used primarily for the treatment of immune-mediated disease in dogs.

Dosage Forms
1. Imuran tablets, azathioprine (50 mg)
2. Imuran, azathioprine injection

Adverse Side Effects. Adverse side effects are related to bone marrow suppression. Long-term use may predispose to infection.

Cyclosporine
Cyclosporine is a substance isolated from a fungus that inhibits proliferation of T-lymphocytes (Boothe, 2001). It was approved for use in humans for prevention of organ transplant rejection; however, it has also been used to treat several immune-mediated diseases (e.g., uveitis, Graves' disease, psoriasis, and pemphigus). It has been used in veterinary medicine for the prevention of organ transplant rejection, for treating immune-mediated skin disorders, and for the management of keratoconjunctivitis sicca (KCS) in dogs.

Clinical Uses. Clinical use of cyclosporine in practice is limited mainly to ophthalmic application for treatment of KCS in dogs.

Dosage Forms
1. Optimmune ointment
2. Sandimmune, cyclosporine gelatin capsules
3. Sandimmune, cyclosporine oral solution
4. Sandimmune, cyclosporine for injection

Adverse Side Effects. In humans, these may include nephrotoxicity, hepatotoxicity, nausea, vomiting, anaphylaxis (intravenous form), and others.

> *Technician's Notes*
> Monitor the eyes for irritation or infection if cyclosporine is being used for KCS.

Metronidazole
Metronidazole is a substance that has antibacterial, antiprotozoal, and immunosuppressive activities. It may be used in conjunction with corticosteroids to enhance its immunosuppressive effects.

Clinical Uses

1. Treatment of lymphocytic-plasmacytic enteritis in dogs
2. Treatment of giardiasis
3. Treatment of anaerobic bacterial infections

Dosage Forms

1. Flagyl, metronidazole tablets
2. Flagyl, metronidazole powder for injection
3. Flagyl IV, injectable

Adverse Side Effects. These may include gastrointestinal upset, neurologic disturbances, and lethargy.

Technician's Notes

Clients must be warned about the potential severe side effects of this drug.

Cyclophosphamide

Cyclophosphamide is an alkylating agent that is used as an antineoplastic agent and an immunosuppressant (see the earlier section on antineoplastic agents). Cyclophosphamide may be accompanied by serious side effects (e.g., hemorrhagic cystitis, bone marrow suppression, and gastroenteritis). It is an injectable agent sold under the trade name Cytoxan.

Clinical Uses. Cyclophosphamide is used primarily as an immunosuppressant.

Dosage Form

Cytoxan

Adverse Side Effects. These include bone marrow suppression, gastrointestinal signs, alopecia, and hemorrhagic cystitis.

Corticosteroids

Corticosteroids exert antiinflammatory and immunosuppressive effects through their inhibitory influence on neutrophils, T-lymphocytes, blood vessels (decreased permeability), and cellular messengers (e.g., prostaglandin). They are generally considered to be antiinflammatory at lower doses and immunosuppressive at higher doses. Corticosteroids are often used in combination with other immunosuppressant/antineoplastic agents.

Other Immunosuppressive Agents

1. Tacrolimus
2. Sirolimus
3. Mycophenolate mofetil

REFERENCES

Barton CL: Chemotherapy. In Boothe DM, editor: Small animal clinical pharmacology and therapeutics, Philadelphia, 2001, WB Saunders Co.

Boothe DM: Immunodulators or biologic response modifiers. In Boothe, DM, editor: Small animal clinical pharmacology and therapeutics, Philadelphia, 2001, WB Saunders Co.

Crow SE and Walshaw SO: Placement and care of intravenous catheters. In Crow SE and Walshaw SO, editors: Manual of clinical procedures in the dog and cat, Philadelphia, 1987, JB Lippincott Co.

Dickinson KL and Ogilvie GK: Safe handling and administration of chemotherapeutic agents in veterinary medicine. In Kirk RW and Bonagura JD, editor: Current veterinary therapy XII: small animal practice, Philadelphia, 1995, WB Saunders Co.

Ganong WF: Endocrine function of the kidneys, heart, and pineal gland. In Ganong WF: Review of medical physiology, ed 21, New York, 2003, McGraw-Hill.

Grant CK and Shelton GH: Biological response modifiers. In Kirk RW and Bonagura JD, editors: Current veterinary therapy X: small animal practice, Philadelphia, 1989, WB Saunders Co.

Jenkins WL: Chemotherapeutic agents affecting host cellular functions: antineoplastics and immunomodulators. In Brander GC et al, editors: Veterinary applied pharmacology and therapeutics, ed 5, London, 1991, Bailliere Tindall.

Kruth SA: Biologic response modifiers: interferons, interleukins, recombinant products, liposomal products. In Boothe DM, editor: The veterinary clinics of North America, small animal practice, Philadelphia, 1998, WB Saunders Co.

MacEwen EG and Rosenthal RC: Approach to treatment of cancer patients. In Ettinger SJ, editor: Textbook of veterinary internal medicine, ed 5, Philadelphia, 2000, WB Saunders Co.

Norsworthy GD: Clinical aspects of feline blood transfusions, Comp Cont Educ Pract Vet 14:470, 1992.

Papich MG: Handbook of veterinary drugs, Philadelphia, 2002, WB Saunders Co.

Plumb DC: Veterinary drug handbook, ed 4, Ames, Iowa, 2002, Iowa State University Press.

Pugh DM: Blood formation, coagulation, and volume. In Brander GC et al, editors: Veterinary applied pharmacology and therapeutics, ed 5, London, 1991, Bailliere Tindall.

REVIEW QUESTIONS

1. Anemia in baby pigs can be treated by the administration of _____.
2. A 10-year-old cocker spaniel is brought to the veterinary clinic with polyuria/polydipsia and mild anemia. What is a potential cause of these signs, and what may be used to treat the anemia? _____
3. Why are hematinics not indicated for cases of acute blood loss? _____
4. What is the anticoagulant of choice for collecting blood for hematologic studies?
   _____
5. How can you explain the fact that clots may form in the vascular system with no external trauma to blood vessels?
   _____
6. You have accidentally cut the quick of a rottweiler puppy's nail. What would you use to stop the bleeding, and how does this agent work? _____
7. A 3-month-old chow is brought to the pet emergency clinic, because it has eaten a box of rat poison. What drug would the veterinarian use to treat this condition, and by what route would it be administered?
   _____
8. An 8-year-old male Persian cat is brought to the veterinary clinic with an early onset of apparent rear leg paralysis and tachycardia. What agent may be used to treat this condition? _____
9. Briefly describe the phases of the cell cycle.
   _____
10. List the six categories of the antineoplastic drugs, and give an example of each.
    _____
11. A 12-year-old Labrador retriever has been through a treatment protocol for lymphoma, and the owner has opted for the use of a BRM. What agent could be used in this case?
    _____

12. List four indications for the use of immunosuppressive agents.
    _____
13. Why should you be very careful to avoid extravasation of antineoplastic drugs?
    _____
14. List eight precautions that should be taken when handling antineoplastic drugs.
    _____
15. Where is erythropoietin produced in the body? _____
16. What drug may be used to treat the anemia associated with chronic renal failure?
    _____
17. _____ digests fibrin threads and other clotting products to cause clot lysis and the release of fibrin degradation products into the circulation.
18. Which anticoagulant may be used to treat DIC? _____
19. Why should heparin not be used as an anticoagulant when collecting blood for performing a differential count?
    _____
20. How does EDTA work as an anticoagulant?
    _____
21. What are some potential adverse side effects associated with the use of antineoplastic drugs? _____
22. What is the dosage that most antineoplastic agents are based on?
    _____
23. Corticosteroids have a lympholytic action, which makes them useful for treating _____.
24. A substance with antitumor, antiviral, and immunoregulatory effects is _____.
25. Cardiomyopathy is a potential side effect of what antineoplastic agent?
    _____

PRINCIPLES OF VACCINATION
COMMON VACCINE TYPES THAT
  PRODUCE ACTIVE IMMUNITY
Inactivated
Live
Modified Live
Recombinant
Toxoid
COMMON VACCINE TYPES THAT
  PRODUCE PASSIVE IMMUNITY
Antitoxin
Antiserum
OTHER TYPES OF VACCINES
Autogenous Vaccine
Mixed Vaccine
ADMINISTRATION OF VACCINES
BIOLOGIC CARE AND VACCINE
  FAILURE
ADVERSE VACCINATION RESPONSES
VACCINATIONS FOR PREVENTIVE
  HEALTH PROGRAMS
   Canine
   Equine
   Feline
   Bovine
   Others
IMMUNOTHERAPEUTIC DRUGS
Immunostimulants
   Complex Carbohydrates
   Immunomodulatory Bacterins

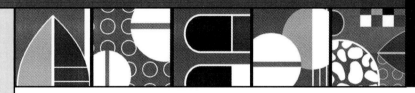

CHAPTER **17**

Immunologic Drugs

LEARNING OBJECTIVES

After studying this chapter, you should be able to:

1. Understand the principles associated with vaccination
2. Understand the differences between vaccine types
3. Be familiar with the advantages and disadvantages of the different types of vaccines
4. Know common diseases that have available vaccines
5. Understand the different routes of administration of vaccines
6. Be familiar with drugs used in immunotherapy

KEY TERMS

ACTIVE IMMUNITY Immunity that occurs by an animal's own immune response after exposure to foreign antigen.

ADJUVANT A substance given with an antigen to enhance the immune response to the antigen. Adjuvants may form a localized granuloma at the injection site or produce systemic hypersensitivity. Adjuvants have received much attention as a result of a possible (but not proven) link with the increased incidence of fibrosarcomas in vaccinated cats. Examples of adjuvants are aluminum hydroxide, aluminum phosphate, aluminum potassium sulfate, water in oil, saponin, and diethyl-aminoethyl (DEAE) dextran.

ANAPHYLAXIS A systemic, severe allergic reaction.

ANTIBODY An immunoglobulin molecule that combines with the specific antigen that induced its formation.

ANTIGEN Any substance that can induce a specific immune response, such as toxins, foreign proteins, bacteria, and viruses.

AVIRULENT The inability of an infectious agent to produce pathologic effects.

BACTERIN A killed bacterial vaccine.

MONOVALENT A vaccine, antiserum, or antitoxin developed specifically for a single antigen or organism.

PASSIVE IMMUNITY Immunity that occurs by administration of antibody produced in another individual.

POLYVALENT A vaccine, antiserum, or antitoxin active against multiple antigens or organisms; mixed vaccine.

PRESERVATIVE A substance, such as an antibiotic, antiinfective, or fungistat, added to a product to destroy or inhibit multiplication of microorganisms.

RECOMBINANT DNA TECHNOLOGY A process that removes a gene from one organism or pathogen and inserts it into the DNA of another. This may also be referred to as gene splicing.

VIRULENCE The ability of an infectious agent to produce pathologic effects.

PRINCIPLES OF VACCINATION

Keeping animals healthy through the proper use of immunization programs is an important aspect in veterinary medicine. Veterinary technicians must have knowledge concerning vaccine types and the diseases animals are vaccinated against. Clients ask many questions regarding this aspect of their pet's care. It should be remembered that immunization should never take the place of regularly scheduled, routine veterinary checkups. As animals age into their geriatric years, regular laboratory profiles should be done to determine the health of major organ systems. Preventive medicine also includes a good physical examination along with taking a complete history on the animal. Therefore immunization programs are only one aspect of the overall health care that should be afforded companion animals. Livestock should also be properly immunized to achieve a healthy herd.

Vaccinations are an important part of the preventive health care program for companion animals and food animals alike. Vaccines are given to lessen the chance for a particular disease to occur. A patient's response is determined by several factors, such as (1) the health and age of the patient, (2) the type of vaccine given, (3) the route of administration, (4) concurrent incubation of infectious disease, (5) exposure to an infectious disease before complete immunity is reached, and (6) drug therapy. The ideal vaccine would be safe, effective on challenge, and have no undesirable side effects. Immunology is a very complex field of study. This chapter outlines only the basics of common vaccines and immunostimulants. Reference to an immunology textbook may be helpful if further information is desired.

The future of vaccination is looking into the development of protocols that individualize vaccine schedules instead of having every animal vaccinated for every disease. There is also research that will hopefully provide optimal revaccination intervals. Some studies have suggested that with some vaccines, protective immunity may last for years and annual revaccination may not be necessary. With new information and technology, the 21st century will see many changes in vaccines.

COMMON VACCINE TYPES THAT PRODUCE ACTIVE IMMUNITY

 ## Inactivated

In the manufacture of inactivated vaccines, organisms are treated most commonly by chemicals that kill the organisms, but very little change occurs in the **antigens**, which stimulate protective immunity. Inactivated vaccines are also referred to as *killed*, or *dead*, vaccines.

Advantages
1. Inactivated vaccines are usually very safe.
2. They are stable in storage.
3. They are unlikely to cause disease through residual virulence.

Disadvantages
1. Inactivated vaccines require repeated doses to achieve adequate protection.
2. Adjuvants may cause severe local reactions.
3. If repeated doses are required, costs may be higher.
4. Inactivated vaccines contain **preservatives**, such as penicillin, streptomycin, and fungistats.

Examples
Leukocell 2: Feline leukemia virus
Duramune Cv-K: Rabies virus
Vibo-5/Somnugen: *Campylobacter fetus*, leptospirosis, *Haemophilus somnus*, **bacterin**

 ## Live

A live vaccine is prepared from live microorganisms or viruses. These organisms may be fully **virulent** or **avirulent.** Few vaccines of this origin are in use, with the exception of several poultry vaccines.

Advantages
1. Live vaccines necessitate fewer doses to achieve an immune response.
2. Adjuvants are unnecessary, but the vaccine may contain preservatives.
3. Live vaccines pose less risk of allergic responses.
4. They are inexpensive.

Disadvantages
1. Live vaccines may be contaminated with unwanted organisms.
2. They require careful handling. For example, accidental injection, ingestion, or exposure through a cut or the mucous membranes of brucellosis vaccine can cause undulant fever in humans.
3. They do not store as well as inactivated vaccines.
4. They may possess residual virulence.

Examples
Brucella abortus vaccine: *Brucella abortus* strain RB-51
Ovine ecthyma vaccine: Ovine ecthyma virus or sore mouth infection
Chick Ark Bronc: Infectious bronchitis (Massachusetts and Arkansas types)
Protex-Bb: *Bordetella bronchiseptica*

 ## Modified Live

In modified live vaccines, organisms undergo a process (attenuation) to lose their virulence so that when introduced to the body via inoculation they cause an immune response instead of disease.

Advantages
1. Effective vaccines for many viruses can be developed through attenuation of the causative virus.
2. Immunity is comparable in response and longevity to killed products.

Disadvantages
1. Modified live vaccines may cause abortion when given to pregnant animals.
2. Some vaccines can cause mild immunosuppression.

3. Residual virulence can cause a mild form of the disease.
4. These vaccines contain preservatives, such as penicillin, gentamicin, thimerosal, or a fungistat.

Examples
Eclipse 3: Feline rhinotracheitis, calicivirus, and panleukopenia
BoviShield 4: Infectious bovine rhinotracheitis (IBR) virus, bovine virus diarrhea (BVD), parainfluenza 3 (PI3) virus, bovine respiratory syncytial virus

 ## Recombinant

In recent years, vaccines produced by **recombinant DNA technology** have become available for veterinary medicine. These vaccines are recognized as being safe, highly specific, potent, pure, and efficacious. These attributes may be the reason recombinant vaccines are more desirable than any other vaccine type. Recombinant vaccines are divided into three categories:

Type I recombinant (subunit) vaccines—These vaccines are derived by inserting a foreign gene from a specific pathogen into a recombinant organism (e.g., yeast, bacterium, or a virus). The recombinant organism multiplies, and the product of the gene is extracted, purified, and prepared for administration as a vaccine.

Type II recombinant (gene-deleted) vaccines—The manufacturing of these vaccines involves deletion of specific genes from a pathogenic organism. This manipulation produces a vaccine that has a low risk of producing disease but can still stimulate a protective immune response.

Type III recombinant (vectored) vaccines—These vaccines are derived from the insertion of specific pathogenic genetic material into a non-pathogenic or gene-deleted organism (e.g., poxvirus). This altered organism is then propagated in vitro and used to manufacture the vaccine (Van Kampen, 1998).

Advantages
1. These vaccines produce fewer adverse effects.
2. They provide effective immunity.

3. Type I and Type III vaccines cannot revert to virulence because of the way they are manufactured.
4. Some of these vaccines can be administered orally.

Disadvantages
1. Currently there are not many recombinant vaccines available.
2. New technology often brings with it a higher cost.

Examples
Type I
RM Recombitek Lyme: *Borrelia burgdorferi*

Type III
RM Recombitek C4: Canine distemper, adenovirus type 2, parainfluenza, and parvovirus
Raboral V-RG: oral vaccine for rabies virus (used in baiting devices for wildlife)
Newcastle disease—fowl pox vaccine (recombinant): Newcastle disease and fowl pox
Trovac-AIV H5: Avian influenza subtype H5 and fowl pox

 ## Toxoid

A toxoid is a vaccine for producing immunity to a toxin rather than a bacterium or a virus. The toxin is treated with heat or chemicals to destroy its damaging properties without eliminating its ability to stimulate **antibody** production.

An anaculture combines toxoid and killed bacteria in a single dose prepared from highly toxigenic cultures and culture filtrates.

Characteristics
1. Toxoids and anacultures provide protection for up to 1 year.
2. Toxoids may contain adjuvants.
3. Many toxoids contain preservatives, such as phenol, thimerosal, and formaldehyde solution.

Examples
Tetanus toxoid: *Clostridium tetani*
Tetnogen: *C. tetani*

Fermicon CD/T: *Clostridium perfringens* types C and D, and *C. tetani*

COMMON VACCINE TYPES THAT PRODUCE PASSIVE IMMUNITY

Antitoxin

An antitoxin is a specific antiserum aimed at a toxin that contains a concentration of antibodies extracted from the blood serum or plasma of a hyperimmunized, healthy animal (usually a horse).

Characteristics
1. An antitoxin neutralizes toxins produced by microorganisms.
2. It may contain preservatives, such as thimerosal, phenol, or oxytetracycline.
3. Antitoxins produce immediate **passive immunity.**
4. Immunity is short lived (about 7 to 14 days).
5. Biologic products of equine origin may be associated with the development of equine serum hepatitis (Theiler's disease). This link has not been proven, but clients should be made aware of this possible risk before these products are administered.

Examples
Clostratox BCD: *C. perfringens* types C and D
Tetanus antitoxin: *C. tetani*

Antiserum

An antiserum is a serum containing specific antibodies extracted from a hyperimmunized animal (usually a horse) or an animal that has been infected with microorganisms containing antigen.

Characteristics
1. An antiserum kills living, infectious antigens.
2. It may contain preservatives, such as phenol, thimerosal, or oxytetracycline.
3. An antiserum produces immediate passive immunity.

4. Do not vaccinate within 21 days after giving antiserum. For example, if a calf is treated with a *Corynebacterium–Escherichia coli–Pasteurella–Salmonella* antiserum, then that calf should not be vaccinated with BVD, IBR, PI_3, *H. somnus*, or *Pasteurella haemolytica* within 21 days of receiving the antiserum.
5. Immunity is short lived.

Examples
Erysipelothrix rhusiopathiae serum antibodies: *E. rhusiopathiae*
E.-Colicin-B: *E. coli*
Septi-Serum: *Salmonella typhimurium*

OTHER TYPES OF VACCINES

Autogenous Vaccine

An autogenous vaccine contains organisms isolated from an infected animal on a farm where a disease problem is occurring. This carefully prepared vaccine contains antigens needed for protection at that particular location.

Mixed Vaccine

A mixed vaccine contains a mixture of different antigens. It is also referred to as a **polyvalent** vaccine (Figure 17-1). Each component of a mixed vaccine is required to achieve an immune response comparable with a vaccine containing a single antigen (**monovalent** vaccine).

ADMINISTRATION OF VACCINES

The intramuscular and subcutaneous routes are by far the most common methods for vaccine administration. These routes are easily accessible and provide systemic immunity, which is important in many diseases. Some diseases also respond well to local immunity. Vaccines against feline rhinotracheitis and calicivirus, canine infectious tracheobronchitis, and infectious bovine rhinotracheitis

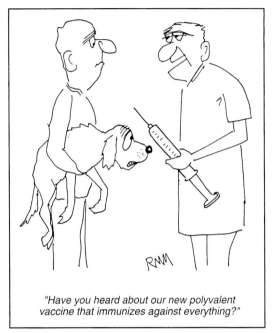

"Have you heard about our new polyvalent vaccine that immunizes against everything?"

FIGURE 17-1
(From Vet Forum, 16:11, 1994.)

are examples of vaccines that may be administered intranasally, or in some cases, intraocular administration may be used to provide local immunity. After administration of these vaccines, the animal may experience a slight bout of watery eyes and occasional sneezing for a few days.

All of the previously mentioned routes of vaccine administration necessitate that each animal be handled individually. When a large number of animals require vaccination, these routes may not be feasible. Some vaccines may be mixed with drinking water or feed. Others can be aerosolized and inhaled by the animal. For example, on mink ranches, vaccine for canine distemper and mink enteritis may be administered in this manner; or poultry houses may vaccinate for Newcastle disease by aerosolization. There is a greater margin for incomplete vaccination when using aerosolization or mixing with feed or water. Some animals may not drink or eat enough to provide adequate protection, or the aerosolized vaccine may not distribute equally

throughout the room. Vaccine failure may be implicated if these animals contract the disease, whereas in reality the animal did not receive enough vaccine to provide adequate immunity.

When using conventional measures for vaccination, it is very important to carefully read the insert provided with the vaccine. Some vaccines may be administered intramuscularly or subcutaneously, but others may be administered by only one route. For example, some rabies vaccines require an intramuscular route to be most effective. Subcutaneous injections should be given according to the manufacturer's instructions. Care should be used when vaccinating a cat to prevent vaccine-induced tumors. The following sites are recommended for feline vaccination: rhinotracheitis-calici-panleukopenia—right front leg; rabies—right rear leg; feline leukemia—left rear leg. Intrascapular injection should also be avoided (McCurnin, 2002).

If a vaccine requires reconstitution, it should be done with the diluent provided by the manufacturer. The vaccine should not be reconstituted until just before it is administered (see Chapter 2 for the proper reconstitution procedure). The full recommended dose should be given. Splitting a vaccine dose may cause an animal to fail to develop an adequate immune response and may lower its protection.

Mixing different vaccines is not recommended to minimize the number of injections the animal receives. This procedure can cause antigen blocking, resulting in one component's interfering with the action of another so that the animal does not receive adequate antigen to promote an effective immune response. Mixing different vaccines may also cause an increased chance of an allergic response. When administering different types of vaccines, each vaccine should be administered in a separate site. It is also advisable to note the locations of administration and vaccine lot numbers on the patient's medical record. If a reaction or problem develops later, a reference will be available to aid in evaluating the problem.

When vaccinating food animals, several things must be considered. Almost all vaccine labels contain information advising not to vaccinate within 21 days of slaughter. Vaccines such as those for *B. abortus* are under federal limitations and regulations, and complete records are maintained on the administration of these vaccines. Brucellosis vaccines are restricted to use by or under the direction of a licensed veterinarian. Carcass destruction is also a factor concerning food animal producers. Injection site lesions may cause damage to muscle tissue, requiring that area to be trimmed and discarded. If a vaccine may be administered either intramuscularly or subcutaneously, the subcutaneous route would produce less tissue reaction and eliminate muscle damage. This is important when dealing with animals used for meat consumption. Most vaccines on the market today can be given subcutaneously.

BIOLOGIC CARE AND VACCINE FAILURE

Biologics (especially modified live and live vaccines) are sensitive to inactivation by heat or sunlight. Clients purchasing vaccines should be provided with a cold pack if needed and should be warned against leaving such biologics in vehicles or in sunlight, where they may become warm and inactivated. Even the performance of killed products can be altered if proper handling and storage measures are not practiced. When these vaccines are shipped from the manufacturer, cold packs are put in the box to provide some refrigeration during shipment. In some areas it may be advisable to anticipate how much vaccine may be needed during the hot summer months and to stock up on that amount during early spring to prevent shipments from overheating during summer transportation. Once a shipment is received, it should be quickly unpacked and placed under refrigeration. Vaccines should never be frozen because cells may rupture when the vaccine thaws, releasing toxins that can damage tissue or cause tissue death.

Inappropriate care of vaccines may lead to inactivation of the vaccine and may be perceived as a vaccine failure. Actual vaccine failure is relatively uncommon. If vaccines are purchased from a reputable manufacturer, one can be fairly sure that the vaccine provided is good. Failure usually occurs because of improper handling, storage, or administration.

Live vaccines, especially, are affected by concurrent antibiotic therapy. Live and modified live vaccines can be inactivated by chemicals used to clean or sterilize syringes and by use of excessive alcohol or other disinfectants to swab the skin before injection. As mentioned earlier, the route of administration may affect the ability of an animal to achieve an adequate immune response. Immunosuppressed, parasitized, stressed, or malnourished animals, or those incubating disease are not able to mount an adequate immune response to prevent disease. Clients should always be advised that such problems can occur. In most cases, an adequate immune response is not achieved before 10 to 14 days. An 8-week-old puppy may not develop a strong immune response to protect against an infectious disease if challenged by maternal antibodies, because it is not feasible to check immune titers to determine the presence of maternal antibodies. Therefore it is recommended that puppies receive boosters every few weeks until about 4 to 5 months of age. Boosters allow vaccines to produce an optimum immune response. Clients often find it difficult to understand why they need to bring their pet in for boosters. If the reasons are explained and if clients are advised about why they should isolate their pet from animals with questionable vaccination histories, many cases of infectious diseases would be prevented among young animals. Clients often perceive one vaccine to be enough or do not understand that their animal is not protected immediately after an injection. Technicians should include this information when educating clients on animal and pet care.

ADVERSE VACCINATION RESPONSES

The most notable risks involving vaccination include residual virulence and toxicity, allergic reactions resulting from hypersensitivity, disease in immunosuppressed animals, possible effects on a fetus, or abortion. The veterinarian assesses these risks before a vaccine is administered. In most cases, the benefits of vaccination far outweigh the risks, but it may occasionally be necessary to omit or delay vaccination because of some of the factors mentioned.

One of the most common reactions noticed with vaccine administration is the sting felt by the animal after injection. This is most often a result of inactivating agents used in manufacturing the vaccine. Manufacturers are constantly researching ways to decrease these undesirable effects and still produce a quality product. This stinging reaction is short lived and does not usually cause a problem unless the animal reacts violently. Other common but not usually serious reactions include a slight fever, lethargy, and soreness at the injection site. These usually subside within 1 day. Hypersensitivity may be caused by several factors, including the immunizing antigens, antigens acquired during the manufacturing of the vaccine, and reactions to **adjuvants** used in the vaccine. Some animals may have an anaphylactic shock reaction after receiving a vaccine, although this is uncommon. Clinical signs of **anaphylaxis** include vomiting, salivation, dyspnea, and incoordination. Epinephrine is usually the antidote of choice in cases of anaphylactic shock. Other adverse side effects that are possible include vaccine-associated fibrosarcoma in cats and immune-mediated hemolytic anemia in dogs (Ford, 1998). The possible etiologies for these effects are under investigation.

VACCINATIONS FOR PREVENTIVE HEALTH PROGRAMS

Canine

As stated earlier, vaccination is an important part of any preventive health program. Many vaccines may be available as a monovalent or polyvalent product. For dogs, a common polyvalent vaccine includes canine distemper (D), respiratory diseases caused by adenovirus type 2 (A_2), canine parainfluenza (P), leptospirosis (L), and canine parvovirus (P). This vaccine may be referred to as DA_2PLP. Many different combinations and product names are available. Most veterinarians choose a particular manufacturer from which to buy vaccine products. This helps to lessen the confusion caused by different names used to designate the manufacturers' products. Other canine vaccines available include those for canine infectious bronchitis (*B. bronchiseptica*), canine coronavirus, rabies, and Lyme disease (*B. burgdorferi*). Manufacturer recommendations should be followed regarding age, route of administration, and follow-up boosters needed for each individual vaccine. Table 17-1 provides an example of a vaccination program for dogs.

Equine

Many horse vaccines are available, including those for tetanus, equine encephalomyelitis (may include Eastern, Western and/or Venezuelan strains), equine rhinopneumonitis, equine influenza, *Streptococcus* (strangles), equine viral arteritis, equine monocytic ehrlichiosis (Potomac horse fever), anthrax spore, and rabies. Tetanus antitoxin is used in wounded horses with no history of recent tetanus toxoid vaccination. It provides immediate immunity, which lasts for about 2 weeks. Tetanus toxoid may be given to a horse to boost its immunity and provide longer protection. Manufacturer recommendations should be followed regarding age, route of administration, and follow-up boosters needed for each individual vaccine. Table 17-2 provides an example of a general preventive health program for horses.

Feline

A common polyvalent vaccine for cats is for the prevention of feline viral rhinotracheitis (FVR), feline calicivirus (C), and feline panleukopenia (P). This combination may be referred to as *FVRCP*. Other vaccines available include those for feline chlamydiosis, feline leukemia, feline infectious peritonitis, *Bordetella*, and rabies. Manufacturer recommendations should be followed regarding age, route of administration, and follow-up boosters needed for each vaccine. Table 17-3 provides an example of a vaccination program for cats.

Bovine

Many vaccines in many different combinations are available for cattle. Vaccine schedules for cattle vary depending on the type of cattle-raising

Table 17-1 General Outline of a Preventive Health Program for Dogs

I. First office visit for health program—usually at 6 wk of age
   A. Conduct a general physical examination and record body weight
   B. Check for external parasites and dermatophytes, and initiate appropriate therapy
      1. Fleas, ticks, ear mites (*Otodectes cynotis*)
      2. Mange mites, especially *Demodex canis* and *Sarcoptes scabiei*
      3. Dermatophytes, particularly *Microsporum* spp. and *Trichophyton mentagrophytes*
   C. Conduct fecal examination including both direct smear and flotation
   D. Initiate administration of heartworm preventive management
   E. Administer an anthelmintic for hookworms and roundworms and, if tapeworms are present, administer praziquantel or epsiprantel
   F. Vaccinate with DA$_2$PL-PC* and, possibly, with kennel cough vaccine,[†] canine Lyme borreliosis vaccine, and *Giardia* vaccine
   G. Advise on nutrition and routine grooming
   H. Provide owner with client education pamphlets on topics such as the following:
      1. Identification, treatment, and control of fleas, ticks, and ear mites
      2. Benefits of preventive management for canine heartworm disease
      3. Management of normal and abnormal puppy behaviors
      4. Skin, nail, and ear care
      5. "How to" on grooming and nutrition
   I. Fill in the puppy's health record for the owner
II. Second office visit for health program—usually at 9 wk of age
   A. Conduct a general physical examination and record body weight
   B. Check for external parasites and dermatophytes, and initiate appropriate therapy
      1. Fleas, ticks, ear mites (*O. cynotis*)
      2. Mange mites, especially *D. canis* and *S. scabiei*
      3. Dermatophytes, particularly *Microsporum* spp. and *T. mentagrophytes*
   C. Conduct fecal examination including both direct smear and flotation
   D. Adjust dosage of heartworm preventive according to body weight

   E. Administer an anthelmintic for hookworms and roundworms and, if tapeworms are present, administer praziquantel or epsiprantel
   F. Vaccinate with DA$_2$PL-PC* and, possibly, with kennel cough vaccine, canine Lyme borreliosis vaccine, and *Giardia* vaccine
   G. Adjust nutrition according to health needs, and, if needed, change the grooming procedures
   H. Provide owner with client education pamphlets on topics such as the following:
      1. Identification, treatment, and control of fleas, ticks, and ear mites
      2. Benefits of preventive management for canine heartworm disease
      3. Dental, skin, nail, and ear care
      4. "How to" on grooming and nutrition
      5. Management of normal and abnormal puppy behaviors
      6. Exercise and its importance
   I. Fill in the puppy's health record for the owner
III. Third office visit for health program—usually at 12 wk of age
   A. Conduct a general physical examination and record body weight
   B. Check for external parasites and dermatophytes, and initiate appropriate therapy
      1. Fleas, ticks, ear mites (*O. cynotis*)
      2. Mange mites, especially *D. canis* and *S. scabiei*
      3. Dermatophytes, particularly *Microsporum* spp. and *T. mentagrophytes*
   C. Conduct fecal examination, including both direct smear and flotation
   D. Adjust dosage of heartworm preventive according to body weight
   E. Administer an anthelmintic for hookworms and roundworms and, if tapeworms are present, administer praziquantel or epsiprantel
   F. Vaccinate with DA$_2$PL-PC* and rabies vaccines, and possibly with kennel cough vaccine,[†] canine Lyme borreliosis vaccine, and *Giardia* vaccine
   G. Adjust nutrition according to health needs and, if needed, change grooming procedures
   H. Provide owner with client education pamphlets on topics such as the following:
      1. Identification, treatment, and control of fleas, ticks, and ear mites

Continued on next page

Table 17-1 General Outline of a Preventive Health Program for Dogs—Cont'd

2. Dental, skin, nail, and ear care
3. "How to" on grooming and nutrition
4. Management of normal and abnormal puppy behaviors
5. Recommendations for spaying and castration
6. Exercise and its importance
I. Fill in the puppy's health record for the owner
IV. Subsequent visits for health program—usually annual visits‡
   A. Conduct a general physical examination and record body weight
   B. Check for external parasites and dermatophytes, and initiate appropriate therapy
      1. Fleas, ticks, ear mites (O. cynotis)
      2. Mange mites, especially D. canis and S. scabiei
      3. Dermatophytes, particularly Microsporum spp. and T. mentagrophytes
   C. Conduct fecal flotation and occult heartworm examination, or all tests for intestinal and heartworm infection screen

D. Adjust dosage of heartworm preventive according to body weight
E. Administer an anthelmintic according to fecal examination findings
F. Vaccinate with DA₂PL-PC* and rabies and possibly with kennel cough vaccine,† canine Lyme borreliosis vaccine, and Giardia vaccine
G. Adjust nutrition according to health needs and, if needed, change grooming procedures
H. Provide owner with client education pamphlets on topics such as the following:
   1. Identification, treatment, and control of fleas, ticks, and ear mites
   2. Dental, skin, nail, and ear care
   3. "How to" on grooming and nutrition
   4. Management of normal and abnormal behaviors
   5. Exercise and its importance
I. Fill in the dog's health record for the owner

*This refers to the use of a vaccine to protect against the following: D—canine distemper; A₂ (canine adenovirus type 2)—infectious canine hepatitis: P—canine parainfluenza; L—leptospirosis; P—canine parvovirus type 2 disease; and C—canine coronavirus disease.
†This refers to the use of vaccine to protect against canine *Bordetella bronchiseptica*–induced disease. Puppies may be vaccinated with either an intranasal vaccine or a parenteral vaccine.
‡A fourth office visit may be desirable at 15 wk of age for an additional parvovirus-2 vaccine booster in some puppies, especially high-risk breeds, such as Doberman pinscher, rottweiler, Labrador retriever, and other presumed high-risk breeds.
From McCurnin DM, Bassert JM: Clinical textbook for veterinary technicians, eds, Philadelphia, 2002, WB Saunders.

operation, and a veterinarian can best decide what program an individual operation needs. Examples of common vaccines used include leptospirosis, vibriosis, clostridial combinations, respiratory tract disease, and enteric disease. As with all vaccines, manufacturer recommendations should be carefully followed for the best results. Tables 17-4 and 17-5 provide examples of preventive health programs for beef and dairy cattle.

Others

Vaccines are also available for sheep, poultry, and swine (Table 17-6). These animals may be raised in large numbers on farms, and as for cattle-raising

operations, vaccination schedules may vary according to the type of conditions and location. Ferrets have become common household pets and should be vaccinated for canine distemper according to the schedule used for dogs. Some rabies vaccines are approved for use in ferrets. Public health authorities can require a rabies-vaccinated ferret that bites a human to be euthanized and tested for rabies virus.

IMMUNOTHERAPEUTIC DRUGS

It may often be desirable to use drugs to stimulate the body's immunologic response. Immunotherapy

Table 17-2 General Outline of a Preventive Health Program for Cats

I. First office visit for health program (usually at 8-10 wk of age)
   A. Perform a general physical examination and record body weight
   B. Check for external parasites and dermatophytes, and initiate appropriate therapy for the following:
      1. Fleas and ear mites (Otodectes cynotis)
      2. Mange mites, especially Notoedres cati, Demodex spp., and Cheyletiella spp.
      3. Dermatophytes, particularly Microsporum spp. and Trichophyton mentagrophytes
   C. Perform fecal examination, including both direct smear and flotation
   D. Administer anthelmintics, such as pyrantel pamoate for roundworms and hookworms and praziquantel or epsiprantel for tapeworms (if present)
   E. Vaccinate with FVRC-P,*† Chlamydia,‡ FeLV§ (possibly test for FeLV/FIV before initial FeLV vaccination), FIP,‖ Bordetella, and Giardia vaccines
   F. Advise on nutrition and routine grooming
   G. Provide owner with client education pamphlets on topics such as the following:
      1. Identification, treatment, and control of fleas, ticks, and ear mites
      2. Benefits of vaccination for FeLV infection
      3. Management of normal and abnormal cat behaviors
      4. Grooming "how to" and nutrition
   H. Fill in kitten's health record for the owner
II. Second office visit for health program (usually at 12-14 wk of age)
   A. Perform a general physical examination and record body weight
   B. Check for external parasites and dermatophytes, and initiate appropriate therapy for the following:
      1. Fleas and ear mites (O. cynotis)
      2. Mange mites, especially N. cati, Demodex spp., and Cheyletiella spp.
      3. Dermatophytes, particularly Microsporum spp. and T. mentagrophytes
   C. Perform fecal examination, including both direct smear and flotation
   D. Administer anthelmintics, such as pyrantel pamoate for roundworms and hookworms and praziquantel or epsiprantel for tapeworms (if present)
   E. Vaccinate with FVRC-P,* Chlamydia,‡ FeLV,§ rabies, FIP,‖ Bordetella, and Giardia vaccines
   F. Adjust nutrition and grooming procedures
   G. Provide owner with client education pamphlets on topics such as the following:
      1. Identification, treatment, and control of fleas, ticks, and ear mites
      2. Benefits of vaccination for FeLV infection
      3. Dental, skin, nail, and ear care
      4. Management of normal and abnormal cat behaviors
      5. Exercise and its importance
      6. Recommendations for spaying, castration, and declawing
   H. Fill in kitten's health record for owner
III. Subsequent visits for health program (usually annual visits)
   A. Perform a general physical examination and record body weight
   B. Check for external parasites and dermatophytes, and initiate appropriate therapy for the following:
      1. Fleas and ear mites (O. cynotis)
      2. Mange mites, especially N. cati, Demodex spp., and Cheyletiella spp.
      3. Dermatophytes, particularly Microsporum spp., and T. mentagrophytes
   C. Perform fecal examination (fecal flotation)
   D. Administer an anthelmintic according to fecal examination findings
   E. Vaccinate with FVRC-P,* Chlamydia,‡ FeLV,§ rabies, FIP,‖ Bordetella, and Giardia vaccines

Continued on next page

Table 17-2 General Outline of a Preventive Health Program for Cats—Cont'd

F. Adjust nutrition and grooming procedures
G. Provide owner with client education pamphlets on topics such as the following:
  1. Identification, treatment, and control of fleas, ticks, and ear mites
  2. Benefits of vaccination for FeLV infection
  3. Dental, skin, nail, and ear care
	4. Management of normal and abnormal cat behaviors
	5. Exercise and its importance
	6. Recommendations for spaying, castration, and declawing
	H. Fill in cat's health record for owner

FeLV, Feline leukemia virus; *FIV*, feline immunodeficiency virus; *FIP*, feline infectious peritonitis.

*FVRC-P refers to the use of a vaccine to protect against feline viral rhinotracheitis (FVR); feline calicivirus infection (C); and feline panleukopenia (P).

†Cats being prepared for shipment or entering a boarding kennel, veterinary hospital, or clinic should be vaccinated at least 1-2 wk before admission or shipment.

‡The vaccine currently available apparently produces effective protection only against *Chlamydia psittaci* infections. As with other vaccines for respiratory ailments, complete protection is not afforded; however, clinical signs of conjunctivitis or upper respiratory tract disease, if they do occur, can be restricted to short courses and are mild.

§Refers to the use of a vaccine to protect against FeLV infection. FeLV and FIV are administered subcutaneously in healthy kittens or older cats as two doses, with the second dose given 3 or 4 wk after the first. Annual revaccination with a single dose is recommended.

‖The Primucell-FIP Vaccine (Pfizer Animal Health) is administered intranasally to healthy cats. Primary vaccination with two doses should be given with the second dose administered 3-4 wk after the first, and single-dose annual revaccination is recommended.

From McCurnin DM, Bassert JM: Clinical textbook for veterinary technicians, eds, Philadelphia, 2002, WB Saunders.

involves using drugs to stimulate or suppress the body's immunologic response to diseases or conditions caused by agents such as bacteria, viruses, or cancer cells. Immunostimulants are agents that stimulate the immune response. Immunomodulators are agents used to adjust the immune response to a desired level. Table 17-7 lists some of the drugs commonly used in immunotherapy.

Immunotherapy involves using drugs to stimulate or suppress the body's immunologic response to diseases or conditions caused by agents such as bacteria, viruses, or cancer cells. Immunostimulants are used to stimulate the body's immunologic response. They may do this by stimulating macrophage activity, producing lymphokine, increasing natural killer cell activity, and enhancing cell-mediated immunity. These drugs may be used in the treatment of chronic pyoderma in dogs, equine sarcoids, and bovine ocular squamous cell carcinoma. They may also be used as adjunctive therapy for some other types of cancers, such as canine malignant lymphoma, fibrosarcoma, and feline retrovirus infections. Some immunostimulants may be used to help reduce the clinical signs and mortality associated with some infections, such as *E. coli* diarrhea in calves. Many other immunostimulants, such as interferons, interleukin-1, and interleukin-2, are being investigated for potential use in veterinary medicine. Immunosuppressive drugs are used to suppress the body's immunologic response. They are used in veterinary medicine to treat various immune-mediated disorders. Further information on immunosuppressive drugs may be found in Chapter 16.

 Immunostimulants

Complex Carbohydrates

Acemannan: This is a complex carbohydrate derived from aloe vera.

Table 17-3 General Outline of a Preventive Health Program for Horses

First Quarter: January-March

All Horses

Deworm at least every 8 wk. Exercise care in choice of anthelmintics for mares in the third trimester. Begin deworming foals at 2 mo of age.

Trim feet every 6 wk; more frequently in foals requiring limb correction.

Dentistry: check twice yearly and float teeth as needed. Remove wolf teeth in 2-yr-olds and retained caps in 2-, 3-, and 4-yr-olds.

Immunize for respiratory disease: influenza, strangles, and rhinopneumonitis.

In southeastern United States immunize for equine encephalitis.

Stallions

Perform complete breeding examination. Maintain stallions under lights if being used for early breeding.

Pregnant Mares

Immunize with tetanus toxoid, and open sutured mares 30 days prepartum. Develop a colostrum bank. Ninth-day breeding only for mares with normal foaling history and normal reproductive tract. Wash udders of foaling mares.

Open Mares

Maintain under lights if being used for early breeding. Perform daily teasing. Perform reproductive tract examination during estrus. Mares should not be too fat but in gaining condition during breeding season.

Newborn Foals

Dip navel in disinfectant.

Carefully, give a cleansing enema at birth.

Administer tetanus prophylaxis if indicated by history.

Perform immunoglobulin test at 12-24 hr.

Second Quarter: April-June

All Horses

Deworm at least every 8 wk.

Trim feet every 6 wk. Do not forget the foals and yearlings.

Dentistry: check teeth and remove or float teeth as needed.

Immunize for equine encephalomyelitis. Administer appropriate vaccine boosters.

Stallions

Maintain an exercise program.

Monitor the semen quality.

Broodmares

Palpate at 21, 42, and 60 days after successful breeding.

Foals

Creep-feed the foals and provide free-choice minerals. Immunize at 3 mo of age.

Group foals by gender and size when weaned.

Third Quarter: July-September

All Horses

Deworm at least every 8 wk. Clip and sweep the pastures.

Trim feet every 6 wk. Continue corrective trimming on foals.

Dentistry: check teeth and remove or float teeth as needed.

Stallions

Maintain an exercise program.

Broodmares

Administer rhinopneumonitis boosters to pregnant mares according to manufacturer's labeled directions. Administer appropriate vaccine boosters to foals and yearlings.

Check condition of mare's udder at weaning, and reduce amount of feed given until milk flow is reduced.

Foals

Administer all appropriate immunizations. Provide free-choice minerals. Maintain a protein supplement in creep feeders.

Fourth Quarter: October-December

All Horses

Deworm at least every 8 wk. Select anthelmintics appropriate for season.

Trim feet every 6 wk. Continue corrective trimming on foals.

Dentistry: check teeth and remove or float teeth as needed.

Stallions

Continue exercise program.

Check immunizations.

Perform breeding examination.

Broodmares

Confirm pregnancy.

Begin treating open mares.

Check immunizations.

From McCurnin DM, Bassert JM: Clinical textbook for veterinary technicians, eds, Philadelphia, 2002, WB Saunders.

Table 17-4 General Outline of a Preventive Health Program for Beef Cattle

Cow-Calf Herd Recommendation*

At Birth

Ingestion of colostrum within the first few hours after birth is an important factor in baby calf survival. Immunize with oral bovine rotavirus and coronavirus enteric disease vaccine if a calf diarrhea problem exists in the herd.

1- to 3-Mo-Old Calves

Immunize with a seven-way clostridial disease product. Deworm with commercial product that is safe for calves.

Preweaning Calves

Deworm with broad-spectrum commercial dewormer, and immunize as follows:

Immunizing Vaccine	Age for Vaccine Administration
Brucella abortus, strain RB-51 (calfhood vaccination—replacement heifers only)	4-12 mo
Clostridial diseases:	
Clostridium perfringens types C and D, *C. Chauvoei, C. novyi, C. septicum, C. sordellii*	5-6 mo
IBR and PI-3 respiratory diseases (inactivated vaccines only)	5-6 mo, booster at 12-13 mo
BVD (inactivated vaccines only)	5-6 mo, booster at 12-13 mo
BRSV	5-6 mo, booster at 12-13 mo

Weaning Calves

Deworm with broad-spectrum commercial dewormer, and treat for lice and grubs. Castrate the bull calves. Immunize with *Pasteurella* (optional) and *Haemophilus* (optional) vaccines.

Prebreeding Replacement Heifers

Deworm with broad-spectrum commercial dewormer and treat for lice. Immunize as follows:

Immunizing Vaccine	Time of Vaccine Administration
IBR and PI-3 respiratory diseases	10-12 mo
Clostridial diseases:	10-12 mo
C. perfringens types C and D, *C. novyi, C. septicum, C. sordellii, C. chauvoei*	
BVD	10-12 mo
BRSV	10-12 mo
Leptospirosis	10-12 mo
Campylobacteriosis	10-12 mo

Prebreeding Cows

Deworm with broad-spectrum dewormer and treat for lice. Immunize for leptospirosis and campylobacteriosis.

Precalving Cows

Immunize as follows:

Immunizing Vaccine	Time of Vaccine Administration
IBR and PI-3 respiratory diseases (inactivated vaccines only)	Before calving
BVD (inactivated vaccine only)	Before calving
BRSV	Before calving
Bovine rotavirus and coronavirus enteric diseases	Before calving
Escherichia coli enteric disease	Before calving
Clostridial diseases:	Before calving
C. perfringens types C and D, *C. chauvoei, C. novyi, C. septicum, C. sordellii*	

Bulls

Deworm annually with broad-spectrum dewormer, and treat for lice and grubs. Immunize as recommended for prebreeding replacement heifers annually (see the above section).

Table 17-4 General Outline of a Preventive Health Program for Beef Cattle—Cont'd

Feedlot Recommendations[†]

On Arrival into the Feedlot

Deworm with a broad-spectrum dewormer and immunize for IBR, PI-3, BVD, BRSV, and clostridial diseases (use seven-way vaccine). Inactivated IBR, PI-3, and BVD vaccines are the safest.

3-4 Wk After Arrival into the Feedlot

Implant a commercial implant product. Treat for lice and grubs. Administer booster immunizations if necessary. Abort the heifers if necessary. Castrate and dehorn if necessary.

BRSV, Bovine respiratory syncytial virus; *BVD*, bovine virus diarrhea; *IBR*, infectious bovine rhinotracheitis; *PI-3*, parainfluenza-3.

*Other optional vaccines that may be incorporated into the immunization program, depending on individual herd needs and diseases endemic to the area, include anthrax and anaplasmosis.

[†]Other optional vaccines that may be incorporated into the immunization program, depending on individual herd needs and diseases endemic to the area, include *Haemophilus somnus*, *Pasteurella* spp., leptospirosis, and anthrax.

From McCurnin DM, Bassert JM: Clinical textbook for veterinary technicians, eds, Philadelphia, 2002, WB Saunders.

Clinical Uses. Acemannan is used as an aid in the treatment of fibrosarcoma in cats and dogs. It has also been used for stimulating wound healing and in treatment of FeLV- and FIV-infected cats.

Dosage Form

Acemannan Immunostimulant

Adverse Side Effects. None.

Immunomodulatory Bacterins

Staphylococcus Phage Lysate (SPL): This is prepared by lysing *Staphylococcus aureus* with a polyvalent bacteriophage.

Clinical Uses. SPL is used in the treatment of canine pyoderma and related skin infections with a staphylococcal component.

Dosage Form

1. Staphage Lysate (SPL)

Adverse Side Effects. These include malaise, fever, chills, and injection site irritation.

Propionibacterium Acnes Bacterin: This is prepared from killed *Propionibacterium acnes*.

Clinical Uses. *P. acnes* is used in the treatment of chronic recurrent pyoderma and as an adjunct therapy in the treatment for equine respiratory disease complex. It has also been used as an adjunctive therapy in the treatment of feline retrovirus infections.

Dosage Forms

1. Immunoregulin
2. Eqstim

Adverse Side Effects. These include malaise, fever, and chills.

Mycobacterial Cell Wall Fraction: This is an emulsion of cell wall fractions that are modified to reduce their toxicity and allergic effects.

Clinical Uses. These include the treatment of equine sarcoids and bovine ocular squamous cell carcinoma. It is also used in the treatment of mixed mammary tumors and mammary adenocarcinoma in dogs.

Dosage Forms

Regressin-V

Nomagen

Table 17-5 General Outline of a Preventive Health Program for Dairy Cattle*

Calves

At Birth

Immunize with bovine rotavirus and coronavirus enteric disease vaccine,[†] and administer *Escherichia coli* enteric disease vaccine orally.

Weaning Age (about 2 mo) to Breeding Age (about 15 mo)

Immunizing Vaccine	Age for Vaccine Administration
Brucella abortus, strain RB-51 (calfhood vaccination—replacement heifers only)	4-12 mo
Clostridial diseases:	2-4 mo, booster in 2 wk
Clostridium perfringens types C and D, *C. chauvoei*, *C. novyi*, *C. septicum*, *C. sordellii*	
IBR and PI-3 respiratory diseases	4-6 mo, booster at 12-13 mo
BVD	6-8 mo, booster at 12-13 mo
BRSV	6-8 mo, booster at 12-13 mo
Leptospirosis	4-6 mo, booster in 2 wk
Campylobacteriosis	4-6 mo, booster at 12-13 mo

Fresh Cows and Heifers

Immunizing Vaccine	Time of Vaccine Administration
IBR and PI-3 respiratory diseases (inactivated vaccines only)	30 days postpartum
BVD (inactivated vaccines only)	30 days postpartum
BRSV	30 days postpartum
Leptospirosis	30 days postpartum
Campylobacteriosis	30 days postpartum

Dry Cows and Bred Heifers

The goal of dry cow immunization is to provide optimal protection for the newborn calf.

Immunizing Vaccine	Time of Vaccine Administration
Leptospirosis	At time of dry-off
Bovine rotavirus and coronavirus enteric diseases[†]	At time of dry-off, booster in 2-3 wk
Escherichia coli enteric disease[†]	At time of dry-off, booster in 2-3 wk
Clostridial diseases:	At time of dry-off, booster in 2-3 wk
C. perfringens types C and D, *C. chauvoei*, *C. novyi*, *C. septicum*, *C. sordellii*	

BRSV, Bovine respiratory syncytial virus; BVD, bovine virus diarrhea; IBR, Infectious bovine rhinotracheitis; PI-3, parainfluenza-3.

*Other vaccines that may be incorporated into the vaccination program, depending on individual herd needs and diseases endemic to the area, include *Haemophilus somnus*, *Pasteurella* spp., *Salmonella* spp., *Clostridium haemolyticum*, anthrax, and anaplasmosis.

[†]Use if problem of neonatal calf diarrhea exists on the farm.

From McCurnin DM, Bassert JM: Clinical textbook for veterinary technicians, eds, Philadelphia, 2002, WB Saunders.

Table 17-6 General Outline of a Preventive Health Program for Swine

Prebreeding Recommendations for Boars

Purchase boars 60 days before intended use. Quarantine new boars for 30 days, then allow fence line contact with gilts and sows for 30 days before breeding. Immunize boars for leptospirosis and erysipelas. Treat for external and internal parasites before breeding.

Prebreeding Recommendations for Sows and Gilts

Immunize for leptospirosis, porcine parvovirus infection,* and pseudorabies* 2-4 wk before breeding. Flush gilts by increasing feed (energy) intake before breeding to increase ovulations. Treat for external and internal parasites before breeding.

Prefarrowing Recommendations for Sows and Gilts

Limit feed intake to about 4 lb per head per day or feed according to condition to avoid overweight sows or gilts at farrowing. Immunize for colibacillosis,* atrophic rhinitis, erysipelas, transmissible gastroenteritis (TGE), porcinc rotavirus infection,* and *Clostridium perfringens* type C* according to manufacturer's labeled instructions. Treat for external and internal parasites before farrowing with approved products.

Farrowing Recommendations

Gradually increase feed intake so lactating swine are receiving full feed at peak milk production. (Rule of thumb: Feed daily 1 lb of feed for every pig being nursed [e.g., a lactating sow with a litter of 12 pigs should receive at least 12 lb of feed daily].)

General Recommendations for Pigs

At Birth

Perform newborn pig procedures (e.g., clip needle teeth, dock tails, castrate, ear-notch, and inject iron dextran).

1 Wk of Age

Immunize for TGE,* rotavirus,* and atrophic rhinitis.

4-5 Wk of Age

Weaning occurs at this time. Immunize for atrophic rhiritis, erysipelas, and *Actinobacillus* infection.*

6-8 Wk of Age

Treat for external and internal parasites with approved products.

Older Than 8 Wk of Age

Repeated treatments for external and internal parasites with approved products may need to be done during the growing-finishing period.

*Dependent on problems in the individual swine herd.

From McCurnin DM, Bassert JM: Clinical textbook for veterinary technicians, eds, Philadelphia, 2002 WB Saunders.

Table 17-7 Immunotherapeutic Drugs and Indications for Their Use

Product Name and Manufacturer	Product Type	Product Indications
Acemannan Immunostimulant (Carrington)	A complex carbohydrate derived from aloe vera; stimulates macrophage activity	An aid in the treatment of fibrosarcoma in cats and dogs, and feline leukemia; also for stimulating wound healing (Tizard, 2000)
Staphage Lysate (SPL) (Delmont)	*Staphylococcus aureus* phage lysate	Treatment for canine pyoderma and related skin infections with a staphylococcal component
Rubeola Virus Immunomodulator (Eudaemonic)	Inactivated rubeola virus with histamine phosphate	Treatment of equine chronic myofascial inflammation
Nomagen (Fort Dodge)	A mycobacterial cell-wall fraction immunostimulant	Treatment of equine sarcoids and bovine ocular squamous cell carcinoma
Immunoregulin (Immuno Vet)	*Propionibacterium acnes* immunostimulant	Chronic recurrent pyoderma in dogs
CL/Mab 231 (Synbiotics)	Canine lymphoma monoclonal antibody	Adjunctive therapy for dogs with lymphoma

Adverse Side Effects. These include malaise, fever, and decreased appetite.

Technician's Notes
The effects of immunotherapy may be decreased with the administration of immunosuppressive drugs.

REFERENCES

Ford RB: Vaccines and vaccinations: issues for the 21st Century, Suppl Compend Contin Educ Pract Vet 20(8C):19-24, 1998.

McCurnin DM and Bassert J, editors: Clinical textbook for veterinary technicians, ed 5, Philadelphia, 2002, WB Saunders Co.

Tizard I: Veterinary immunology: an introduction, ed 6, Philadelphia, 2000, WB Saunders Co.

Van Kampen KR: Recombinant technology, Suppl Compend Contin Educ Pract Vet 20(8):28-32, 1998.

REVIEW QUESTIONS

1. Immunizations should never take the place of regularly scheduled

   _____.

2. What are six factors that may determine an animal's response to immunization?

   _____

3. What is an inactivated vaccine?

   _____

4. What is a live vaccine?

   _____

5. What is a modified-live vaccine?

   _____

6. What is a toxoid? _____

7. What is an antitoxin?

   _____

8. When a shipment of vaccine arrives at a veterinary facility, what should occur immediately? _____

9. What is immunotherapy?

   _____

10. _____ is a complex carbohydrate derived from aloe vera.

ALTERNATIVE MEDICINES
Chondroprotectives
  Polysulfated Glycosaminoglycans
Nutraceuticals
  Glucosamine and Chondroitin Sulfate
  Echinacea
  Garlic
  Ginseng
  Fatty Acids
  Brewer's Yeast
  Probiotics
  Bioflavonoids
  Fiber
  Ginkgo
  St. John's Wort
  Saw Palmetto
  Superoxide Dismutase
  Coenzyme Q
  Aloe Vera
  S-Adenosylmethion (SAMe)
Miscellaneous Antidotes
  Activated Charcoal
  Calcium EDTA
  Methylene Blue
  Acetylcysteine
  Dimercaprol
  Pralidoxime Chloride
  Penicillamine
  Sodium Thiosulfate
  Ethanol
  Fomepizole
  Antivenin Polyvalent (Crotalidae)/
    Antivenin (*Micrurus fulvius*) Coral
    Snake
  Vitamin K-1 (Phytonadione)
  Thiamine HCl
Reversal Agents
  Atipamezole HCl
  Flumazenil
  Naloxone HCl
  Tolazoline HCl
  Yohimbine HCl
Lubricants

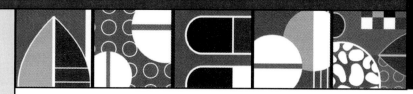

CHAPTER **18**

Miscellaneous Therapeutic Agents

LEARNING OBJECTIVES

After studying this chapter, you should be able to:

1. Develop a knowledge of polysulfated glycosaminoglycans and how they act as chondroprotectives
2. Develop a general knowledge about the uses and adverse side effects of common antidotes
3. Understand the use of naloxone and yohimbine HCl as reversal agents
4. Be familiar with the names of common lubricants
5. Be able to define neutraceutical and discuss the uses of neutraceuticals in veterinary medicine

KEY TERMS

CHELATING AGENT An agent used in chemotherapy for metal poisoning.

METHEMOGLOBINEMIA The presence of methemoglobin in the blood caused by injury or toxic agents that convert a larger-than-normal proportion of hemoglobin into methemoglobin, which does not function as an oxygen carrier.

NUTRACEUTICAL Any nontoxic food component that has scientifically proven health benefits.

ALTERNATIVE MEDICINES

Chondroprotectives

Chondroprotectives are substances that are able to decrease the progression of osteoarthritis by providing support to cartilage and promoting its repair.

Polysulfated Glycosaminoglycans

Polysulfated glycosaminoglycan (PSGAG) consists of a repeating chain of hexosamine and hexuronic acid (Boothe, 2001). The complex nature of the molecule allows water to be trapped in hyaline cartilage to provide resistance to compression and resiliency to the proteoglycan and collagen matrix. It is extracted for commercial use from the tracheal tissue of the bovine. After intramuscular (IM) injection, PSGAG is deposited in articular cartilage and preferentially taken up by osteoarthritic cartilage (Plumb, 2002). When used to treat degenerative joint conditions, these PSGAGs increase synovial fluid viscosity, and inhibit enzymes that damage cartilage matrix within joints. PSGAGs also reduce inflammation by inhibiting prostaglandin released in joint injury.

Adverse Side Effects. Adverse side effects are minimal with use of this product.

Clinical Uses. PSGAG is used in the treatment of noninfectious degenerative or traumatic joint dysfunction and associated lameness of the carpal joints in horses. It has also been used to treat degenerative joint disorders in dogs and lameness in swine.

Dosage Forms
1. Adequan I.A., for intraarticular injection
2. Adequan I.M., for intramuscular injection
3. Adequan Canine
4. Legend

> *Technician's Notes*
>
> 1. Amikacin may be used concurrently with intraarticular use to prevent infection resulting from possible contamination.
> 2. PSGAG should not be used in horses intended for food.
> 3. Safety in breeding animals is undetermined.

Nutraceuticals

A **nutraceutical** has been defined as any nontoxic food component that has scientifically proven health benefits, including disease treatment and prevention. The popularity of these products, which may have characteristics of nutrients and pharmaceuticals, has seen tremendous growth in use by people in recent years. The medical community has acknowledged that some of them may have treatment or preventive effects (Boothe, 1997). Products such as niacin, beta-carotene, calcium, fiber, and antioxidants have widespread use for therapeutic purposes or prevention of selected medical conditions in people.

As people have become more aware of alternative medical options for themselves, they have come to expect similar options for their pets. Veterinarians and their clients can be expected to use nutraceuticals as treatment options to complement traditional medicine or when traditional treatment options have been exhausted.

The North American Veterinary Nutraceutical Council has defined a veterinary nutraceutical as "a nondrug substance that is produced in a purified or extracted form and administered orally to provide agents required for normal body structure and function with the intent of improving the health and well-being of animals." Even though the definitions listed for nutraceutical and veterinary nutraceutical seem straightforward, a great deal of confusion exists over what is actually a nutraceutical. It has been stated that the term nutraceutical was developed to refer to a product marketed under the premise of being a dietary supplement but with the real intent of preventing or treating a disease (Fascetti, 1998).

The question often asked about these products is "is it a food (nutrient) or a drug?" If it is a food, then it is not subject to FDA approval; if it is a drug, it must go through the FDA approval process at a great deal of expense to the manufacturer. A product is usually determined to be a drug if its label has a claim that indicates a therapeutic or preventive intent. If a product is determined to be a food, it is usually determined to be "generally regarded as safe (GRAS)" by the FDA.

The Dietary Supplement Health and Education Act (DSHEA) of 1994 listed dietary supplements as vitamins, minerals, amino acids, herbal products, and substances that supplement the diet by increasing total dietary intake. This action made these products "food" and excluded them from FDA regulation. The act does require, however, that the manufacturer show a disclaimer on the label after the product claim that says "this statement has not been evaluated by the Food and Drug Administration. This product is not intended to diagnose, treat, cure, or prevent any disease." Because of concerns about potential residues and the potential differences in response across species, the Center for Veterinary Medicine (CVM) of the FDA has stated that the DSHEA does not apply to animals or animal feeds.

Since nutraceuticals have not been through an extensive evaluation process to validate their purity, safety, and efficacy, it is up to the veterinarian to evaluate the suitability of particular products for use in companion animals and to promote their use in the context of a valid veterinarian-client-patient relationship. Some questions that should be answered when evaluating a nutraceutical product include the following:

1. What controlled studies have been done to determine whether the product does what it claims to do and who performed the studies?
2. Does the product contain what it says it does, and is that product bioavailable?
3. Is the label easily understandable with all ingredients listed in the same units?
4. Is the dosage appropriate?

The following is a partial list of the substances marketed as nutraceuticals.

Glucosamine and Chondroitin Sulfate

Glucosamine is an amino sugar manufactured by animal cells from glucose and used by the body in the synthesis of glycoproteins and polysulfated glycosaminoglycans. Chondroitin sulfate is a glycosaminoglycan that combines with hyaluronic acid, proteins, and other glycosaminoglycans to from the basic cartilage matrix. Glucosamine and chondroitin sulfate are believed to act synergistically (Davidson, 2000) to exert a positive effect on cartilage metabolism and an inhibition of cartilage breakdown. They have been used extensively in the treatment of osteoarthritis in dogs and horses. Four to six weeks of administration may be necessary for a therapeutic effect to be seen. A common veterinary product containing these substances is called Cosequin, which is composed of glycosaminoglycan derived from the chitin of crab shell and chondroitin sulfate from bovine trachea. Glyco-Flex and Syno-Flex derive their glycosaminoglycan from the *Perna canaliculus* mussel.

Echinacea

Echinacea is a commonly used remedy for colds and flu in people in the United States and Europe where research has been done demonstrating that it is an immunostimulant. It is derived primarily from the

American coneflower. No major side effects have been reported other than the occasional allergic reaction (Fascetti, 1998).

Garlic

Garlic is a perennial bulb in the lily family that is related to the onion. This plant has been used for centuries for its reported medicinal value. People have claimed that it produces disinfectant, diuretic, and/or expectorant effects. There is some evidence that it does lower cholesterol values in people. There is no evidence, however, that garlic has any value in the treatment of parasites in animals. Garlic can produce a Heinz body anemia in cats and possibly in dogs at high dosages.

Ginseng

Ginseng is made from the dried roots of several species of plants from the Panax family. The Chinese believe that ginseng increases vitality and overall strength, possibly by improving aerobic metabolism. Side effects may include hypertension, nervousness, and excitement.

Fatty Acids

The omega-6 and omega-3 fatty acids are the ones most often found in commercial veterinary fatty acid supplements. Omega-6 fatty acids have double bond 6 carbons from the methyl end, whereas omega-3 fatty acids have double bond 3 carbons from the methyl end. Fatty acid supplementation has been shown to be useful in treating certain dermatologic conditions in dogs and cats because of their antiinflammatory effects. Omega-3 fatty acids are normally found in low concentrations in the cellular plasma membrane compared with omega-6 fatty acids, but the omega-3 level can be increased by a food or supplement enriched in this substance (Roudebush, 2000). The breakdown products of the omega-3 acids are apparently less powerful mediators of the inflammatory response than those derived from the omega-6 fatty acids. The omega-3 and omega-6 fatty acids also may be helpful in treating heart disease, cancer, autoimmune disease, and rheumatoid arthritis. The proper ratio of omega-6 to omega-3 fatty acids in a product has apparently not been determined and is often debated. Fish oil and plant oils are common sources of these fatty acids. Side effects may include increased bleeding times and possible decreased immune function.

Brewer's Yeast

The claim has been made that brewer's yeast given to a pet will cause fleas to be repelled. No controlled studies have shown this effect to be true. Brewer's yeast is a good source of the B vitamins.

Probiotics

Probiotics are substances that competitively inhibit enteropathogens. They have been used to treat inflammatory bowel disease, food allergy, chronic antibiotic use, and diarrhea.

Bioflavonoids

Bioflavonoids are plant chemicals (phytochemicals) also called bioflavins or vitamin P. They are found in citrus pulp and a variety of other plants. They are known for their potential antioxidant activity.

Fiber

Soluble fiber from fruits and insoluble fiber from vegetables and whole grains are known for their ability to soften stool. Fiber is used to treat constipation and diabetes mellitus.

Ginkgo

Ginkgo biloba is thought to increase circulation to the brain and extremities and has been reported to improve memory and symptoms of senile dementia in people.

St. John's Wort

St. John's wort is a plant that has reported (anecdotal) antianxiety and antidepression effects in people.

Saw Palmetto

Saw palmetto plant extract may be of value in treating benign prostatic hyperplasia because of its possible ability to reduce testosterone formation.

Superoxide Dismutase

Superoxide dismutase from protein sources is an oxygen radical scavenger that has been used as an antiinflammatory agent for musculoskeletal problems.

Coenzyme Q

This substance is an enzyme co-factor of mitochondrial membranes that is important in electron transport and ATP formation. It is used in the treatment of cardiovascular problems.

Aloe Vera

The aloe vera plant is known to contain substances with immunomodulator activity.

S-Adenosylmethion (SAMe)

The SAMe SD4 is a molecule produced in the body from methionine and ATP by the enzyme SAMe synthetase (Davidson, 2002). It is recommended for veterinary use as a dietary supplement to support normal structure and function of the liver.

 Miscellaneous Antidotes

Activated Charcoal

Activated charcoal is a fine, black, odorless, tasteless powder used to adsorb certain drugs or toxins to prevent or reduce their systemic absorption from the upper gastrointestinal tract.

Clinical Uses. These include oral administration to prevent or reduce the systemic absorption of certain drugs or toxins.

Dosage Forms
1. Toxiban Suspension
2. Toxiban Granules
3. Activated charcoal powder (generic) (for reconstitution with water)

Adverse Side Effects. These include vomiting after very rapid administration of activated charcoal. Activated charcoal can also cause either constipation or diarrhea, and the stool is black.

Technician's Notes
1. Activated charcoal is not considered effective against heavy metals (e.g., lead, mercury, and inorganic arsenic), mineral acids, caustic alkalis, nitrates, sodium, chloride/chlorate, ferrous sulfate, or petroleum distillates.
2. Other oral therapeutic agents should not be administered within 3 hours after activated charcoal therapy.
3. Dairy products and mineral oil reduce activated charcoal's adsorptive properties.

Calcium EDTA

Calcium EDTA (CaEDTA) is a heavy metal **chelating agent** available commercially (human) as an injection. It may also be referred to as edetate calcium disodium, calcium disodium edetate, calcium edetate, calcium disodium ethylenediaminetetraacetate, and sodium calcium edetate.

Clinical Uses. In veterinary medicine, calcium EDTA is used for the treatment of lead poisoning.

Dosage Forms
1. Calcium Disodium Versenate injection (human label)
2. Meta-Dote

Adverse Side Effects. These include renal toxicity, depression (dogs), and vomiting/diarrhea (dogs). Zinc deficiency may occur from chronic therapy.

Technician's Notes
1. Calcium EDTA should not be used in anuric patients, and caution should be exercised when it is used in patients with renal insufficiency.
2. Calcium EDTA should not be administered orally.
3. Do not confuse with edetate disodium, which may cause severe hypocalcemia.
4. Magnesium sulfate (Epsom salt) or sodium sulfate may be used orally to prevent further intestinal absorption of lead.

Methylene Blue

Methylene blue is a thiazine dye that appears as dark green crystals or crystalline powder with a bronzelike luster. It is an oxidating agent that helps to convert methemoglobin (a compound formed from hemoglobin by oxidation of the iron atom) from the ferrous (Fe^{2+}) to the ferric (Fe^{3+}) state. It does not function as an oxygen carrier to hemoglobin.

Clinical Uses. Methylene blue is used for treatment of **methemoglobinemia** resulting from oxidative agents (e.g., nitrites, nitrates, and chlorates) in ruminants. It may be used for cyanide toxicity in ruminants. It can be used in dogs to intraoperatively stain pancreatic islet cell tumors preferentially and for treatment of acetaminophen poisoning.

Dosage Forms
1. Methylene blue injection (generic) (human label)
2. Methylene blue tablets (generic)
3. Methylene blue powder (generic)

Adverse Side Effects. These include the development of Heinz body anemia or morphologic changes in red blood cells and decreased red blood cell life span. Methemoglobinemia may occur but is usually dose- and species-dependent. Tissue necrosis may occur with subcutaneous administration or extravasation during intravenous injection.

Technician's Notes
1. Methylene blue is usually contraindicated in cats.
2. Dogs and horses may show greater occurrence of side effects than ruminants.
3. Methylene blue should not be used in patients with renal insufficiency.
4. Safety during pregnancy is unknown.

Acetylcysteine

Acetylcysteine is a white crystalline powder that is soluble in water or alcohol. It may also be referred to as *N*-acetylcysteine or *N*-acetyl-L-cysteine.

Clinical Uses. These include oral therapy for acetaminophen poisoning in dogs and cats. It may also be used as a mucolytic agent for pulmonary (via nebulization) or ophthalmic (via topical application) conditions.

Dosage Forms
1. Mucomyst (human label)
2. Mucosil (human label)
3. Acetylcysteine (human label)

Adverse Side Effects. These include nausea, vomiting, and occasionally urticaria (hives) when administered orally. Chest tightness, bronchoconstriction, bronchial or tracheal irritation, and acetylcysteine hypersensitivity are rare but are possible side effects when administered into the pulmonary tract. Acetylcysteine may cause bronchospasm in some patients receiving treatment via the pulmonary tract.

Technician's Notes
1. Acetylcysteine is incompatible with amphotericin B, chlortetracycline hydrochloride, erythromycin lactobionate, oxytetracycline hydrochloride, ampicillin sodium, tetracycline hydrochloride, iodized oil, hydrogen peroxide, chymotrypsin, and trypsin.
2. Activated charcoal may adsorb acetylcysteine, reducing its effectiveness in treating acetaminophen toxicity.
3. Carefully monitor patients that have bronchospastic diseases and that receive pulmonary treatment.
4. Oral solution has a bad taste, and a masking agent (e.g., colas, juices) may be used.
5. Open vials should be refrigerated and discarded after 96 hours.

Dimercaprol

Dimercaprol is a dithiol chelating agent that occurs as a colorless or nearly colorless viscous liquid with a disagreeable odor. The commercial solution may be cloudy or may contain small amounts of flaky material or sediment. This is normal and does not indicate deterioration of the product. It may also be referred to as BAL, British antilewisite, dimercaptopropranol, or dithioglycerol.

Clinical Uses. Dimercaprol is primarily used for the treatment of toxicity resulting from arsenic compounds but may be used for lead, mercury, or gold toxicity.

Dosage Forms
1. Dimercaprol injection 100 mg/ml (human label)
2. BAL in oil (human label)

Adverse Side Effects. Intramuscular injections are painful. Vomiting and seizures may occur with high doses. It is potentially nephrotoxic. Most side effects subside quickly because of rapid elimination of the drug.

Pralidoxime Chloride

Pralidoxime chloride is a quaternary ammonium oxime cholinesterase reactivator. It reverses the action of cholinesterase inhibitors, such as certain organophosphates. It may also be referred to as a 2-PAM chloride or 2-pyridine aldoxime methyl chloride.

Clinical Uses. Pralidoxime chloride is used for oral treatment of organophosphate poisoning. It may be used in conjunction with atropine and supportive therapy.

Dosage Form
1. Protopam injection (human label)

Adverse Side Effects. These are uncommon, but rapid intravenous injection may cause tachycardia, muscle rigidity, transient neuromuscular blockade, and laryngospasm.

Technician's Notes
1. Pralidoxime, like other anticholinesterases, may potentiate the action of barbiturates.
2. Patients with impaired renal function require a lower dose and careful monitoring.

Penicillamine

Penicillamine is a chelating agent of metals, such as copper, lead, iron, and mercury. It is a degradation product of penicillins but does not have antimicrobial activity. It may also be referred to as D-penicillamine, B, B-dimethylcysteine, or D,3-mercaptovaline.

Clinical Uses. Penicillamine is used for copper-associated hepatopathy and for long-term oral treatment of lead poisoning and cystine urolithiasis.

Dosage Forms
1. Depen Titratabs, tablets (human label)
2. Cuprimine capsules (human label)

Adverse Side Effects. These include nausea and vomiting. Other rare side effects include fever, lymphadenopathy, skin hypersensitivity reactions, or immune-complex glomerulonephropathy.

Technician's Notes
Absorption of penicillamine may be reduced by concurrent administration of food, antacids, or iron salts.

Sodium Thiosulfate

Sodium thiosulfate uses the enzyme rhodanese to convert cyanide to a nontoxic thiocyanate ion, which is excreted in the urine.

Clinical Uses. Sodium thiosulfate is used in the treatment of cyanide poisoning in horses and ruminants. It may be used in combination with sodium molybdate for the treatment of copper poisoning in ruminants. It has also been used for treatment of arsenic poisoning. When applied topically, sodium thiosulfate has antifungal properties.

Dosage Forms
1. Cya-dote Injection
2. Sodium Thiosulfate for Injection 25% (human label)

Adverse Side Effects. These are uncommon.

> ### Technician's Notes
> When administering sodium thiosulfate intravenously, it should be given slowly.

Ethanol

Ethanol is an alcohol that is a competitive inhibitor of ethylene glycol metabolism. It may also be referred to as pure grain alcohol, grain alcohol, or ethyl alcohol.

Clinical Uses. Ethanol is used to treat ethylene glycol (antifreeze) poisoning.

Dosage Form
Ethanol

Adverse Side Effects. Ethanol reduces body temperature and can be fatal if overdosed.

> ### Technician's Notes
> 1. A 20% to 50% solution of pure ethanol is administered intravenously until the animal is comatose and does not respond to a toe pinch. Administration is repeated as needed to maintain a comatose state for 3 days.
> 2. Sodium bicarbonate is usually administered to control metabolic acidosis.

Fomepizole

Fomepizole is competitive inhibitor of alcohol dehydrogenase. Its action prevents the conversion of ethylene glycol into glycoaldehyde and other toxic metabolites. This allows ethylene glycol to be excreted primarily unchanged. It may also be referred to as 4-methylpyrazole (4-MP).

Clinical Uses. Fomepizole is used to treat ethylene glycol (antifreeze) poisoning in dogs.

Adverse Side Effects. Clinical signs of possible anaphylaxis include tachypnea, gagging, excessive salivation, and trembling.

Dosage Form
Antizol-Vet

> ### Technician's Notes
> 1. Fomepizole must be diluted with 0.9% NaCl before intravenous injection.
> 2. Dogs treated within 8 hours of ingestion have a better prognosis than those treated 10 to 12 hours after ingestion (Plumb, 2002).

Antivenin Polyvalent (Crotalidae)/ Antivenin (Micrurus fulvius) Coral Snake

These products are concentrated serum globulins collected from horses vaccinated with different types of snake venoms.

Clinical Uses. These products are used in the treatment of snakebite in domestic animals from many of the poisonous snakes of North America. A bottle of Crotalidae antivenin may cost $100 per vial, and one to five vials may be needed for treatment. The coral snake product (human label) may cost more than $150 per vial (Plumb, 2002).

Dosage Forms
1. Antivenin—Fort Dodge. Approved for use in dogs.
2. Antivenin (Crotalidae) Polyvalent Equine Origin (human label)—Wyeth-Ayerst
3. Antivenin (Micrurus fulvius)—Wyeth-Ayerst

Adverse Side Effects. Anaphylaxis may occur.

Vitamin K-1 (Phytonadione)

Vitamin K-1 is necessary for the synthesis of blood coagulation factors II, VII, IX, and X by the liver.

Clinical Uses. The main use of this product is for the treatment of anticoagulant rodenticide poisoning.

Dosage Forms
1. Phytonadione. Numerous veterinary-approved products are available, including oral capsules and an aqueous colloidal solution for injection.

2. Phytonadione (human label). Mephyton oral capsules and Aqua-Mephyton injectable.

Adverse Side Effects. Anaphylaxis may occur with intravenous injection. The intramuscular route is usually recommended.

Thiamine HCl

Thiamine HCl is a water soluble B vitamin used for the treatment or prevention of thiamine deficiency.

Clinical Uses. Thiamine HCl is used for thiamine deficiency in several species. It is used to treat polioencephalomalacia in cattle, sheep, and goats, and thiamine deficiencies associated with dietary lack or thiamine-destroying compounds in the diet.

Dosage Form
Thiamine HCl. Numerous veterinary and human-label products are available.

Adverse Side Effects. Hypersensitivity or muscle soreness may be seen.

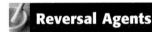

Reversal Agents

Atipamezole HCl

Atipamezole acts as a reversal agent for alpha$_2$-adrenergic agonists by competitively inhibiting alpha$_2$-adrenergic receptors.

Clinical Uses. Atipamezole HCl is used for the reversal of medetomidine (Domitor). It has also been used in the treatment of amitraz toxicity.

Dosage Form
Antisedan

Adverse Side Effects. These include vomiting, diarrhea, hypersalivation, tremors, and apprehension.

Technician's Notes

Pain perception returns after administration of atipamezole.

Flumazenil

Flumazenil acts as a benzodiazepine antagonist by acting as a competitive blocker of benzodiazepines at benzodiazepine receptors.

Clinical Uses. Flumazenil is used for the reversal of benzodiazepines.

Dosage Form
Romazicon (human label)

Adverse Side Effects. Seizures may occur.

Naloxone HCl

Naloxone is a narcotic antagonist. It is structurally related to oxymorphone and may be referred to as *N*-allylnoroxymorphone HCl.

Clinical Uses. Naloxone is used for the treatment, prevention, or control of narcotic depression.

Dosage Forms
1. P/M Naloxone HCl injection
2. Narcan (human label)

Adverse Side Effects. These are uncommon.

Technician's Notes
1. Intravenous injection provides the quickest response.
2. A repeat dose may be necessary if the action of the narcotic outlasts the action of naloxone.
3. Naloxone also reverses the effects of butorphanol (Torbugesic), pentazocine (Talwin-V), and nalbuphine (Nubain).

Tolazoline HCl

Tolazoline is a competitive alpha$_1$- and alpha$_2$-adrenergic receptor blocking agent that reverses the effects of alpha$_2$-adrenergic agonists.

Clinical Uses. Tolazoline HCl is used in horses for the reversal of xylazine (Rompun).

Dosage Form
Tolazine

Adverse Side Effects. These include transient tachycardia, peripheral vasodilation, licking lips, piloerection, clear lacrimal and nasal discharge, muscle fasciculations, and apprehension.

Technician's Notes
1. Tolazoline is not approved for use in food-producing animals.
2. Tolazoline has a short duration and may require repeated doses.

Yohimbine HCl
Yohimbine is an alpha$_2$-adrenergic receptor antagonist that reverses the effects of alpha$_2$-adrenergic agonists.

Clinical Uses. Yohimbine is used to reverse the effects of xylazine (Rompun). This action usually occurs within 1 to 3 minutes. It is approved for use in dogs and deer but is also effective in other species.

Dosage Forms
1. Yobine
2. Antagonil (approved for deer)

Technician's Notes
1. Normal pain perception remains after administration of yohimbine.
2. Caution should be exercised when using in epileptic or seizure-prone patients.
3. Yohimbine should not be used in food-producing animals.
4. Safety in pregnant or breeding animals is unknown.

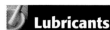

Lubricants

Lubricants are used to lubricate hands, arms, or instruments before gynecologic and rectal examinations.

Dosage Forms
1. K-Y Jelly
2. Lube Jelly
3. Lubri-Nert
4. Lubrivet

Adverse Side Effects. Adverse side effects are uncommon.

Technician's Notes
Petroleum jelly (Vaseline) is not recommended for use as a lubricant because it is not water-soluble and is not easily rinsed from instruments.

REFERENCES

Boothe DM: Antiinflammatory drugs. In Boothe DM: Small animal clinical pharmacology and therapeutics, Philadelphia, 2001, WB Saunders Co.

Boothe DM: Nutraceuticals in veterinary medicine: part I definitions and regulations. Compend Contin Educ Prac Vet 19(11):1248-1255, 1997.

Davidson G: S-adenosylmethionine, Compend Contin Educ Prac Vet 24(8):600-603, 2002.

Davidson G: Glucosamine and chondroitin sulfate, Compend Contin Educ Prac Vet 22(5):454-458, 2000.

Fascetti AJ: Nutraceuticals and food faddism, World Wide Web document, http://www.avma.org/noah/default.asp, 1998.

Plumb DC: Veterinary drug handbook, ed 4, Ames, Iowa, 2002, Iowa State University Press.

Roudebush P and Freeman LM: Nutritional management of heart disease. In Bonagura JD, editor: Kirk's current veterinary therapy small animal practice, XIII, Philadelphia, 2000, WB Saunders Co.

REVIEW QUESTIONS

1. A 2-year-old beagle has clinical signs of lead toxicity and a history to support the diagnosis. Which agent would be the drug of choice for treating this condition?
   a. Yohimbine HCl
   b. 2-PAM
   c. Calcium EDTA
   d. Methylene blue

2. A client calls and says that she has been giving her cat Tylenol for a limp. Now the cat is breathing fast, its face is swollen, and it is not active. You should tell the client to:
   a. Give the cat hydrogen peroxide orally
   b. See whether she can get the cat to eat
   c. Bring the cat to the hospital to start treatment with hydrogen peroxide
   d. Bring the cat to the hospital to start treatment with acetylcysteine

3. Yohimbine HCl is a reversal agent for:
   a. Rompun
   b. Acepromazine
   c. Pentothal
   d. Oxymorphone

4. Penicillamine should be administered
   a. With food
   b. On an empty stomach
   c. With antacids
   d. With copper

5. Name four drugs that naloxone effectively reverses.

   _____

   _____

   _____

   _____

6. BAL has been administered to a 4-year-old, mixed-breed dog for arsenic poisoning. Results

of which of the following laboratory tests should be monitored closely?
   a. Packed cell volume (PCV)
   b. Blood urea nitrogen (BUN)
   c. White blood cell count (WBC)
   d. Alanine aminotransferase (ALT)

7. Glycosaminoglycans occur naturally in what part(s) of the body?

   _____.

8. What role do glycosaminoglycans (GAGs) provide in the treatment of degenerative joint conditions? _____

9. Define nutraceutical. Give an example.

   _____

10. True or False: A product is usually determined to be a drug if its label has a claim that indicates a therapeutic or preventive intent.

    _____

11. What Act made dietary supplements as vitamins, minerals, amino acids, herbal products, and substances that supplement the diet by increasing total dietary intake "food" and excluded them from FDA regulation?

12. _____ supplementation has been shown to be useful in treating certain dermatology conditions in dogs and cats.

13. What are two possible side effects for using fatty acids as a dietary supplement?

    _____

14. What is activated charcoal used for?

    _____

15. In veterinary medicine, calcium EDTA is used primarily for the treatment of

    _____.

16. Petroleum jelly is not recommended as a lubricant because it is not

    _____.

17. _____ is a narcotic antagonist used for the treatment, prevention, or control of narcotic depression.

18. Yohimbine is used to reverse the effects of _____.

19. A dietary supplement for support of normal structure and function of the liver is _____.

20. Grain alcohol may be used to treat what poisoning? _____

INTRODUCTION
INVENTORY
The Time Equation
Turnover
   Calculating Turnover Rate
CONTROLLING INVENTORY
A Proactive Inventory Control System
Keeping Accurate Records
Inventory Records
   Reorder Quantity
   Rabies Vaccine
Organizing Inventory
   Pharmacy and ICM office
   Organizing Inventory in the Veterinary
     Hospital
   Staff Memos
   Special Conditions
Physical Inventory
   Monthly Inventory Versus Rotating
     Inventory
Purchasing Information
   Incoming Freight
   FOB Rules
   Receiving Freight
   Stocking Shelves
   Vendors
   Communicating With Sales
     Representatives
   DEA Forms
   Special Orders
   Human Pharmacy
Computers and Inventory
The Job of ICM

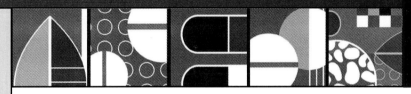

CHAPTER **19**

Inventory: The Veterinary Technician's Role

LEARNING OBJECTIVES

After studying this chapter, you should be able to:

1. Understand why having an inventory control system is important
2. Know ways in which inventory control benefits a business
3. Understand why inventory turnover is important
4. Know ways of becoming an efficient inventory control manager
5. Become familiar with various inventory record-keeping systems
6. Understand the differences in vendor types
7. Understand good communication techniques to use with sales representatives
8. Understand ways veterinary management computer software aids pharmaceutic inventory

KEY TERMS

AVERAGE COST OF INVENTORY ON HAND Average cost of inventory on hand is determined by adding the year's beginning inventory to the year's ending inventory and dividing by 2.

DEA FORM An official federal government carbon form used for ordering controlled substances.

DELAYED BILLING A benefit some companies offer the buyer purchasing increased amounts of merchandise. The date the statement must be paid is usually greater than 30 to 60 days.

FOB Acronym for "free on board."

FOB DESTINATION Title of possession passes from the pharmaceutical company to the buyer (i.e., the purchaser) when the shipment is delivered to the buyer's business destination (i.e., the veterinary facility).

FOB SHIPPING POINT Title passes from the pharmaceutical company to the purchaser when the vendor places the goods in the possession of the carrier (e.g., United Parcel Service, Federal Express, Averitt Express, etc.).

FULL-SERVICE COMPANY A pharmaceutical company offering full service (e.g., the company employs sales representatives (reps) who visit veterinary facilities), usually with a limited number of products.

INVENTORY The amount of goods or assets a veterinary facility possesses requiring proactive control to keep supplies stable and current.

ICM (INVENTORY CONTROL MANAGER) A person (many times a licensed veterinary medical techni-cian [LVMT]) responsible for monitoring, ordering, and maintaining inventory in a veterinary facility.

INVOICE A form generated by a company documenting the quantity and the price of each item ordered by the inventory control manager.

MAIL-ORDER DISCOUNT HOUSES A company accepting orders from the buyer by telephone; a good source for ordering items such as gauze, cotton, isopropyl alcohol, or paper towels.

MARKUP The amount of money over cost that a product sells for. Markup percentages vary from practice to practice, but all markups reflect a retail value over wholesale value.

PACKING SLIP A document supplied by the vendor accompanying a purchase. A packing slip generally reflects quantities ordered, not prices.

STATEMENT A document generated by the vendor that details the quantity and pricing of all goods purchased (usually in 1 month) by the buyer. The total balance is generally expected to be paid in full within 30 days.

TURNOVER The number of times a product is sold or used up in a veterinary facility. The minimum turnover rate should be established at four times a year.

VETERINARY SUPPLY DISTRIBUTOR An intermediate company (i.e., not full service, not mail order) that generally stocks a large inventory and employs sales representatives who visit veterinary facilities.

INTRODUCTION

Controlling inventory is an important concern for companies both large and small, and veterinary businesses are no exception. Proactively maintaining pharmaceutic inventory is an ongoing endeavor for veterinary hospitals (Figure 19-1). Deciding how much trade- or generic-name product to buy, keeping expired items off the shelves, and performing a physical inventory are all integral parts of keeping a veterinary facility functioning as a healthy business. When product is depleted before the next order arrives, it is frustrating for both the veterinary staff and clientele. When product is not available, it cannot be sold and no profit can be made. Deciding which employee to entrust with this responsibility is an important decision for veterinary practice owners and should be made with careful consideration. Therefore the employee chosen for this job should treat the position with respect and make every effort to be frugal with the employer's money.

The veterinary technician is often the employee chosen to perform this job. Therefore knowledge of pharmaceutic products and the ability to observe amounts of product used within a month are important talents the veterinary technician must possess.

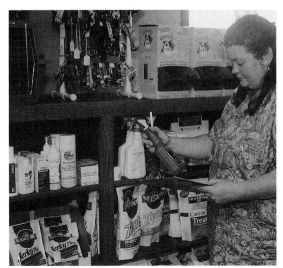

FIGURE 19-1
A veterinary technician taking inventory.

In our technologically advanced society, pharmaceutic products change rapidly, and new products are constantly being developed. The veterinary technician charged with being the ICM must be willing to learn about new products and pass this information on to the whole veterinary staff. Communication and good people skills are useful when dealing with pharmaceutic sales representatives. Sales reps are invaluable to veterinary practices, because they are armed with all available information about drugs, both old and new.

The ICM has many responsibilities, some of which include keeping the staff informed regarding discontinued items, knowing the dates on which back-ordered items will be released from the vendor, packing in boxes those goods awaiting return to the vendor (e.g., expired items), rotating stock correctly, maintaining current prices on all products, organizing inventory for easy location and counting, receiving and inspecting orders upon arrival at the veterinary facility, and learning about new products. These are only a few of the responsibilities the ICM will meet daily. Inventory should be handled as a continuing process. Each day inventory must be visually counted, and physical inventory must be done at least once a month.

INVENTORY

Accounting of inventory items is very important in the event of a fire or natural disaster. Veterinary practices providing an accurate inventory of their business assets are assured that their insurance companies will reimburse the business accurately should a disaster occur. This is but one of the many reasons inventory should be taken seriously.

Inventory is an ongoing process, and trends within the practice must be observed daily. The ICM must be able to recognize the products each veterinarian in the practice uses and dispenses to ensure items are on hand when needed. Nothing is more frustrating than needing a drug or other inventory item to treat a patient with only to find it is not in stock. Computer software designed for the veterinary business can help tremendously with tracking trends within the practice. Most software has the ability to provide printouts of day-by-day, week-by-week, month-by-month, and yearly sales trends (Figure 19-2).

By establishing a workable inventory control system within a realistic budget, expenses can be kept at a minimum.

Date: 05-21-03

INVENTORY REPORT

Code	Description	U/M	Price	On hand	Avg cost	Stock value	Unit cost	Pkg. cost	Codes	Cls	Last sold	Document
ANTHELMINTICS						0.00						
CANINE VACCINES												
1008	Bordetella (Injection)	Ds	0.00	14	0.000	0.00	0.000	0.000		1		
	Qty sold, Last 12 Months											
	May Jun Jul Aug Sep Oct Nov Dec Jan Feb Mar Apr May											
1009	Bordetella (Intra-nasal)	Ds	0.00	1	0.000	0.00	0.000	0.000		0		09-28-01
	Qty sold, Last 12 Months											
	May Jun Jul Aug Sep Oct Nov Dec Jan Feb Mar Apr May											
9010	DA2PP/CV	Ds	0.00	15	0.000	0.00	0.000	0.000		0		
	Qty sold, Last 12 Months											
	May Jun Jul Aug Sep Oct Nov Dec Jan Feb Mar Apr May											
9052	Rabies Vaccine	Ds	0.00	21	0.000	0.00	0.000	0.000		1		
	Qty sold, Last 12 Months											
	May Jun Jul Aug Sep Oct Nov Dec Jan Feb Mar Apr May											
CANINE VACCINES						0.00						
MISCELLANEOUS ITEMS												
1007	Large Garbage Sacks	Box	0.00	0	0.000	0.00	0.000	0.000		1		
	Qty sold, Last 12 Months											
	May Jun Jul Aug Sep Oct Nov Dec Jan Feb Mar Apr May											
7022	Small Garbage Sacks	Box	0.00	0	0.000	0.00	0.000	0.000		1		
	Qty sold, Last 12 Months											
	May Jun Jul Aug Sep Oct Nov Dec Jan Feb Mar Apr May											
7023	Computer Printer Paper	PACK	0.00	0	0.000	0.00	0.000	0.000		1		
	Qty sold, Last 12 Months											
	May Jun Jul Aug Sep Oct Nov Dec Jan Feb Mar Apr May											

FIGURE 19-2
AVI-mark veterinary software management system.

After determining and implementing a realistic budget based on the mission statement of the facility and practice needs, and implementing that budget, there will be no danger of running out of inventory items, because there will always be sufficient numbers of product on hand. An annual inventory evaluation is beneficial when developing a vision for the practice and its potential growth.

The Time Equation

When dealing with inventory, no equation is more important than:

$$Time = Money$$

Although it is important to have merchandise on hand for retail sale, a fine balance exists in order to keep products from sitting too long on the pharmacy shelves. Products staying on the shelf for too long will not make money for the veterinary practice. Instead, it is like placing money in a jar and burying it in the back yard; the money is there, but it is not earning interest and it is not working for you. So it is with inventory products. A fine inventory balance is crucial to the financial health of a business. Besides, clients do not like to buy products that have been sitting on the pharmacy shelves for a long time, because the labels become smudged and dusty.

A periodic evaluation of inventory is crucial to keeping the balance in fine adjustment. Items not selling well or used infrequently within the practice should be deleted from the inventory master list and not ordered in the future. This is where turnover becomes an important issue.

Turnover

Technician's Notes

Turnover is the number of times a product is sold or used in-house on an annual basis.

Since there are 12 months in a year, the ideal situation is to use all inventory each month and reorder in time to begin the next month. However, in the real world, this simply does not happen.

Technician's Notes

Four turnovers is a workable goal, while 12 turnovers may be set as the ideal goal. A mean turnover rate of eight turns per year is acceptable for most veterinary practices.

Calculating Turnover Rate

The following equation determines turnover rate:

$$Turnover\ Rate = \frac{Yearly\ inventory\ expense}{Average\ cost\ of\ inventory\ on\ hand}$$

Example:

$$\frac{\$100,000}{\$20,000} = 5$$

The following equation determines the **average cost of inventory on hand:**

$$Average\ cost\ of\ inventory\ on\ hand = \frac{Year's\ beginning\ inventory + Year's\ ending\ inventory}{2}$$

Example:

$$\frac{\$150,000 + \$35,000}{2} = \$92,500$$

CONTROLLING INVENTORY

Establishing effective inventory control in a veterinary practice necessitates placing a person in charge of ordering and stocking supplies. An additional person trained as a backup is a must, because when the ICM goes on vacation or is sick, someone else must be knowledgeable about the system. These two people can work effectively as a team to keep product supplies on hand.

The duties of the ICM are intense. This person is responsible for keeping an adequate supply of all products used, dispensed, and sold; organizing inventory items for easy location; recognizing when products need to be reordered; keeping accurate inventory records; ordering, receiving, and inspecting shipments; and maintaining price and price updates for all items. The ICM also is responsible for rotating stock, keeping expired items off the shelves, learning about new products, and keeping the practice owner apprised of the specials suppliers may offer. This responsibility must be acted upon every day. The veterinary technician accepting the role of ICM must be able to perform clinical and nursing skills and keep an eye on inventory levels.

Technician's Notes

The objectives of an inventory control system are twofold:

1. To make certain items are on hand when needed.
2. Being able to purchase needed items while staying within a budgeted amount.

A Proactive Inventory Control System

In order for an inventory control system to be workable, it must be easy to use and have a turnover rate of at least four turns per year. It is the inventory control manager's job to make sure all supplies are on hand when needed. Expenses can be reduced when amounts of inventory are ordered properly.

Proper handling of DEA substances is an important concern.

Technician's Notes

Controlled substances (e.g., Sleepaway, diazepam) must be kept in a locked cabinet that has been bolted to the floor, and all amounts used must be correctly recorded in the controlled substance log.

DEA forms (Figure 19-3) must be filled out properly by including the correct spelling of the substance to be ordered, documenting the exact amount and milligrams, and obtaining the signature of the veterinarian. No liquid paper may be used on these forms, and no strikeouts are allowed. In addition, these forms must be filled out using an ink pen or a typewriter.

Each **invoice** (Figure 19-4) arriving at the veterinary hospital should be checked to verify amounts ordered and prices the practice is charged. A packing slip (Figure 19-5), an invoice, and a statement (Figure 19-6) are three different forms. Mistakes can be made on these forms unintentionally by the product vendor, but it may fall to the ICM to audit these mistakes and notify the vendor so the account can be adjusted to receive proper credit.

Back-ordered items can present problems. Back-ordered items are those items not on hand at the vendor for any number of reasons. Sometimes the product may be on back order because of manufacturing reasons, while another reason may be that the manufacturer is redesigning the product's label. Buyouts of large pharmaceutic corporations can also cause product to be on back order until all minor details are worked out concerning the merger.

Identification of expired items may be one of the most frustrating experiences an ICM may face.

Technician's Notes

Most products have an expiration date on the label, and these must be checked frequently in order to remove them from the pharmacy.

Veterinary practice management systems software can be an invaluable aid in tracking expired items. When products are received, the *earliest* expiration date should be the one that is recorded in the computer system. Therefore at the beginning of each month, the computer will reflect those products expiring first, and the ICM can print a list of the "old" drugs and quickly remove them from the pharmacy. As soon as the "old" products have been removed from the pharmacy shelves, the next

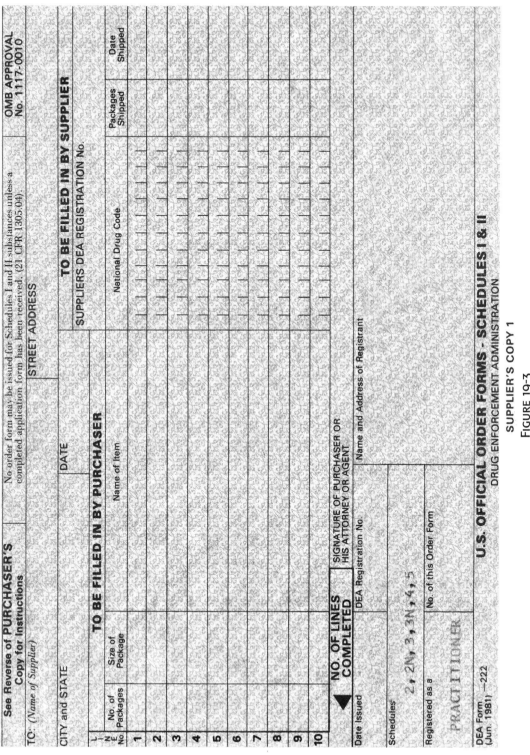

FIGURE 19-3
An example of a DEA form.

The Phamaceutical Warehouse
1546 Warehouse Road
Plains, Georgia 36945

INVOICE

Ship To:

All Pets Veterinary Hospital
1785 Lawrenceville Road
Lawrenceville, Georgia 37965

Bill To:

All Pets Veterinary Hospital
1785 Lawrenceville Road
Lawrenceville, Georgia 37965

Bill To	Invoice Total
A7796	$335.10
Invoice Number	**Invoice Date**
953146-000	06-03-03
Customer Account Number	**Ship To**
198531	Lawrenceville, Georgia

Item Code	Unit/Size	Description/ Strength	Quantity Ordered	Quantity Shipped	Item Status	Unit Price	Extension	Box No.	REM
15637	18/box	Vetrap	3	3	Sent	$54.95	$164.85	1	
15937	9/pack	Gauze bandage rolls	5	5	Sent	$25.65	$128.25	1	
13465	Each	Roll Cotton	12	12	Sent	$ 3.50	$ 42.00	1	

- *Please note that late payments are subject to a 1.5% monthly finance charge*

Merchandise Total
$335.10

Invoice Total
$335.10

* Please pay within thirty days of receipt of this invoice.

FIGURE 19-4
A sample invoice.

The Phamaceutical Warehouse

PACKING LIST

Ship To:
All Pets Veterinary Hospital
1785 Lawrenceville Road
Lawrenceville, Georgia 37965

Bill To:
All Pets Veterinary Hospital
1785 Lawrenceville Road
Lawrenceville, Georgia 37965

Customer Account Number		Ship To	
198531		Lawrenceville, Georgia	

Item Code	Unit/Size	Description/ Strength	Quantity Ordered	Quantity Shipped	Item Status	Unit Price	Extension	Box No.	REM
15637	18/box	Vetrap	3	3	Sent	$54.95	$164.85	1	
15937	9/pack	Gauze bandage rolls	5	5	Sent	$25.65	$128.25	1	
13465	Each	Roll Cotton	12	12	Sent	$ 3.50	$ 42.00	1	

FIGURE 19-5
A sample packing slip. (Some vendors don't record prices on their packing slips.)

earliest expiration date is recorded in the computer. Some pharmaceutic companies have policies that entitle the practice to free replacement of expired items. However, other vendors do not concur with this arrangement, and therefore the ICM must be able to distinguish which expired product will produce a free product refund and which will not. There are some pharmaceutic companies that prefer to credit the facility's account instead of sending replacement merchandise, while others offer no reimbursement whatsoever for expired items.

Hopefully, pilferage will not occur in the veterinary facility. However, an effective inventory control system will deter employees who may elect to steal, because they know that inventory is counted on a regular basis. Likewise, merchandise displayed (e.g., leashes, collars, shampoo, or groom-ing brushes) in the reception area of a veterinary facility can be enticing to some clients who may decide to "pick up" an item instead of paying for it. This is another reason why proper inventory control plays an important role.

 Keeping Accurate Records

An orderly way of keeping track of data concerning inventory should be employed. Most veterinary facilities in this age of computer technology use software designed especially for the veterinary business. Remember, when dealing with computers, the old adage—"garbage in, garbage out" "GIGO" — can detract from the quality of information a computer contains.

The Phamaceutical Warehouse
1546 Warehouse Road
Plains, Georgia 36945

STATEMENT

0100000034569786221321313213213132456654

Statement Date	Account Number	Due Date
06-03-03	198531	07-03-03
New Balance	**Indicate Amount Enclosed**	
$335.10		

The Pharmaceutical Warehouse
1546 Warehouse Road
Plains, Georgia 36945

Please detach here and return the above portion with your payment

Questions? Call 1-800-897-3679

Account Name	Account Number	Statement Date	Statement Number	Page
All Pets Veterinary Hospital	198531	06-03-03	3596342	1 of 1

BALANCE SUMMARY

Previous Balance	Add Purchases	Payments	Credits	Late Charge	Adjustments	Balance Due
$120.00	$335.10	$120.00	0.00	0.00	0.00	$335.10

ACCOUNT AGING

1-30 Days Past Due	31-60 Days Past Due	61-90 Days Past Due	91-120 Days Past Due	>120 Days Past Due	Current Balance
0.00	0.00	0.00	0.00	0.00	$335.10

FIGURE 19-6
A sample statement.

Inventory Records

There are many types of inventory records that may be used in a veterinary facility. At least some of the following should be used, although some practices may elect to use them all.

A reorder log, sometimes called a "want book" (Figure 19-7), is an effective way to track products to be ordered. Each member of the veterinary staff can use this log to record items that need to be ordered.

Technician's Notes

All veterinary personnel should know the importance of maintaining inventory and make every effort to record in the reorder log any product that has been depleted.

Re-order Log

Date of Order	Amount	Item Description	Catalog Number	Cost		Extended Cost	
3-14-03	6	Sharps' containers	796029	$ 3	79	$ 22	74
3-15-03	3 boxes	Tuberculin syringes	194356	$ 9	59	$ 28	77
3-15-03	6 boxes	Needles 22ga. x 3¼"	355796	$ 7	50	$ 45	00

FIGURE 19-7
An example of a reorder log.

In a busy practice this habit is of utmost importance, because once supplies have been exhausted, obtaining interim product from the neighboring veterinary facility becomes an "emergency." Afterwards the amounts borrowed must be replaced or paid for.

Technician's Notes
The reorder point is the level reached that necessitates a product reorder.

It is the responsibility of the ICM to set the reorder point. If orders are placed each week, then a minimum of a 3-week supply should be kept in stock. Larger veterinary hospitals, emergency clinics, or colleges of veterinary medicine may require that inventory be ordered via a purchase order. A purchase order is a written form accompanied by a purchase order number. Generally the form is mailed, although it may be faxed to the vendor who will then send the merchandise.

Technician's Notes
In keeping basic order records, it is imperative to keep a copy of each order.

Regardless of whether a purchase order form is mailed to the vendor or an order is given over the phone, all of the following items should be recorded: order date, order amount, order size, name of the product, vendor(s), product catalog number, unit cost, total cost, receive date, amount received, and discount or special cost (i.e., if this applies). By keeping the above items in a written form, an inaccurate order can be corrected easily by contacting the company involved.

An inventory master list provides endless amounts of information. Each veterinary practice should strive to keep a current list of all products in stock. An inventory master list provides information such as name of the product, item number code, usage, order status, and price. Some veterinary management software includes information regarding the seasonal use of products. One category in which this may be important is the area of flea and tick products. Today's computer software designed for veterinary business has the ability to reflect the months containing the highest amount of product sold. For instance, it may be that flea and tick shampoo is purchased more during the months of March through September, as compared with other times of the year. By using this information, the ICM can better predict how much merchandise needs to be ordered. The master list also reflects trade names, generic names, unit size, strength, name of the product's manufacturer, phone numbers, addresses, practice account numbers, order information, unit price, and a formula for calculating markup. (Some of these items are optional.)

Technician's Notes
Markup is the amount of money (usually a percentage) over cost that an item is sold for.

There is a difference between cost and retail value. Cost is what the practice pays for an item. *Total cost* is the amount the item costs plus tax. The retail price is the amount the practice charges a client for an item. Retail price usually includes a profit margin (i.e., markup). Each practice has a way of figuring markup, and the percentages used may vary. A common way to figure total cost is to multiply the product's cost by the appropriate tax. After obtaining the total cost of an item and multiplying by two, a 100% markup (i.e., retail price) is the result. This is illustrated below.

Equation to Figure Total Cost

$$\text{Cost} + \text{Tax} = \text{Total Cost}$$

Example:

Amoxicillin (100 mg, 100-count bottle) cost = $26.75
Tax (@ 10%) = .100
$26.75 × .100 = $2.675
$26.75 + $2.675 = $29.425

To Find Retail Price @ 100% Markup

Total cost of the item × 2 = Retail Price @ 100% markup
$29.43 × 2 = $58.86

Then: $58.86 divided by 100 tablets in the bottle =
.5886 or $0.59 each

So, each tablet can be retailed for $0.59 (or $0.60 to make accounting easier)

Reorder Quantity

When determining the reorder quantity, a good idea is to set the amount equal to a 1-month supply. By ordering a 1-month supply of product, the ICM will not have to micromanage inventory. The reorder quantity can be posted on the computer's master inventory list.

Rabies Vaccine

Records concerning rabies vaccine are very important. Each rabies certificate reflects the vaccine's expiration date and serial number (Figure 19-8). Therefore the ICM must make certain the certificates reflect those numbers by ensuring that the serial number and expiration date are posted correctly in the computer. This is not optional; it *must* be done.

 Organizing Inventory

Pharmacy and ICM Office

> **Technician's Notes**
> Establishing a room in the veterinary facility to serve as the pharmacy office and ICM office provides a place to organize catalogs, journals, magazines, and sales lists.

Other items also can be stored in the pharmacy office, such as DEA order records, OSHA manuals, material safety data sheets (MSDSs), and suppliers' catalogs.

Organizing Inventory in the Veterinary Hospital

The ideal situation for organizing inventory in the veterinary hospital is to establish a centrally located pharmacy area. In this manner all pharmaceutics can be easily counted.

> **Technician's Notes**
> Inventory within the pharmacy area can be arranged in a variety of ways. The most common ways to arrange products are alphabetically, by therapeutic use, or classification of the drug.

An easy way to organize inventory is to print the master inventory list and stock products on the shelf in the same way they are listed on the master list. In this way, when it is time to perform inventory, the products are arranged on the pharmacy shelves in the same order they appear on the master inventory list—thereby enabling inventory to be carried out in a timely fashion.

Staff Memos

> **Technician's Notes**
> The ICM should designate a bulletin board for memos to the veterinary staff.

Memos attached to a bulletin board can alert all the hospital staff of company buyouts, discontinued items, and back-ordered items. Use of a bulletin board provides the ICM with freedom from frustrating interruptions by office staff concerning inventory questions. Additionally, this bulletin board is a good location for the reorder log (i.e., "want book").

CERTIFICATE OF VACCINATION

Date of rabies vaccination	29 APR 03
Next rabies vaccination on	29 APR 04
Certificate number	N/A
Previous rabies vaccination	N/A
Best Veterinary Hospital	
Taylor Lane, DVM	
621 Banner Street	
Camden, Arkansas 71701	
501-836-8390	
Owner's name	**Best Veterinary Client**
Owner's address	**1313 Schnauzer Lane Camden, Arkansas 71701**
County of owner's residence	Ouachita

This is to certify...
That I have vaccinated against rabies the animal described below:

Patient's name	Tangent
Species	Canine
Breed	Mix
Gender	Male/Neutered
Color and markings	Brindle/White on chest
Tag number	N/A
Weight	101.4 lbs.
Age	2 years

Signed:_____
         Taylor Lane, DVM

Vaccinations administered:

RV/DA2PP/CV/*Bordetella*

Manufactured by	Pfizer Animal Health
Serial number	A232705A
Lot expiration date	26 AUG 03
Administration of vaccine	SC on right side

FIGURE 19-8
A sample rabies certificate.

Special Conditions

Some special conditions must be recognized when arranging inventory. Products needing refrigeration have only a limited amount of storage space in the refrigerator. Therefore care should be taken to avoid ordering too large a quantity of these items, because the available amount of refrigeration may not be able to contain the order amount. DEA substances should be kept in a locked cabinet that has been bolted to the floor. Therefore the space within the cabinet should be considered before ordering increased amounts of merchandise.

 Physical Inventory

Monthly Inventory Versus Rotating Inventory

Deciding when and how often to perform this necessary function is the question. One effective method is to perform a rotating inventory. A rotating inventory necessitates the division of like products into categories. The categories are given a number of one through four. For example, each category designated as one is counted during the month of January. Each category designated as two is counted during the month of February, three is counted in March, and four in April. During the month of May, the inventory begins again starting with those categories designated with number one. Thus each category is counted three times a year (Figure 19-9). While this may not be acceptable to all veterinary practice owners, it certainly can be an efficient way to perform a physical inventory. Many times only one person is responsible for inventory control within the veterinary facility, and counting every item stocked in a practice may take a single person 1 to 2 days to complete. If inventory is done on a monthly basis (i.e., all items counted each month), the ICM cannot perform other nursing or technical skills the day inventory is taken. By using a rotating method, a smaller amount of inventory is counted each month, thereby enabling the ICM to have available time for other job duties.

Technician's Notes

Nothing is as effective as performing a physical inventory.

Some practice owners may require a monthly inventory count. However, performing inventory on a rotational 3- to 4-month cycle makes the ICM's job easier. Because of the many functions a veterinary technician may hold in a veterinary practice, allowing a rotating inventory will ensure an accurate count and good use of the veterinary technician's nursing skills.

 Purchasing Information

In a busy veterinary facility an ideal situation is to deal with as few suppliers as possible. The ICM will constantly be involved in an appointment with sales representatives if various vendors are used. Dealing with as few suppliers as possible releases the ICM to assume regular nursing and technical duties also associated with their employment. By asking sales reps to make an appointment, the ICM will know when to expect a visit and better prepare their normal work schedule around the visit. The ICM should be sure that sales representatives are aware of lunch breaks and quitting time; otherwise they may just "pop in" to make a sale and not consider the ICM's schedule.

When dealing with pharmaceutic and supplier sales representatives, it is advantageous to be aware of several things. (Knowledge of the following information will make the ICM more effective in the responsibility of inventory maintenance.) Quantity and assortment discounts are ways that pharmaceutic companies can offer increased quantity of goods. Usually the company will offer a discount for buying in increased amounts, but there are several conditions that must be considered by the ICM. First, how fast can increased amounts of the product be sold in the practice? Remember time is money, and product left sitting in the pharmacy for extended periods will end up costing the practice money even though the merchandise may have been bought at a discounted rate. Also, where will

Anthelmintics (1)

Dry Goods (1)

In-house Products (1)

Anesthetics (1)

Bovine Vaccines (1)

Equine Vaccines (1)

Equine Products (1)

Large Animal Sprays (2)

Flea Products and Shampoo (2)

Large Animal Powders (2)

Otic Products (2)

Ophthalmics (2)

Lab Test Kits (3)

Small Animal Pharmacy (3)

Dietary Items (3)

Heartworm Preventive (3)

Porcine Vaccines (3)

Large Animal Injectables (4)

Large Animal Gallons (4)

Large Animal Products (4)

Small Animal Vaccines (4)

Vitamins (4)

Start rotating inventory in January, by counting all items with a #1 beside them. In February, count all items with a #2 beside them. Proceed in the same manner for the rest of the year and thus, all inventory will be counted three times a year.

FIGURE 19-9
An example of how to divide inventory.

the overstock be stored? Does the practice have sufficient room to store increased quantities of product? Sometimes quantity discounts are not what they appear to be.

Delayed billing is another feature some pharmaceutic and supplier companies may offer. When discounts for quantity buying are offered to the veterinary practice, many times the statement will reflect a delayed billing option (i.e., the statement does not have to be paid within the usual 30-day span). Instead the option of paying within a 60- to 90-day period will extend the discount. Usually no interest is charged the buyer, and the practice owner may be able to purchase increased amounts of stock at a reduced rate without the trial of coming up with funds to pay for it all within a 30-day limit. Consideration must still be given to whether or not there is sufficient room for storage of overstock and how soon the product can be sold.

When placing an order, many companies waive the shipping fee if the veterinary practice orders a minimum amount of product. For example, if the minimum order amount is $250 per order, the ICM can save the practice shipping fees by ordering the minimum amount. Keep in mind that a shipping fee of $10 when multiplied over 10 orders adds up to $100. Shipping costs multiplied by 12 months could buy other products instead of being spent on shipping fees.

Some pharmaceutic and supplier companies offer discounts for early payment. Veterinary practices can save money by paying the **statement** early. This too is a way to save the practice money. On the flip side, penalties may be imposed for statements paid after the 30-day time limit. The amount paid in penalties can also buy product instead of being spent on late fees. Every practice should endeavor to pay within 30 days.

The ICM should also be familiar with each vendor's return policy. Items that are expired may need to be returned along with any item not selling well. Some vendors will allow product to be returned and the practice's account will be credited accordingly. Items that have expired may be picked up by a sales representative and replaced. It should be noted that expired controlled substances cannot be picked up by the sales representative for return to the pharmaceutic company.

Incoming Freight

The inventory control manager must be alert to possible damage incurred to freight during shipping.

Technician's Notes

At the time freight is being unloaded at the veterinary facility, the ICM should visually check for damage by noting any boxes that are not intact. Wetness to the cardboard container may indicate breakage of the contents, and the boxes should be counted and compared with the number of containers listed on the **packing slip**.

As soon as freight arrives, it should be opened and any damages should be noted. Evidence of damage should be reported to the vendor as soon as possible to receive credit and/or replacement of damaged items. Some companies have a 24-hour reporting period (i.e., all damaged items must be reported within 24 hours from time of arrival). The damaged goods should be returned to the vendor, from which they were ordered, in the original shipping carton along with the damaged goods inside. In this way the vendor can assess the damage and apply the correct credit to the veterinary facility's account.

FOB Rules

A vendor delivers freight to the purchaser. The veterinary facility may make an order with a telephone representative, sending or faxing a purchase order, or making an order with the sales representative during his or her appointment at the veterinary facility.

A vendor uses a form of transportation to send the required items to the veterinary hospital (e.g., UPS [United Parcel Service], Averitt Express, Federal Express, or United States Postal Service). Once the vendor releases freight to the carrier, the freight becomes subject to **FOB** (free on board) rules. There are two FOB rules: FOB destination and FOB shipping point.

Receiving Freight

If the order is incorrect, the person who placed the order will know it immediately, whereas a person unpacking freight who did not place the order will not know what is correct. There are several important questions to ask when unpacking an order, such as: "Did I get exactly what I ordered?"; "Did I get the right drug form (i.e., capsules, tablets, or powder)?"; "Did I receive the correct size and/or strength?"; "Is the product's expiration date a long way into the future?"; "Does the invoice list the price I was quoted by the phone rep, or sales rep?"; "Does this order cost more than the last order of the same items?"; "Is anything backordered, and if so, when will that item be shipped?"; "Is any freight damaged or missing?"; "Is the order correct, and if so, can the bill be paid?" (SmithKline, 1993). By asking all these questions, the ICM is assured the veterinary facility will be fairly treated by the vendor.

Stocking Shelves

By rotating stock in this manner, the facility is assured that the product is sold or used by the hospital before the expiration date. When stocking shelves, it is good to record expiration dates. The earliest date should be the one recorded in the computer in order for the software to present an accurate list of expired items when the command is given to print an expired items list. Stocking shelves also presents a convenient time to dust and wipe off labels and lids on products that have been sitting on the shelf for extended periods. It should be noted that after cleaning, products should be replaced in specific locations to facilitate accurate inventory.

Vendors

There are several different types of vendors. The ICM must have adequate knowledge of these types to correctly place an order. Some vendors allow ordering by phone while others require the order be given to a sales rep. Still others require a faxed order or an order sent through the mail.

Full-service companies are those that send a sales rep to visit the veterinary facility and offer full service. A technical staff, usually made up of veterinarians, is employed. Full-service companies usually carry a limited product line. Some of the products may be newly developed products that still retain a patent with the federal government and cannot be ordered through a distributorship. A full-service company has sales reps who call on the veterinary hospital and take orders. Most full-service companies will replace outdated product with new or credit the hospital's account accordingly.

> ## Technician's Notes
> The sales rep may not pick up expired controlled substances, as these must be mailed back to the company.

A full-service company may have several "deals" the ICM must decide to accept or decline. Examples of full-service companies include Pfizer Animal Health, Pharmacia-Upjohn, Schering Animal Health, and Fort Dodge Animal Health. These companies employ veterinarians as technical support staff, and their product lines are often limited as compared with distributorships. However full-service companies are forerunners in the development of new drugs protected under US patent laws, in which case they may not be sold under a generic name until the patent expires.

Mail-order discount houses provide a good source for ordering items such as gauze, syringes, needles, paper towels, paper drapes, and even isopropyl alcohol. Ordering from this type of vendor occurs over the telephone, as most do not employ sales reps to visit the hospital—although catalogs may be supplied and mailed to the buyer.

Veterinary supply distributors constitute the most common way for acquiring supplies for the veterinary facility. A distributor is an intermediate between a full-service company and the mail-order discount house. If a full-service company gives its approval and a contract is signed between two companies, some products normally sold only through a full-service company may be obtained from a distributor. Many times the products sold by the full-service company to the distributor are those with a patent about to expire or those with an already expired patent. The distributor may elect to sell under a generic name instead of the full-service company's trade name. A distributorship usually maintains a huge inventory and employs sales reps that call on veterinary facilities. Products ordered from a distributorship should be documented carefully. Should expired product need to be returned, the ICM may need to provide invoice numbers proving which distributorship the product was purchased from before credit is applied to the facility's account.

Communicating With Sales Representatives

It is important for the ICM to be certain that sales reps who visit the facility are aware of certain things. The sales reps should know the ICM's scheduled lunch and quitting times. Additionally, the ICM should make sure the sales representative is aware that all emergencies take priority over scheduled sales appointments. It is usually best to schedule an appointment with a visiting sales rep, as this is much easier than having to drop other responsibilities in order to talk to the representative.

DEA Forms

Dealing with **DEA (U.S. Drug Enforcement Administration) forms** can be a frustrating experience if not handled correctly. However, by keeping in mind certain rules, ordering controlled substances need not be stressful.

> ## Technician's Notes
> All veterinarians have a **DEA number** assigned to them and their veterinary license. This number is private and should never be given out for any reason.

The form must be ordered from the U.S. Drug Enforcement Administration and kept in a secure location once mailed to the veterinarian. A DEA form is a multicopy form (i.e., carbon copies are made). The veterinarian keeps a copy of the order for his or her records. All the information contained on these forms must be correct. Important considerations to keep in mind when filling out these forms include no markouts, no Liquid Paper, using correct spelling, citing the correct strength, and that the veterinarian must sign the form. These forms must be filled out using an ink pen or typewriter.

Special Orders

Many times there may be clients who require a "special order." The client must be made aware that once a "special order" is made for them, it must be purchased. If this is not understood, the veterinary facility may be "stuck" with a slow-moving item, or one that is never sold at all. Once this "special order" has been received by the hospital, the ICM should call the client to make them aware the item has arrived. It is best to place these "special orders" near the receptionist's desk, as the ICM may be busy with other duties when the client arrives to pick up their order.

Human Pharmacy

At various times, the veterinary practitioner may need to use a human pharmacy to supply drugs for their clients' pets. A veterinarian may call the order into the pharmacy or provide the order on a written prescription. Keeping a good working relationship between pharmacist and veterinarian is important, because a pharmacist can supply unlimited knowledge about pharmaceutic products.

Computers and Inventory

The advent of computer software technology has made inventory easier for all businesses. There are many veterinary management software program choices. Most programs offer features including provisions for entering client information, inventory control, printout of common forms (e.g., rabies certificates), medical history, and accounting information. It is important to enter all inventory products used on each patient because the software has the ability to automatically subtract inventory amounts used. This is where "GIGO" is very important. Although each employee has good intentions, the ICM may find discrepancies in the total amount

of product on hand. Staff meetings represent a good time to remind employees how important "GIGO" is. All newly received inventory items must be added to amounts already posted in the computer. Bar coding is available on most pharmaceutic products. Using a device capable of reading bar codes greatly enhances the counting and maintaining of inventory.

Additionally, most software contains the ability to produce automatic expiration lists from computer files each month. The total amount of money spent on inventory in a day, week, month, or year can be obtained when using computer software systems.

The Job of ICM

It cannot be overemphasized how important inventory control is to the veterinary facility. The veterinary technician who is willing to take on this added responsibility will find himself or herself an invaluable member of the staff. Keeping in mind that inventory is the second-highest expense for the veterinary hospital will enable the ICM to use care when considering sales offers. Understanding the practice's mission is crucial in inventory control. Remember that time is money, and product left sitting on the shelf for extended periods does not benefit the facility. Keeping a turnover of at least four turns per year is a minimum goal. Training a backup person to monitor inventory during times of vacation or sickness experienced by the ICM is crucial. Reminding employees during staff meetings of the importance of "GIGO" and documenting outages on the reorder log will enable the facility to never run out of needed product. DEA products must be controlled by effective documentation of their use in a log book solely for this purpose (e.g., controlled substance log book).

Establishing a formula for markup is critical. The way inventory is arranged within the pharmacy has a great deal to do with the ease of counting it. No better method to count inventory can replace doing a physical inventory. Keep sales reps abreast of lunch breaks and leaving times. Carefully observe all freight for damage and report claims as soon as possible after receiving the product. Always rotate product on shelves so that the oldest product is sold first. Be knowledgeable about the different types of vendors. Decide which method of inventory counting is most advantageous to your particular situation by deciding whether to count all inventory monthly or on a rotating basis. Keep a good relationship with a local pharmacy, as these businesses provide a good source of knowledge and enable the veterinarian to order human products not normally sold through veterinary vendors. Decide whether a manual or computerized system is best for your facility. In this age of technology, it is best to use a computer system to facilitate efficient work flow.

REFERENCES

Lukens RL and Landon RM: A guide to inventory management for veterinary practices: effective inventory control, Westchester, Pa, 1993, Smith Kline Beecham Animal Health.

McCurnin DM and Bassert J, editors: Clinical textbook for veterinary technicians, ed 5, Philadelphia, 2002, WB Saunders Co.

Locklar CF Jr and Locklar MS: Personal interview, March 12, 2003.

McAllister Software Systems: AVI-Mark Veterinary Software System, Piedmont, Mo, avimark@semo.net.

REVIEW QUESTIONS

1. What is inventory? _____
2. Name the five principles used to control expenses:
   a. _____
   b. _____
   c. _____
   d. _____
   e. _____
3. When dealing with inventory, it is crucial to remember: time is _____.
4. What is turnover? _____
5. Calculate the turnover rate by using the following information: Yearly inventory expense = $125,000; average cost of inventory on hand = $31,250.
   _____
6. Calculate the average cost of inventory on hand by using the following information: Year's beginning inventory = $75,000; year's ending inventory = $130,000.
   _____
7. Name two objectives of an inventory control system.
   a. _____
   b. _____

8. What is a packing slip?
   _____
9. What is an invoice?
   _____
10. What is a statement?
    _____
11. What is the reorder point?
    _____
12. Why is recording the expiration date and serial number for rabies vaccine so important?
    _____
13. Once the reorder point is reached, a basic rule of thumb is to order a _____-month supply.
14. Name some materials that may be kept in the pharmacy library. _____
15. List some rules for filling out a DEA form.
    a. _____
    b. _____
    c. _____
    d. _____
    e. _____
    f. _____

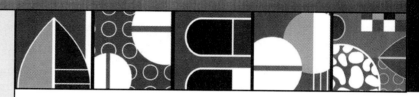

APPENDIX **A**

Common Abbreviations Used in Veterinary Medicine

AD	right ear	NPO	nothing by mouth (nil per os)
ad lib	freely, as wanted (ad libitum)	O	pint
A.L.	left ear (auris laeva)	O.D.	right eye (oculus dexter)
A.M.	morning	O.S.	left eye (oculus sinister)
AMA	against medical advice	O.U.	both eyes (oculi unitas)
ASAP	as soon as possible	oz	ounce
A.U.	each ear (aures unitas)	p.c.	after meals (post cibum)
b.i.d.	twice daily (bis in die)	per os or PO	by mouth, orally
bol.	large pill, bolus	Phos	phosphorus
Bute	phenylbutazone	p.r.n.	as needed (pro re nata)
c̄ (cum)	with	PTA	prior to administration
caps	capsule	pwd	powder
cc	cubic centimeters	q2h	every 2 hours (quaque secunda hora)
cwt.	hundredweight		
DDx	differential sulfoxide	q4h	every 4 hours (quaque quarta hora)
DES	diethylstilbestrol		
DMSO	dimethyl sulfoxide	q.d.	every day (quaque die)
DS	dose or days not acceptable	q.h. or o.h.	every hour (quaque hora)
D/S or D-S	dextrose in saline	q.i.d.	four times a day (quater in die)
D₅W or D5W	5% dextrose with water	q.o.d.	every other day
Dx	diagnosis	R or rt	right
e.o.d	every other day	Rx	take thou of (prescription)
g or gm	gram	s̄ (sine)	without
gal	gallon	SC or SQ	subcutaneous
GI	gastrointestinal	s.i.d.	once a day (semel in die)
gtt	drops (guttae)	sig.	directions, instructions
GU	genitourinary	SOB	shortness of breath
h or hr	hour	SR	sustained release
IM	intramuscular	stat.	immediately (statim)
IP	intraperitoneal	Sx	surgery
IV	intravenous	T, Tbs, Tbsp	tablespoon
IVP	intravenous pyelogram	t, tsp	teaspoon
K	potassium	Tab	tablet
l or lt	left	t.i.d.	three times a day (ter in die)
l or L	liter	TLC	tender loving care
LA	long acting	TR	trace
lb	pound	Tx	treatment
LRS	lactated Ringer's solution	U	unit
mcg or μg	microgram	UG	urogenital
mEq	milliequivalent	μl	microliter
mg	milligram	ung.	ointment
mm	millimeters	Ut dict.	as directed (ut dictum)
Na	sodium	V-D	vomiting/diarrhea
non repetat.	do not repeat (non repetatur)	X	times, multiply

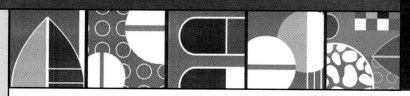

APPENDIX **B**

Weights and Measures

TABLE OF LIQUID MEASURES

1 cup = 8 ounces
2 cups = 1 pint = 16 ounces
2 pints = 1 quart = 32 ounces
4 quarts = 1 gallon = 128 ounces

Metric	*Approximate Apothecary Equivalent*
1000 milliliters (ml or cc)	= 1 quart
500 ml	= 1 pint
30 ml	= 1 ounce = 8 drams

WEIGHT EQUIVALENTS

Metric	*Approximate Apothecary Equivalent*
30 grams	= 1 ounce
4 grams	= 60 grains
1 gram	= 15 grains
60 milligrams	= 1 grain

TABLE OF AVOIRDUPOIS WEIGHT

16 drams = 1 ounce
16 ounces = 1 pound
100 pounds = 1 hundredweight (cwt.)
2000 pounds = 1 ton
2240 pounds = 1 long ton

TABLE OF APOTHECARIES' WEIGHT

20 grains = 1 scruple
3 scruples = 1 dram
8 drams = 1 ounce
12 ounces = 1 pound

TABLE OF TEMPERATURE EQUIVALENTS

$F = (C \times 9/5) + 32$
$C = (F - 32) \times 5/9$

Fahrenheit:	*Celsius*
98.6	37.0
99.0	37.2
100.0	37.7
101.0	38.3
102.0	38.8
103.0	39.4
104.0	40.0
105.0	40.5
106.0	41.1

TABLE OF WEIGHT EQUIVALENTS

kilogram (kg) = pound ÷ 2.2
pound (lb) = kilogram × 2.2

pound:	kilogram
5	2.27
10	4.5
15	6.8
20	9.0
25	11.4
30	13.6
35	15.9
40	18.2
45	20.5
50	22.7
55	25.0
60	27.3
65	29.5
70	31.8
75	34.1
80	36.4
85	38.6
90	40.9
95	43.2
100	45.5

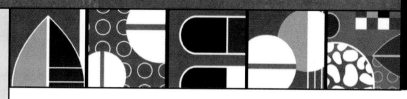

APPENDIX C

Resource Information

Drug Information Resources

Subject	Phone Number	Website
Animal blood banking	See Chapter 6, Table 6-2	
Adverse drug reactions	888-FDA-VETS	www.fda.gov/cvm
Associations		
American Academy of Veterinary Consultants		tpvec.unl.edu/public/avc.avc.htm
American Academy of Veterinary Pharmacology and Therapeutics		www.vet.purdue.edu/depts/bms/ aavpt/index.htm
American Animal Hospital Association		www.acmepet.com/aaha
American College of Veterinary Clinical Pharmacology		www.acvcp.org/
American Veterinary Medical Association	800-248-2862	www.avma.org
Governmental agencies		
Drug Enforcement Agency Office of Diversion Control, Registration Section	800-238-7332	http://www.usdoj.gov/dea
Food and Drug Administration		www.fda.cvm
Center for Veterinary Medicine	301-594-1755	www.fda.gov/cvm
Office of Management and Communications	301-594-1752	
Offce of New Animal Drug Evaluation	301-594-1620	
Office of Surveillance and Compliance	301-827-6644	
Office of Research	301-827-8010	
Communications Staff	301-827-6514	
United States Department of Agriculture		
Animal and Plant Health Inspection Service		www.aphis.usda.gov
Centers for Disease Control and Prevention		www.cdc.gov
Center for Epidemiology and Animal Health	800-545-8732 (voice response only)	www.aphis.usda.gov/vs/ceah
Center for Health Monitoring		www.cdc.gov/cdc.htm
Interstate Shipping		www.aphis.usda.gove/vs/sregs
Center for Animal Health Monitoring		www.aphis.usda.gov/vs/ceah/ cahm
Occupational Safety and Health Administration		www.osha.gov
Clinical pharmacology education		
Clinical Pharmacology Online		www.cponline.gsm.com
First Course in Pharmacokinetics and Biopharmaceutics		www.ouhsc.edu
Kinetics: KinetiClass		www.vetmed.vt.edu/Research/ Research/Informatics
Internet Self Assessment in Pharmacology (ISAP)		www.cs.umn.edu/Research/ GIMME/isap.html
Therapeutic Drug Monitoring		
Clinical Pharmacology Laboratory, Texas A&M University		www.cvm.tamu.edu/vcpl
Pharmacokinetic and Pharmacodynamic Resources		www.boomer.org/
Velterinary Information Network (subscriptions)	800-700-4636	vingram@aol.com
Compounding and compounding pharmacies		
Professional Compounding Pharmacy		www.rx-compound.com/info.htm
Professional Compounding Centers of America	800-331-2498	

Subject	Phone Number	Website
Formularies and drug databases		
Antibiotics: Medical College of Wisconsin Antibiotic Guide		www.intmed.mcw.edu/ AntibioticGuide.html
Internet Drug Index RxList		www.rxlist.com/
Formulary Medical College of Wisconsin		
Governmental agencies		
Drug Enforcement Agency Office of Diversion Control, Registration Section	800-238-7332	www.usdoj.gov/dea
Green Book, Freedom of Information		www.fda.gov/cvm
Physicians GenRx (by subscription only)		www.mosby.com/Mosby/ phyGenRx/
Jag's Apothecary (conversions)		www.ourworld.compuserve.com/ homepages/jbaluri/home.HTM
DoseCalcu Online (dose calculations)		www.meds.com/Dchome.html
Health sciences information gateway sites		
Animal Health Institute		www.ahi.org
Martindale's Health Science Guide		www-sci.lib.uci.edu/HSG/Vet.html
The Virtual Veterinary Center		www-sci.uci.edu/HSG/Vet.html
The Virtual Pharmacy Center		www-sci.lib.uci.edu/HSG/ Pharmacy.html
WWW Virtual Library: Pharmacy		www.pharmacy.org/
National Library of Medicine		www.nlm.nih.gov
Medical Sciences Bulletin		www.pharminfo.com/pubs/msb/ msbmnu.html
Poisoning antidotes ($50 consultation fee)	888-426-4435	www.aspca.org/apcc
Research information		
Morris Animal Foundation		www.MorrisAnimalFoundation.org
Vaccines		
Rabies control		www.avma.org/pubhlth/ rabprev.html www.avma.org/pubhlth/ rabcont.html
Small Animal Vaccination Schedule		www.avma.org/care4pets/ genvacs.htm

From Booth DM: Small animal clinical pharmacology and therapeutics, Philadelphia, 2001, WB Saunders.

Veterinary Pharmaceutic Companies, Distributors, and Other Important Numbers

Company Name	Telephone	Website
Abbott Laboratories	888-299-7416	www.abbott.com
AgriPharm/Dealer Distribution of America	901-366-4442	
Alpharma, Inc. Animal Health Division	201-228-5074	www.alpharma.com
Animal Blood Bank	800-243-5759	
Aspen Veterinary Resources, Ltd.	816-413-1444	
Bayer Corp. Agriculture Division, Animal Health	800-633-3796	www.bayerus.com/ah
Biopure Corp.	617-234-6500	www.biopure.com
Boehringer Ingelheim Vetmedica, Inc.	800-821-7467	www.bi-vetmedica.com
Bowie Cattle City Calf Jack	800-831-0960	
The Butler Co.	614-761-9095	www.wabutler.com
C.E. Kord Animal Disease Laboratory Nashville, Tenn.	615-360-0125	
Columbus Serum Co.	800-848-1090	
Durvet, Inc.	816-229-9101	www.durvet.com
DVM Pharmaceuticals, Inc.	800-367-4902	www.DVMPharmaceuticals.com
Elanco Animal Health	800-428-4441	www.elanco.com
EVSCO Pharmaceuticals	856-691-2411	www.evscopharm.com
Fort Dodge Animal Health	800-533-8536	www.ahp.com/fortdodge.htm
G.C. Hanford Manufacturing Co.	800-234-4263	www.hanford.com
Halocarbon Laboratories	800-338-5803	www.halocarbon.com
Heska Corp.	800-GO-HESKA	www.heska.com
Hills Pet Nutrition, Inc.	800-354-4557	
IDEXX Laboratories, Inc.	800-248-2483	
Intervet Inc.	800-247-4838	
Lloyd Laboratories, Inc.	800-831-0004	www.lloydinc.com
Luitpold Pharmaceuticals, Inc.	800-458-0163	www.luitpold.com
Merial, Ltd.	888-637-4251	www.merial.com
Merritt Veterinary Supplies, Inc.	800-972-4744	
Nasco West	800-558-9595	
Neogen Corp.	800-525-2022	www.neogen.com
Novartis Animal Health US, Inc.	800-332-2761	www.ah.novartis.com
Orthopedic Foundation for Animals (OFA)	573-442-0418	www.offa.org
Pet-Ag, Inc.	800-323-6878	www.petag.com
Pfizer Inc., North American Region, Animal Health Group	800-733-5500	www.pfizer.com/ah
Pfizer Animal Health	800-793-0596	www.pfizer.com/ah/
Phoenix Pharmaceutical, Inc.	800-759-3644	www.phoenixpharmaceutical.com
Phoenix Scientific, Inc.	816-364-3777	
PRN Pharmacal	800-874-9764	
Schering-Plough Animal Health Corp.	800-648-2118	www.sp-animalhealth.com
Sunbelt Veterinary Supply	800-476-4343	
Vedco, Inc.	816-238-8840	www.vedco.com/dvmonly/
Vet-A-Mix, a division of Lloyd, Inc.	800-831-0004	www.lloydine.com
Veterinary Products Laboratories	800-720-0032 ext. 2158, 2283, or 2284	www.vpl.com
Vetus Animal Health	800-92-BURNS	www.burnsvet.com
Vortech Pharmaceuticals, Ltd.	800-521-4686	
Webster Veterinary Supply	800-225-7911	
Wildlife Pharmaceuticals, Inc.	970-484-6267	www.wildpharm.com
Zinpro Corp.	800-445-6145	www.zinpro.com

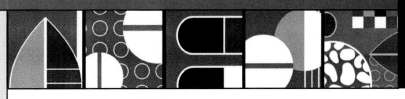

APPENDIX **D**

Controlled Substances Information Summary

The comprehensive Drug Abuse Prevention and Control Act was passed by Congress in 1970 and became effective in May 1971. This law placed narcotics and other drugs with potential for abuse into schedules and called for the registration of professionals who administer or prescribe these drugs in their practices. In 1973, the U.S. Drug Enforcement Administration (DEA) was established through the merger of the Bureau of Narcotics and Dangerous Drugs with other agencies. The DEA was established to control the abuse of dangerous drugs through prevention and enforcement.

The drugs that are under the control of the controlled substances act are placed into five schedules, or classes, according to the potential for abuse. The schedule is designated by a C with a Roman numeral (I, II, III, IV, or V) inside the C.

Schedule I substances have no (or controversial) accepted medical use and a high potential for abuse. LSD, heroin, crack cocaine, marijuana, and peyote are substances in this class. The use of medicinal marijuana in human medicine is controversial but may be permitted in some states.

Schedule II drugs have accepted medical uses but have a high potential for abuse. A partial list of schedule II drugs includes morphine, meperidine, codeine, cocaine, oxymorphone, amphetamines, and pentobarbital.

Schedule III substances have less potential for abuse than those in schedule II and include Hycodan, paregoric, barbiturates such as thiamylal or thiopental, and anabolic steroids.

Schedule IV drugs have lower abuse potential than those in schedule III. Included in this class are phenobarbital, diazepam, and pentazocine.

Schedule V drugs are the lowest on the scale of abuse potential and include mostly antidiarrheal and anticough medications. Lomotil and Robitussin with codeine are in this schedule.

Any veterinarian who administers, dispenses, or prescribes a controlled substance must be registered with the DEA. A registry number issued to the veterinarian is used when ordering controlled substances. Schedule II drugs also require a special order form (DEA form 222). Registry must be renewed every 3 years. Registration may be suspended or revoked for noncompliance with the Comprehensive Drug Abuse and Control Act.

An inventory of all controlled substances on hand must be taken on the date that the registered veterinarian first begins the practice and every 2 years thereafter. The inventory should include the following:

1. The name, address, and DEA registration number
2. The date and time the inventory is taken
3. The inventory information
4. The signature of the person taking the inventory

The inventory records of schedule II drugs must be kept separate from all other records in the practice. Schedule III, IV, and V drug records must be kept separate or must be readily retrievable. All inventory records must be kept 2 years.

Controlled substances should be kept in a locked, substantially constructed cabinet.

More detailed information about the Comprehensive Drug Abuse and Control Act may be found in *Veterinary Pharmaceuticals and Biologics* (Veterinary Medicine Publishing Company) or in the *Veterinary Drug Handbook* (Pharma Vet Publishing).

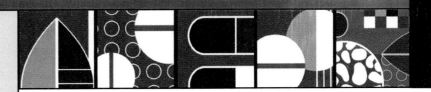

BIBLIOGRAPHY

Ahrens AA: Pharmacology, the national veterinary medical series for independent study, Philadelphia, 1996, Lippincott Williams & Wilkins.

Anderson KN, Anderson L, editors: Mosby's pocket dictionary of medicine, nursing, and allied health, St. Louis, 1998, Mosby.

Anonymous: White paper: rogue Internet pharmacies, http://www.avma.org/noah/members/scientific/prescribing/white_paper.asp, 2001.

Barragry TB: Cardiac disease: veterinary drug therapy, Philadelphia, 1994, Lea & Febiger.

Bill R, editor: Pharmacology for veterinary technicians, Goleta, Calif, 1993, American Veterinary Publications.

Birchard S and Sherding R, editors: Saunders manual of small animal practice, Philadelphia, 1994, WB Saunders Co.

Beech J, Bistner S, Boothe DM, et al: The Bristol veterinary handbook of antimicrobial therapy, ed 2, Trenton, NJ, 1987, Veterinary Learning Systems Co.

Blankenship J and Campbell JB, editors: Laboratory mathematics: medical and biological applications, St. Louis, 1976, Mosby.

Bonagura JD, editor: Kirk's current veterinary therapy XIII: small animal practice, Philadelphia, 2000, WB Saunders Co.

Boothe DM: Nutraceuticals in veterinary medicine: part I: definitions and regulations, Compend Contin Educ Prac Vet 19(11):1248-1255, 1997.

Boothe DM: Small animal clinical pharmacology and therapeutics, Philadelphia, 2001, WB Saunders Co.

Boothe DM, editor: The veterinary clinics of North America, small animal practice, Philadelphia, 1998, WB Saunders Co.

Brander GC, Pugh DM, Bywater RJ et al, editors: Veterinary applied pharmacology and therapeutics, ed 5, London, 1991, Bailliere Tindall.

Carter GR et al, editors: Essentials of veterinary microbiology, Baltimore, 1995, Williams & Wilkins.

Coppoc GL: Drug residue avoidance. In class notes for BMS 513, http://www.vet.purdue.edu/bms/courses/bms513/scavma97.htm, 2003.

Cowgill LD: Managing renal disease and hypertension, 1991, Harmon-Smith.

Davidson G: Pharmacy update: new FDA policy gives clear guidance for compounding, Vet Tech 18(3):195-201, 1997.

Crow SE and Walshaw SO, editors: Manual of clinical procedures in the dog and cat, Philadelphia, 1987, JB Lippincott Co.

Davidson G: S-adenosylmethionine, Compend Contin Educ Prac Vet 24(8):600-603, 2002.

Davidson G: Glucosamine and chondroitin sulfate, Compend Contin Educ Prac Vet 22(5):454-458, 2000.

DeLahunta A, editor: Veterinary neuroanatomy and clinical neurology, Philadelphia, 1983, WB Saunders Co.

DeNovo RC: Chronic vomiting in the cat and dog, Proc Am Vet Med Assoc, Nashville, Tenn, 2002.

DiBartola SP, editor: Fluid therapy in small animal practice, ed 2, Philadelphia, 2000, WB Saunders Co.

Dowling PM: Respiratory drugs. In proceedings of the annual meeting of the American Veterinary Medical Association, Boston, 2001.

Ettinger SJ, editor: Pocket companion to textbook of veterinary internal medicine, Philadelphia, 2001, WB Saunders Co.

Ettinger SJ, editor: Textbook of veterinary internal medicine, ed 3, Philadelphia, 1989, WB Saunders Co.

Ettinger SJ, editor: Textbook of veterinary internal medicine, ed 5, vol I and II, Philadelphia, 1993, WB Saunders Co.

Fascetti AJ: Nutraceuticals and food faddism, World Wide Web document, http://www.avma.org/noah/default.asp, 1998.

Ford RB: Vaccines and vaccinations: issues for the 21st Century, Suppl Compend Contin Educ Pract Vet 20(8C):19-24, 1998.

Foushee LL: Omeprazole, Compend Contin Educ Pract Vet 22(8):746-749, 2000.

Ganong WF: Review of medical physiology, ed 21, New York, 2003, McGraw-Hill.

Gelatt KN: Textbook of veterinary ophthalmology, Philadelphia, 1981, Lea & Febiger.

Giovanoni R and Warren RG: Principles of pharmacology, St. Louis, 1983, Mosby.

Hall JA and Washabau RJ: Gastrointestinal prokinetic therapy: dopaminergic antagonist drugs, Compend Contin Pract Vet 19(2):214-219, 1997.

Hamlin RL: Cardiovascular system, introduction. In proceedings of the Music City Veterinary Conference, Nashville, Tenn, 2003.

Hand MS et al, editors: Small animal clinical nutrition, ed 4, Topeka, 2000, Mark Morris Institute.

Haskins SC: Fluid overload: how to identify and manage. Proceedings of the International Veterinary Emergency and Critical Care Symposium, Orlando, Fla, 2000.

Hendrix CM et al, editors: Diagnostic veterinary parasitology, ed 2, St. Louis, 1998, Mosby.

Hoffman AM: What's new with aerosol medications in the horse. In Proceedings of the annual meeting of the American Veterinary Medical Association, Boston, 2001.

Kamerling SG: Pain recognition and relief. In Proceedings of the annual meeting of the American Veterinary Medical Association, Boston, 2001.

Kirk RW, editor: Current veterinary therapy VIII: small animal practice, Philadelphia, 1983, WB Saunders Co.

Kirk RW and Bonagura JD, editors: Current veterinary therapy X: small animal practice, Philadelphia, 1989, WB Saunders Co.

Kirk RW and Bonagura JD, editors: Current veterinary therapy XII: small animal practice, Philadelphia, 1995, WB Saunders Co.

Lane DR and Cooper BC, editors: Veterinary nursing, ed 2, Oxford, England, 1999, Butterworth-Heinemann.

Langston VC and Mercer HD: Nonsteroidal antiinflammatory drugs. In Proceedings of the 17th Seminar for Veterinary Technicians, The Western Veterinary Conference, Las Vegas, 1988.

Lavoie JP: Inhalation therapy for equine heaves, Comp Contin Educ Prac Vet 23(5):475-477, 2001.

Locklar CF Jr and Locklar MS : Personal interview, March 12, 2003.

Lukens RL and Landon RM: A guide to inventory management for veterinary practices: effective inventory control, Westchester, Pa, 1993, Smith Kline Beecham Animal Health.

McAllister P: McAllister Software Systems: AVI-Mark Veterinary Software System, Piedmont, Mo, avimark@semo.net.

McCurnin DM and Bassert JM, editors: Clinical textbook for veterinary technicians, ed 5, Philadelphia, 2002, WB Saunders Co.

McKiernan B: Respiratory therapeutics. In proceedings of the 17th Seminar for Veterinary Technicians, The Western Veterinary Conference, Las Vegas, 1988.

Mealey KL: Clinically significant drug interactions, Compend Contin Educ Proc Pract Vet 24(1):10-22, 2002.

Muir WW and Hubbell JA: Handbook of veterinary anesthesia, ed 3, St. Louis, 2000, Mosby.

Muller GH, Kirk RW and Scott DW: Small animal dermatology, ed 4, Philadelphia, 1989, WB Saunders Co.

Norsworthy GD: Clinical aspects of feline blood transfusions, Comp Cont Educ Pract Vet 14:470, 1992.

Paddleford RR: Manual of small animal anesthesia, Philadelphia, 1999, WB Saunders Co.

Papich MG: Handbook of Veterinary Drugs, Philadelphia, 2002, WB Saunders Co.

Parker AR: Domperidone, Compend Contin Educ Pract Vet 23(10):906-908, 2001.

Pasquini C, Spurgeon T, and Pasquini S, editors: Anatomy of domestic animals, ed 7, Pilot Point, Texas, 1995, Sudz Publishing.

Plumb DC: Veterinary drug handbook, ed 4, Ames, Iowa, 2002, Iowa State University Press.

Quinn PJ et al, editors: Microbial and parasitic diseases of the dog and cat, London, 1997, Saunders.

Robertson SA: Systemic uptake of buprenorphine after buccal administration in cats. In Proceedings of the annual meeting of the American College of Veterinary Anesthesiologists, New Orleans, 2001.

Scott DW, Miller WH, and Griffin CE: Dermatologic therapy. In Small animal dermatology, ed 5, Philadelphia, 1995, WB Saunders Co.

Shull EA: Psychopharmacology in veterinary behavioral medicine. Annual Conference for Veterinarians and Technicians, Knoxville, Tenn, 1998, UT-CVM.

Simpson BS and Simpson DM: Behavioral pharmacotherapy: part I: antipsychotics and antidepressants, Compend Contin Educ Pract Vet 18(10):1067-1081, 1996.

Simpson BS and Simpson DM: Behavioral pharmacotherapy: part II: anxiolytics and mood stabilizers, Compend Contin Educ Proc Vet 18(11):1203-1210, 1996.

Smith P: New studies, products fuel heartworm debate, Veterinary Product News 11(4):34-36, 1999.

Spinelli JS and Enos LR, editors: Drugs in veterinary practice, St. Louis, 1978, Mosby.

Snyder S, editor: Drugs and the brain, New York, 1986, Scientific American Library.

Swaim SF and Gillette RL: An update on wound medications and dressings, Compend Cont Educ Prac Vet 20(10):1133-1145, 1998.

Tilley LP and Smith WK: The 5-minute veterinary consult canine and feline, ed 2, Baltimore, 2000, Lippincott Williams & Wilkins.

Tizard I: Veterinary immunology: an introduction, ed 4, Philadelphia, 1992, WB Saunders Co.

Upson DW: Handbook of clinical veterinary pharmacology, ed 4, Manhattan, Kan, 1988, Dan Upson Enterprises.

Ware WA: Problems in chronic heart failure management. Proceedings of the American Veterinary Medical Association annual conference, Nashville, Tenn, 2002.

Webb AI and Aeschbacher G: Animal drug container labels: a guide to the reader, JAVMA, 202:1591-1599, 1993.

Williams BR and Baer C, editors: Essentials of clinical pharmacology in nursing, Springhouse, Pa, 1990, Springhouse Corp.

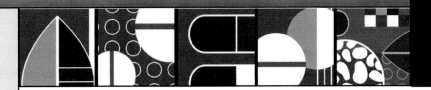

Review Question
Answers

ANSWERS TO CHAPTER 1

1. **a.** An agonist is a drug that has affinity for a receptor and stimulates the receptor to action.
   b. A contraindication is a reason not to use a drug in a particular situation.
   c. Efficacy is the degree to which a drug produces its desired effects in a patient.
   d. An over-the-counter drug is one that may be purchased and used without a prescription from a veterinarian.
   e. A prescription drug is one that must be used under the supervision of a veterinarian.
   f. A receptor is a group of specialized molecules on or in a cell that binds with a drug to cause an effect.
   g. The therapeutic index expresses the relationship between a drug's therapeutic and harmful effects.
   h. The withdrawal time is the amount of time that must elapse between the end of drug therapy and the elimination of that drug from the patient's tissues or products.
   i. The veterinarian-client-patient relationship is the relationship that must exist between the veterinarian, his or her patient, and the patient's owner before prescription drugs may be dispensed.

2. Four sources for veterinary drugs are animal products, plant materials, minerals, and synthetic products.

3. A drug regimen includes the dose, the route of administration, the frequency of administration, and the duration of administration.

4. For a valid veterinarian-client-patient relationship to exist, (1) the veterinarian must assume responsibility for making clinical judgments in relation to the health of the animal, (2) the veterinarian must have recently seen the animal and be acquainted with its care, and (3) the veterinarian must be available for follow-up care of the animal.

5. It is a technician's responsibility to carry out the veterinarian's orders correctly. The technician should read the drug label three times to ensure that the proper drug is being administered and should take care to administer the correct dose by the correct route. The technician should also be aware of the expected effects and potential adverse side effects to be able to monitor the patient in a responsible way. In a large animal practice, the technician should be aware of withdrawal times and potential residue problems.

6. A drug is first absorbed (or directly placed) into the bloodstream. In the blood, the drug may bind with a plasma protein or exist in the free state. The circulating blood distributes the drug to the capillary level, where the drug leaves the circulation and enters the interstitial fluid. The interstitial fluid bathes the cell and allows the drug to enter the cell or bind with surface receptors. The drug then exits the cell (or its surface), moves back into the interstitial fluid, reenters the circulation, and is then transported to the liver for metabolism. After it is metabolized, the metabolite is transported to the kidneys for excretion.

7. **(1)** The oral route provides a simple route of administration. Many factors may influence the rate of absorption, and the oral route may not be appropriate if the animal is vomiting.
   (2) Subcutaneous administration of drugs is usually a simple procedure. Absorption from subcutaneous sites may be slow, and hypertonic solutions should not be given by this route.
   (3) The intramuscular route produces faster absorption than the subcutaneous route, but care must be taken with many drugs not to inject them into blood vessels.
   (4) The intravenous route allows immediate access to the bloodstream and the dilution of irritating drugs. A toxic or allergic reaction can be a side effect.
   (5) The intraperitoneal route may be used to administer fluids and some other solutions when other routes are not available. Absorption from the peritoneal cavity is slow, however.
   (6) The intraarterial route is a seldom used route that may produce seizures or death.

(7) The intracardiac route is used primarily for administering emergency drugs or for euthanasia.

(8) The intramedullary route may be used to administer fluids or blood to small animals or those with damaged veins.

(9) The inhalation route is used to administer drugs to the respiratory system. Special equipment may be required.

(10) The topical route may be used to place drugs on skin or mucous membranes and may be facilitated by using carrier substances in some instances.

(11) The intradermal route is used primarily for allergy testing and for diagnosing tuberculosis.

8. The absorption of a drug may be influenced by (1) the method of absorption, (2) the pH of the drug and its ionization status, (3) the absorptive surface area, (4) the blood supply to the area, (5) the solubility of the drug, (6) the dosage form, (7) the status of the gastrointestinal tract, and (8) interactions with other drugs.

9. b. Liver

10. a. Kidneys

11. Receptors

12. Proprietary/trade

13. The six items that must be on a drug label are the drug names (generic and trade), the drug concentration and quantity, the name and address of the manufacturer, the controlled substance status, the manufacturer's control or lot number, and the drug's expiration date.

14. The government agencies that regulate the development, approval, and use of animal health products are the FDA, EPA, and USDA.

15. Many veterinary clinics dispense rather than prescribe drugs because of the profit earned from selling the products.

16. Veterinary pharmaceuticals may be purchased directly from the manufacturer, from distributors, or from generic mail-order companies. In some instances, drugs may be sold under one label to graduate veterinarians and under another as an over-the-counter product.

17. The Green Book

18. FARAD provides resources concerning the avoidance of drug residues in animals.

19. AMDUCA (Animal Medicinal Drug Use Clarification Act)

20. Compounding refers to the diluting or combining of existing drugs.

21. Drug residues in animal products may cause allergic reactions or neoplasia in people, and they may cause the development of antibiotic resistant strains of bacteria.

22. Pharmacodynamic, pharmacokinetic, and pharmaceutic

23. Liver

24. An "ethical" product is one sold only through veterinarians as a policy of the manufacturer rather than by FDA requirement.

25. Metabolite

ANSWERS TO CHAPTER 2

1. Drugs for oral administration, drugs for parenteral administration, drugs for inhalation, drugs for topical administration

2. Large; balling gun

3. Injections, implants

4. Single-, multi-

5. Sharps container

6. Right patient, right drug, right dose, right route, right time and frequency

7. Vomiting

8. Rapid

9. 72

10. Large

11. Date, owner's name, patient's name, drug name, amount dispensed or administered, name(s) of personnel administering the drug to the patient

12. The plastic syringe may absorb the drug, which may cause it to be less effective.

13. Luer-lok, slip-tip, eccentric, catheter-tip

14. 1

15. Insulin syringe

ANSWERS TO CHAPTER 3

Ratios

1. 1:4; 0.25
2. 75:100; $\dfrac{75}{100}$
3. 4:1000; $\dfrac{4}{1000}$
4. $\dfrac{1}{80}$; 0.0125
5. 9:1000; 0.009
6. $\dfrac{1}{32}$; 0.031

Proportions

1. 50
2. 8
3. 2.5
4. 5
5. 200 mg
6. 37.5 mg
7. 31.25 mg
8. 118.25 ml
9. 5 ml
10. 1.25 tablets

Problems Using the Metric System

1. 0.15 g
2. 2000 ml
3. 2.25 g
4. 5000 mg
5. 3 L
6. 2000 g
7. 500 g
8. 0.005 kg
9. 0.00125 g
10. 4 mg
11. 2.05 mg
12. 0.01 g
13. 500 ml
14. 0.75 L
15. 0.3 mg
16. 2500 µg

Problems Using the Apothecary and Household Systems

1. 3 pt
2. 1.5 gal
3. 1 Tbsp
4. 12 cups
5. 6 pints
6. 4 Tbsp
7. 128 oz
8. 16 oz
9. 3 qt

Problems Combining Both Systems

1. 480 ml
2. 30 ml
3. 15 cc
4. 16 oz
5. 0.013 pt
6. 25 tsp
7. 45 ml
8. 33 lb
9. 0.52 pt
10. 150 ml
11. 15.9 kg

Problems Measuring Oral Medications

1. 2 tablets
2. 1.5 tablets
3. 4 tablets
4. 2.5 tablets
5. 1.5 tablets; 7.5 tablets
6. 20 tablets
7. 200 mg; 100 mg; 50 mg/ml; 4 ml; 2 ml; 44 ml
8. 2.5 tablets; 25 tablets
9. 0.25 tablet; 5.25 tablets
10. 0.5 tablet; 4.5 tablets
11. 6.8 kg; 68 mg; 0.75 tablet; 31.5 tablets
12. 120 ml mebendazole; 5 oz Combot
13. 100 oz or 3.125 qt (containing 3 oz powder per quart of water)
14. 0.5 tablet; 7 tablets
15. 66.67 mg; 17.7 ml

Problems Measuring Parenteral Medications

1. 0.4 ml
2. 3.7 ml
3. 17 ml
4. 1.5 ml
5. 525 mg; 1.75 ml
6. 2 ml

7. 15 mg
8. 0.74 m^2; 0.37 mg; 0.37 ml
9. 2500 mg; 25 ml; 2.5 bottles
10. 54 mg; 0.54 ml
11. 3.5 ml
12. 0.1 ml
13. 47.5 mg; 1.9 ml
14. 30 ml
15. 1.5 ml

Injection Problems
1. 2 ml
2. 5 ml
3. 1.5 ml
4. 3.75 ml
5. 0.25 ml
6. 2 ml
7. 0.75 ml
8. 7.5 ml
9. 0.6 ml
10. 0.22 ml

Preparing Solutions
1. $V1 \times C1 = V2 \times C2$
   $V1 \times 100 = 100 \times 10$
   $V1 \times 100 = 1000$
   $V1 = 10$
   10 ml 37% formaldehyde + 90 ml water
2. $V1 \times C1 = V2 \times C2$
   $V1 \times 50 = 1000 \times 5$
   $V1 \times 50 = 5000$
   $V1 = 100$
   100 ml $D_{50}W$ + 900 ml 0.9% NaCl
3. $V1 \times C1 = V2 \times C2$
   $V1 \times 50 = 100 \times 5$
   $V1 \times 50 = 500$
   $V1 = 10$
   10 ml $D_{50}W$ + 90 ml water
4. $V1 \times C1 = V2 \times C2$
   $V1 \times 0.9 = 500 \times 0.45$
   $V1 \times 0.9 = 225$
   $V1 = 250$
   250 ml 0.9% NaCl + 250 ml D_5W
5. $V1 \times C1 = V1 \times C2$
   $V1 \times 50 = 2000 \times 2.5$
   $V1 \times 50 = 5000$
   $V1 = 100$

100 ml $D_{50}W$ + 1900 ml lactated Ringer's solution
6. $V1 \times C1 = V2 \times C2$
   $V1 \times 50 = 50 \times 5$
   $V1 \times 50 = 250$
   $V1 = 5$
   5 ml $D_{50}W$ + 45 ml water
7. $V1 \times C1 = V2 \times C2$
   $V1 \times 50 = 500 \times 2.5$
   $V1 \times 50 = 1250$
   $V1 = 25$
   25 ml $D_{50}W$ + 475 ml 0.45% NaCl
8. Remember: 10% solution = 100 mg/ml packets containing 50 gm = 50,000 mg
   $V1 \times C1 = V2 \times C2$
   $V1 \times 50,000 = 1000 \times 100$
   $V1 \times 50,000 = 100,000$
   $V1 = 2$
   2 packets of 50 g GG powder + 1000 ml water
9. Remember: 8% solution = 80 mg/ml
   One 5 g vial contains 5000 mg
   $V1 \times C1 = V2 \times C2$
   $1 \times 5000 = V2 \times 80$
   $5000 = V2 \times 80$
   $62.5 = V2$
   62.5 ml needs to be added to one 50-g vial to prepare an 8% solution
10. Remember:
   2% solution = 20 mg/ml
   $V1 \times C1 = V2 \times C2$
   $V1 \times 100 = 5 \times 20$
   $V1 \times 100 = 100$
   $V1 = 1$
   1 ml of Sandimmune (cyclosporine) + 4 ml virgin olive oil
11. Remember:
   37% formaldehyde = 100% formalin
   $V1 \times C1 = V2 \times C2$
   $V1 \times 100 = 50 \times 2$
   $V1 \times 100 = 100$
   $V1 = 1$
   1 ml 37% formaldehyde + 49 ml water

Problems Calculating IV Drop Rates
1. 42 gtt/min or approximately 0.69 gtt/sec
2. 60 gtt/min or 1 gtt/sec
3. 30 gtt/min or 1 gtt/2 sec

4. 0.15 ml/min or 9 gtt/min
5. 0.5 ml/min or 30 gtt/min

ANSWERS TO CHAPTER 4

1. An agonist is a drug that combines with a receptor to bring about an action, whereas an antagonist combines with a receptor and blocks the action.
2. A neurotransmitter is a chemical substance released by a nerve ending at the synapse. It acts on the adjacent neuron to stimulate, inhibit, or change its activity.
3. b. Thalamus
4. Interrupting the generation or conduction of nerve impulses; interfering with
5. Epinephrine or norepinephrine
6. Mimicking neurotransmitters, interfering with neurotransmitter release, blocking the attachment of neurotransmitters to receptors, and interfering with the breakdown of neurotransmitters
7. To control vomiting, to treat urinary retention, to stimulate gastrointestinal activity, to treat glaucoma, and to aid in the diagnosis of myasthenia gravis
8. Cholinergic blocking agents (anticholinergic)
9. Adrenergic (sympathomimetic)
10. d. Beta blocker
11. Bradycardia and hypotension may be antagonized by using atropine; respiratory depression or excessive CNS depression may be antagonized by using yohimbine.
12. Thiobarbiturates are very soluble in fat, which acts like a sponge to take the barbiturate out of the circulation and away from the CNS. Thin animals have reduced fat levels, which means that more of the thiobarbiturate remains in the bloodstream and may cause excessive depression of the CNS.
13. Analgesia, increased muscle tone, maintenance of pharyngeal/laryngeal reflexes, muscle tremors, and loss of the blink reflex
14. Respiratory depression, cardiac depression, agitation, excitement, or seizures
15. Naloxone and nalorphine

16. Because of its tendency to precipitate out of solution when stored
17. Doxapram (Dopram) may be administered on or under the tongue, into the umbilical vein, or by intramuscular injection
18. Some pentobarbital euthanasia agents have a red dye added to distinguish them from pentobarbital agents that may be used for anesthesia. Since these agents are easily identified as euthanasia agents, they have less potential for abuse.
19. Neurotransmitter
20. Burning
21. Propofol
22. GABA
23. Diazepam
24. Clomicalm
25. Anipryl

ANSWERS TO CHAPTER 5

1. Nostrils, nasal cavity, pharynx, larynx, trachea, bronchi, and bronchioles
2. The four functions of the respiratory system are oxygen-carbon dioxide exchange, regulation of acid-base balance, body temperature regulation, and voice production.
3. Structures in the nasal passages filter, warm, and humidify inspired air. The cough, sneeze, and reverse sneeze attempt to remove foreign material that has entered the respiratory system. The mucociliary mechanism also removes foreign material from the respiratory system. Macrophages and immunoglobulins inactivate or destroy invasive organisms.
4. The three important principles of respiratory therapeutics are control of secretions, control of reflexes, and maintenance of normal airflow.
5. Productive
6. Through the breakdown of disulfide chemical bonds
7. Acetylcysteine is administered by nebulization.
8. Through depression of the cough center in the brain
9. Schedule V

10. Release of acetylcholine, release of histamine, and blockade of beta-2-adrenergic receptors
11. Epinephrine and albuterol
12. Phosphodiesterase
13. Treatment of insect bites and treatment of heaves in horses
14. –amine
15. Treatment of respiratory depression associated with anesthesia and stimulation of respiration in newborn animals
16. 22.7 kg × 0.22 mg/kg = 4.9 mg; 5 mg tablets are available. Dispense 14 tablets.
17. 1. As a mucolytic agent. 2. As an antidote for acetaminophen toxicity.
18. E
19. 1 to 5 microns
20. Albuterol

ANSWERS TO CHAPTER 6

1. Kidneys, ureters, bladder, urethra
2. Rompun and Ketaset
3. Prerenal, renal, postrenal
4. Diuretics work by removing excess extracellular fluid by increasing urine flow and sodium excretion, and decreasing hypertension
5. Potassium (K)
6. Angiotensin II
7. Struvite
8. Erythropoietin, decrease
9. Loop diuretics inhibit the tubular reabsorption of sodium
10. The posterior pituitary gland

ANSWERS TO CHAPTER 7

1. The right atrium and right ventricle serve functionally as one pump for ejecting blood to the lungs, and the left atrium and left ventricle pump blood to the systemic circulation.
2. Syncytium (interconnected mass)
3. Sodium (Na^+), calcium (Ca^{2+}), potassium (K^+)
4. Refractory period

5. *Chronotropic* refers to the rate of contraction, whereas *inotropic* refers to the force or strength of contraction.
6. Preload is the volume of blood in the ventricles at the end of diastole (the amount of blood that must be pumped out). Afterload is the resistance in the arteries that the ventricle must overcome to pump blood.
7. Increasing the heart rate, increasing the stroke volume, increasing the efficiency of the heart muscle, and heart enlargement
8. Control rhythm disturbances, maintain or increase cardiac output, relieve fluid accumulations, increase the oxygenation of blood, and provide oxygen/sedatives
9. Beneficial effects include improved cardiac contractility, decreased heart rate, antiarrhythmic effect, and decreased signs of dyspnea. A toxic effect is vomiting.
10. Stimulation of cardiac contraction in cardiac arrest
11. Conditions that cause hypoxia; electrolyte imbalances; increased levels or sensitivity to catecholamines; certain drugs such as digitalis, barbiturates, and others; and cardiac trauma or disease
12. Class IA—quinidine; class IB—lidocaine; class IC—flecainide; class II—propranolol; class III—bretylium; class IV—diltiazem
13. Hydralazine—arteriolar dilator; nitroglycerin—venodilator; prazosin—combined; enalapril—combined
14. Lasix is called a *loop diuretic* because it inhibits reabsorption of sodium in the loops of Henle.
15. Potassium
16. Bronchodilation, oxygen therapy, sedation, aspiration, and centesis
17. Depolarization
18. Cardiac output
19. Congestive heart failure
20. Angiotensin I to angiotensin II
21. Wear gloves; rotate application sites; do not pet the animal at the application site; measure the dosage in inches; and contact the veterinarian if a rash appears at the application site.
22. Lasix

23. An abnormally low potassium level in the blood

24. The primary goals are (1) sodium restriction and (2) maintenance of good body weight and condition (reduction of obesity or cachexia). In some instances specific nutrient deficiencies, concurrent disease, and/or electrolyte disorders may need addressing.

25. (1) Increased force of contraction; (2) An increase in blood pressure; (3) Elevated blood glucose levels

ANSWERS TO CHAPTER 8

1. Entry of food and fluid into the body, absorption of nutrients, and excretion of waste products

2. Dogs, cats, and primates

3. Ruminants have a system of forestomachs, including the reticulum, rumen, and omasum, which allows them to digest coarse plant material, as well as a true stomach (abomasum).

4. Regurgitation is a normal process of ruminants that permits them to bring up partially digested foodstuff for rechewing. Vomiting is the forcible expulsion of gastric contents and is generally considered to be pathologic.

5. Microorganisms in the rumen

6. The automatic nervous system, hormonal control, and chemical (histamine, prostaglandin, and others) control

7. Bacterial endotoxins may increase the permeability of intestinal blood vessels, resulting in increased fluid loss. They may also induce fever and initiate shock.

8. Chemical substances (digitalis compounds, urea, ketone bodies, and others) and impulses from the inner ear

9. Centrally acting—apomorphine and xylazine; peripherally acting—syrup of ipecac and mustard

10. Antiemetics

11. Reducing the secretion of hydrochloric acid by gastric mucosal cells

12. Cimetidine and ranitidine

13. Peristalsis (A wave of contraction) and segmentation (a mixing action)

14. Withholding food for 12 to 24 hours

15. Rats and horses

16. By retaining water osmotically in the gut, these agents cause softening of the stool.

17. Psyllium

18. By mimicking the effect of acetylcholine

19. Metronidazole

20. C.E.T., Nolvadent, Oral Dent, and Oxydent

21. Peristalsis refers to a wave of contraction that moves contents along, and segmentation refers to intestinal constrictions that mix contents.

22. False

23. 80%

24. By forming a pastelike barrier over the surface of gastric ulcers

25. Felines

ANSWERS TO CHAPTER 9

1. Releasing factors (RFs) are messengers made by the hypothalamus in response to its detection of hormone levels in the blood. RFs send messages to the pituitary to stimulate this gland to manufacture trophic hormones. Trophic hormones, in turn, stimulate a specific tissue or gland to produce the hormone in question.

2. The major endocrine glands are the pituitary, the thyroid, the ovaries, the testicles, the adrenals, and the pancreas.

3. To correct a deficiency and to obtain a desired effect

4. In the body; external

5. The pituitary gland is located at the base of the brain ventral to the hypothalamus, and its primary function is to control the activity of the other endocrine glands.

6. A negative feedback mechanism occurs when the hypothalamus senses a high level of a specific hormone in the blood and in response reduces the amount of releasing factor (RF) for this hormone. A reduced amount of RF causes a decreased amount of trophic hormone to be produced by the pituitary, and this results in

decreased production of the hormone by the target organ.

A positive feedback mechanism occurs when the hypothalamus senses a low level of the hormone in question and increases its production of RF. Increased RF causes an increase in trophic hormone and a resulting increase in activity of the target organ.
7. Neurohormonal reflex
8. Gonadotropin
9. Progestins
10. Estrus synchronization, to induce abortion, and to induce estrus
11. Pregnant; asthmatics
12. Estrogen and progesterone
13. The reproductive tract has been examined for blockage or torsion.
14. Triiodothyronine (T_3) and tetraiodothyronine (T_4)
15. Soloxine and Synthroid
16. Short acting (regular/Semilente), intermediate acting (NPH/Lente), long acting (PZI/Ultralente)
17. Regular/Semilente
18. NPH/Lente
19. Weakness, ataxia, shaking, and seizures
20. Breeding purposes
21. Because of the potential for abuse by human athletes
22. Pheromones
23. Wear gloves and/or avoid getting the drug on the skin.
24. Residues of DES were shown to have a likely link to cervical cancer in women.
25. Corpus luteum

ANSWERS TO CHAPTER 10

1. Dilate
2. Glaucoma, keratoconjunctivitis sicca
3. Pupillary
4. Ophthalmic stains are used as diagnostic aids for detecting disease in both the anterior and posterior segments and in the nasolacrimal system.
5. Fluorescein
6. Aural
7. Topical ophthalmics (e.g., ointments, drops)
8. Since the eye secretes tears, the medication may be quickly diluted and thus reapplication becomes necessary
9. To provide local anesthesia to the eye
10. False

ANSWERS TO CHAPTER 11

1. Three, integumentary
2. Proper nutrition
3. Protection, temperature regulation, storage, immunoregulation, secretion, vitamin D production, and sensory perception
4. Five to ten
5. Antiseborrheic
6. Inflammatory, debridement, repair, maturation
7. Has drying and cleansing properties
8. True
9. Systemic
10. To keep the animal from excessive self-licking and/or mutilation

ANSWERS TO CHAPTER 12

1. Gram
2. Blue
3. Red
4. Naxcel
5. Tetracyclines
6. Tetracycline
7. Oto-, nephro-
8. Dermatophytosis
9. Spectrum
10. True

ANSWERS TO CHAPTER 13

1. Predator-prey, commensalism, mutualism, phoresis, parasitism

2. Parasitiasis occurs when an animal is infected with parasites, but no clinical signs can be observed.
3. Parasitosis occurs when an animal is infected with parasites and clinical signs can be observed.
4. Ectoparasites infest the outside of the body.
5. Endoparasites infect the inside of the body.
6. Infected; infested
7. An anthelmintic is administered to rid the body of endoparasites.
8. Organophosphate
9. Insect growth regulators
10. Tapeworms

ANSWERS TO CHAPTER 14

1. Nociceptors
2. Increased heart rate, increased respiratory rate, vocalization, guarding the painful site, restlessness, salivation, failure to groom, unresponsiveness, abnormal gait, abnormal stance, and rolling.
3. Cox-2
4. Gastrointestinal ulceration and/or bleeding
5. Cats metabolize aspirin very slowly.
6. False
7. Fentanyl
8. False
9. These substances regulate electrolyte and water balance in the body.
10. Alternate day dosing may help prevent iatrogenic hypoadrenocorticism; administration should be tapered off gradually; very large doses may be used in certain emergency situations; corticosteroids should be avoided when treating corneal ulcers; use aseptic technique when injecting into joints.
11. Caused by the doctor
12. Short-term effects of corticosteroid use include polyuria, polydipsia, polyphagia, and delayed healing. Long-term effects include thinning of the skin, gastric ulcers, osteoporosis, and iatrogenic Cushing's disease.
13. Local anesthetics prevent generation and conduction of nerve impulses by peripheral nerves.

14. Local anesthetics are used for infiltrating into local areas for suturing wounds, for nerve blocks (lameness examination), for antiarrhythmic effects, for topical use, and others.

ANSWERS TO CHAPTER 15

1. Hyperkalemia is an excess of potassium in the blood.
2. b. 5%
3. A fluid solution is balanced if it resembles extracellular fluid in composition.
4. mEq/L, Mosm/L, and g/100 ml
5. c. 300
6. Sensible losses are primarily represented by urine losses. (In a research setting, fecal losses might be considered sensible because they can be measured.) Insensible losses include fecal, sweat, and respiratory losses.
7. Obese animals
8. 500, 1000
9. Hydration deficit, maintenance requirement, and ongoing losses
10. 2520 ml
11. 26 gtt/min
12. First check the bag to ensure that the solution is clear. Inspect the container's insertion port cover to make sure that it is intact and then remove the cover, being careful not to contaminate it. Close the flow clamp on the administration set and remove the cover from the set spike. Wipe the port with an alcohol swab and insert the spike into the insertion port. Hang the bag and fill the administration set line, clearing all the bubbles in the process. Close the flow clamp and attach the line adapter to the intravenous catheter using sterile technique. Open the flow clamp and adjust the flow rate.
13. Draw 50 ml from the bottle of 50% dextrose solution and add it to 450 ml of water.
14. Lactate is added to help correct acidosis in a patient. Lactate is converted to bicarbonate (alkaline) by the liver.
15. An esophageal feeder is used to provide oral electrolytes to neonatal calves. It consists of a

tube (with a hollow ball on its end) attached to a heavy plastic bag. Oral electrolytes are placed in the bag, and the tube is passed into the esophagus of the calf. The ball on the end of the tube prevents entry into the trachea.
16. Hypertonic
17. Lactated Ringer's solution (balanced); saline (unbalanced)
18. Osmolality
19. 300
20. Isotonic
21. Every 6 to 12 hours
22. 72 hours
23. Avoid hypertonic or irritating solutions and avoid placing so much fluid at one site that the skin is dissected from its blood supply causing a slough of tissue.
24. Saline (0.9% sodium chloride)
25. Calcium

ANSWERS TO CHAPTER 16

1. Iron compounds
2. Chronic renal failure; erythropoietin
3. Because a patient's response to hematinics does not occur quickly enough
4. EDTA
5. Because of the existence of an intrinsic clotting mechanism
6. A silver nitrate stick; through coagulation of blood proteins
7. Vitamin K_1; SC or IM
8. A fibrinolytic agent such as streptokinase
9. G_0, resting; G_1, presynthesis preparation; S, DNA synthesis; G_2, RNA production; and M, mitosis
10. Alkylating agents—cyclophosphamide; antimetabolites—methotrexate; plant alkaloids—vincristine; antibiotics—Adriamycin; hormonal—prednisolone; and miscellaneous—biologic response modifiers
11. Canine lymphoma monoclonal antibody
12. Treatment of autoimmune hemolytic anemia, treatment of lymphocytic-plasmacytic enteri-

tis, treatment of rheumatoid arthritis, and treatment of lupus erythematosus
13. Because most antineoplastic drugs are very irritating to tissue and may cause sloughing
14. Designate a specific location for handling. Wear nonpermeable latex gloves when handling. Cover work surfaces with a disposable, plastic-backed sheet. Wear an appropriate laboratory coat and mask. Reconstitute all materials carefully to avoid aerosolization. Clean reconstituted material of any contamination, and properly mark and date it. Dispose of contaminated material in leak-proof, puncture-resistant containers. Wash hands thoroughly.
15. In the kidney
16. Epogen (erythropoietin)
17. Plasmin
18. Heparin
19. It may distort the white blood cells making identification difficult.
20. It chelates (binds with) calcium.
21. Anaphylactic reactions, immunosuppression, vomiting, diarrhea, hair loss, cystitis, pain associated with administration, and tissue damage from extravasation.
22. Body surface area
23. Lymphoid neoplasia
24. Interferon
25. Doxorubicin

ANSWERS TO CHAPTER 17

1. Routine checkups
2. Health/age, type of vaccine administered, route of administration, concurrent incubation of infectious disease, exposure to an infectious disease before immunity is reached, drug therapy
3. An inactivated vaccine has organisms commonly treated by chemicals to kill the organism, but very little change occurs in the antigens that stimulate protective immunity.
4. A live vaccine is prepared from live microorganisms or viruses.

5. Modified-live vaccine has organisms that have undergone a process (attenuation) to lose their virulence so that when inoculated into the body, they cause an immune response instead of disease.
6. A toxoid is a vaccine used in producing immunity to a toxin rather than bacterium or virus.
7. An antitoxin is a specific antiserum aimed against a toxin that contains a concentration of antibodies extracted from blood plasma of a hyperimmunized, healthy animal (usually a horse).
8. The contents should be unpacked and placed in the refrigerator.
9. Using drugs to stimulate the body's immune response to disease
10. Acemannan

ANSWERS TO CHAPTER 18

1. c. Calcium EDTA
2. d. Bring the cat to the hospital to start treatment with acetylcysteine.
3. a. Rompun
4. b. On an empty stomach
5. Oxymorphone, Torbugesic, Talwin-V, and Nubain
6. b. Blood urea nitrogen (BUN)
7. Articular cartilage and connective tissue
8. GAG's act as chondroprotective agents.
9. A neutraceutical is any nontoxic food component that has scientifically proven health benefits, including disease treatment and prevention. Glucosamine/chondroitin sulfate.
10. True
11. The Dietary Supplement Health and Education Act of 1994
12. Omega-6 and omega-3 fatty acids.
13. Increased bleeding time and possible decreased immune function.
14. To prevent or reduce the systemic absorption of ingested drugs or toxins.
15. Lead poisoning.

16. Water soluble.
17. Naloxone
18. Xylazine
19. S-adenosylmethione
20. Ethylene glycol (antifreeze)

ANSWERS TO CHAPTER 19

1. Inventory is the quantity of goods present in the veterinary facility.
2. Develop a budget; keep abreast of expenses on a regular basis; once a system has been put in place, keep it active; budget analysis should mirror the practice's philosophy; analyzing expenses provides a comprehensive view of the condition of the practice and helps shape its future endeavors.
3. Money
4. The number of times a product is used and replenished each year.
5. 4 Turns
6. $102,500
7. Make sure items are on hand when needed and minimize the expense of keeping items in stock.
8. A packing slip is found in the carton in which freight is shipped. It documents how many of each item is shipped. It may or may not include the prices of the item(s), although most commonly it does not.
9. An invoice is documentation of an order shipped to the veterinary hospital. It may or may not accompany the packing slip in the shipping carton.
10. A statement is most commonly mailed to the veterinary practice. It documents the items received by the hospital and the amount due on account. Commonly it must be paid within 30 days in order that no late fees are incurred by the business.
11. The point at which a product is allowed to be sold or used in-house before new product is ordered.
12. This number is included on the rabies certificate given to the client; also rabies is a zoonotic disease, and the veterinarian must account for

the expiration date of the vaccine and the serial number.

13. 1

14. DEA inventory and usage, OSHA manuals, MSDS sheet, supplier's catalogs

15. All information on the form must be correct, no mark outs are allowed, no liquid paper can be used, must have correct spelling, must have correct strength, and the veterinarian must sign the form.

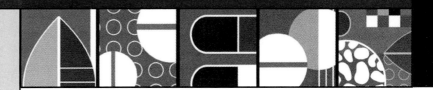

INDEX

A

Abbokinase, 323
Abbreviations, used in veterinary medicine, 389-390
Abdominocentesis, 141
Absorbine Veterinary Liniment, 215
Absorption, 7-9
    formulation of drug affecting, 9
    passive and active, 8
    by pinocytosis, 8
Acarexx, 200
Acemannan, 212, 329, 346, 349
Acemannan immunostimulant, 351t
Ace-Otic Cleanser, 200
Acepromazine, 79
Acepromazine maleate, 80
Acetaminophen, 276
    toxicity: treatment of, 360
Acetazolamide, 118, 193
Acetic acid, 200, 211
Acetylcholine, 77
    release of, 106
Acetylcholinesterase, 77, 92
Acetylcholinesterase inhibitors, 159-160
Acetylcysteine, 104, 360
Acid citrate dextrose (ACD) solution, 322
Acidified Copper sulfate, 216
Acral lick dermatitis, canine, 216
Actimmune, 329
Activase, 323
Activated charcoal, 156, 359
Active immunity, vaccine types producing, 337-339
Active transport, 8
Acyclovir, 237
Adalat, 137
Additives, for IV fluids, 306-309
Adenovirus type 2, 338
Adequan, 277-278, 356
Adrenalin, 78
Adrenergic agents
    adverse side effects, 78-79
    clinical uses, 78
    dosage forms, 78
Adrenergic antagonists, for renal dysfunction, 119
Adrenergic blocking agents, alpha and beta blockers, 79
Adrenergic nervous system receptors, 75-76
Adrenocorticotropic hormone, 167, 282
Adriamycin, 328

Adsorbents, for GI tract, 156
Adspec Sterile Solution, 233
Adulticides, melarsomine dihydrochloride, 257, 259
Advantage, 263
Adverse drug reaction, definition of, 14
Aerosolization, of vaccines, 340
Aerosols, 33
Afrin, 108
Afterload, cardiac, 129
Age, effect on drug biotransformation, 11
Agonist, definition of, 13
Airflow, normal, maintenance of, 103
Akarpine, 77
Albendazole, 253, 256-257
Albon, 234
Albuterol, 78, 107
Alcohols
    as antiseptics, 210
    mode of action of, 237-238
Aldosterone antagonists, 117
Alferon N, 329
Alkaban-AQ, 327
Alkalis, 241
Alkaloids
    examples of, 3
    plant, 327
Alkeran, 327
Alkylating agents, 325-327
Allerseb-T Shampoo, 206
Allopurinol, 121
Aloe vera, 359
Alopecia, feline psychogenic, 216
Alpha blockers
    adverse side effects, 79
    dosage forms, 79
Alpha Keri Therapeutic Bath Oil, 209
Alpha-adrenergic antagonists, 119
Alprazolam, 94
Alteplase, 323
Alternative medicines
    chondroprotectives, 356
    lubricants, 364
    miscellaneous antidotes, 359-363
    nutraceuticals, 356-359
    reversal agents, 363-364
Altrenogest, 173
Aluminum acetate, mixed with water, 209
Aluminum hydroxide, 154
Alveoli, functions of, 101-102
Amikacin, 230

Aminoglycosides
    pharmacodynamics of, 229-230
    pharmacokinetics of, 229
Aminopentamide, 77, 156
Aminopentamide hydrogen sulfate, 151
Aminophylline, 107
Amiodarone, 136
Amitraz, 265
Amitriptyline, 94, 123, 216
Amlodipine, 137
Ammonium chloride, 120
Amoxicillin, 224
Amoxicillin + clavulanate potassium, 225
Amphetamines, 92
Amphoteracin B, 235
Ampicillin, 224-225
Amprolium, 256
Ampules, breaking of, 27
Amtech Prostamate, 174
Anabolic steroids, 185-186
Anabolism, tissue, 171
Anafranil, 94
Analgesia, produced by phenothiazine derivatives, 80
Analgesics
    narcotic, 155-156
    opioid, 278-279
    in pain control, 270-271
    urinary tract, 123
Anaphylaxis, clinical signs of, 342
Anaprime ophthalmic solution, 196
AnaSed, 78, 81
Anatomy
    GI system, 144-147
    heart, 126-129
    nervous system, 69-73
    pain, 271-272
    pituitary gland, 166-168
    respiratory system, 100-102
    skin, 204-206
Ancobon, 236
Androgens, 171-172, 318
Anemia
    iron deficiency, 317
    normocytic, normochromic, 121
Anesthesia
    inhalant gas as, 44
    spinal, 7
Anesthetics
    inhalant, 88-90
    local, regional, and topical, 284-286
    topical, 194

Angiogenesis, 212
Angiotensin-converting enzyme
    inhibitors, 119-120, 139
Animal Medicinal Use Clarification
    Act (AMDUCA), 20-21
Animal safety trials, in drug
    development, 20
Animax Ointment, 235
Anipryl, 95
Anorexia, fluid therapy for, 297t
ANS. see Autonomic nervous
    system
Antacids, 154
Antagonil, 364
Antagonist, definition of, 13
Anthelmintics, 245, 253-257
Anthocaine Injection, 286
Antianxiety agents
    azapirones, 94
    benzodiazepines, 93-94
Antiarrhythmic drugs, 133-137
    class IA, 134
    class IB, 135
    class II, 135-136
    class III, 136
    class IV, 136-137
Antibacterial agents
    ophthalmic, 195
    topical, 213-214
Antibiotics
    antineoplastic agents, 327-328
    fluoroquinolone ophthalmic, 195
    metronidazole, 160
    as preservative, 33
Anticestodal drugs, 255-256
Anticholinergic drugs
    as antiemetics, 151
    for diarrhea, 156
    for renal dysfunction, 118-119
Anticholinesterase agents, 77
Anticoagulants
    acid citrate dextrose (ACD)
        solution, 322
    antiplatelet drugs, 322
    citrate phosphate dextrose adenine
        (CPDA-1), 322
    coumarin derivatives, 321
    ethylenediamine tetraacetic acid
        (EDTA), 321
    heparin, 319-320
Antidepressants
    monoamine oxidase-B inhibitors,
        94-95
    serotonic reuptake inhibitors, 94
    synthetic progestins, 95
    tricyclics, 94

Antidiarrheal medications
    anticholinergics/antispasmodics,
        156
    narcotic analgesics, 155-156
    protectants/adsorbents, 156
Antidiuretic hormone, for renal
    dysfunction, 120
Antidotes
    acetylcysteine, 360
    activated charcoal, 359
    antivenin, 362
    calcium EDTA, 359
    dimercaprol, 360-361
    ethanol, 362
    fomepizole, 362
    methylene blue, 360
    penicillamine, 361
    pralidoxime chloride, 361
    sodium thiosulfate, 361
    thiamine HCl, 363
    vitamin K-1, 362-363
Antiemetics, 149-152
    anticholinergics, 151
    antihistamines, 151
    butyrophenones, 152
    phenothiazine derivatives, 150
    procainamide derivatives, 150-151
Antifoaming agents, for ruminants,
    161
Antifungal agents
    antimetabolic, 236
    imidazole, 235-236
    ophthalmic, 195
    polyene, 235
    superficial, 236
    topical, 214
Antihistamine Injection, 280
Antihistamines, 108
    as antiemetics, 151
    for pain, 279-280
Antiinfectives
    aminoglycosides, 229-230
    antifungal drugs. see Antifungal
        agents
    antiviral drugs. see Antiviral agents
    bactericidal or bacteriostatic, 220
    cephalosporins, 225-227
    chloramphenicol, 231-232
    disinfectants/antiseptics, 237-241
    florfenicol, 232
    fluoroquinolones, 231
    macrolides and lincosamides,
        232-233
    nitrofurans, 234
    penicillins, 222, 224-225
    polymyxin B and bacitracin, 234

Antiinfectives (Continued)
    spectinomycin, 233
    sulfonomides, 234
    susceptibility testing for, 221-222
    tetracyclines, 227-229
    topical ophthalmic, 195
    topical otic, 197-199
    vancomycin, 233
Antiinflammatory agents
    for bowel disease, 161
    topical ophthalmic, 196
Antilirium, 77
Antimetabolic antifungal agents,
    236
Antimetabolites, 327
Antinematodal drugs, 253-255
Antineoplastic drugs, 323-325
Antiparasitics
    invermectin, 199-200
    pyrethrins, 199
    rotenone, 199
Antiphlogistine Poultice, 215
Antiplatelet drugs, 322
Antiprotozoal drugs, 256-257
Antipruritics, 209-210
Antiseborrheics, topical, 206, 208
Antisedan, 79
Antiseptics
    dermatologic, 210-211
    and disinfectants, 237-241
Antiserum, 339
Antispasmodics, 156
Antitoxin, 339
Antitrematodal drugs, 256
Antitussives
    butorphanol, 104
    codeine, 105
    dextromethorphan, 106
    hydrocodone bitartrate, 104-105
    temaril-P, 106
Antiulcer medications
    antacids, 154
    gastromucosal protectants, 154
    H$_2$ receptor antagonists, 152-153
    prostaglandin E-1 analogs, 155
    proton pump inhibitors, 153-154
Antivenin
    coral snake (Micrurus fulvius), 362
    polyvalent (Crotalidae), 362
Antiviral agents
    acyclovir, 237
    interferon alfa-2A human
        recombinant, 237
    ophthalmic, 195
Antizol-Vet, 362
Anxiety, sedation for, 141

APL, 171
Apomorphine, 86, 148-149
Apothecary system, units used in, 55-56
Apresoline, 120
AquaMEPHYTON, 323
Arachidonic acid, 214
Aristocort, 109
Arquel granules, 278
Arrhythmias, 128, 130
Arsenic toxicity, treatment of, 361
Artificial tear products, 196-197
Asparaginase, 328
Aspirin, 274, 322
    used in heart disease, 141
Astramorph PF, 278
Astringents, 210
Atapryl, 95
Atarax, 280
Atenolol, 79, 136
Atipamezole, 79
Atipamezole hydrochloride, 363
Ativan, 94
Atracurium, 93
Atrophate, 192
Atropine, 77-78
Atropine sulfate, 191
Aurimete, 199
Autogenous vaccine, 339
Autonomic nervous system, 73-76
    adrenergic agents, 78-79
    adrenergic blocking agents, 79
    anticholinergic agents, 77-78
    cholinergic agents, 76-77
    regulation of GI system, 147
Avermectins, 254-255
Avian Bluelite, 310
Avian influenza subtype H5, 338
Axons
    electric-like messages carried by, 70-71
    preganglionic and postganglionic, 73
Azapirones, 94
Azathioprine, 161, 331
Azium, 283
Azulfidine, 161

B
Babesia, drugs for treating, 257
Baby pig anemia, 317
Bacillus Calmette-Guerin (BCG), 330
Bacitracin, 195, 234
Bacteria, staining properties of, 220

Bacterin, 337
Bacterins, immunomodulatory, 349, 352
Bactoderm, 213
Baking soda. see Sodium bicarbonate
BAL in oil, 361
Balling gun, 35f
Banamine, 275
Barbioc, 136
Barbiturates
    long-acting, 82-83
    short-acting, 83
    ultrashort-acting, 83
Barriers, to drug movement, 10
Bath oils, 209
Baytril Otic, 200
Beaucoup, 240
Beclomethasone dipropionate, 109
Behavioral pharmacotherapy, 93-95
Belladonna alkaloids, 77
Benadryl, 108, 280
Benazepril, 120
Bendiocarb, 265
Benzalkonium chloride, 211
Benzimidazoles, 253
Benzodiazepine antagonist, 363
Benzodiazepine derivatives, 80-81
Benzodiazepines, 93-94
Benzoic acid, 236
Benzoyl peroxide, 208
Benzyl benzoate, 266
Benzylpenicillin, 225
Beta blockers
    adverse side effects, 79
    class II antiarrhylmics as, 135-136
    dosage forms, 79
Beta-2-adrenergic agonists, 107
Beta-adrenergic antagonists, 119
Betadine, 211, 239
Beta-lactamase, 224
Betapace, 136
Betasone, 283
Bethanechol, 77, 118
Beuthanasia-D, 95
BIGEOIL, 215
Biguanide compounds, 240-241
Bioavailability
    digoxin, 132
    factors affecting, 8
BioDres, 212
Bioflavonoids, 358
Biologic response modifiers, 329-330
Biologics, care of, 341
Biolyte, 310
Bion tears, 197
Biopsy needles, 32f

Biotransformation, factors affecting, 10-11
Bipyridine derivatives, 133
Birds, digestive system of, 147f
Bisacodyl, 158
2,3,4,5-Bis(2-butenylene)tetrahydro-2-furaldehyde, 266
Bismuth subsalicylate, 156
Bladder, neuropathic, 122
Bleeding needles, 32f
Bleomycin, 328
Blistering stage, of counterirritation, 215
Bloat Guard, 161
Blood levels, factors affecting, 4, 6
Blood substitutes, 318-319
Blood supply, affecting drug absorption, 9
Blood-brain barrier, 10
Blood-modifying drugs/agents
    alkylating agents, 325-327
    antibiotic antineoplastic agents, 327-328
    anticoagulants, 319-322
    antimetabolites, 327
    asparaginase, 328
    biologic response modifiers, 329-330
    fibrinolytic (thrombolytic) drugs, 323-325
    glucocorticoids, 328-329
    hematinics, 316-319
    hemostatics/anticoagulant antagonists, 322-323
    immunosuppressive drugs, 330-332
    plant alkaloids (mitotic inhibitors), 327
    platinum drugs, 328
Body fat
    metabolism of, 179
    thiobarbiturates and, 83
Body water, distribution of, 290-291
Body weight, conversion to body surface area for dogs, 325t
Boldenone undecylenate, 186
Bolus
    administration of, 27
    with indwelling IV catheter, 41
    IV direct, 40
    using Y injection site, 43
Bone marrow, injection directly into, 7
Bonine, 280
Bordetella bronchiseptica, 337
Boric acid, 200
Borrelia burgdorferi, 338

Bo-Se, 312
Bovilene, 174
Bovine respiratory syncytial virus, 338
Bovine somatotropin, 185
Bovine virus diarrhea, 338
BoviShield 4, 338
Bradyarrhythmias, 130
Bradycardia
    atropine-resistant, 133
    medetomidine-induced, 82
Brain, pharmacologically important areas of, 72-73
Bran mush, 157
Brethine, 78
Bretylium, 136
Brevane, 83
Brewer's yeast, 358
Bromide, 88
Bromocriptine, 176
Bronchoconstriction, definition of, 101
Bronchodilators
    beta-2-adrenergic agonists, 107
    categories of, 106
    cholinergic blockers, 107
    for heart failure, 141
    methylxanthines, 107
Broth dilution susceptibility test, 221-222
Brucella abortus Vaccine, 337
Bulk-producing agents, 157
Bunamidine, 255
Bupivacaine, 285-286
Buprenex, 279
Buprenorphine, 86
Buscopan, 119
Buspirone, 94
Butazolidin, 274
Butorphanol, 279
Butorphanol tartrate, 86, 104
Butoxypolypropylene glycol, 266
Butyl hyoscine, 119
Butyrophenones, 152

C
Caffeine, 92, 107
Calcium channel blockers
    class IV antiarrhythmics as, 136-137
    for renal dysfunction, 120
Calcium Disodium Versenate, 321
Calcium disodium versenate injection, 359
Calcium EDTA, 359

Calcium supplements, as fluid additive, 308
Calf scours, 309
CALF-oid implant, 185
Cambendazole, 253
Campylobacter fetus, 337
Canine acral lick dermatitis, 216
Canine distemper, 338
Canine Lymphoma Monoclonal Antibody 231 (CL/MAb 231), 329
Cannula
    intraosseous, 43-44
    J-12 teat infusion, 36
Cantharide, 215
Capoten, 120
Capsules
    advantages of, 27
    procedure for administration of, 34-36
Captopril, 120, 139
Carafate, 154
Carbacel, 193
Carbachol, 193
Carbam, 260
Carbamates, 265
Carbamylcholine, 77
Carbaryl, 265
Carbenicillin, 225
Carbimazole, 178-179
Carbonic anhydrase inhibitors, 118, 193
Carboplatin, 328
Cardiac conduction system, 127f
Cardiac glycosides, 131-132
Cardiomyopathy
    dilated, 130
    hypertrophic, 130
Cardiovascular drugs
    antiarrhythmic, 133-137
    diuretics, 139-140
    positive inotropic, 131-133
    vasodilator, 137-139
Cardiovascular system
    compensatory mechanisms of, 129-131
    disease, treatment objectives, 131
Cardizem, 120
Carfentanil, 86
Carlytene, 119
Carmustine, 327
Carprofen, 276
Carravet Wound Dressing, 212
Carvedilol, 136
Castor oil, 158

Catecholamines, 119, 132-133
Catheter, IV
    changing of, 38
    indwelling, 41
Cationic detergents, 240
Cats
    avoidance of phosphate enemas in, 157
    cisplatin contraindicated in, 328
    excessive self-licking, 216
    external parasites, 251t
    facial pheromones, 176-177
    heartworm disease, 257, 259
    ibuprofen side effects in, 277
    internal parasites, 246t
    metabolizing capability, 10
    oral administration procedures for, 34-36
    preventive health programs for, 345-346t
    vaccinations for preventive health programs, 342
Cattle
    external parasites, 252t
    internal parasites, 248t
    preventive health program for, 348-349t
    vaccinations for preventive health programs, 342, 344
Caustics, dermatologic use of, 216
Cefaclor, 227
Cefadroxil, 227
Cefazolin, 227
Cefepime, 227
Cefotaxime, 227
Cefotetan, 227
Cefoxitin, 227
Ceftazidime, 227
Ceftiofur, 227
Cell cycle-nonspecific drugs, 324
Cell cycle-specific drugs, 324
Central nervous system
    dissociative agents, 84
    drug effects on, 79-80
    drugs for control or prevention of seizures, 87-88
    inhalant anesthetics, 88-90
    miscellaneous drugs, 91-92
    neuroleptanalgesics, 87
    opioid agonists, 84-86
    opioid antagonists, 86-87
    stimulants, 92-93
    tranquilizers, 80-83
Central sensitization, 272
Centrine, 77, 156
Cephalexin, 227

Cephalic vein, for long-term IV therapy, 38
Cephalosporins, 225-227
Cephalothin, 227
Cephradine, 227
Cephulac, 157
Cerumen, softening of, 46
Cerumite, 199
Cestex, 256
Charcoal, activated, 156, 359
Chemoreceptor trigger zone, 148-152
Chemotherapy, 323-324
Cheque Drops, 172
Chick Ark Bronc, 337
Chloral hydrate/magnesium sulfate, 91-92
Chlorambucil, 327
Chloramphenicol, 195, 198, 231-232
Chlora-Otic, 198
Chlorhexidene, 236, 238t
ChlorhexiDerm Maximum Shampoo, 210
Chlorhexidine, 210-211
Chlorinated hydrocarbons, 265
Chlorines, 239
Chloromycetin, 232
Chlorothiazide, 117
Chlorpheniramine maleate, 280
Chlorpromazine, 150
Chlorpromazine hydrochloride, 80
Chlorpropamide, 120
Chlorpyrifos, 265
Chlortetracycline, 228
Chlor-Trimeton, 280
Choledyl SA, 107
Cholinergic agents
    adverse side effects, 77
    clinical uses, 76
    direct, 159
    direct- and indirect-acting, 77
Cholinergic agonists, for renal dysfunction, 118
Cholinergic blocking agents
    adverse side effects, 78
    clinical uses, 77
    dosage forms, 77-78
Chondroitin sulfate, and glucosamine, 357
Chondroprotectives, polysulfated glycosaminoglycans, 356
Chorionic gonadotropin, 170-171
Chorulon, 171
Chronotropic effects, on heart, 128
Chyme, 146
Cimetidine, 152-153, 280
Ciprofloxacin, 195, 231

Cisapride, 159
Cisplatin, 328
Citrate phosphate dextrose adenine (CPDA-1), 322
Clavamox, 225
Clavulanate potassium, amoxicillin with, 225
Cleaning agents
    otic, 200
    wound, 212
Clemastine, 108
Clidinium/chlordiazepoxide, 156
Client education, by technician, 48
Clindamycin, 233
Clinical trials, in drug development, 20
CL/Mab 231, 351t
Clomicalm, 94
Clomipramine, 94
Clopidol, 175
Cloprostenol sodium, 175
Clorazepate, 88
Clorox bleach, 239
Clorsulon, 256
Closed-angle glaucoma, 192
Clostratox BCD, 339
Clostridium perfringens, 339
Clostridium tetani, 338, 339
Clot formation, 319
Clotisol (ferric sulfate), 322
Clotting factors, 321t
Cloxacillin, 225
Coal tar, 208
Coccidia, drugs for treating, 256
Codeine, 86, 105, 278
Coenzyme Q, 359
Collagen, 211
Collagen shields, 195
Collamend, 212
Colloid solutions, 305-306
Colon, physiology of, 146-147
Combinations, with undesired consequences, 15t
Commensalism, type of parasitic relationship, 244
Compazine, 80
Compensatory mechanisms, cardiovascular system, 129-131
Complex carbohydrates, acemannan, 346, 349
Compliance policy guidelines (CPGs), 21
Compounding, and FDA regulations, 21-22
Compudose, 184

Concentration gradient, definition of, 10
Concentrations
    calcualtions involving, 58-59
    expressions of, 57
Congenital anomalies
    ectopic ureter, 122
    heart, 130
Congestive heart failure, 130-131
    fluid therapy for, 297t
Conjunctivitis, 195
Conofite, 214, 236
Constant rate infusion problems, calculations for, 59-60
Controlled substances
    Beuthanasia-D, 95
    information summary, 397-398
    inventory records of, 4, 47-48, 372
    label identification of, 18
    opioid agonists, 278-279
Conversion, between metric units, 53-55
Copper sulfate, 216
Copper-associated hepatopathy, treatment of, 361
Coral snake antivenin, 362
Cordarone, 136
Cortaba, 274
Cort-Astrin Solution, 284
Corticosteroids, 176, 332
    for inflammation, 281-284
    for respiratory conditions, 108-109
    systemic, 213
    topical dermatologic, 210
    topical ophthalmic, 196
Corticotropin-releasing factor, 282
Cortisate-20, 283
CortiSpray, 284
Cosequin, 278
Coumadin, 321
Coumaphos, 253
Coumarin derivatives, 321
Counterirritant
    definition of, 33
    stages of irritation due to, 215
Crystalloid solutions
    2.5% dextrose in half-strength saline/K added, 305
    dextrose 5% in water, 305
    lactated Ringer's solution, 304
    multisol-R/Normosol-R, 305
    Normosol-M in 5% dextrose, 305
    physiologic saline, 304
    Plasma-Lyte/Plasma-Lyte M in 5% dextrose, 305
    Ringer's solution, 305

C-Stat, 212
Cuprimine capsules, 361
Curare, 93
Curatrem, 256
Cya-dote Injection, 361
Cyanide poisoning, treatment of, 361
Cyanocobalamin, 311
Cyclic adenosine monophosphate, 107
Cyclogyl, 192
Cyclopentolate hydrochloride, 192
Cyclophosphamide, 327, 332
Cycloplegic agents
    atropine sulfate, 191-192
    cyclopentolate hydrochloride, 192
    homatropine hydrobromide, 192
Cyclosporin A, 196
Cyclosporine, 196, 331
Cycrin, 173
Cyproheptadine, 108
Cystorelin, 170
Cythioate, 265
Cytobin Tablets, 178
Cytokines, 271
Cytosar-U, 327
Cytosine arabinoside, 327
Cytoxan, 327, 332

D

D-128, 240
Dacarbazine, 327
Dactinomycin, 328
Dakin's solution, 212
Danocrine, 171
Darbazine, 80
Datril, 276
Debridement phase, wound healing, 211
Deca-Durabolin, 318
Decamethonium, 93
Decongestants, 108
Decoquinate, 256
Defend ExSpot Insecticide, 264
Defense mechanisms, respiratory, 102
Dehorning Paste, 216
Dehydration
    clinical signs of, 298t
    fluid therapy for, 297t
Delayed billing, 383
Delta opioid receptors, 85
Demecarium, 77
Demerol, 85, 278
Dendrites, electric-like messages carried by, 70-71
Depen Titratabs, 361

Depolarization, cardiac, 127-128
Depolarizing agents, 92
Depo-Medrol injection, 213, 283
Depo-Provera, 95, 173
Depot
    definition of, 6
    in relation to drug formulation, 9
Depo-Testosterone, 171
Deracoxib, 277
Deramaxx, 277
Dermacide, 211
DermaCool-HC, 210
Dermal Dry, 200
Dermal Wound Gel, 213
Dermalone Ointment, 235
Dermathycin, 178
Dermatologic therapy
    fatty acid supplements, 214
    systemic corticosteroids, 213
    topical antibacterial agents, 213-214
    topical antifungal agents, 214
Dermcaps, 214
Detergents
    anionic, 241
    cationic, 240
Detomidine hydrochloride, 81-82
Detrusor muscle, 121-122
Dexamethasone, 109
    injection, 213, 283
Dexasone, 283
Dexatrim, 78
Dex-A-Vet Injection, 283
Dextrans, in fluid therapy, 305-306
Dextromethorphan, 106
Dextrose
    50%, 308-309
    crystalloid solutions, 305
Diabetes mellitus
    drugs for treatment of, 179-183
    fluid therapy for, 297t
Diagnostic method, for choosing drug, 3
Diamox, 193
Diarrhea
    antidiarrheal medications, 155-156
    fluid therapy for, 297t
Diazepam, 81, 87, 94, 216
Diazinon, 265
Diazoxide, 183-184
Dibenzyline, 79, 119
Dichlorphenamide, 118, 193
Dichlorvos, 253, 265
Diclazuril, 256
Diclofenac sodium, 196
Dicloxacillin, 225

Dietary management, heart disease, 140-141
Diethylcarbamazine citrate, 260
Diethylstilbestrol, 171
Difloxacin, 231
Digestive enzymes, 160
Digitalis, 131-132
Digoxin, 132
Dihydrotachysterol, 121
Dilantin, 87-88
Diltiazem, 120, 137
Dimenhydrinate, 280
Dimercaprol, 360-361
Dimetapp DM, 106
Dimethyl sulfoxide
    as drug vehicle, 7
    as NSAID, 275-276
Dinoprost tromethamine, 174
Di-n-propyl isocinchomeronate, 266
Dipentum, 161
Diphenhydramine, 108
Diphenhydramine hydrochloride, 280
Diphenoxylate, 86, 156
Dips, for ectoparasites, 262, 265
Direct-acting hormones, 168
Disc susceptibility test, 221
Disclosing solution, 162
Disease processes, interference with drug distribution, 10
Disinfectants, 237-241
Dispensing, by veterinary clinics, 22
Disseminated intravascular coagulation (DIC), 319
Dissociative agents, 84
Diuretics
    for heart failure, 139-140
        furosemide, 139-140
        spironolactone, 140
        thiazides, 140
    for renal dysfunction
        carbonic anhydrase inhibitors, 118
        loop, 117
        osmotic, 117
        potassium-sparing, 117-118
        thiazide, 117
D-Limonene, 266
DMSO. see Dimethyl sulfoxide
Dobutamine, 78, 133
Dobutrex, 78
Docusate calcium, 158
Docusate sodium, 158
Dogs
    body weight conversion to body surface area, 325t
    dog appeasing hormone, 177

Dogs (Continued)
  excessive self-licking, 216
  external parasites, 251t
  heartworm disease, 257-260
  ibuprofen side effects in, 277
  internal parasites, 246t
  keratoconjunctivitis sicca, 196-197
  oral administration procedures for,
    34-36
  preventive health programs for,
    343-344t
  vaccinations for preventive health
    programs, 342
Dolophine, 86
Domeboro, 209
Domitor, 82
Domperidone, 159
Donnatal, 156
Dopamine, 78, 120, 133
Dopaminergic antagonists, 158-159
Doramectin, 255
Dormosedan, 81
Dorzolamide, 193
Dosage calculations, 56-57
  antineoplastic agents, 324-325
Dosage forms
  implants, 33
  microencapsulation, 33
  oral preparations, 26-27
  parenteral injection, 27
  topical medications, 33
Dose-response curve, 13
Doxapram, 92
Doxapram hydrochloride, 109
Doxorubicin hydrochloride, 328
Doxycycline, 228
Doxylamine, 108
D-Phenothrin, 264
Dramamine, 280
Dressings, wound, 212-213
Droncit, 256
Drontal Plus, 255
Droperidol, 79, 87, 152
Drug administration, five rights of,
    34
Drug development
  federal laws relating to, 20-22
  preliminary and preclinical trials,
    20
  regulatory agencies, 18-20
Drug distribution, process of, 9-10
Drug Enforcement Administration
    (DEA) forms, 372, 385
Drug interactions, 14-15
  absorption and, 9
  cimetidine with other drugs, 153

Drug interactions (Continued)
  classification of, 15
  theophylline with other drugs, 108
Drug sources, 3
Drying agents, otic, 200
D-trans allethrin, 264
Dulcolax, 158
Duocide spray, 264
Durabolin, 121
Duragesic, 278
Durakyl, 264
Duramorph, 85
Duramune Cv-K, 337
Duramycin powder, 229
Duricol Chloramphenicol 1%
    Ophthalmic Ointment, 232
Dusting powders, 33
Dusts, for ectoparasites, 262, 265

E
E.-Colicin-B, 339
Ear Mite Lotion, 266
Ears
  antiparasitics, 199-200
  cleaning agents, 200
  cleaning of, 46
  drying agents, 200
  silver sulfadiazine, 200
  topical otic antiinfective agents,
    197-199
  tris-EDTA, 200
Echinacea, 357-358
Echodids, 193
Echothiophate iodide, 193
Eclipse 3, 338
Ectokyl IGR Pressurized Spray, 264
Ectoparasites
  application systems, 260, 262-264
  insecticides, 264-266
Ectopic ureter, 122
Ectropion, 190
Edema, reduction with
    counterirritants, 215
Edrophonium, 77
Effector organs, 76
Efficacy, definition of, 13
Elavil, 94, 123
Eldepryl, 95
Electrolytes
  disorders of, 297t
  distribution of, 290-291
  mineral sources of drugs including,
    3
  oral, preparations of, 309-310
Elixer, definition of, 27
Elmiron, 123

Elpak-G Electrolyte Gel, 310
Elspar, 328
Emetics
  centrally acting, 148-149
  locally acting, 149
Emodin, 158
Empirical method, for choosing drug,
    3
Emulsifiable concentrates
  dips, 262
  yard and kennel sprays, 262
Emulsion, definition of, 27
Enacard, 120
Enalapril, 120, 139
Endocrine system
  control of, 168-169
  pituitary gland, 166-168
Endometrium, 171
Endoparasites
  anthelmintics for, 245, 253-257
  anticestodal drugs, 255-256
  antinematodal drugs, 253-255
  antiprotozoal drugs, 256-257
  antitrematodal drugs, 256
Endothelial layer, of blood vessel,
    319
Endotoxic shock, fluid therapy for,
    297t
Endotoxins
  diarrhea induced by, 155
  effect on GI activity, 148
Enemas, phosphate, 157
Enrofloxacin, 231
Enrofloxin, 199
Entrolyte, 310
Entropion, 190
Enzymes, digestive, 160
Ephedrine, 78, 108
Epidural Injection, 286
Epidural/subdural route, 7
Epifrin, 192
Epinephrine, 78-79, 107, 132-133,
    192, 286
Epi-Soothe, 209
Epithelialization, 212
Epoetin Alfa for Injection, 318
Epogen, 121, 318
Epsiprantel, 256
Epsom salt, 209
Equidone, 159
Equimate, 175
Equine Bluelite, 310
Equine Psyllium, 157
Equine Thyroid Supplement, 178
Equipalazone Powder, 275
Equi-Phar Phenylbutazone, 275

Equi-Phar Proud Blue Liquid, 216
Equipoise, 318
Equipose, 186
Equiproxen, 277
Equ-Lin, 215
Ergot, 176
Erysipelothrix rhusiopathiae, serum
    antibodies, 339
Erythro, 232
Erythromycin, 159
Erythropoietin, 316
    recombinant human, 121
    treatment of anemia, 318
Escherichia coli, 339
Escort, 265
E-SE, 312
Eserine, 77
Esmolol, 136
Essential fatty acids, 214
Estradiol, 184-185
Estradiol cypionate, 171
Estrogen, 171, 184
Estrumate, 175
Estrus cycle, control of, 169-170
Ethacrynic, 117
Ethanol, in treatment of ethylene
    glycol poisoning, 362
Ethylene glycol poisoning, treatment
    of, 362
Ethylene oxide, 238-239
Ethylenediamine tetraacetic acid
    (EDTA), 321
Etodolac, 277
EtoGesic, 277
Etorphine, 86
Euthanasia-6, 95
Euthanasia agents, 95
Excretion, by kidneys, 11-12
Expectorants, 103-104
Extracellular fluid, 290-292
Extralabel use, 3
    drugs prohibited for, 21
Eyes
    external structures of, 191f
    ophthalmic agents for, 190-197

F

Facial pheromones, feline, 176-177
Factrel, 170
Famotidine, 153
Fatal-Plus, 95
Fat-soluble vitamins, 312
Fatty acid supplements, 214, 358
Febantel, 254-255
Febendazole, 253
Feces, drug excretion by, 12

Feedback control mechanisms,
    endocrine system, 168-169
Felaxin, 158
Felbamate, 88
Feline leukemia virus, 337
Feline psychogenic alopecia, 216
Feline rhinotracheitis, 338
Feliway, 176-177
Fenoxycarb, 266
Fenprostalene, 174
Fentanyl, 86-87
    transdermal use, 278-279
Fenthion, 265
Fermicon CD/T, 339
Ferrodex 100, 317
Fertagyl, 170
Fever, purpose of, 271
Fiber, soluble, 358
Fibrinolytic drugs. *see* Thrombolytic
    agents
Filaribits Plus, 260
Filgrastrim, 330
Finadyne, 275
Finaplix-H, 185
Fipronil, 263
First-pass effect, 9
Flagyl, 160, 256, 332
Flaxedil, 93
Flea and tick control
    product comparison, 261t
    products for monthy use, 263-264
Flo Vent, 109
Florfenicol, 232
Flucort Solution, 283
Flucytosine, 236
Fluid therapy
    composition of solutions used in,
        293-294t
    determining amount of fluid to
        administer, 296, 298
    fluid balance, 296
    indications for, 295-296
    monitoring fluid administration,
        301-302
    patient information regarding, 296
    preparing equipment for, 302-304
    rate of fluid administration,
        300-301
    routes of fluid administration,
        298-300
    types of solutions used in, 304-309
Fluids
    administration of, calculations
        involving, 59-60
    balance of, 296
    disorders of, 297t

Fluids (*Continued*)
    piggyback setup of, 303f
    tonicity of, 292, 295
Flumazenil, 363
Flunixin meglumine, 275
Fluorescein stain, 194
Fluoride products, 162
Fluoroquinolone ophthalmic
    antibiotics, 195
Fluoroquinolones, 231
Fluorouracil, 327
Fluoxetine, 94, 216
Fluprostenol, 174-175
Flurbiprofen sodium, 196
Flushing, ear canal, 200
Fluticasone propionate, 109
Fluvoxamine, 94
Foggers, for ectoparasites, 263
Follicle-stimulating hormone, 167,
    169-170
Follicle-stimulating hormone-
    pituitary, 171
Follutein, 170
Fomepizole, 362
Food Animal Residue Avoidance
    Databank (FARAD),
    18-19
Food animals, vaccination of,
    340-341
Forane, 90
Formaldehyde, 239
Formamidines, 265
Formula 911 (powder), 310
Formulations, prolonged- or
    sustained-release, 9
Forte Topical, 214, 234
Fortekor, 120
Fowl pox vaccine, 338
Free on board (FOB) rules,
    383-384
Freight
    incoming, 383
    receiving, 384
Fresh-Ear, 200, 211
Frick speculum, 35
Frontline Top Spot, 263
FSHP, 171
Fulvicin-U/F, 236
Fungizone, 235
Furosemide, 117, 139-140

G

Gallamine, 93
Gallimycin, 232
Garlic, 358
Gastrogard, 154

Gastrointestinal tract
  anatomy and physiology, 144-147
  drugs absorbed from, 9
  effects of NSAIDs, 273-274
  prokinetics/stimulants, 158-160
  regulation of, 147-148
Gastromucosal protectants, 154
Gecolate, 91
Gelfoam absorbable gelatin sponge, 322
Gemini, 81
Gentamicin, 195, 230
Gentamicin sulfate, 197
GentaVed Otic, 197
Gentocin Durafilm, 196
Gentocin Topical Spray, 210
GI. *see* Gastrointestinal tract
Giardia
  drugs for treating, 256
  preventive drugs, 257
Giardia Vax, 257
Ginkgo biloba, 358
Ginseng, 358
Glargine insulin, 183
Glaucoma, closed- and open-angle, 192
Gleptosil, 318
Glipizide, 183
Glomerular filtration, 11-12, 113, 114f
Glucocorticoids, 273, 328-329
Glucophage XR, 183
Glucosamine, and chondroitin sulfate, 357
Glucose, 117
Glucotrol, 183
Glutaraldehyde, 238t, 241
Glycerol, 193
Glyceryl guaiacolate, 91
Glycols, added to increase drug solubility, 33
Glycopyrrolate, 77
Glycosaminoglycans, 123
  polysulfated, 356
Glycosides
  cardiac, 131-132
  examples of, 3
Goats
  external parasites, 252t
  internal parasite, 248t
Gonadorelin, 170
Gonadotropin-releasing hormone, 169-170
Gonadotropins, 170-171
Gram stain, 220

Granulation tissue, 211
  exuberant, 7
Granulex-V, 212
Granulocyte Colony Stimulating Factor (G-CSF), 330
Gravity set, for IV fluids administration, 43
Green Book, available on Internet, 20
Griseofulvin, 236
Growth hormone, 167, 185
Growth promoters, hormones acting as, 184-185
Guaifenesin, 91
Guaifenesin (glyceryl guaiacolate), 103-104
Guailaxin, 91

H
H$_1$ blockers, 280
H$_2$ blockers, 280
H$_2$ receptor antagonists
  cimetidine, 152-153
  famotidine, 153
  nizatidine, 153
  ranitidine, 153
Haemophilus somnus, 337
Half-life, definition of, 13
Halogens, 238t
Haloperidol, 152
Halothane, 90
Haloxon, 253
Happy Jack Kennel Dip, 265
Healing stimulators, topical wound dressings as, 212
Heart, anatomy and physiology, 126-129
Heart disease
  categories of, 130
  dietary management of, 140
  individualized treatment for, 126
Heart failure, ancillary treatment of, 141
Heartgard Plus, 259
Heartworm disease
  adulticides, 257-259
  microfilaricides, 259
  preventatives, 259-260
Heatstroke, fluid therapy for, 297t
Hematinics, 316-319
  androgens, 318
  blood substitutes, 318-319
  erythropoietin, 318
  iron compounds, 317-318
Hematuria, 113

Hemopad Absorbable Collagen Hemostat, 322
Hemorrhagic shock, fluid therapy for, 297t
Hemostat Powder (ferrous sulfate powder), 322
Hemostatics/anticoagulant antagonists
  parenteral agents, 322-323
  topical agens, 322
Heparin, 319-320
Heparin sodium injection, 320
Hepatopathy, copper-associated, treatment of, 361
HepLock flush solution, 320
Hespan, 306
Hetastarch, 306
Histacalm, 280
Histamine
  regulation of GI system, 148
  release of, 106, 271
Histavet-P, 280
Homatrocel Ophthalmic, 192
Homatropine hydrobromide, 192
Hormonal drugs, associated with reproduction, 170-177
Hormones
  acting as growth promoters, 184-185
  insect growth, 266
  reasons for administering, 166
  regulation of GI system, 147
  synthesis of, 3
  thyroid, 177-184
  trophic, 167-168
Horn buds, removal with caustics, 216
Horses
  dermatologic counterirritants, 215
  external parasites, 251t
  internal parasites, 247t
  large intestine of, 146f
  preventive health programs for, 347t
  vaccinations for preventive health programs, 342
Household system, units used in, 56
Humalin L, 181
Humalog, 181
Human pharmacy, 386
Humidification, of inspired air, 101
Humilac, 209
Humilin N, 181
Humilin R, 181
Humorsol, 77
Hyalovet, 278

Hyaluronate sodium, 278
Hyaluronidase, added to drugs given SC, 7
Hybridoma, 329
Hycodan, 86
Hydralazine, 120, 138
Hydration status, laboratory tests for, 296
Hydrochlorothiazide, 117
Hydrocodone bitartrate, 86, 104-105
Hydrogen peroxide, 241
Hydro-Plus, 284
Hydroxyurea, 327
Hydroxyzine, 108
Hydroxyzine hydrochloride, 280
Hyoscyamine, 156
Hyperadrenocorticism, fluid therapy for, 297t
Hyperalgesia, 272
Hyperglycemic agents, 183-184
Hyperkalemia, 307
Hyperparathyroidism, renal secondary, 121
Hyperpigmentation, 204
Hypertension, associated with renal dysfunction, 117-121
Hypertensive reactions, from drug interactions, 16
Hyperthyroidism, drugs for treatment of, 178-179
Hypertonic solutions, 306
Hypertrophic cardiomyopathy, 130
Hypoadrenocorticism, fluid therapy for, 297t
Hypodermoclysis. see Subcutaneous (SC) route
Hypoglycemic agents, oral, 183
Hypokalemia, 117, 307
Hyponatremia, 304
Hypophyseal portal system, 167
Hypothalamus, 167-170, 271
Hypothyroidism, drugs for treatment of, 177-178
Hytakerol, 121

I

Ibuprofen, 277
Idiosyncratic drug reaction, 14
Idoxuridine, 195
IGRs, 266
Illotycin, 232
Imidacloprid, 263
Imidazole antifungal agents, 235-236
Imidazothiazoles, 254
Imipramine, 94
Imizol, 257

Immiticide, 257, 259
Immunity
    active, vaccine types producing, 337-339
    passive, vaccine type producing, 339
Immunoregulin, 330, 351t
Immunostimulants
    complex carbohydrates, 346, 349
    immunomodulatory bacterins, 349, 352
Immunosuppressive drugs, 330-332
Immunosuppressive effects, corticosteroids, 282
Immunotherapeutic drugs, 344, 346
    immunostimulants, 346, 349, 352
    indications for usage, 351t
Imodium, 156
Implants
    Ralgro, 185
    SC insertion of, 33
Implus-H, 184
Imuran, 161, 331
In Synch, 174
Inactivated vaccines, 337
Incontinence, urinary, 121-123
Inderal, 79, 119
Indications. see also Contraindications
Indirect-acting hormones. see Hormones, trophic
Infectious bovine rhinotracheitis, 338
Infectious bronchitis, 337
Inflammation
    corticosteroids for, 281-284
    muscle relaxants for, 280-281
    process of, 271
Inflammatory phase, wound healing, 211
Informed consent, for behavioral pharmacotherapeutic agents, 93
Infumorph, 278
Infusion pump, 44
Inhalant anesthetics, 88-90
Inhalation route
    considerations for, 7
    indications for, 44-45
Inhalation therapy, for respiratory disease, 103
Injectables
    corticosteroids, 283
    iron, 317
Innovar-Vet, 87, 152
Inotropic drugs, positive, 131-133
Inotropic effects, on heart, 128

Inotropin, 133
Insecticides
    carbamates, 265
    chlorinated hydrocarbons, 265
    formamidines, 265
    insect growth regulators (IGRs), 266
    organophosphates, 265
    pyrethrins, 264
    repellents, 266
    synergists, 266
    synthetic pyrethroids, 264
Insulin, 179-183
    intermediate-acting, 181
    long-acting, 183
    products, use of, 183
    short-acting, 181
Insulin syringe, 31f, 180f
Interceptor, 259
Interferon, 329
Interferon alfa-2A, human recombinant, 237
Interleukins, 329-330
Intermediate-acting insulin, 181
Internet, role in drug marketing, 23
Interstitial fluid, composition of, 291t
Intraarterial (IA) route, 7
Intraarticular route, 7
Intracardiac route, 7
Intracarotid injection, avoidance of, 7
Intracell, 212
Intracellular fluid, 290-292
Intradermal (ID) route, 7
Intramedullary route, 7
Intramuscular (IM) route, 6, 37f
    administration procedures for, 39
Intraocular pressure, reducing agents, 193-194
Intraosseous cannulation, 43-44
Intraosseous route, for fluid administration, 300
Intraperitoneal (IP) route, 7
    for fluids, 299
Intrathecal route, 7
Intravenous (IV) route, 6, 38f
    direct bolus, 40
    for fluids, 42, 298-304
Intron A, 329
Intropin, 78, 120
Inventory
    computers and, 386
    organizing, 379, 381
    pharmaceutic, 368-387
    physical, 381
    proactive control system, 372, 375

Inventory (*Continued*)
   purchasing information, 381, 383-386
   records, 375-376, 378-379
   reorder log, 377f
   sample invoice, 374f
   sample packing slip, 375f
Inventory control manager, 369, 371-372, 379, 381, 383, 386, 387
Investigational New Animal Drug (INAD), 20
Iodine, 211, 236, 239
   radioactive, 179
   Shampoo, 214
Ipecac, syrup of, 149
Ipodate, 179
Iron compounds, injectable and oral preparations, 317-318
Iron Dextran Complex, 317
Irritants, as laxatives, 158
Isoflo, 90
Isoflurane, 90
Isopropyl alcohol, 215
Isoproterenol, 78, 107, 133
Isoptin, 120
Isopto Carpine, 77
Isopto Homatropine, 192
Isuprel, 78, 107
Itraconazole, 236
Ivermectin, 199-200, 254-255, 259, 266

J

Jugular vein, for long-term IV therapy, 38

K

K9 Advantix, 263
Kanamycin, 230
Kaolin/pectin, 156
Kappa opioid receptors, 85
Kat-A-Lax, 158
Keflin, 227
KeraSolv Gel, 208
Keratitis, 195
Keratoconjunctivitis sicca, treatment agents, 196-197
Keratolytics, 206, 208
Keratoplastics, 206, 208
Ketaset, IM injection, 44
Ketmaine hydrochloride, 84
Ketoconazole, 235-236
Ketofen, 277
Ketone bodies, 179
Ketoprofen, 276-277
Ketorolac, 278

Ketorolac tromethamine, 196
Kidney tubules, secretory role, 113, 115
Kidneys, drug excretion by, 11-12
Konakion, 323
Kopertox, 214
K-Y Jelly, 364

L

Labels
   components of, 16-18
   specific wording of, 3
Lactulose, 157
Lansoprazole, 154
Lantus, 183
Lasix, 117, 140
Laudanum, 85
Lavage, warm water, 212
Laxatives, 157-158
Laxatone, 158
Lead poisoning, treatment of, 361
Lente Iletin II, 181
Lente Purified Pork, 181
Leptospirosis, 337
Leukeran, 327
Leukocell 2, 337
Leukotrienes, 271
Leuprolide, 176
Levamisole, 254, 259, 330
Levophed, 78
Levothyroxine sodium (T_4), 177-178
Levsin, 156
Librax, 156
Lidocaine, 135, 285-286
Lincomycin, 233
Lincosamides, 233
Lindane, 265
Liniments, 33, 215
Lin-O-Gel, 215
Liothyronine sodium, 178
Lipid solubility, 9
Liquichlor, 198
Liquid preparations
   administration procedures for, 35-36
   forms of, 27
Liquifilm Tears, 197
Live vaccines, 337
Liver
   drug excretion by, 12
   and drug interaction, 16
Lixotinic, 317
Loading dose, 4
Local anesthetics, administration routes of, 284-285
Lomotil, 86, 156

Lomustine, 327
Long-acting insulin, 183
Loop diuretics, 117
Loperamide, 156
Lorazepam, 94
Lotensin, 120
L-Se, 312
Lubricants
   for gynecologic and rectal exams, 364
   as laxatives, 157
   ocular, 196-197
Lubrivet, 364
Lufenuron, 263
Lugol's Solution, 211
Lungs, drug excretion by, 12
Lutalyse, 174
Luteinizing hormone, 167, 169-170
Luvox, 94
Lysol I.C. Disinfectant Spray, 240
LyTar, 208

M

M-99, 86
Macrolides, 232
Maduramicin ammonium, 256
Magnesium hydroxide, 154, 157
Magnesium sulfate, 157
   mixed with water, 209
Mammary glands, drug excretion by, 12
Mannitol, 117, 193
Marcaine, 286
Marketing
   Internet role in, 23
   mail order, 22
Markup, figuring, 378-379
Mathematics
   calculations for constant rate infusion problems, 59-60
   concerning solutions, 57
   dosage calculations, 56-57
   fundamentals of, 52-53
   milliequivalents, 59
   percent concentrations, 58-59
   systems of measurement, 53-56
Maturation phase, wound healing, 211-212
Mebendazole, 253
Meclizine, 280
Meclofenamic acid, 278
Medetomidine, 82
Medication orders, written or verbal, 46-47
Medrol, 283
Medrol tablets, 213

Medroxyprogesterone, 95
Medroxyprogesterone acetate, 172-173
Megace, 172
Megestrol acetate, 95, 172
Melarsomine dihydrochloride, 257, 259
Melatonin, as reproductive drug, 176
Melengestrol acetate, 173
Melphalan, 327
Meperidine, 85, 278
Mephyton, 323
Mercuric oxide, 215
Mestinon, 77
Metabolic acidosis, 306
Metabolic alkalosis, 305
Metabolites, inactive or active, 10
Meta-Dote, 359
Metamucil, 157
Metastases, 323
Metformin, 183
Methadone, 86
Methazolamide, 193
Methemoglobin, 316
Methemoglobinema, 360
Methigel, 120
Methimazole, 178
Methionine, 120
Methocarbamol, 280-281
Methohexital, 83
Methoprene, 266
Methotrexate, 327
Methoxychlor, 265
Methoxyflurane, 90
Methscopolamine, 77, 156
Methylene blue, 360
Methylprednisolone
    plus aspirin, 274
    tablets, 283
4-Methylpyrazole. see Fomepizole
Methylxanthines, 107
Meticorten, 283
Metoclopramide, 77, 150-151, 159
Metofane, 90
Metoprolol, 136
Metrazol, 92
Metric system, 53
Metronidazole, 160, 256, 331-332
Mexiletine, 135
MGK 11, 266
Mibolerone, 172
Miconazole, 195, 214, 235-236
Micotil, 232
Micro Pearls Advantage Seba-Moist
    Shampoo, 208

Microencapsulation, drugs
    administered by, 33
Microfilaricides, 259
Microorganisms, 220
Midazolam, 81
Milbemycin oxime, 259
Milliequivalents, 59, 292
Mineral oil, 157
Mineralocorticoid potency, of
    corticosteroids, 281t
Minimal inhibitory concentration,
    221-222
Minimum alveolar concentration
    (MAC), 88
Minipress, 79, 119
Minocycline, 228
Minor Use and Minor Species
    Animal Health Act
    (MUMS), 22
Miotics
    carbachol, 193
    echothiophate iodide, 193
    pilocarpine, 192
Misoprostol, 155
Mitaban, 265
Mita-Clear, 199
Mitaplex-R, 199
Mitotic inhibitors, 327
Mitoxantrone, 328
Mitral disease, 130
Mixed vaccine, 339
Mixing drugs, in same syringe, 16
Modified live vaccines, 337-338
Monensin, 256
Monistat, 236
Monitoring
    fluid administration, 301-302
    patients on IV fluid therapy, 44
    of products, 20
Monoamine oxidase-B inhibitors,
    94-95
Monoclonal antibodies, 329
Monogastric GI configuration, 145f
Monthly inventory, and rotating
    inventory, 381
Morantel tartrate, 254
Morphine sulfate, 85, 278
Motilin-like drugs, 159
Motilium, 159
Moxidectin, 255, 259
Moxisylyte, 119
Mu opioid receptors, 85
Mucolytics, acetylcysteine, 104
Mucomyst, 360
Mucosil, 360
Multidose syringe, 31f

Multisol-R/Normosol-R, 305
Muscarinic receptors, 76
Muscle relaxants, 280-281
Mu-Se, 312
Mutualism, type of parasitic
    relationship, 244
Mycitracin Sterile Ointment, 234
Mycobacterial cell wall fraction, 349,
    352
Mycodex Pet Shampoo, 264
Mycodex Tar and Sulfur Shampoo,
    208
Mycophenolate mofetil, 332
Mycoses, topical and systemic, 235
Mydfrin, 191
Mydriacyl, 192
Mydriatic agents
    atropine sulfate, 191-192
    cyclopentolate hydrochloride, 192
    epinephrine, 192
    homatropine hydrobromide, 192
    phenylephrine hydrochloride, 191
    tropicamide, 192
Myeloma cells, 329
Myelosuppression, 324
Mylepsin, 87
Myocardial disease, 130
Myofibrils, uterine, 175
Myosan Cream, 211
Myotrol, 281

N

Nalbuphine, 279
Nalorphine, 87
Naloxone, 87, 109, 216
Naloxone hydrochloride, 363
Naltrexone, 216
Naming of drugs, 16
Nandrolone, 121
Nandrolone decanoate, 186
Naprosyn, 277
Naproxen, 277
Narasin/nicarbazine, 256
Narcan, 363
Narcotic analgesics, 155-156
Narcotics
    naturally occurring, 85
    synthetic, 85-86
Natamycin, 195
National drug code (NDC) number,
    18
Needles, sizes and styles of, 32f
Nembutal, 83
Neobacimyx Ophthalmic Solution,
    234
Neo-Carbazole, 179

Neomycin, 195, 230
Neomycin sulfate, 198-199
Neo-Predef, 196
Neoral, 196
Neostigmine, 77, 160
Neo-Synephrine, 78, 108
Nerve block, 284-285
Nerve fibers
    ANS, 73
    myelinated and nonmyelinated, 71
Nervous system
    anatomy and physiology, 69-73
    autonomic. see Autonomic nervous
        system
    central. see Central nervous system
    functions of, 68
Neurohormonal reflex, 169
Neuroleptanalgesics, 87
Neuromuscular blocking drugs, 92-93
Neurotransmitters
    for adrenergic and cholinergic
        sites, 76
    mimicked or blocked by drugs, 71f
Neutersol, 176
Newcastle disease, 338
Nexaband, 213
NFZ Puffer, 234
Nicergoline, 119
Nicotinic receptors, 76
Nifedipine, 137
Nitrofurans, 234
Nitrofurazone, 213, 234
Nitrogen balance, positive, 185
Nitroglycerin ointment, 138
Nitrosoureas, 327
Nitrous oxide, 90
Nizatidine, 153
Nizoral, 236
No Sting Barrier Film, 213
Nociceptors, 271
Nolvadent oral cleansing solution,
    161
Nolvalube, 240
Nolvamite, 199
Nolvasan, 240-241
Nolvasan Antiseptic Ointment, 210
Nomagen, 351t
Nonsteroidal antiinflammatory agents
    (NSAIDs), 196
    acetaminophen, 276
    dimethyl sulfoxide, 275-276
    drugs with similar activity, 277-278
    etodolac, 277
    flunixin meglumine, 275
    mechanism of action, 272-273
    propionic acid derivatives, 276-277

Nonsteroidal antiinflammatory agents
    (NSAIDs) (Continued)
    pyrazolone derivatives, 274-275
    salicylates, 274
    tepoxalin, 277
Nonsteroidal antipruritics, 209-210
Noradrenalin, 78
Norepinephrine, 78
Norfloxacin, 195
Norgestomet, 173
Normosol-M, in 5% dextrose, 305
Norvasc, 137
Novolin L, 181
Novolin N, 181
Novolin R, 181
Novolog, 181
NPH (isophane) insulin/lente, 181
Nubain, 279
Nuflor Injectable Solution, 232
Numorphan, 85-86, 278
NuSal-T Shampoo, 206
Nutraceuticals, 356-359
    aloe vera, 359
    bioflavonoids, 358
    brewer's yeast, 358
    coenzyme Q, 359
    echinacea, 357-358
    fatty acids, 358
    fiber, 358
    garlic, 358
    ginkgo biloba, 358
    ginseng, 358
    glucosamine and chondroitin
        sulfate, 357
    probiotics, 358
    S-adenosylmethion (SAMe), 359
    saw palmetto, 358
    St. John's wort, 358
    superoxide dismutase, 359
Nutrition. see also Dietary
    management
    importance of, 112-113
    parenteral, 310
    while administering acidifying diet,
        121
NutriVed T-4, 178
Nylar, 266
Nystatin, 235

O

N-Octyl bicycloheptene
    dicarboximide, 266
Ocular lubricants, 196-197
Ofloxacin, 195
Ointments, 33
    nitroglycerin, 138

Olsalazine, 161
Omega fatty acids, 214
Omeprazole, 154
Oncovin, 327
Ondansetron, 152
Open-angle glaucoma, 192
Ophthaine, 194
Ophthaine Solution Veterinary,
    286
Ophthalmic agents
    antibacterial, 195
    antifungals, 195
    application of, 45-46
    collagen shields, 195
    miotics, 192-193
    mydriatics and cycloplegics,
        191-192
    ophthalmic stains, 194
    for reducing intraocular pressure,
        193-194
    as solutions or ointments, 190
    topical anesthetics, 194
    topical antiinfectives, 195
    topical antiinflammatory, 196
    for treatment of
        keratoconjunctivitis sicca,
        196-197
Ophthalmic stains, 194
Ophthetic, 286
Opioid agonists, 84-86, 278-279
Opioid analgesics, 278-279
Opioid antagonists, 86-87
Opioid partial agonists, 279
Opium, 85, 156
Optimmune Ophthalmic Ointment,
    196, 331
Oragrafin, 179
Oral electrolyte preparations,
    309-310
Oral health products
    dentifrice and cleansing, 161-162
    fluoride and perioceutic agents,
        162
Oral hypoglycemic agents, 183
Oral preparations
    corticosteroids, 283-284
    procedure for administration of,
        34-36
    types of, 26-27
Oral route
    absorption of drugs administered
        by, 6
    for fluid administration, 299
Ora-Lyte, 310
Orap, 152
Organic mercury compounds, 241

Organophosphate compounds
    antinematodal use of, 253
    as insecticides, 77, 265
    poisoning from: antidote for, 361
Orgotein, 278
Ornade, 78, 108
Orudis, 277
Osmoglyn, 193
Osmolality, 292
Osmolarity, 292, 295
Osmotic diuretics, 117
Osmotic pressure, 292, 295
Otic drugs
    antiparasitics, 199-200
    cleaning agents, 200
    drying agents, 200
    silver sulfadiazine, 200
    topical antiinfective agents,
        197-199
    tris-EDTA, 200
Oti-Clens, 200, 212
Otomax, 197
Ototoxicity, 198
Ovaban, 95, 172
Overhydration, signs os, 301
Over-the-counter drugs, 4
Ovine Ecthyma Vaccine, 337
Oxfendazole, 253
Oxibendazole, 253
Oxybarbiturates, 82-83
Oxydent, 161
OxyDex, 208
Oxygen, nitrous oxide given with,
    90
Oxygen therapy, for heart failure,
    141
Oxyglobin (hemoglobin glutamer-
    200), 319
Oxymetazoline, 108
Oxymorphone, 85-86, 278
Oxypolygelatin, 306
Oxytetracycline, 195, 228
Oxytocin, 175

P

Pain
    anesthetic agents for, 284-286
    antihistamines for, 279-280
    assessment in animals, 270
    deep, 272
    NSAIDs for, 272-278
    opioid analgesics for, 278-279
Palosein, 278
2-PAM, 77
Pamine, 156
Panalog, 199, 214, 235

Pancrelipase, 160
Pancuronium bromide, 93
Panmycin, 229
Panteck Cleanser, 240
Parainfluenza 3 virus, 338
Paraplatin, 328
Parasites
    ectoparasites, 260-266
    endoparasites, 245, 253-257
    filarial nematodes, 257-260
    types of symbiotic relationships,
        244
Parasiticide treatment
    external parasites
        cattle, sheep, and goats, 252t
        dogs and cats, 251t
        horses, 251t
        swine, 253t
    internal parasites
        cats and dogs, 246t
        cattle, sheep, and goats, 248t
        horses, 247t
        reptiles, 250t
        swine, 249t
Parasympathetic nervous system, 70,
    75-76
Paravertebral block, 285
Paregoric, 85, 156
Parenteral agents, hemostatic,
    322-323
Parenteral injection
    administration procedures for,
        36-44
    androgens, 121
    drugs given by, 6-7
    forms of, 27-33
Parenteral nutrition, 310
Parenteral vitamin/mineral products,
    310-312
Parepectolin, 156
Parietal cells, gastric, 152-153
Paroxetine, 94
Partial pressure, inhalant anesthetic
    in brain, 88
Partition coefficient
    inhalant agents, 88
    lipid, 9
Parvovirus, 338
Passive immunity, vaccine type
    producing, 339
Passive transport, 8
Paxil, 94
Penicillamine, 361
Penicillin G, 225
Penicillinase. see Beta-lactamase
Penicillin-binding proteins, 222, 224

Penicillins
    indications and antagonists
        drugs, 223-224t
    pharmcodynamics, 222, 224-225
    pharmcokinetics, 222
Pentazocine, 86, 279
Pentobarbital, 87
Pentobarbital sodium, 83, 95
Pentosan polysulfate sodium, 123
Pentothal, 83
Pentylenetatrazol, 92
Percent, definition of, 52
Percent concentrations, 58-59
Percorten-V, 283
Periactin, 108
Perioceutic agents, 162
Peristalsis, 146
Permethrin, 263-264
Pet Tabs FA liquid, 214
Pet Tinic, 317
Pet-Derm III, 283
Petrolatum, 158
Petroleum distillate, 266
Petroleum jelly, 364
P.G. 600, 170
pH, drug absorption and, 8
Pharmaceutic drug interaction, 15
Pharmacodynamics, 13-14
    aminoglycosides, 229-230
    cephalosporins, 226-227
    fluoroquinolones, 231
    penicillins, 222, 224-225
    tetracyclines, 228-229
Pharmacokinetics, 4-13
    aminoglycosides, 229
    biotransformation, 10-11
    cephalosporins, 226
    drug absorption, 7-9
    drug distribution, 9-10
    drug excretion, 11-13
    fluoroquinolones, 231
    penicillins, 222
    routes of administration, 6-7
    tetracyclines, 228
Pharmacotherapeutics, 3-4
    antianxiety medications, 93-94
    antidepressants, 94-95
    euthanasia agents, 95
    renal failure complications, 121
Phenazopyridine, 123
Phencyclidine, 84
Phenergan, 106, 280
Phenobarbital, 82-83, 216
Phenolics, 238t, 240
Phenothiazine derivatives, 80, 150
Phenoxybenzamine, 79, 119

Phenylbutazone, 274-275
Phenylephrine, 78
Phenylephrine hydrochloride, 191
Phenylpropanolamine, 78, 108
Phenylzone Paste, 274
Phenytoin sodium, 87-88
Pheromones, 176-177
Phlebitis, avoidance of, 6
Phoresis, type of parasitic
    relationship, 244
Phosmet, 265
Phosphodiesterase, 107
Phospholine iodide, 193
Photosensitivity, 14
Physiologic saline, 304
Physiology
    GI system, 144-147
    heart, 126-129
    nervous system, 69-73
    pain, 271-272
    pituitary gland, 166-168
    respiratory system, 100-102
    skin, 204-206
Physostigmine, 77
Phytonadione, 323, 362-363
Pilocarpine, 77, 192
Piloptic, 192
Pimozide, 152
Pindolol, 136
Pinocytosis, 8
Pipa-tabs, 255
Piperazine, 255
Piperonyl butoxide, 266
Pip-pop 320, 255
Pirsue aqueous gel, 233
Pitressin, 120
Pituitary gland, anatomy and
    physiology of, 166-168
Plant alkaloids, 327
Plasma, composition of, 291t
Plasma-Lyte, 305
Platinol, 328
Platinum drugs, 328
P/M Naloxone HCl injection, 363
Polioencephalomalacia, treatment of,
    363
Polishing paste, 162
Polydipsia, 120
Polyene antifungal agents, 235
Polymyxin B, 234
Polymyxin B sulfate, 195
Polysulfated glycosaminoglycan,
    277-278
Polysulfated glycosaminoglycans, 356
Polyuria, 120
Polyvalent vaccine, 339

Ponazuril, 256
Pontocaine, 194
Pontocaine hydrochloride, 194
Positive inotropic drugs
    bipyridine derivatives, 133
    cardiac glycosides, 131-132
    catecholamines, 132-133
Postganglionic fibers, ANS, 73
Potassium chloride, for injection,
    307
Potassium citrate, 121
Potassium-sparing diuretics, 117-118
Povidone, 239
Powders
    dusting, 33
    oral electrolytes packaged as, 309
    Viokase-V, 160
Pralidoxime, 77
Pralidoxime chloride, 361
Praziquantel, 255-256
Prazosin, 79, 119, 139
Predator-prey, type of parasitic
    relationship, 244
Predef, 283
Prediluted sprays, for ectoparasites,
    260, 262
Prednisolone acetate, 196
Prednisolone generic tablets, 284
Prednisolone sodium phosphate, 196
Prednisolone sodium succinate, 109
Prednisone, 161, 213, 284
Preganglionic fibers, ANS, 73
Preliminary trials, in drug
    development, 20
Preload, cardiac, 129
Preservatives
    in fluid therapy, 305
    for parenteral drugs, 33
Prevacid, 154
Preventatives, heartworm, 259-260
Preventic Tick Collar, 265
Primatene, 108
Primidone, 87
Primor, 234
Pro-Banthine, 77, 119, 156
Probahist Syrup, 108, 280
Proban, 265
Pro-Bute, 275
Procainamide, 134
    derivatives of, 150-151
Procaine hydrochloride, 286
Prochlorperazine, 150
Prochlorperazine/isopropamide, 80
Prodine solution, 214
Progesterone, 184-185

Progestins, 172-173
    synthetic, 95
Proglycem, 183-184
Program Tablets, 263
ProHeart, 259
Prokinetic drugs, to increase GI
    motility, 158-160
Prolactin, 167
Prolamine, 78
Promace, 80
Promazine hydrochloride, 80
Promethazine, 280
Propantheline, 77, 119, 151, 156
Proparacaine hydrochloride, 194
Propionibacterium acnes, 330
Propionibacterium acnes bacterin,
    349
Propionic acid derivatives, 276-277
Propofol, 91
Proportion, definition of, 52-53
Propoxur, 265
Propranolol, 79, 119, 135-136, 179
Propylene glycol, 210
Propylthiouracil, 179
Prostaglandin E-1 analogs, 155
Prostaglandins, 173-176, 271
Prostamate, 174
Prostigmine, 77
Protamine sulfate, 322
Protamine zinc insulin (PZI), 183
Protectants
    for GI tract, 156
    in wound healing, 213
Protein binding, 10
Protex-Bb, 337
Proton pump inhibitors, 153-154
Protopam, 77
Protopam injection, 361
Protozoans, drugs for treating, 256
Proud flesh, 7, 216, 271
Proudsoff, 216
Proventil, 78, 107
Provera, 173
Prozac, 94
Pruritis, 213
Pseudoephedrine, 108
Psyllium, equine, 157
Purchasing information, 381
    communicating with sales
        representatives, 385
    DEA forms, 385
    FOB rules, 383-384
    human pharmacy, 386
    incoming freight, 383
    receiving freight, 384
    special orders, 385-386

Purchasing information (*Continued*)
  stocking shelves, 384
  vendors, 384-385
Purified Pork R, 181
Purina Cattle Dust, 265
Pyoben, 208
Pyoderma, 204
Pyrantel pamoate, 254-255
Pyrantel tartrate, 254
Pyrazolone derivatives, 274-275
Pyrethrins, 199, 264
  synergists for, 266
Pyridostigmine, 77
Pyrilamine, 108
Pyrilamine maleate, 280
Pyrogen, fever initiated by, 271

Q

Q-Cide, 240
Quaternary ammonium compounds,
  238t, 240
Quinidine, 134

R

Rabies vaccine
  certificate of vaccination, 380f
  records concerning, 379
Rabies virus, 337, 338
Raboral V-RG, 338
Radioactive iodine, 179
Ralgro implants, 185
Ranitidine, 153, 160, 280
Rapinovet, 91
Rate of administration, for fluid
  therapy, 300-301
Ratio, definition of, 52
Receptor binding, by drugs, 13
Recombinant DNA technology, 3,
  338
Reconstitution
  of medication, 29f
  vaccines requiring, 340
Re-Covr Injection, 280
Reflex arc, parts of, 71-72
Reflexes, respiratory, control of,
  103
Regimen, components of, 3
Reglan, 77, 159
Regular crystalline insulin/semilente,
  181
Regu-Mate, 173
Releasing factors, 167
Releasing hormones, 167
Relief Shampoo, 209
Renal dysfunction
  adrenergic antagonists for, 119

Renal dysfunction (*Continued*)
  angiotensin-converting enzyme
    inhibitors for, 119-120
  anticholinergic drugs for, 118-119
  antidiuretic hormone for, 120
  cholinergic agonists for, 118
  diuretic drugs for, 117-118
  urinary acidifiers for, 120-121
  urinary alkalizers for, 121
  vasodilators and calcium channel
    blockers for, 120
  xanthine oxidase inhibitors for,
    121
Renal failure, 116
  complications, pharmacotherapy
    of, 121
  fluid therapy for, 297t
Renal insufficiency, dosage
  modifications in, 116b
Repair phase, wound healing, 211
Repellents, as insecticides, 266
Repolarization, cardiac, 128
Reproductive system, control of,
  169-170
Reptiles
  drug toxicity in, 10
  internal parasites, 250t
Residues, in animal products, 12
Resmethrin, 264
Re-Sorb, 310
Resource information, 393-395
Respiratory drugs
  antihistamines, 108
  antitussives, 104-106
  bronchodilators, 106-107
  corticosteroids, 108-109
  decongestants, 108
  expectorants, 103-104
  mucolytics, 104
  respiratory stimulants, 109
Respiratory system
  anatomy and physiology, 100-102
  defense mechanisms, 102
  disease, inhalation therapy for, 103
  drugs. see Respiratory drugs
  therapeutics, principles of, 102-103
Revalor-S, 185
Reversal agents
  atipamezole HCl, 363
  flumazenil, 363
  naloxone HCl, 363
  tolazoline HCl, 363-364
  yohimbine HCl, 364
Revolution, 260, 264
Rimadyl, 276
Ringer's solution, 304, 305

Ringworm, 214
Ritrol, 310
RM Recombitek C4, 338
RM Recombitek Lyme, 338
Robaxin-V, 280-281
Robenidine hydrochloride, 256
Robinul-V, 77
Robitussin DM, 106
Rocaltrol, 121
Roccal-D Plus, 240
Rodenticide poisoning, treatment of,
  362-363
Roferon-A, 237, 329
Rompun, 78, 81
Rotenone, 199, 266
Routes of administration
  of anesthetics, 284-285
  of fluids, 298-300
  inhalation, 7
  oral, 6
  parenteral, 6-7
  topical, 7
  of vaccines, 339-341
Rubefaction stage, of
  counterirritation, 215
Rubeola virus immunomodulator,
  351t
Ruminant animals, GI system, 145

S

S-Adenosylmethion (SAMe), 359
Safe handling, antineoplastic agents,
  325b
Sales representatives, communicating
  with, 385
Salicylates, 274
Salicylic acid, 200, 236
  as antiseborrheic, 206, 208
Saline solutions, hypertonic, 306
Saline/hyperosmotic agents, 157
Salmeterol, 107
Salmonella typhimurium, 339
Sandimmune, 196, 331
Saponated cresol, 240
Saw palmetto, 358
Scarlet Oil, 212
Scolaban, 255
Scopolamine, 77
SebaLyt Shampoo, 206, 208
Sebolux Shampoo, 206
Seborrheic dermatitis, 213
Secretions, respiratory, control of,
  103
Sedation, as ancillary treatment for
  heart failure, 141
Sedazine, 81

Segmentation, pattern of intestinal constrictions, 146
Seizures, drugs for control or prevention of, 87-88
Selamectin, 260, 264
Seldane, 108, 280
Selegiline, 95
Selenium and vitamin E, 278
Selenium sulfide, 208
Seletoc, 278, 312
Self-mutilation, resulting from counterirritants, 215
Selsun Blue, 208
Semisynthetic phenols, 240
Sentinel, 259, 263
Septi-Serum, 339
Serevent, 107
Sermion, 119
Sernylan, 84
Serotonergic drugs, 159
Serotonin receptor antagonists, 152
Serotonin reuptake inhibitors, 94
Serotonin syndrome, 16
Sertraline, 94
Sevoflurane, 90
Sex steroids, 184-185
Shampoo
    for ectoparasites, 262
    types of, 205-206
Sheep
    external parasites, 252t
    internal parasite, 248t
Shin-O-Gel, 215
Short-acting insulin, 181
Sigma opioid receptors, 85
Silvadene, 200
Silver nitrate, 216
Silver nitrate sticks, 322
Silver sulfadiazine, 199-200
Sirolimus, 332
Skin
    anatomy and physiology, 204-206
    antifungals, 214
    antipruritics, 209-210
    antiseptics, 210-211
    astringents, 210
    caustics, 216
    counterirritants, 215
    fatty acid supplements, 214
    medications mixed with water, 209
    systemic corticosteroids, 213
    topical antibacterial agents, 213-214
    topical antiseborrheics, 206-208
    wound healing, 211-213
Skin turgor test, 296

Sleepaway, 95
Slo-bid, 107
Small intestine
    absorptive surface area of, 8
    sections of, 145-146
Snakebite antivenin, 362
Soaps, as disinfectants, 241
SOA/Sex, aerosol, 176
Sodium bicarbonate, 121
    as fluid additive, 306-307
Sodium hypochlorite, 239
Sodium phosphate salts, 157
Sodium thiosulfate, 361
Soloxine, 177
Solubility, affecting drug absorption, 9
Solu-Delta-Cortef, 283
Solutes
    crossing cell membrane, 292
    definition of, 291
Solutions
    general discussion of, 57
    used in fluid therapy
        composition of, 293-294t
        types of, 304-309
Solvents, for parenteral drugs, 33
Somatotropin, bovine, 185
Sore mouth infection, 337
Sotalol, 136
Spansule, in relation to drug formulation, 9
Sparine, 80
Spasgesic, 281
Special orders, important points regarding, 385-386
Spectam, 233
Spectinomycin, 233
Spinal reflex, 72
Spironolactone, 118, 140
Sporanox, 236
Sprays, prediluted, for ectoparasites, 260, 262
St. John's wort, 358
Stadol, 279
Stains, ophthalmic, 194
Stanisol, 210
Stanozolol, 185-186
Staphage lysate, 351t
Staphylococcal Protein A, 330
Staphylococcus phage lysate, 349
Starvation, fluid therapy for, 297t
Steroids
    anabolic, 185-186
    formation of, 283
    sex, 184-185
Stiglyn, 77, 160

Stimulants
    CNS, 92
    to increase GI motility, 158-160
    respiratory, 109
Stocking shelves, 384
Stomach tube, 35
Storage tissues, 10
Streptase, 323
Streptokinase, 323
Stroke volume, 129
Subcutaneous (SC) route, 6-7, 38f
    administration procedures for, 39
    for fluids, 299
Sublimaze, 86
Succinylcholine chloride, 93
Sucralfate, 154
Sudafed, 108
Sulfadimethoxine, 256
Sulfasalazine, 161
Sulfonamides, 234
Sulfonylureas, 183
Sulfur, as antiseborrheic, 206
SU-PER Poultice, 215
SU-PER Sweat, 215
Superficial antifungal agents, 236
Superoxide dismutase, 359
Supplements
    calcium, 308
    fatty acid, 214, 358
    vitamin, 309
Surfactants/stool softeners, 158
Surgical Absorbable Hemostat, 322
Susceptibility testing, 221-222
Suspension, definition of, 27
Sustain III Cattle Bolus, 234
Swine
    external parasites, 253t
    internal parasites, 249t
    preventive health program for, 351t
Symbiotic relationships, among parasites, 244
Sympathetic nervous system, 70, 73, 75-76
Sympathomimetic agents. see Adrenergic agents
Symptomatic method, for choosing drug, 3
Synalar, 284
Syncro-Mate-B, 173
Syncurine, 93
Synergistic drug interaction, 15
Synergists, for pyrethrins, 266
Synotic, 276
Synovex, 184
Synthetic pyrethroids, 264

Synthroid, 178
Syringes
  insulin, 31f
  multidose, 31f
  tuberculin, 30-31f
Syrup of ipecac, 149
Systemic corticosteroids, 213
Systemic mycosis, 235

T

T-61, 95
Tablets
  procedure for administration of,
    34-36
  scored, 26
Tachyarrhythmias, 130
Tacrolimus, 332
Tagamet, 280
Taktic, 265
Talwin, 86
Talwin-V, 279
Tanisol, 210
Tannic acid, 200
Tanni-Gel, 210
Tapazole, 178
Tavist, 108
Telazol, 84
Telodendron, 70-71
Temaril-P, 106, 109, 283
Tempra, 276
Tensilon, 77
Tepoxalin, 277
Terbutaline, 78
Terfenadine, 108, 280
Testosterone, 184-185
Testosterone cypionate, 171-172
Testosterone enanthate, 121, 171-172
Testosterone propionate, 171-172
Tetanus antitoxin, 339
Tetanus toxoid, 338
Tetnogen, 338
Tetracaine, 194
Tetracaine hydrochloride, 194
Tetracyclines, 227-229
Tetrahydropyrimidines, 254
Tetraiodothyronine (T_4), 168
Tetramethrin, 264
Theobromine, 107
Theo-Dur, 107
Theophylline, 107
Therabloat, 161
Therapeutic fluids, composition of,
    291-292
Therapeutic index, 13
Therapeutics, respiratory, principles
    of, 102-103

Thiabendazole, 236, 253
Thiamine hydrochloride, 311, 363
Thiazide diuretics, 117, 140
Thiobarbiturates, 83
Thiola, 121
Thiopental, 83
Thoracocentesis, 141
Thorazine, 80
Thromboembolism, 320
Thrombogen topical thrombin
    solution, 322
Thrombolytic drugs
  alkylating agents, 325-327
  antibiotic antineoplastic agents,
    327-328
  antimetabolites, 327
  antineoplastic drugs, 323-325
  asparaginase, 328
  biologic response modifiers,
    329-330
  glucocorticoids, 328-329
  immunosuppressive drugs, 330-332
  plant alkaloids (mitotic inhibitors),
    327
  platinum drugs, 328
Thrombus, 319
Thrush, 214
Thuja-Zinc Oxide Ointment, 213
Thyro-Form, 178
Thyroid hormones, 177-184
Thyroid-stimulating hormone,
    167-168, 178
Thyrozine Tablets, 178
Thytropar, 178
Ticarcillin, 225
Tightener, 215
Tiletamine hydrochloride, 84
Time equation, in inventory
    management, 371
Timolol, 79
Timolol maleate, 193
Timoptic, 79, 193
Tiopronin tablets, 121
Tissue uptake, anesthetic agent, 88
Tissuemend, 213
Tocainide, 135
Tofranil, 94
Tolazine, 364
Tolazoline hydrochloride, 363-364
Tolnaftate, 236
Tonicity, of fluids, 292, 295
Topical administration
  anesthetics, 194
  considerations for, 7
  corticosteroids, 284
  decongestants, 108

Topical administration (Continued)
  DMSO, 275-276
  forms of medication for, 33
  procedures for, 45-46
  treatments for skin conditions,
    206-211
  wound dressings, 212-213
Topical agents, hemostatic, 322
Topical mycosis, 235
Torbugesic, 279
Torbutrol, 86, 279
Total body water, 290
Total nutrient admixture, 310
Toxiban, 359
Toxoids, 338-339
Tracrium, 93
Tranquilizers
  acting as alpha blockers, 79
  benzodiazepine derivatives, 80-81
  detomidine hydrochloride, 81-82
  medetomidine, 82
  phenothiazine derivatives, 80
  xylazine hydrochloride, 81
Transdermal administration
  considerations for, 7
  fentanyl, 278-279
Trenbolone, 184
Tresaderm, 199
Triamcinolone, 109, 283
Triamterene, 118
Tribrissen, 234
Trichlorfon, 253
Tricyclic antidepressants, 94, 123, 216
Trifluridine, 195
Triiodothyronine (T_3), 168
Tri-Otic, 197
Tripelennamine, 108
Tripelennamine hydrochloride, 280
Tris-EDTA, 200
Tritop, 199
Trophic hormones, 167-168
Tropicamide, 192
Trovac-AIV H5, 338
Tuberculin syringe, 30-31f
d-Tubocurarine chloride, 93
Tubular secretion, 11-12
Tumil-K, 310
Turnover rate, for inventory, 371
Tussigon, 86
Tylan, 232
Tylenol, 276
Tylocine, 232
Tylosin, 232
Type I diabetes, 179
Type I recombinant (subunit)
    vaccines, 338

Type II diabetes (NIDDM), 179
Type II recombinant (gene-deleted) vaccines, 338
Type III recombinant (vectored) vaccines, 338

U

Ultralente insulin, 183
Urecholine, 77, 118
Uremia, 115
Urethral obstruction, fluid therapy for, 297t
Urinary acidifiers, 120-121
Urinary alkalizers, 121
Urinary incontinence, pharmacotherapy of, 121-123
Urinary system, functions of, 112
Urinary tract infection, 121
Urine, formation of, 113
Urocit-K, 121
Uroeze, 120
Urogenital system, 112-113f
Urokinase, 323
Uterine contractility, drugs affecting, 175-176

V

Vaccination
    adverse responses to, 341-342
    for preventive health programs, 342-344
    principles of, 336-337
    rabies, certificate of, 380f
Vaccine types
    producing active immunity, 337-339
    producing passive immunity, 339
Vaccines
    administration of, 339-341
    autogenous, 339
    failure, biologic care and, 341
    mixed (polyvalent), 339
    rabies: records concerning, 379
Valacyclovir, 237
Valbazen, 253, 256-257
Valium, 81, 94, 216
Valvular disease, 130
Vanceril, 109
Vancocin, 233
Vancomycin, 233
Vapona, 265
Vapor pressure, inhalant agents, 88
Vasodilators
    for heart failure, 137-139
    for renal dysfunction, 120

Vasopressin, 120
Vasotec, 139
Vatronol, 78
Vazepam, 81
Vecuronium bromide, 93
Vedalyte 8X, 310
Velosef, 227
Vendors
    full-service companies, 384-385
    mail-order discount houses, 385
    veterinary supply distributors, 385
Ventolin, 107
Verapamil, 120
Verapamil hydrochloride, 136
Versed, 81
Vesication stage, of counterirritation, 215
Vetalar, 84
Vetalog, 109, 210, 213
Vetalog Oral Powder, 284
Vetalog Parenteral, 283
Vetaplasma, 306
Veterinarian-client-patient relationship, 3-4
Veterinary Feed Directive (VFD), 22
Veterinary hospital, organizing inventory in, 379
Veterinary medicine, abbreviations used in, 389-390
Vet-Shield 72, 195
Vibo-5/Somnugen, 337
Vidarabine, 195
Vinblastine sulfate, 327
Vincristine sulfate, 327
Viokase-V powder, 160
VIP Flea Dip, 266
Virosan, 241
Vita-Jec Thiamine HCl, 311
Vitamin A, 312
Vitamin B$_1$, 311
Vitamin B$_{12}$, 311
Vitamin B complex, 311
Vitamin D, 312
    supplements, 121
Vitamin E, 312
Vitamin K, 312
Vitamin K$_1$, 362-363
Vitamin K$_1$ (phytonadione), 321, 322-323
Vitamin supplements, as fluid additive, 309
Vitamins
    fat-soluble, 312
    parenteral products, 310-312
    water-soluble, 311

Volume control system, 302
Vomiting
    antiemetics, 149-152
    antiulcer medications, 152-155
    control of, 148
    emetics for induction of, 148-149
    fluid therapy for, 297t

W

Warts, removal with caustics, 216
Wartsoff, 216
Waste gases, anesthetic agents, 88, 90
Water-soluble vitamins, 311
Web sites
    Green Book, 20
    pharmaceutic companies, 396
    resource information, 394-395
Weights and measures, 391-392
White Liniment, 215
Wildnil, 86
Winstrol-V, 186, 318
Wound healing
    stages of, 211-212
    topical antibacterial agents in, 213-214
    topical dressings in, 212-213

X

Xanax, 94
Xanthine oxidase inhibitors, 121
Xenodine Spray, 211
Xylazine, 78, 149, 286
    yohimbine as reversal agent for, 364
Xylazine hydrochloride, 81

Y

Y injection site, bolus using, 43
Yard and kennel sprays, for ectoparasites, 262
Yobine, 79, 109, 364
Yohimbine, 79
Yohimbine hydrochloride, 364

Z

Zantac, 160, 280
Zeranol, 184
Zinc oxide, 212
Zofran, 152
Zoloft, 94
Zoonotic potential, parasites, 245
Zovirax, 237
Zubrin, 277
Zyloprim, 121